HANDBOOK OF
MALARIA

Professor Azza Fahmy

ALLIED
HEALTH
PRESS

Handbook of Malaria

Author: **Professor Azza Fahmy**

Allied Health Press
4164 Lakeshore Road
Burlington ON L7L 1A4
Canada
www.alliedhealthpress.com
Email: orders@arclereducation.com

ISBN: 978-1-77956-793-2

ABOUT THE AUTHOR

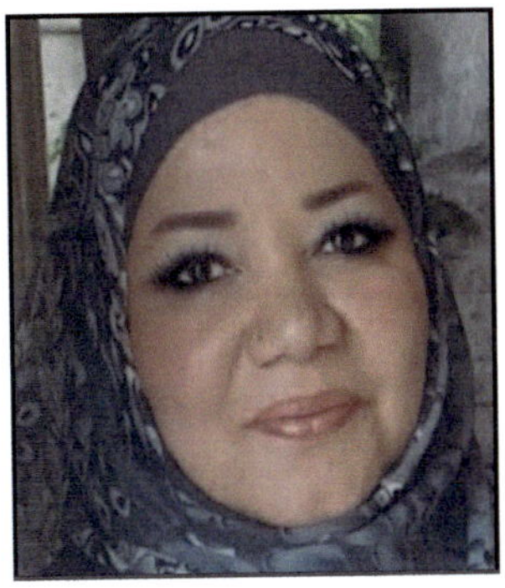

Professor Azza Fahmy is a distinguished Egyptian parasitologist and senior academic at the Theodore Bilharz Research Institute, with a PhD in Comparative Physiology and a distinguished record of contributions to parasitic disease research, diagnostics, and experimental therapy. Her work has significantly advanced both laboratory and clinical approaches to parasitic infections, with a focus on novel therapeutics, smart diagnostics, and host-pathogen interactions.

Professor Fahmy has authored numerous peer-reviewed publications covering a wide range of research themes, including:

- Experimental therapies for schistosomiasis, trichinellosis, cryptosporidiosis, toxoplasmosis, and giardiasis using agents such as GABA, Lepidium sativum, Albendazole, Mefloquine, and Commiphora molmol.
- Nanotechnology-based drug delivery systems in cancer therapy.
- The role of the microbiome in human health, and the immunomodulatory effects of parasitic antigens.
- Stem cell-based interventions for hepatic granuloma reversal in schistosomiasis models.
- Evaluations of plant-derived antiparasitic compounds (e.g., Cyperus rotundus, Syzygium aromaticum).
- Public health and policy-focused studies on antihypertensive medication adherence and its economic burden.
- Pioneering reviews on AI applications in healthcare, including the early diagnosis of diabetic foot ulcers and chronic disease prediction.

Her diagnostic innovations, such as antigen-based ELISAs, have improved the detection of various parasitic infections. She also engages in molecular diagnostics, immunopathology, and host-parasite interaction studies, enriching the field with both basic and translational insights.

An active reviewer for several leading parasitology and biomedical journals, Professor Fahmy contributes to maintaining rigorous academic standards across disciplines. She is committed to professional development and global collaboration, frequently presenting at international symposia and fostering research partnerships.

Brief Table of Contents

Detailed Table of Contents

CHAPTER 3

Vector Biology of Mosquitoes 77

CHAPTER 4

Pathophysiology of Malaria 117

CHAPTER 5

Clinical Manifestations of Malaria 155

CHAPTER 6

Diagnosis of Malaria 193

CHAPTER 7

Treatment Guidelines and Antimalarials 229

CHAPTER 10

CHAPTER 11

CHAPTER 14

Malaria in Special Populations 487

CHAPTER 15

Health Systems and Malaria Control 519

LIST OF FIGURES

LIST OF ABBREVIATIONS

ACT	Artemisinin-Based Combination Therapies
AL	Artemether-Lumefantrine
AMR	Antimicrobial Resistance
AQ	Amodiaquine
AQAS	Amodiaquine-Artesunate
ARDS	Acute Respiratory Distress Syndrome
AS-AQ	Artesunate-Amodiaquine
AS-MQ	Artesunate-Mefloquine
AS-SP	Artesunate-Sulfadoxine-Pyrimethamine
AUFI	Acute Undifferentiated Febrile Illness
CHIKV	Chikungunya Virus
CHMTs	Council Health Management Teams
CHW	Community Health Workers
CLE	Cutaneous Lupus Erythematosus
CNN	Convolutional Neural Network
CSP	Circumsporozoite Protein
CYP2B6	Cytochrome P450 2B6
DHA-PPQ	Dihydroartemisinin-Piperaquine
DHIS2	District Health Information System 2
EARS	Early Aberration Reporting System
eMIS	Electronic Malaria Information System
EV	Extracellular Vesicle
FAST	Framework for the Application of Systems Techniques
GAP	Genetically Weakened Parasites

GHIs	Global Health Initiatives
GIS	Geographic Information Systems
GSK	Glaxosmithkline
HBsAg	Hepatitis B Surface Antigen
HCQ	Hydroxychloroquine
HLC	Human Landing Catches
HRP2	Histidine-Rich Protein 2
IIT	Incompatible Insect Technique
IPM	Integrated Pest Management
IPTp	Intermittent Preventive Treatment in Pregnancy
IRS	Indoor Residual Spraying
ITN	Insecticide-Treated Net
ITT-C	Ifakara Tent Trap
IVM	Integrated Vector Management
JAK/STAT	Janus Kinase/Signal Transducer and Activator of Transcription
K13	Kelch 13
LAMP	Loop-Mediated Isothermal Amplification
LDH	Lactate Dehydrogenase
LED FM	Light Emission Diode Fluorescence Microscopy
LLIN	Long-Lasting Insecticidal Net
LSM	Larval Source Management
MCDA	Multi-Criteria Decision Analysis
MFT	Multiple First-Line Therapies
mHealth	Mobile Health
MM-MP	Medical Mission Malaria Program
mNGS	Metagenomic Next-Generation Sequencing
NSAID	Non-Steroidal Anti-Inflammatory Drug
ORN	Olfactory Receptor Neuron
PAM	Pregnancy-Associated Malaria
PCR	Polymerase Chain Reaction
PDMC	Post-discharge Malaria Chemoprevention
PET-PCR	Photo-Induced Electron Transfer PCR
PfCRT	Chloroquine Resistance Transporter Gene
PfKRS	*Plasmodium falciparum* Lysyl-tRNA Synthetase
PKC	Protein Kinase C

PREFACE

Malaria continues to be a significant danger to global health, infecting millions of individuals annually across the globe. Malaria is brought on by *Plasmodium parasites* spread through bites by infected female *Anopheles* mosquitoes and presents with fever, chills, and anemia; in its most severe forms, it results in organ failure or death. Despite advances in medical treatment and public health campaigns, malaria continues to be a considerable obstacle for under-resourced populations, hence inhibiting social and economic growth. The parasite's life cycle, which is complex and alternates between humans and mosquitoes, poses tremendous hurdles to prevention and treatment and therefore necessitates ongoing coordination between clinicians, scientists, and policymakers.

Malaria needs to be understood both in biological terms of its foundations as well as in social determinants. Genomic diversity between the *Plasmodium* species determines drug sensitivity and disease virulence, while ecological conditions dictate the habitat and breeding grounds of mosquitoes. At the same time, access to diagnostic facilities, steady drug supplies, and efficient vector control programs differ vastly between one area and another. In most endemic areas, poor healthcare infrastructure and financial resources represent significant challenges for the implementation of control programs. This evolving landscape necessitates a tool that not only distills current knowledge but also focuses on actual steps toward the reduction of transmission, improved patient outcomes, and progress toward the long-term objective of complete eradication.

The *Handbook of Malaria*, with contributions from leading experts in parasitology, entomology, clinical medicine, epidemiology, and public health, offers a coherent collection ranging from basic scientific principles to applied practice. The book aims to offer concise and lucid instruction, supplemented by detailed discussion, to enable readers to grasp key concepts as well as examine detailed results. Whether people are learning about malaria for the first time or expanding on what they already know, this handbook's users will discover authoritative information presented in a readily accessible way.

The first chapter introduces the historical context and current global burden of malaria, setting the stage for subsequent exploration. Chapter 2 examines the cellular and molecular biology of *Plasmodium parasites*, from invasion mechanisms to sexual reproduction, while Chapter 3 focuses on mosquito vector biology, covering species identification, life cycles, and environmental influences. Chapter 4 will apprise readers of the interaction of the parasite with human physiology to generate inflammatory responses and tissue injury. Chapter 5 presents the wide range of clinical presentations, from uncomplicated fever to severe complications, and includes criteria for staging disease severity.

Chapter 6 focuses on the issue of diagnosis, including an overview of microscopy, rapid diagnostic tests (RDTs), molecular techniques, and new biomarkers. Chapter 7 follows with a discussion of current treatment regimens and outlines the characteristics of antimalarial drugs, including their modes of action, dosage intervals, and safety profiles. Chapter 8 deals with the increasingly problematic issue of drug resistance, describing genetic markers associated with decreased susceptibility and strategies for ensuring the long-term efficacy of pharmacological interventions. Chapter 9 covers epidemiological trends and determinants of transmission severity, while Chapter 10 provides a model for surveillance systems, data collection approaches, reporting structures, and the use of geographic information systems.

Chapters 11 and 12 turn to response and prevention, with Chapter 11 examining practices and principles engaged in outbreak investigations and Chapter 12 evaluating vector control interventions, such as insecticide-treated nets (ITNs), indoor residual spraying, and new strategies. Chemoprevention strategies and vaccine development, such as clinical trials, immunological targets, and implementation implications, are discussed in Chapter 13. Chapter 14 is a detailed examination of vulnerable groups, namely pregnant women, infants, travelers, and those with comorbidities. Then, Chapter 15 places malaria control in the context of the overall health system, including governance arrangements, financing, integration with primary health care services, and approaches to sustainable elimination.

The book is written for general readership. Graduate students and trainees in tropical medicine and public health departments will appreciate clarification of fundamentals and the focus on recent developments. Clinicians practicing in endemic nations or treating returning travelers can utilize the diagnostic and treatment chapters as ready reference. Researchers in laboratories and entomologists are exposed to current information on parasite biology and vector ecology, whereas program managers and policymakers can look at discussions on surveillance, outbreak response, and health system-related elements. This collection seeks to bring together the varied viewpoints into one comprehensive volume, with the hope of facilitating parallel efforts at local, national, and international levels to reduce the burden of malaria and to accelerate progress towards the eradication of the disease.

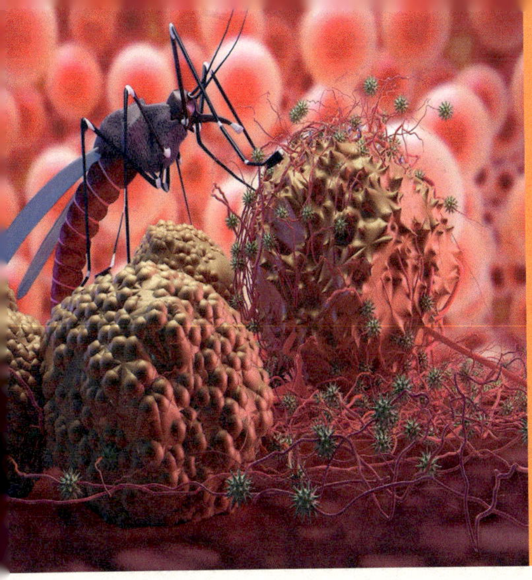

Chapter 1

INTRODUCTION TO MALARIA

Contents

Introduction

Malaria is a parasitic disease that's spread when infected female *Anopheles* mosquitoes bite people. You'll usually encounter it in tropical, wet areas where mosquitoes can breed pretty much unfettered. The illness is brought on by many *Plasmodium* species, *Plasmodium falciparum* and *Plasmodium vivax* are the worst culprits, with each species producing a variation on the theme of mischief. Human beings tend to develop fever, chills, and headache, in certain instances, even the disease results in neurological complications and, in very severe cases, death. Despite there being progress in avoiding and treating malaria, the disease remains an unyielding disease, mostly in underprivileged communities with lesser access. Knowing how the disease is spread and presents itself is quite important to establishing better ways of stemming it. Apart from how precisely it transmits from person to person, the mechanisms of malaria proper are a real nuisance, especially given the *Plasmodium parasites* have the potential to become drug-resistant. Resistance can disrupt treatment plans, making it harder to keep the disease on the backburner of global health problems. Most often, this resistance is quite similar to what takes place with bacteria that start to ignore antibiotics, something that underlines the need for an overall approach to handle all sorts of infections in one go (Murray et al., 2022). In areas mostly plagued by malaria, where hospitals are already strained, the problem adds to the burden. It requires methods that synthesize prevention, quick diagnoses, effective treatments, and ongoing follow-up for resistance into one overall strategy. Malaria's effects don't remain in the domain of health alone but have an impact "ripple" into social and economic life as well. High infection rates usually lead to time off from work, adding further burden to already beleaguered healthcare systems. The cyclical pattern of malaria, with repeated attacks tending to weaken an individual's immune system and even trigger long-term complications, can make it a challenging situation to break the cycle of spread. It should also be noted that supportive treatment plays its part; treatments for co-morbid conditions like anemia or even neurological disorders can radically change patient outcomes, though sometimes in an unpredictable manner. Further, general public health efforts, such as better standards of living, sanitation, and access to more education—are also a key component in fighting malaria. Like many of the hard problems that involve multiple approaches to a solution (Livingston et al., 2020), understanding what malaria is helpful in directing resources where they will be most beneficial and in developing policy that does make a difference (Figure 1.1).

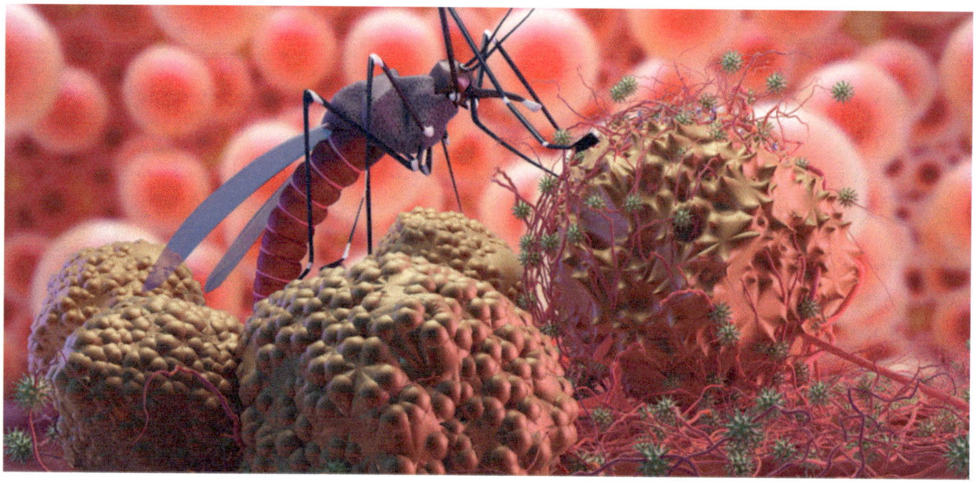

Figure 1.1. Overview of malaria.

Source: DiagNear. (n.d.). *Malaria.* https://external-content.duckduckgo.com/iu/?u=https%3A%2F%2Fdiagnear.com%2Ffiles%2Fblog_images%2F1050x500%2FMALARIA.png&f=1&nofb=1&ipt=2f39c818dd0bb315ff9d14e81bb93835c796f37571ad64dcb7a5cb4b637fd927.

Explanation of Malaria as a Disease

Pathogens and our immune system share a sort of capricious association that decides how severely diseases affect us. Take malaria, for example, when the female *Anopheles* mosquito infected with *Plasmodium* bites, the parasite enters the blood. It infiltrates liver cells, goes through its sinister lifecycle, subsequently lurches onto red blood cells (RBCs). All of this back-and-forth comes to leave us with those recurring fever cycles and even anemia. The body's response – an inflammatory burst attempting to attack the invader – at times can rebound and trigger further complications. For the most part, it's all a matter of sorting through this complicated association between the pathogen and our immune defense so that we can come up with treatments and prevention strategies that work. In the world scenario, malaria's touch is difficult to miss. In the tropics, where the climate is conducive to mosquito breeding, malaria can creep in unnoticed as a low-grade fever or climb to as grave an illness as cerebral malaria, which may even claim the life of the patient or leave them with permanent brain damage if not attended to in time. Early detection and immediate treatment are usually necessary, for letting things drag on normally tends to worsen results.

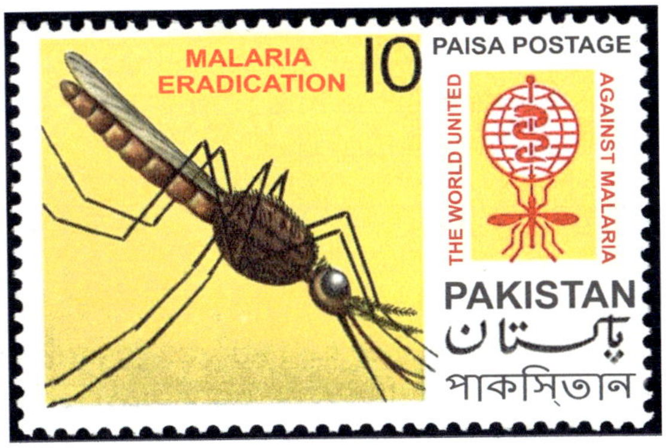

Figure 1.2. What is malaria?

Source: By Wellcome Images - +L0074987 Malaria eradication : the world united against malariaWellcome Library, London. Wellcome Imagesimages@wellcome.ac.ukwellcomeimages.org, Public Domain, https://commons.wikimedia.org/w/index.php?curid=47072528

And drug resistance, more and more troublesome – a reality to which global health organizations refer – strikes in the same vein as problems faced with other infectious diseases. It would seem that only getting the many facets of malaria, from how diverse its symptoms can be to how challenging it is to treat, is imperative in lowering its overall effect. As with other infections, malaria provokes a complex immune response that plays a significant role in shaping the severity of the disease. In most instances, when central communicators of immunity such as cytokines are out of control, the case can spiral into further danger, with some inflammatory signals even predicting a more severe course. Research in this area, sometimes identifying markers like interleukin-6 in situations like respiratory issues —continues, leaving us with hopeful signs of better ways of controlling the disease (Gubernatorova et al., 2020). At its general level, through the tuning of the body's overactive immune systems, we can subdue the overlying damage without losing the worth of its protective fight, offering a more balanced treatment approach (Figure 1.2).

Historical Context and Significance

Malaria's course through history isn't a tale of medicine only, it is a tale of nature and human choices crossing in unexpected ways. Think of all those ancient Egyptian accounts and the hasty scribbles of Greek physicians; they imply an era when the disease wasn't merely making people sick but also directing communities to reevaluate where they resided, staying out of areas infested with mosquitoes. Individuals used to relocate their dwellings from such buzzing threats, which means that the disease had an impact on both a health level and an economic-social one. Oftentimes such epidemics even had effects on wars and migrations, silently shaping political developments. For the most part, long before science was able to pinpoint its causes or identify a cure, malaria was already a part of the narrative of human evolution. Its reach goes beyond biology into the heart of cultural life. Ancient customs, like the Jia Cai Festival, for instance, emerged in part as a reaction to malaria's perpetual presence; individuals even turned to religious fasting and ritualistic behaviors in hopes of some kind of divine defense against the disease (Kamnoi, 2024). This mixing of religious belief and practical reality helped to integrate the disease into everyday life, bringing people together in hard times. Interestingly enough, the whole process converted malaria from a threat—it became a symbol of cultural adaptation and a sign of community resilience that still resonates in collective memory. From the perspective of scientific progress, the history of malaria is an evolution from folklore to hands-on exploration. Medical scrolls and anecdotal accounts initially gradually gave way to more guarded, formalized research that ultimately gave rise to modern epidemiology. Notably, studies on the development of special libraries and information systems among researchers in light of not being directly related to malaria explain how trading organized knowledge has played a crucial role in fighting extensive health problems (de Young and Raju, 2024). Enhancing research tools as well as informal communication networks eventually allowed researchers worldwide to approach malaria more wisely. To summarize, malaria is a two-fold symbol: one that not only indicates the rise of biomedical science but also highlights just how important a strong network of knowledge is in the face of global health threats.

Global Prevalence and Impact

Malaria still hits hard around the world, it is not just an issue of human illness but of nature itself. Wherever the weather and environment are exactly right, the disease takes root. Sub-Saharan Africa, for example, generally bears the brunt, with heat, rainfall, and dense vegetation conspiring to create a hospitable home for the parasite-carrying *Anopheles* mosquitoes. Nigeria, over the last 20 years or so, has shown a kind of patchy pattern of cases - with the northern regions sometimes having alarmingly high numbers. Environmental features like the Enhanced Vegetation Index and land surface temperature seem to be key players here, affecting both the mosquito population and how the parasite develops. On the other hand, increased use of insecticide-treated nets (ITNs) has been linked, albeit tenuously, with fewer cases—meaning that focused control measures can indeed reap benefits. Following these changes on maps and in data not only shows how high the global burden is but also educates smarter deployment of resources (Ogunsakin et al., 2024). The effects of malaria reach far beyond human health; the disease even wreaks havoc on the natural world. Some birds, even birds of prey that many individuals consider to be nature's barometers of ecosystem well-being, are not completely outside the reach of malaria. One Thai study found that both diurnal and nocturnal raptors carry the malaria parasite, albeit at low levels, although even these low levels are sufficient to result in stress enough to affect survival or bring on other complications. What is intriguing is that when the habitats are more humid, something which appears to favor mosquito breeding, the birds also appear to be more likely to be infected.

This would mean that the same environmental conditions feeding mosquito populations could spill over to induce malaria across a range of species, indicating a broader impact on global biodiversity as well as overall ecosystem stability (Subaneg et al., 2024). In spite of unprecedented success in the fight against malaria, the disease continues to be a significant public health challenge. Environmental factors combine with socio-economic issues in a complex association that dictates where and how badly malaria manifests. Generally, the disease imposes a heavy toll on healthcare, economic growth, and community health, particularly in regions where malaria is perennial. Plotting its ups and downs over time has given glimpses of shifting hotspots and emerging risk factors, which seem key to slightly more targeted prevention. In the meantime, bringing in lessons from ecology is a reminder that the effect of malaria does not end with humans—it also struggles with wildlife and the environment. In large part, this broader perspective is key to developing sustainable solutions for lowering the global malaria burden (Ogunsakin et al., 2024; Subaneg et al., 2024).

1.1. Life Cycle of the Malaria Parasite

Malaria's global toll is wrapped up in the strangely complex *Plasmodium parasite* life cycle. It starts when a bitten human is infected by an *Anopheles* mosquito carrying sporozoites and injects them right into the blood. These sporozoites, quitely, travel to the liver where they enter what we can call a resting, sort of covert, phase. In the liver, they develop into schizonts—a silent but super-critical process in that it primes downstream pathways. When the schizonts then rupture, merozoites are released into the blood, a shift to the red blood cell (RBC) phase. This stage, by its rapid asexual reproduction, is the one that will usually cause the fever and chills we all associate with malaria and, in some cases, produces more serious complications, especially among vulnerable populations (Roth et al., 2018). Soon not all *parasites* follow the asexual stage; some mature into sexual forms called gametocytes.

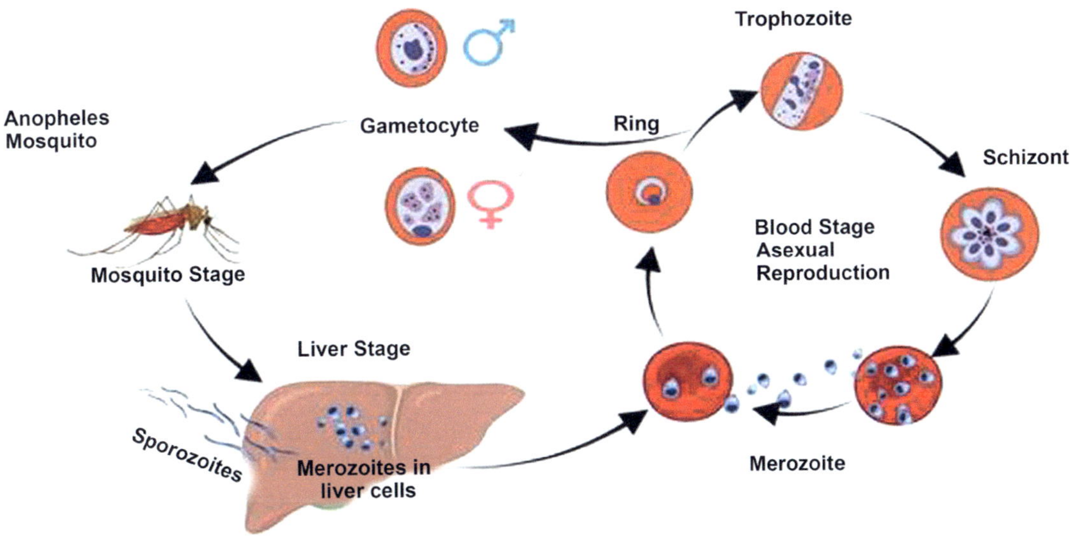

Figure 1.3. Life cycle of the malaria parasite.

Source: Simoiu M, Codreanu R, Corlatescu A-D, Pauna AM, Cilievici SE. Camillo Golgi's Impact on Malaria Studies. *Cells*. 2023; 12(17):2156. https://doi.org/10.3390/cells12172156

This process is a kind of surprise in the narrative: when the other mosquito (or occasionally mosquitos) takes blood, it receives these gametocytes. They develop into gametes gradually in the midgut of the mosquito so that fertilization and ookinete development can take place. These ookinetes invade the gut wall of the mosquito to develop oocysts. Upon development, the oocysts burst and release a myriad of sporozoites that find their way into the salivary glands of the mosquito—abiding in wait to infect another human, thus perpetuating the cycle haphazardly adrift (Vos et al., 2017). Appreciating every turn of the parasite's life cycle becomes the key when developing control measures and treatments. Overall, there's a target for every stage: the liver stage may present with no symptoms but an early diagnosis may be vital, and the blood stage is all physical symptoms of the infection and where most of the treatments are focused. There are the gametocytes, naturally, which are critical because they amplify the transmission, so they're also an optimal target if we want to break the chain. Such multi-layered complexity makes vaccine design a real challenge and compels public health professionals to navigate many interventions, ranging from vector control to prophylactic drugs and diligent patient treatment, especially as collective health trends shift with declining infectious deaths and rising chronic morbidity (Vos et al., 2017; Roth et al., 2018) (Figure 1.3).

1.1.1. Description of Plasmodium Species

Malaria is a challenging disease to pin down, at least partly because its parasite family—the *Plasmodium* species—is so heterogeneous. A number of different species have their own unique characteristics that define how the disease manifests itself and is spread. These tiny protozoa have a complex life cycle that jumps from *Anopheles* mosquitoes to mammalian hosts subsequently undergoes morphological changes to survive in each setting.

For instance, *Plasmodium falciparum* is known for its rapid replication and can infect any age group of RBCs, making the disease very virulent. *Plasmodium vivax*, however, prefers reticulocytes, and the clinical picture is marked by a relapsing picture due to its latent phases in the liver. You can see these distinctions in the various stages—trophozoites, schizonts, and gametocytes, which have been so much under microscopic scrutiny, testing us to combine old approaches with new molecular technology (Sallum et al., 2020). Even apart from a general appearance, the difficulty of establishing these *parasites* is aggravated by their genetic diversity and commonalities. In a good number of cases, laboratory examinations dependent solely on morphology are not sufficient. Overall, molecular diagnostics have been revolutionary, allowing scientists to identify differences at the DNA level when the visual cues are ambiguous or indistinct. This is significant because sometimes hidden species or cryptic forms can affect the effectiveness of treatments and even mosquito behavior. Additionally, strain differences in distribution regionally are part of the reason that it is hard to institute monolithic interventions. For the most part, understanding how each of the *Plasmodium* species operates with the many types of *Anopheles* mosquitoes, each with its own degree of proficiency, is an important part of the malaria control scenario, something provided clarification by modern molecular taxonomy (Sallum et al., 2020). Subsequently there is our own body's war strategy, in which the spleen is the behind-the-scenes hero cleansing blood and coordinating immune defense.

The moment that these *parasites* invade the blood stream, they set in motion a chain reaction of immune reactions: antigens are marched around and lymphocytes get busy in the spleen's maze-like kingdom. However, *Plasmodium* has evolved evasive strategies to counteract these defenses, with sometimes by hiding infected RBCs or even manipulating the signals that would otherwise activate our immune system. These devious strategies not only allow the infection to persist but also mislead efforts at useful vaccines and therapies. Researchers continue to try to fully unravel this interaction since a better grasp of these evasive maneuvers is crucial in designing more effective anti-malaria drugs (Figure 1.4).

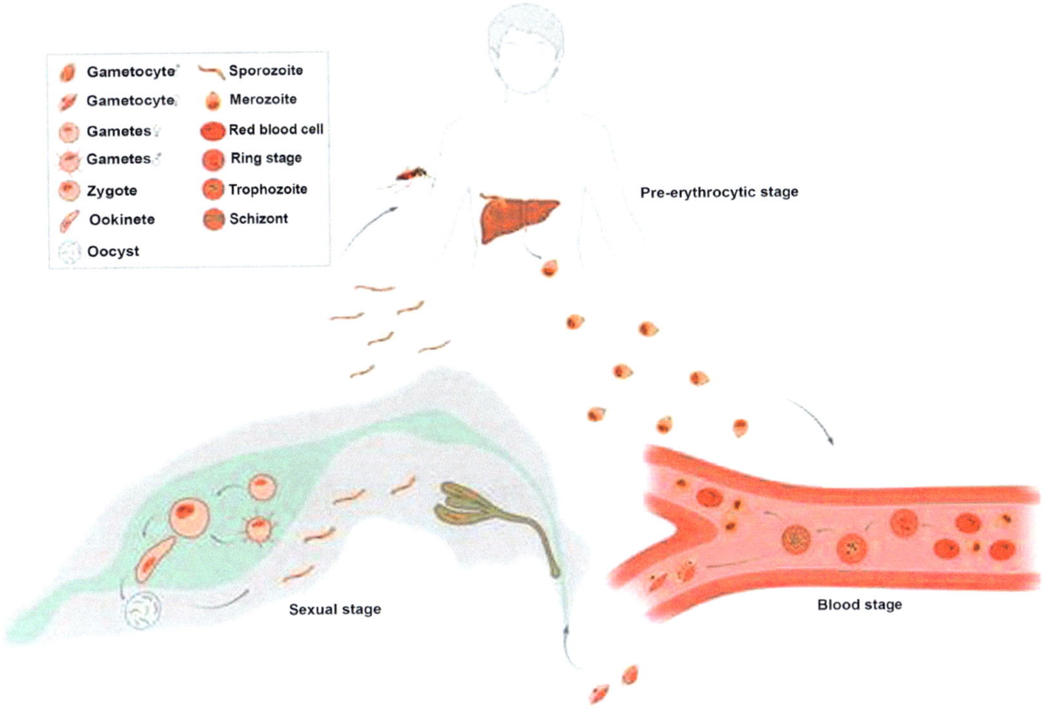

Figure 1.4. Description of *Plasmodium* species.

Source: Chen J, Wang Q, He X, Yang B. Malaria Vaccines: Current Achievements and Path Forward. *Vaccines*. 2025; 13(5):542. https://doi.org/10.3390/vaccines13050542

1.1.2. Stages of the Parasite's Life Cycle

Malaria *parasites* go on a wild ride the moment an infected *Anopheles* mosquito bites a human host, injecting *Plasmodium* sporozoites into the bloodstream. The sporozoites rush towards the liver where they enter hepatocytes and start multiplying asexually and end up churning out thousands of merozoites. It is a comparatively quiet phase—no obvious symptoms, but significant because it lays up a tremendous parasite load before these invaders spill over into the blood. Soon after, the merozoites infect RBCs, beginning the phase when symptoms first become evident. Inside these cells, the parasite randomly shifts between rings, trophozoites, and finally to schizonts, bursting open host cells to release even more merozoites; the cycle then continues from there. In most cases, knowing what happens in both the liver and blood stages has been crucial in directing attempts to halt such important proteins as the SUB1 protease, which is essential in assisting the parasites in exiting cells (Puszko et al., 2025). The life cycle in RBCs not only gets the individual ill—it also forms gametocytes, or structures needed for the parasite to hitch a ride back through mosquitoes. These male and female structures are necessary if the parasite is going to keep its life cycle going. If an infected individual is bitten by a mosquito, it will ingest the gametocytes that will mature in the midgut before they unite to form zygotes. Next thing you know, these zygotes are already ookinetes and even become oocysts, where sporozoites form; these proceed to migrate into the salivary glands, poised to infect the next human. This cycle of constantly shifting antigens on the surface makes it a monkey wrench for vaccine development and remains a hard nut to crack. Recently, scientists have been testing multistage vaccines that are able to trigger stronger immune responses at various stages of this cycle (Tiwari et al., 2023). Battling malaria is about attacking the parasite at many stages simultaneously. Take the SUB1 protease, for example, it plays an important role in both the liver stage and blood stage, helping *parasites* escape from host cells. Recent drug studies that enhanced compound permeability and inhibitory activity against SUB1 have shown encouraging *in vitro* results, suggesting a mechanism for retarding the parasite's advancement in the human body (Puszko et al., 2025). In addition, with the parasite's sinuous life cycle, from mosquito to liver, blood, and even sexual stages, a single-hit strategy just won't do. Rather, vaccines are mixed, chemotherapies targeted, and vector control measures mixed, which seems to be the way forward, particularly as our increasing knowledge of each phase is offering new perspectives for combating malaria's continued worldwide effects (Tiwari et al., 2023) (Figure 1.5).

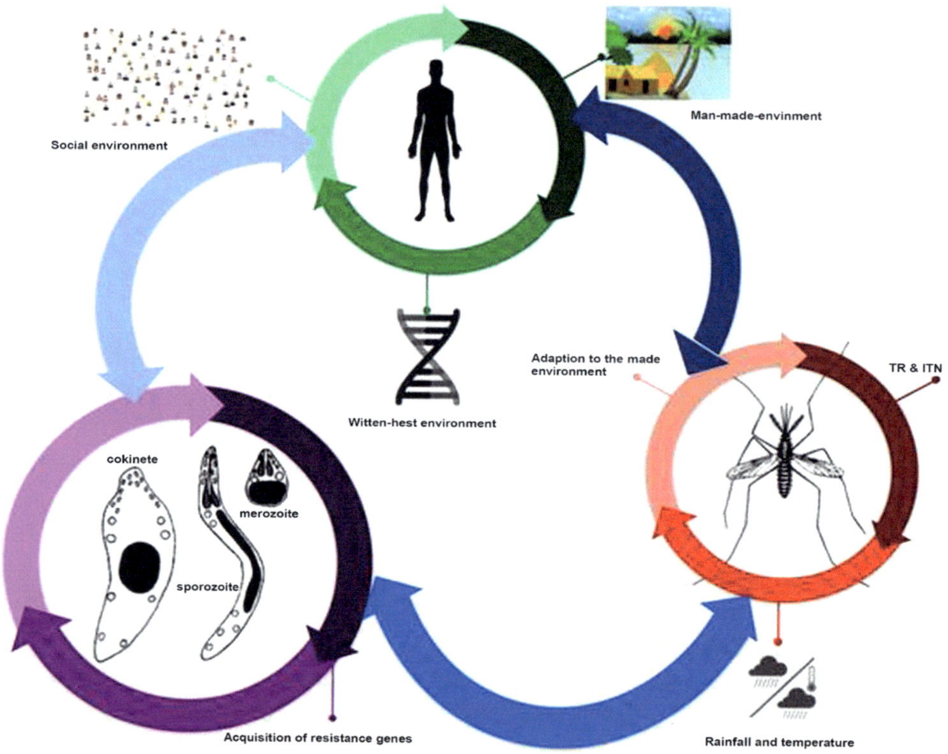

Figure 1.5. Stages of the malaria *parasites* life cycle.

Source: Savi MK. An Overview of Malaria Transmission Mechanisms, Control, and Modeling. *Medical Sciences*. 2023; 11(1):3. https://doi.org/10.3390/medsci11010003

1.1.3. Role of the Anopheles Mosquito

Transmission of malaria simplifies to one main culprit: the mosquito. *Anopheles* is usually the *Plasmodium parasite*-carrying mosquito which causes malaria in most instances. Its habits, wheredwelldetermine how often humans get bitten. Every now subsequently, you see such mosquitoes shift from their indoor nighttime feeding to a bit more outdoor or early evening pattern, and this wreaks havoc on something like long-lasting insecticidal nets (LLINs). General studies suggest that when mosquito behavior changes and resistance to insecticides grows, LLINs don't work, so control strategies must keep up with what the mosquitoes are doing (Briët & Chitnis, 2013). Environmental conditions outside play an enormous part in all of this, too. The weather around homes—temperature, humidity, and other microclimatic features—can change where and how often mosquitoes bite. For example, *Anopheles arabiensis* bites outdoors as indoor spaces get relatively warmer, behavior that may compromise indoor-focused solutions such as coated walls or bed nets. *Anopheles funestus*, on the other hand, seems to disregard climatic changes, and it bites at a consistent rate all year round. These minor behavioral shifts force us to include local environmental data in our monitoring, since changing climates may mean seasonally fluctuating highs and lows in risk of bites (Ngowo et al., 2017). It all adds up to a pretty complicated problem to fight malaria. The interplay of adaptive biting behavior and rising insecticide resistance creates a two-fold barrier to vector control. Some epidemiologic models, , despite their own peculiarities, suggest that crepuscular feeding cycles by mosquitoes in subsequent rounds of feeding can suppress LLINs nearly as much as straightforward insecticide resistance. More bizarre, these two mechanisms never occur in the same batch of mosquitoes; they seem to evolve independently, so solutions for each will differ. Whereas LLINs are still economical for most settings, in situations where we have extremely high transmission or severe resistance, we must keep developing our strategy in order to be ahead of the battle against malaria (Briët & Chitnis, 2013) (Figure 1.6).

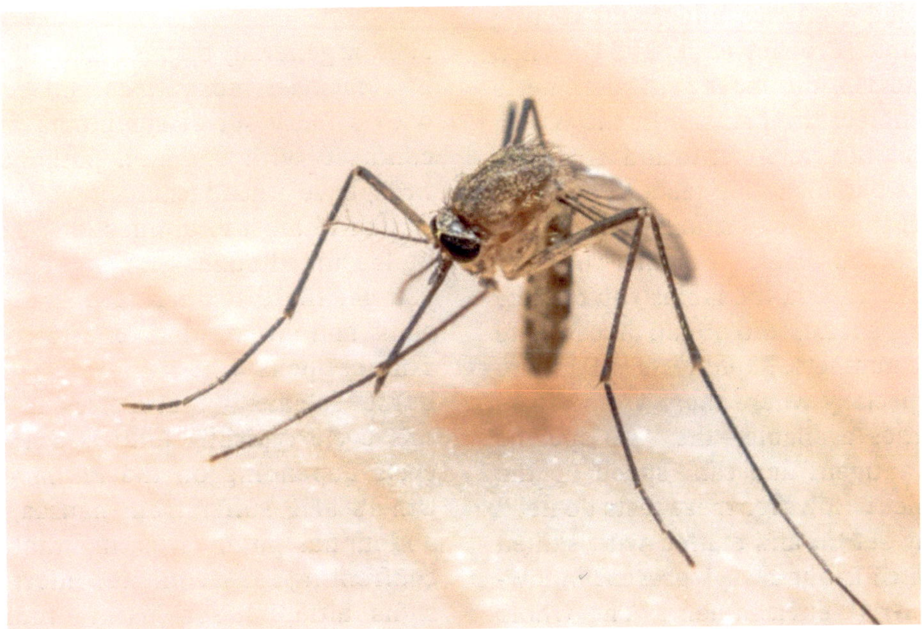

Figure 1.6. *Anopheles* mosquito.

Source: InfoEscola. (2016). *Anopheles Mosquito.* https://external-content.duckduckgo.com/iu/?u=https%3A%2F%2Fwww.infoescola.com%2Fwp-content%2Fuploads%2F2016%2F04%2F*Anopheles*_376047214.jpg&f=1&nofb=1&ipt=f47b66af7a39dac6075ce39ccad3ed2e6df064cc543822bb5db70044e4ede3b8.

1.2. Symptoms and Diagnosis

Malaria has so many varying presentations, that it's hard to catch and have treated early. It tends to start with some relatively mild symptoms – a bit of fever somewhere, a bit of shivering somewhere, and generally just not quite feeling right – that are simply mistaken for other common infections in those areas. With time, the condition may deteriorate, with the manifestations of anemia, spells of vomiting, and diarrhea suddenly arising, all pointing to a body-wide infestation by the *Plasmodium parasites*. In some cases, especially in children who are admitted to rural Malawian hospitals, the illness takes a lethal turn whereby about half of the children not only get anemia but also develop serious brain complications. These contradictory clues contribute to the difficulty for doctors trying to rule out malaria from other fevers, or added vigilance and rapid testing are indispensable (Crowley et al., 2024). When diagnosing malaria, the most critical thing is to be able to detect the parasite in the blood. Healthcare practitioners prefer to add what they observe with a patient to lab tests to be quite confident with the outcomes, and microscopic inspection of blood smears remains the gold standard in this respect. It enables you to view the *Plasmodium* species and obtain an estimate of the *parasite* numbers. Rapid tests (RDTs) are useful too, especially where there are no fixed medical facilities available—they are specific to particular antigens and can speed up the start of treatment. However these tests do need to be properly set up and staffed with skilled personnel, which is not always present in low-resource, high-risk environments. The whole process becomes even more difficult when malaria imitates symptoms of other conditions, like hookworm, and therefore a detailed clinical examination alongside laboratory findings is crucial (Shooraj & Mahdavi, 2022). It is also important to add that social and economic factors mainly decide how malaria will spread and how quickly it will be diagnosed. Issues like poor sanitation, unrelenting temperatures in the tropics, and limited healthcare infrastructure have a tendency to pave the way for higher rates of infection and delayed diagnosis. These challenging conditions not only worsen the effects of the disease – enhancing the chances of side effects like anemia and cerebral manifestations – but also disproportionately impact vulnerable groups such as children and pregnant women. At most, early identification of the symptoms and use of proper diagnostic methods will make a significant difference in reducing the risks, whereas more general public health measures based on local co-infection patterns and local epidemiology are most crucial to ensure that the patients receive proper treatment in time (Shooraj & Mahdavi, 2022; Crowley et al., 2024).

1.2.1. Common Symptoms of Malaria

Malaria generally begins quietly. It is transmitted by *Anopheles* mosquitoes and becomes active with a fuzzy set of symptoms that are easily confused with common pathogens—you are tired, have a headache, and your muscles hurt, similar to most viral infections. As the parasite builds up, though, things get more detailed: you get these temperature spikes, along with chills and sweats that tend to come in waves. This happens when infected red blood cells burst, releasing merozoites into the blood; this cycle typically follows a 48- to 72-hour cycle depending on the *Plasmodium* species. Others also suffer from nausea, vomiting, or abdominal pain, reflecting that the body is confronting a disseminated infection. The early signs, although serious as predictors, are at times mistaken for other illnesses – an acute challenge to trigger corrective action in poor-resource settings (Riaz et al., 2024). As the illness matures, the case takes a totally different dimension. High-grade fever continues, and you typically recognize severe anemia due to the destruction of infected RBCs, which presents a patient with pallor and weakness. Visible hepatosplenomegaly—a swelling reaction from body cleaning mechanisms leading to tissue congestion—is possible to observe. Interestingly enough, chills and shudders that come just before the fever crest seem to be the body's desperate attempt to push away the parasite. In more serious infections, neurologic complications like confusion, seizures, or even coma may manifest, pointing to cerebral malaria, a highly dangerous condition most frequently linked to *Plasmodium falciparum*. In most cases, all these overlapping presentations necessitate a careful, nuanced approach to diagnosis and treatment, which underscores just how challenging malaria is (Riaz et al., 2024).

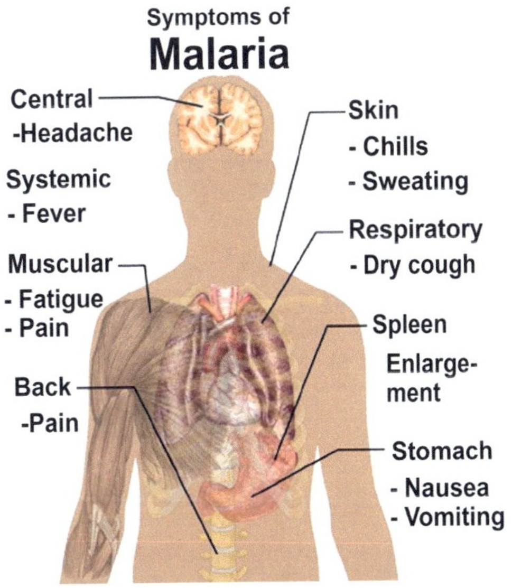

Figure 1.7. Symptoms of malaria.

Source: By Mikael Häggström.When using this image in external works, it may be cited as:Häggström, Mikael (2014). "Medical gallery of Mikael Häggström 2014". WikiJournal of Medicine 1 (2). DOI:10.15347/wjm/2014.008. ISSN 2002-4436. Public Domain.orBy Mikael Häggström, used with permission. - All used images are in public domain., Public Domain, https://commons.wikimedia.org/w/index.php?curid=6557991

To further complicate things, malaria's symptoms are extremely easily mistaken for other infections, especially during times of larger outbreaks. During the COVID-19 outbreak, for example, fever and chills typical of malaria were sometimes mistakenly attributed to coronavirus infection as well, and treatment was consequently delayed. This kind of overlap demonstrates how closely looking at the symptoms and making a proper differential diagnosis is essential, particularly in regions where multiple infections exist side by side. In addition, starting antimalarial treatment without a confirmatory parasitological diagnosis exposes one to complications like resistance or relapse, and this is a specific worry with *Plasmodium vivax*. These risks, as seen in the large public health emergencies, remind us of that careful symptom identification and corroborative analysis are needed for successful malaria control programs (Jaski et al., 2023) (Figure 1.7).

1.2.2. Diagnostic Methods Used in Healthcare

Getting the diagnosis right is crucial, especially in something like malaria where other fevers might look the same. Microscopy has long been the method for detecting the parasite in blood smears—it's a nice picture and counts the *parasites* down to a fine level of detail. But it takes skilled hands, serviced machines, and time, which can be a real nuisance in the less-resourced places. Because of these challenges, simpler instruments have appeared. RDTs like the MAL Card test come on to the field with rapid, easy-to-read results without the full lab setup. These technologies most commonly have taken diagnosis out of big hospitals and into communities, speeding up treatment and cutting down on disease spread (Mahajan et al., 2025). However, while these rapid tests are handy, their true deployment in the field is accompanied by an entire array of issues. Research in nations such as Nigeria shows that factors such as the tests' availability, the patients awaiting being tested in a queue, and even the level of experienced and confident health workers can change the efficacy of these tests. Workers can delay following a test finding if they are not completely sure about it—which can lead them to take several antimalarial drugs and eventually become drug-resistant. Patients, in the same way, can refuse to go for the test, either because they are nervous about needles or have muddy thoughts about malaria. Generally speaking, although rapid tests make things easier, an effective strategy has to deal with both the problem of operations and individuals' emotions regarding the process (Omale, 2024). Comparing both microscopy and rapid tests simultaneously makes one realize that there needs to be a single solution. Speed tests are usually very sensitive and specific , the MAL Card test worked well in distant hospitals, proving a godsend for preliminary tests , but occasionally they will return false positives. That is, in some cases, another test by microscopy would be prudent to firm up the diagnosis. Such a multi-level approach enables health workers to move fast without compromising accuracy. Most contemporary health programs integrate both: expanding the use of quick tests for instant information but still investing in good-quality microscopy training and capabilities. In the end, integrating these strategies works to the advantage of healthcare systems in managing malaria, especially when finances are low and malaria is widespread (Omale, 2024; Mahajan et al., 2025) (Figure 1.8).

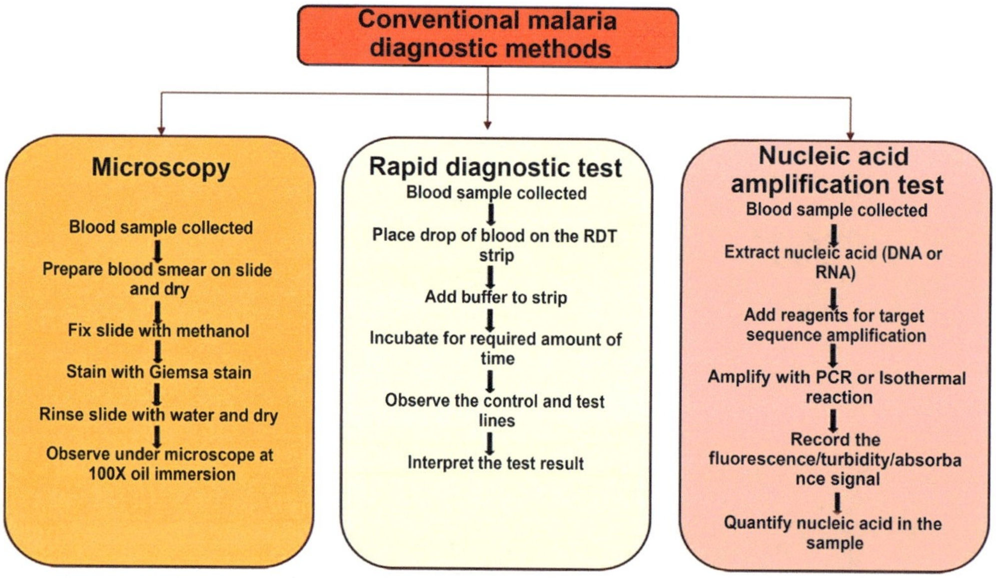

Figure 1.8. Malaria diagnostic methods.

Source: Chatterjee, S., & Chakraborty, A. (2020). Malaria and climate change: Review of the current global scenario and a glimpse of the Indian perspective. *Tropical Medicine and Infectious Disease, 5*(4), 102.

1.2.3. Challenges in Accurate Diagnosis

In regions where malaria is not normally found, doctors struggle to diagnose the disease. Fever, chills, and muscle pains occur often in malaria – but these exact same symptoms occur in dengue fever, so it is easy to get them mixed up. One urban example from Indonesia was when a patient with both *Plasmodium vivax* and *Plasmodium malariae* was misdiagnosed with dengue because the symptoms seemed so similar and not many practitioners were used to seeing malaria outside of areas where it was endemic. Asking for the patient's travel history and doing a detailed blood smear test cleared up the matter. Such a situation, in most cases, brings to the fore why neglecting subtle signs and travel histories would delay proper treatment and why enhancing clinician perception and training is so important (Andrean et al., 2025). Problems of data quality and technology constraints further throw a spanner into malaria diagnosis, particularly in lower-resourced settings. While deep learning and computer-aided diagnostic systems have produced some promising results , with good accuracy as well as scalability , problems like biased datasets as well as regional biases come to wreak havoc with how well such systems function. A model that is trained on a particular demographic can seriously fail when faced with alternative forms of parasites or clinical patterns in a different region, and that variability tends to lower performance. Techniques such as synthetic data augmentation and domain adaptation (consider transfer learning) have managed to enhance data heterogeneity and system robustness, albeit slightly, but further quality boosts in datasets and algorithm explainability through global data sharing also remain a necessity (Kabore & Guel, 2024). The puzzle gets only more complex when you introduce the parasite's biological features and the oscillating phases of infection that make parasite density sometimes impossible to find. Classic microscopy, much touted as the gold standard, is very much dependent on the skill of the technicians—yet differences in slide preparation or mere human error can instantly sabotage the findings. RDTs, though more accessible, in certain instances do not deliver sufficient sensitivity or specificity, especially in distinguishing between *Plasmodium* species or identifying mixed infections. Such diagnostic imprecision can lead to somewhat incorrect treatments and even to the survival of malaria. It does seem to require the union of clinical experience with local knowledge of epidemiology and advanced diagnostic methods to achieve the proper diagnosis. Overall, developments in explainable AI will be expected to assist clinical decision-making and drive expanded adoption of state-of-the-art technology in the treatment of malaria (Kabore & Guel, 2024; Andrean et al., 2025).

1.3. Transmission and Risk Factors

Malaria is spread in an complex web of the parasite, their insect vectors, and the people they bite. *Plasmodium falciparum*, for instance, is a major player in the tropics where there are plenty of areas where *Anopheles* mosquitoes can breed. Uncontrolled overgrown plants and puddles of standing water are both perfect nurseries for these female mosquitoes, allowing the parasite to keep going around in its circle. Habits and immediate surroundings can worsen, those who reside near water or in forgotten areas of town are more likely to have additional hazards. Research within endemic countries suggests that age and occupation also become involved; kids and employees spending time outside, in the majority of cases, become more exposed. And indeed, how often families make use of nets or engage in other forms of prevention can affect infection probabilities (Sambo et al., 2024). Economic and social hardships place another twist on how malaria takes hold. Conditions of poverty and limited education generally lead to bad sanitation and lesser access to protective gear such as treated bed nets or proper healthcare. Studies, such as in urban centers like Kisangani, point out that garbage piles and areas of standing water around homes aren't just mosquito magnets—they're also symptoms of broader poverty-related problems. Generally speaking, these are closely related environmental issues so better waste disposal and sanitation would go a long way. It is also clear that the poor segments—pregnant women and young children in particular—are more impacted, so social issues and disease susceptibility are connected. Person-by-person, the interrelation of genetic and immunological factors makes some people more prone to malaria than others.

For example, individuals with sickle cell disease have a much higher rate of infection and other health issues to struggle with that can put them at risk and heighten the severity of their illness. Age and gender are just complicating factors; young children and male outdoorsmen have higher rates of infection, perhaps because their daily routines put them out in the elements more. Others even rely on old remedies instead of modern prevention methods, and in so doing can inadvertently help facilitate being at risk. These results overall show the need for not just mass preventive action, but also specific intervention for the most at-risk individuals (Sambo et al., 2024).

1.3.1. Modes of Transmission

The transmission of malaria is closely linked to the interaction of our bodies and mosquitoes, specifically the *Anopheles* subspecies responsible for carrying *Plasmodium*. When an infected female mosquito bites, she injects sporozoites directly into our bloodstream; these microscopic agents usually find themselves in the liver before proceeding further. Even recent studies indicate that saliva from mosquitoes can bring bacteria along for the ride with the parasite. That is, the mix of organisms within a mosquito's mouth may modulate how malaria is spread around. Rather interestingly, when *Plasmodium* gets established, it seems to change the mosquito's internal micro-society, which subsequently could change the way the parasite is transmitted. Overall, it is a sophisticated biological association, which suggests new paths to possibly block malaria at that mosquito-human interface (Accoti et al., 2023). How the public understands malaria also plays an enormous role in how well we are able to fight it. Most people know that bites by mosquitoes, especially those evening bites from *Anopheles*, are the main way the disease is transmitted. But not everyone is aware that breeding grounds show up where one would least expect them, for instance, riverbanks or even animal refuges. This imperfect knowledge of mosquito behavior sabotages efforts to control the environment or cling to individual protection strategies.

And, further, there is usually many unequivocally clear facts and still-haunting myths on what causes malaria and other such diseases. Primarily, expanding education to allay such misconceptions is most critical to galvanizing communities to become more proactive in bringing malaria's spread to an end (Atah et al., 2023).

It is not the mosquitoes themselves only; what is around us and how we do things is just as crucial. Poor drainage of water or not trimming the bushes on our homes gives the mosquitoes perfect breeding conditions to keep the cycle continuous. Even those treated bednets (ITNs) are useless if people don't use them because they don't think it's bad enough. In addition to that, when people are also affected by other illnesses like intestinal *parasites* concurrently, it makes the whole situation more complex. Addressing issues such as poor personal hygiene, symptomless carriers, and ensuring safer behaviors requires interventions that are responsive to the local environment and lifestyles. All these interrelated factors illustrate just how complex malaria transmission is and why we need an all-out, holistic strategy to alleviate the disease's burden (Atah et al., 2023) (Figure 1.9).

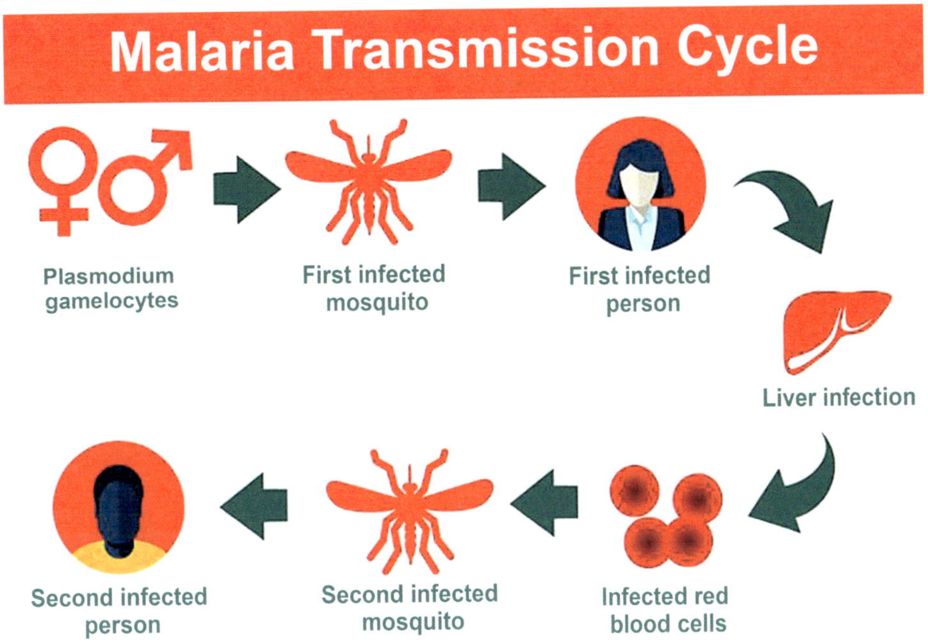

Figure 1.9. Transmission of malaria.

Source: Mosquito Magnet. (n.d.). *Malaria Transmission.* https://external-content.duckduckgo.com/iu/?u=https%3A%2F%2Fimages.mosquitomagnet.com%2Fis%2Fimage%2Fwoodstream%2Fmalaria-transmission-article-3B%3F%24fullpng%24&f=1&nofb=1&ipt=518ed7c2f5ef205d1ec16ae36004dcde43ce959eeafc2d33e36f0c5fcba3a943.

1.3.2. Geographic Regions Most Affected

Malaria is still a major issue around the globe—in most places, its impact falls asymmetrically. In sub-Saharan Africa, for instance, the numbers are especially high; the hot, humid climate there makes it an ideal breeding ground for *Anopheles* mosquitoes, the major vectors of transmission. A hot climate, combined with widespread poverty and an inability to access good healthcare, makes the fight against the disease much more challenging. There are also foci in South Africa and Latin America, where the disease continues due to fragile diagnostic and treatment systems that enable the infection cycle to continue. Largely for the most part, local economic differences and frail public health systems guarantee that prevention mechanisms need to be as unique as the settings in which they are intended to protect. Most of the heavy burden of malaria stems from the coupling of environmental factors with poor health services. Western sub-Saharan Africa, for example, appears to bear the brunt not only because of the parasite but also from treatment complications like drug resistance—complications on which some bacterial infections (Murray et al., 2022) also wreak havoc. Although malaria is, by nature, a parasitic infection, the added complexity of antimicrobial resistance (AMR) also worsens the treatment of secondary infections. Underserved and rural communities, which often lack such basics as ITNs and timely medical care, are the most severely affected. All this calls for an even more urgent appeal for ever-more integrated, locally specific health solutions, measures that not only understand the science, but the social context of the disease as well. Despite international pressures exerting themselves forcefully against malaria, some areas still remain stubborn hotspots, laying bare glaring global health inequities. Some areas of South America and Southeast Asia are still battling high caseloads, with problems arising from many malaria species and rising drug resistance. This calls for region-specific approaches that address every element from diagnosis through treatment and vector control. For instance, controlling *Plasmodium vivax* across much of Asia often requires different strategies than those needed in Africa, where *Plasmodium falciparum* dominates. The crippling impact in poor settings, where childhood deaths are high and health infrastructure is weak, further complicates the lessening of the disease's burden. Local heterogeneity of this sort needs to be understood if investments are to be effectively allocated and worldwide efforts are to tackle malaria's heterogeneous challenges (Figure 1.10).

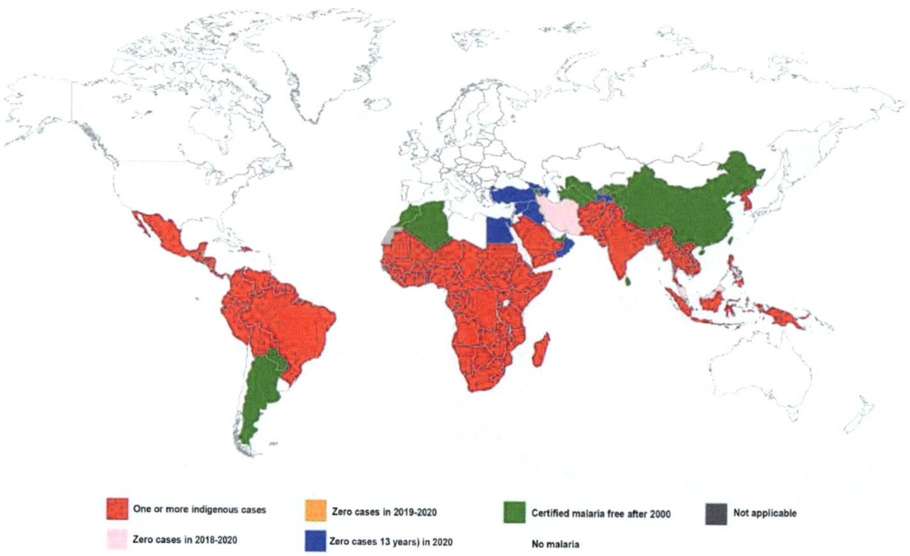

Figure 1.10. Geographic regions most affected of malaria.

Source: Malaria Free World. (2022). *World Map: Malaria 2021 (WHO).* https://external-content.duckduckgo.com/iu/?u=https%3A%2F%2Fmalariafree2030.org%2Fwp-content%2Fuploads%2F2022%2F04%2FWorld-map-malaria-2021-WHO.png&f=1&nofb=1&ipt=d89935faeea890310be3808efe34fe0ba49da702409d6611b58b87d6b942365a.

1.3.3. Socioeconomic Factors Influencing Risk

Populations become vulnerable to malaria because of a combination of factors, and economic challenges seem to be at the center of all things. In most parts of sub-Saharan Africa, parts of the continent where malaria is widely seen, poor households may not have an easy access to such things as ITNs or robust housing materials. Some studies of Nigerian under-five children even provide evidence that dirty living conditions, such as, such as makeshift toilets and walls or ceilings made of poor-quality material (Mhelembe et al., 2025)—are linked with higher malaria rates. Those tough physical surroundings, along with overall economic hardship, may raise exposure to mosquitoes and delay proper treatment. Education of the parent, especially mothers, also proves to influence what health interventions are used in the home. Fundamentally, economic status not only changes the physical boundaries of a home but even colors how families respond when malaria comes knocking on their doors. It is not the house; the way in which families take care of their children also plays an important role. Nutrition, being directly associated with the financial status of a person, has an extreme influence on how susceptible babies are to contracting malaria. In countries like West Africa, a poor diet can greatly impair the immune system, thus indirectly preparing the way for more severe infections (Maina, 2024). When children lack adequate protein and vital micronutrients, their own immune systems are impaired, setting off a vicious cycle where malaria robs them further of their nutritional reserves. Besides these immediate biological impacts, infant diets are shaped by maternal education and local dietary habits in ways that impact malaria risk from infancy through childhood.

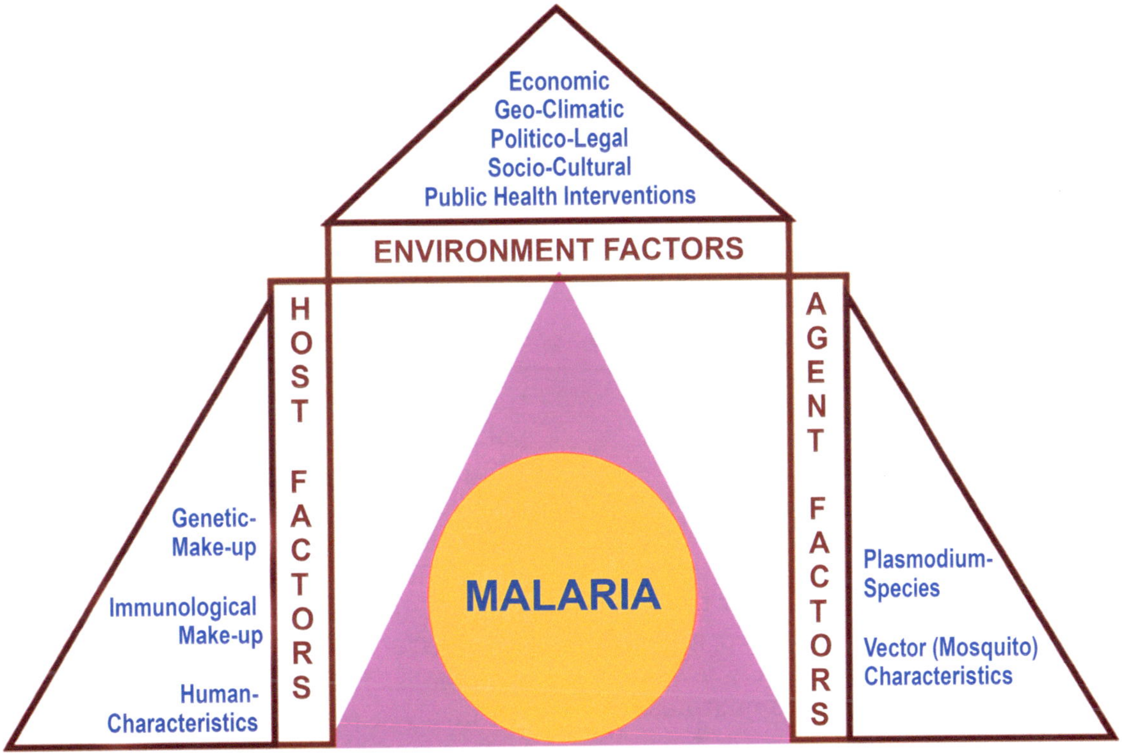

Figure 1.11. Socioeconomic factors influencing risk of malaria.

Source: Ganguly, K. S., Modak, S., & Karmakar, A. K. (2016). Factors of epidemiological triad (i.e., different co-variates), e.g., economic, geo-climatic, politico-legal, socio-cultural, etc. In Forecasting based on a SARIMA model of urban malaria for Kolkata. *American Journal of Environmental and Industrial Development*, *4*(2), 34–41.

The quality of how well infants are fed good breastfeeding and nutritious complementary foods often depends on household resources, caregivers' information, and the influence of local tradition – rendering economic distress even more of a health impediment. Addressing both these economic and nutritional challenges, in many instances, is vital in order to combat malaria successfully. City vs. countryside lines create another dimension to the problem. Urban and rural settings exhibit largely disparate malaria risk patterns, thanks largely to the fact that where you reside intermingles with economic conditions in unforeseen manners. Rural settings are more likely to have a heavy burden of malaria due to poverty, a compromised healthcare system, and limited resources for access to prevention information (Mhelembe et al., 2025). All of these settings simply don't have sufficient resources for proper vector control or rapid diagnosis and treatment. The stark contrast in resources between metropolitan cities and country towns guarantees that less affluent are doubly-troubled—both by their environment and by barriers finding necessary care. And if gender dynamics enter into the picture, girls' and their caregivers' statuses can also affect when assistance is rushed in or how often protection is provided. Socioeconomic status combines in a complex way with social and environmental issues to amplify malaria risks among those already on the margins (Figure 1.11).

1.4. Prevention Strategies

Prevention of malaria does not occur through a single approach. It is a synergy of environmental interventions, killing of mosquitoes, and joined effort on the part of local populations. All too often the struggle starts with mosquito population reduction, specifically, those nuisance *Anopheles* flies that transmit the disease. Simple measures like removing breeding grounds by keeping water sources and sanitation in check can decrease the risk quite dramatically. And with global warming and the introduction of new mosquito species to new places, constant watchful observation is needed; they may erupt in full fury in places they have never appeared in before. In general, this means that public health planning should integrate insect science and local knowledge to see and act on new threats (Volkan & Karanis, 2025). Coming to another key player in the fight, ITNs form a vital barrier. Nets work on a dual front—a physical block and a chemical shield—to keep deadly mosquito bites away from victims at peak-transmission times. Even though they have proven to be effective, challenges still remain in achieving mass application, especially among the poor and rural populace where malaria is prevalent. Social marketing efforts—experimenting with such fundamentals as price, place, product, and promotion—have succeeded in raising both purchase and regular use of ITNs. They don't merely target the distribution of nets; they target behavior as well, making it easier to use while incorporating them into daily habits in a low-key way. Most times, this type of strategy evokes the kind of positive behavioral change that's essential to the decrease in cases of malaria (Chukwuocha et al., 2024). In perspective, there is long-term malaria prevention that needs a One Health approach that relates human, animal, and environmental health. In practice, this means that physicians, veterinarians, policymakers, and residents all collaborate in order to undertake systems of mosquito control and disease surveillance. Recognizing that local environmental conditions and animals might affect transmission pressures One Health projects to become more specific with their methods of control in order to adapt to local conditions. Furthermore, when communities get involved proactively, the interventions are more adaptable, culturally tailored, and easier to scale up, even if sometimes the details are not tidier. Essentially, this broad approach is key to decelerating the transmission of malaria and reducing the burden of vector-borne disease among vulnerable groups (Volkan & Karanis, 2025).

1.4.1. Use of Insecticide-Treated Nets (ITNs)

Malaria is always hanging over the head in most locations, and what one can do to halt its progress is a necessity. One widely adopted method is the application of ITNs – they are both a physical and chemical deterrent to those pesky mosquitoes. Naturally, even if the majority of people have these nets, their application is another matter altogether. In one study done in Berekum East Municipality, for example, approximately 87.6% of the respondents said they had a net, yet only about 28% of them regularly used them daily. Issues of being too hot, the nets being inconvenient, or even allergic reactions to the skin have a cumulative effect, so it becomes a hard habit to keep. Generally, these are signs that more hands-on instructional and behavior-based changes might be needed (Gyaase et al., 2023). Identifying why some people use their nets but others don't is not always easy. Level of education is one of them – people with higher levels of education are likely to be more consistent in their use. The same survey in Berekum East indicated that individuals with tertiary-level schooling were nearly twice as likely to make use of the nets as compared to others with lower schooling. Younger adults, especially the 20s to early 30s age group, also seem more likely to keep themselves covered. Subsequently there are home factors like space configuration and how many people sleep in a given room that can impact the level of effectiveness and comfort the net affords. In most cases, bringing together easy access to informal community and health talks seems to be inevitable to call for change (Gyaase et al., 2023). Pregnant women should also be given a special mention regarding malaria since they are at increased risk. In Malawi, a survey indicated that while most women of reproductive age had nets, barely 53% had slept under one the previous night. Other problems – age, whether or not a woman is pregnant now or has just given birth, and even residence – all combine to impact use. Ironically, pregnant women or women who have just given birth are more cautious, which could be due to reminders during antenatal care visits. Increased vigilance in early and increased antenatal care might be able to push these figures further upwards, illustrating just how critical an integrated health system is in the fight against malaria in this vulnerable group (Figure 1.12).

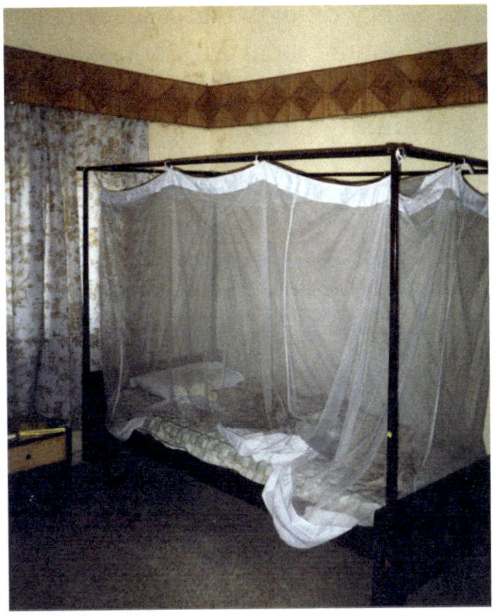

Figure 1.12. Use of insecticide-treated nets (ITNs).

Source: CC BY-SA 3.0, https://commons.wikimedia.org/w/index.php?curid=690992

1.4.2. Vaccination Efforts and Developments

Vaccines have been our main weapon against infectious diseases since time immemorial, as they lower levels of illness and death (Figure 1.13). Take malaria, for example, the parasite infecting us takes a very hidden path, dodging forms and avoiding our immune system. Early vaccine trials only targeted one stage of the parasite life cycle, but its cleverness in dodging defenses used to get in the way. Still, we now have RTS,S/AS01, a genuine breakthrough that even got an approval stamp from regulators. Scientists are now looking into multi-stage vaccines and combination treatments to better mimic the capricious nature of malaria. Looking at overall disease control, it seems that vaccines aren't the panacea. The COVID-19 response showed that many immunization, coupled with interventions like case isolating and contact tracing (Hu et al., 2020), will develop into an outbreak. There's an emerging understanding that vaccines at times give incomplete protection and have plenty of logistical issues. This forces experts to combine them with other approaches, such as preventative treatments and surveillance at the community level.

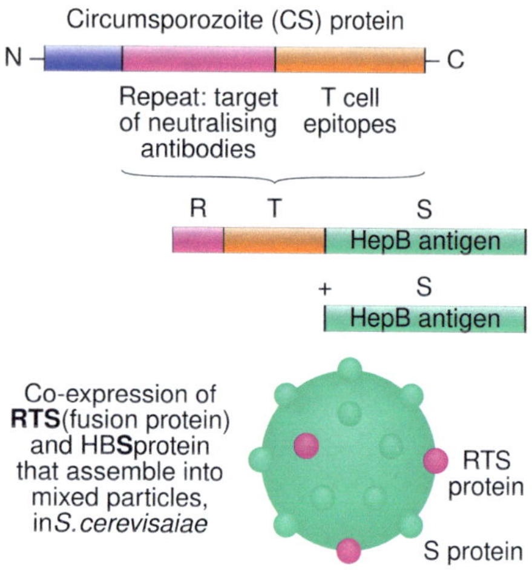

Figure 1.13. Vaccination efforts and developments.

Source: By Cmglee - Own work, CC BY-SA 4.0, https://commons.wikimedia.org/w/index.php?curid=110868231

The way the laboratory experiments and real vaccine distributions fill in for each other illustrates just how important it is to get immunologists, epidemiologists, and public health professionals collaborating. It also shows the need for ongoing funding for both cutting-edge vaccine research and reliable distribution systems, especially in the most malaria-stricken areas. Existing vaccine efforts have been favored, to a large extent, by faster research strategies and trial designs that change as new outbreaks occur (Casamitjana et al., 2020). Ring vaccination, for instance, first used in the Ebola epidemic, now seems to be ready for controlling localized epidemics of malaria and for avoiding high-risk exposures. Apart from that, new advances in adjuvant combinations and novel delivery systems are improving both the strength of effect and the duration of protection. There is a global system within the health community that is introducing these technologies into communities even while it is meeting economic concerns and random scheduling delays. Ultimately, these improvements may not only help cut malaria transmission but also offer clues on how to approach other diseases spread by vectors or jumping from animals to people.

1.4.3. Public Health Initiatives and Education

Malaria control isn't an issue of treatments—it's more of a general, community-based initiative to avoid transmission and enhance general health. Integrated vector management (IVM) is part of that, but it integrates government initiatives with local input in a somewhat unique manner. In a vast number of cases, malaria is not seen as exclusively the domain of the health sector; instead, it needs to be helped by schools, fisheries, forestry, and social services. For example, rural Kenyan primary schools have been mobilized to disseminate the word, and fish farming and tree planting not only increase incomes but also dissipate breeding sites for the disease (Ng'ang'a et al., 2021). Such community-level initiatives, combined with formal interventions, can gradually nudge community practices and environmental care in the right direction. Community education is at the center of the fight—empowering the most vulnerable. Public health workers share simple tips like using ITNs, keeping living spaces clean, and when to seek treatment early. Students in schools often become neighborhood health ambassadors through fun "mosquito days" that spur learning and community pride. This form of learning, sometimes more friendly than austere, strengthens social bonds tighter and bridges the traditional gaps between formal health provision and everyday life. Even limited training for local health volunteers—on vector control and case detection in early stages—gives an extra boost in rendering neighborhoods that much stronger against the epidemic of malaria (Ng'ang'a et al., 2021). Public health training is not enslaved to malaria, however; it intersperses other health concerns as well. Even though there are programs that concentrate on vector control and case management, there is a greater context that skims along issues like cognitive impairment in older people. Generally speaking, simple care routines such as a bit of sensory stimulation, easy infection avoidance, and hydration replicate those initial warning signals and supporting measures in preventing malaria. By integrating malaria lessons with general health promotion activities, communities step-by-step build up their total know-how and resilience. This multi-level, sometimes chaotic approach not only does an excellent job of fending off malaria but also readies communities to handle other health challenges in the future (Ng'ang'a et al., 2021).

1.5. Treatment Options

Quick and accurate diagnosis along with proper treatment is the most effective method of staving off malaria's worst effects. Physicians in many malaria-endemic areas used to rely on symptoms to diagnose because superior testing equipment simply wasn't available. This educated guess approach systematically led to too much antimalarial medication being given, which not only increases costs but, in most cases, also increases the chances of medications losing their effectiveness. More recently, studies have shown that RDTs can be a cost-saving measure, despite incurring some added expense—by avoiding unnecessary treatments. Choices between drug pairs, like artesunate plus amodiaquine or artemether-lumefantrine (AL), eventually merge with these testing methods to affect both health outcomes and economic impacts in malaria control programs (Rolland et al., 2006). While the new testing tools show a lot of promise, the cost of malaria still appears rather high, especially in sub-Saharan Africa where young children are most affected. Costs reveal themselves in two forms: direct medical costs and hidden indirect costs, including lost work time and the devastating cost of premature death. Research that initiated studies in nations like Ghana, Kenya, and Tanzania tends to discover that households ultimately bear a high percentage of these costs, with indirect costs often making up a large percentage. And when illnesses are severe, like cerebral malaria causing ongoing brain issues, the expense and long-term impact on family life escalate exponentially. It is good to have a solid grasp of these economic realities when crafting treatment policy, maintaining aid available and viable (Sicuri et al., 2013). Choosing the appropriate malaria treatment regimen is not simply a question of which medicines work; it also has to be appropriate for the local health infrastructure and economic conditions. While medicines like artesunate-amodiaquine and AL are efficacious, their success is sometimes contingent on the availability of resources and treatment regimen adherence by the patients. RDTs, in addition to improving diagnosis, also improve how treatments are dispensed in that they cut down on drug abuse and conserve resources. A twinning of lowering the costs of RDTs with improving access to affordable drugs could dramatically improve cost-effectiveness overall, with more being able to be treated without the healthcare system going over budget. Put briefly, an array of improved diagnostic methods and effective drug regimens, and their enablement by supportive policies, is more or less the absolute requirement if we are to sustain malaria control and reduce its significant burden on societies (Rolland et al., 2006).

1.5.1. Antimalarial Medications Available

Malaria control is more a question of access to the proper medicines and their proper use. Our treatment of malaria has changed through time—a very long time ago, chloroquine and quinine were the treatments of choice, but these soon developed resistance problems, so more modern, more powerful regimens became dominant. In most cases, artemisinin-based combination therapies (ACTs) are the pillar of treatment now. They pair a fast-acting artemisinin derivative with a concomitant drug that stays longer, quickly clearing *parasites* and decreasing the likelihood of resistance developing. In most of the malaria-endemic world, these are supplemented by RDTs, the dual pair being a central component of the control package. However, getting people available to take these drugs consistently and as directed is a gigantic undertaking, especially in areas where resources are limited and understanding of how malaria is transmitted is thinly spread (Ruberto et al., 2014). All of this generally implies the implementation of measures that integrate drug availability with good public health education. While antimalarial drugs are at the forefront of the war against the disease, their appropriate application at the patient level is not unchallenged. Several studies on fever case management using rapid diagnostic tests (mRDTs) in combination with ACTs have documented variable results. For instance, research in high-transmission settings reported that despite availability of drugs like AL, a good number of the children with fever either did not receive the correct medication after tests came back positive or were administered ACTs even when the test revealed that they were not necessary (Chandler et al., 2017). Health workers prefer the fact that mRDTs can detect malaria quickly but generally have structural barriers, like less time per patient and poor facilities, which make it harder for them to use these tools to the best of their abilities. In most cases, even the stock of drugs might not be enough unless the health systems are flexible and strong enough to facilitate their proper utilization. It also must be kept in mind that the selection of antimalarial drugs is not restricted to ACTs only.

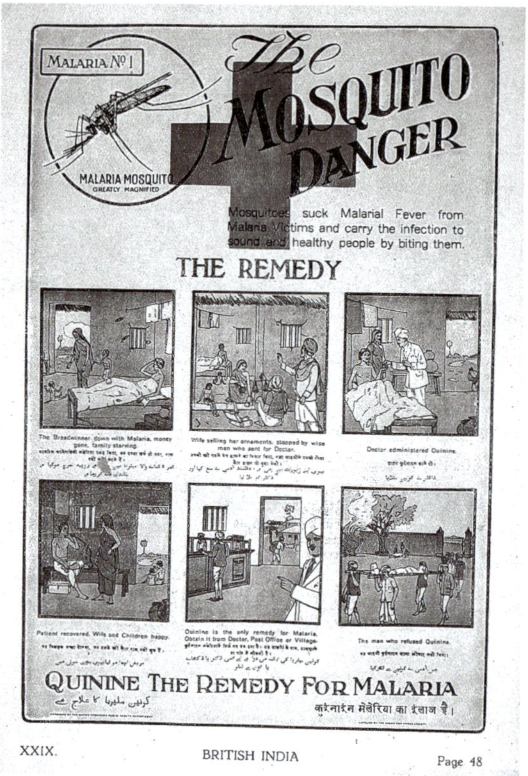

Figure 1.14. Antimalarial medications.

Source: By https://wellcomeimages.org/indexplus/obf_images/ce/b0/96e5a4b06e6d1cc67e4237b4f872.jpgGallery: https://wellcomeimages.org/indexplus/image/L0022443.htmlWellcome Collection gallery (2018-03-21): https://wellcomecollection.org/works/xce2v52p CC-BY-4.0, CC BY 4.0, https://commons.wikimedia.org/w/index.php?curid=35997577

The alternatives also lie in a broader spectrum, addressing varying clinical needs and even prophylaxis. Take the example of primaquine—it is administered to wipe out those latent liver stages of *Plasmodium vivax* and *Plasmodium ovale* infections that do not allow relapse; a similarly well-tolerated option is offered by atovaquone-proguanil, both as prophylaxis and as treatment in certain cases. Combination of drugs that are dissimilar in their activity is another strategy employed to fight back against resistance. However, despite these drug advances, responsible drug management remains a concern. Any antimalarial therapy's success is dependent not only on the availability of the medicine but also on its correct application, this means getting an accurate diagnosis, having patients adhere to their treatment regimens, and screening for potential side effects. In the majority of communities, drug dissemination should be integrated with attempts at enlightening them, while others do not know about the spread of malaria (Ruberto et al., 2014). Based on the current situation, what becomes clear is that the integration of medicine and community enlightenment is necessary to overcome malaria successfully (Figure 1.14).

1.5.2. Resistance Issues and Challenges

Control of malaria has recently encountered some significant setbacks, both the *Plasmodium* parasite and the pesky mosquito vectors have become rather drug-resistant. We've tried the tried-and-true with the widespread use of ITNs and other antimalarial drugs, but these measures are now commonly circumvented by emerging resistance. In the majority of cases, the *parasites* resist several drugs, most notably in regions of high transmission intensity, under which clouds treatment regimens and regretfully magnifies illness and death. Meanwhile, mosquitoes are slowly but surely developing ways to shrug off routine insecticides, which takes away the benefit of indoor spraying. All these complex resistance issues translate into the fact that we do need to get beneath the surface of *parasite* function and what is occurring genetically in the vectors. In most cases, the upsurge in resistance strongly suggests a desperate necessity for fresh thought in drug as well as vector control arenas (Aderoyeje & Ehruanga, 2024). Elsewhere, far away in East Africa, where malaria still runs frighteningly rampant—drug-resistant *Plasmodium* species along with insects that are difficult to control through the use of insecticides are a gigantic public health headache. Local healthcare is usually under attack by mounting caseloads, coupled with the deficiencies of low resources, overall poverty, and even poor education levels. Those might slow down treatment and diagnosis and disrupt the distribution of prevention materials. To put all that on top, altering environmental conditions and volatile climate lead to the expansion of mosquito breeding sites and the prolongation of the transmission periods. In the field, these barriers to resistance are not just biological features; they are combined with a broader mix of social and environmental impediments. Overall, combating malaria here needs a mix of ongoing surveillance of resistance, increased healthcare intervention, and community actions at the grassroots (Ndayishimiye, 2024). Fighting these challenges of resistance is absolutely crucial to any actual attempt at eradicating malaria worldwide, but it requires overcoming some substantial scientific and logistical hurdles. The idea that has shown some promise is using genomic surveillance, watching for resistance mutations in mosquitoes and *parasites* so that treatment and control can be preadjusted. New technologies in controlling mosquito genetics even provide benefits with long-term effects by either eliminating mosquitoes or interfering with the parasite's capacity to transmit. This new opportunity, however, also has its baggage, including having complex regulatory challenges, ethical issues, and needing to win the trust of communities to which things are not always easy. In addition, sound funding and effective international cooperation are required to ensure continued research, practice implementation, and capacity building. Thus, in general, malaria resistance is more of a biological problem—instead, it is a multi-faceted, complicated problem that needs to be addressed with a coordinated, flexible response if we are to progress toward eventually eradicating the disease (Aderoyeje & Ehruanga, 2024; Ndayishimiye, 2024) (Figure 1.15).

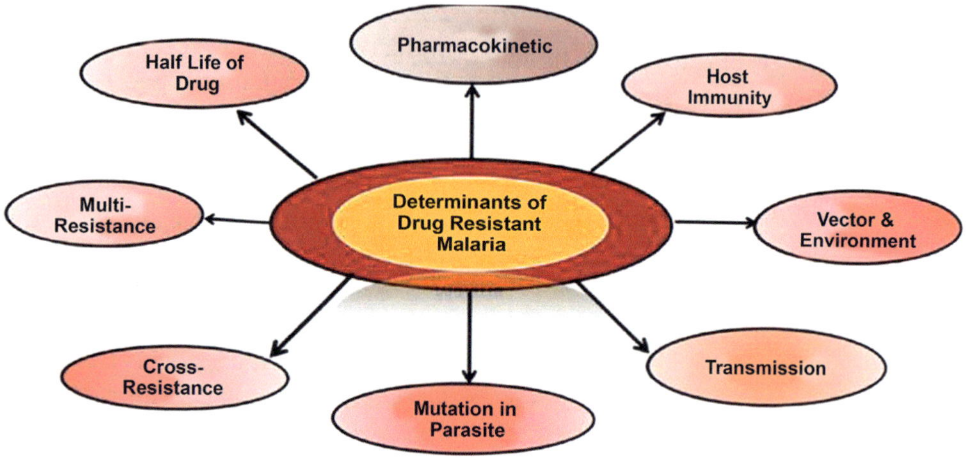

Figure 1.15. Resistance issues and challenges of malaria.

Source: ResearchGate. (2014). Different parameters that contribute to antimalarial resistance. In *Challenges of Drug-Resistant Malaria*.

1.5.3. Importance of Timely Treatment

Malaria gets serious very rapidly after symptoms develop, so it is critical to get help right away. Any delay, even for a short time, can lead to extremely serious problems, like brain involvement, profound anemia, or even multi-organ failure, all of which can greatly raise the risk of death. The parasite multiplies very rapidly in your bloodstream, so strong medicines need to be given promptly to slow it down and limit the damage. Quick treatment not only boosts individual survival rates but also lessens the chances of spreading it around; after all, if the parasite is cleared out fast, there is less for mosquitoes to pick up. It is also beneficial if tests are easily available to individuals and they know the symptoms of early onset. A rapid, more or less organized reaction can even keep other already established problems from deteriorating further, especially important for risk groups like pregnant women and small children. How a health system reacts also plays a tremendous role. If there are waiting lines, incorrect diagnoses, or poor care management, treatment is delayed, aggravating the problem on both the individual and community levels. All too frequently, a lack of resources, like inadequate diagnostic machinery or effective medicines—makes prompt intervention unavailable, especially in poor areas most ravaged by malaria. For the most part, expanding health infrastructures to facilitate quick assessments and treatments is necessary. Health services have to mix good communication with polite patient care and timely follow-up (sometimes a bit untimely, as life happens) to keep patients compliant with treatments. It is this synergy that decreases mortality and creates trust in health services, so people come forward earlier than later. Each of these elements together pushes the system towards the provision of the kind of timely, quality care that can negate the impact of malaria (Livingston et al., 2020). In addition to the immediate medical interventions, quick response to malaria removes a great many wider social and economic stresses. Delays, on the other hand, balloon health costs, thanks to prolonged hospitalization and other complications, and cost communities dearly in the form of lost productivity from work or school days missed. Early treatment keeps patients in their daily routines, generating economic activity and breaking cycles of poverty that the disease might otherwise worsen. Early case management eases the strain on hospitals, as fewer cases need intensive care and long-term resources. Such public health notices that stress the necessity of being treated early can, in the long term, heighten overall community health awareness, which lowers the incidence and also the mortality rate of malaria. By placing such a premium on early treatment, policymakers exhibit concern for individual and public health, a change in attitude that is vital to the control of the disease (Livingston et al., 2020).

1.6. Current Research and Developments

Medical science in recent years has made some bold strides in how we tackle incurable diseases. Consider oncology, for example, nowadays researchers are dedicated to using brain-penetrating tyrosine kinase inhibitors to cure cases of HER2-positive breast cancer that have spread to the brain. This approach, which tends to improve intracranial control and survival overall, implies the greater promise of precision medicine. Interestingly enough, the very same methods are being hunted for in the research of malaria now. In most cases, researchers are looking into new drug targets and even disease-resistant strains of parasites by using advanced molecular tools that occasionally circumvent the drawbacks of traditional therapy. Overall, this interdisciplinary movement seems to usher in a new era—one where several disciplines might be the key to enhancing survival and well-being (Sammons et al., 2024). Quite frequently, these multidisciplinary ideas end up being crucial to speeding effective antimalarial advances. Next-generation diagnostic tools have flipped the script for old-fashioned disease control, especially in such domains as immunotherapy and infectious diseases. For example, the use of standardized patient imaging , take the case of [18F] FDG PET/CT for solid cancers , in a real sense illustrates the way established guidelines can refine the accuracy of response assessments. Such precision is particularly worth its salt when applied to the tuning of patient treatment in real-time, a concept that works hand-in-hand with malaria research in which early diagnosis of parasite resistance is paramount. Global institutions are also, for the most part, working together (with some minor hiccups in between) to revitalize and sustain diagnostic standards, demonstrating a real interest in both clinical excellence and patient care. By coupling modern imaging with molecular diagnostics, researchers are mapping epidemics more accurately and individualizing treatment more accurately, thereby pushing clinical outcomes in the right direction (Lopci et al., 2022). Regular methods, as it turns out, are relatively central to jumping on technological advances in the face of old infectious foes. Today's research is increasingly dedicated to what occurs with patients, marrying real-world data with traditional outcomes to underpin more successful treatment and public health policy. In conditions such as malaria, where socio-economic and environmental factors do have a strong impact upon the spread of the disease and the efficacy of treatments—patient-reported outcomes may sometimes offer surprisingly useful information, even if they appear redundant at first sight. Researchers now recommend collecting a combination of biological samples, be it tissue, blood, or cerebrospinal fluid, in a bid to obtain a comprehensive account of disease dynamics and host-pathogen interactions. Such multi-dimensional investigations tend to uncover new biomarkers identifying disease severity or drug resistance, pushing the development of more effective vaccines and medicines. Learning from some of the recent oncology and immunotherapy trials, malaria science might just adopt these integrative strategies, speeding advances in prevention, diagnosis, and overall treatment—hopefully lopping the global disease burden in the process (Lopci et al., 2022; Sammons et al., 2024) (Figure 1.16).

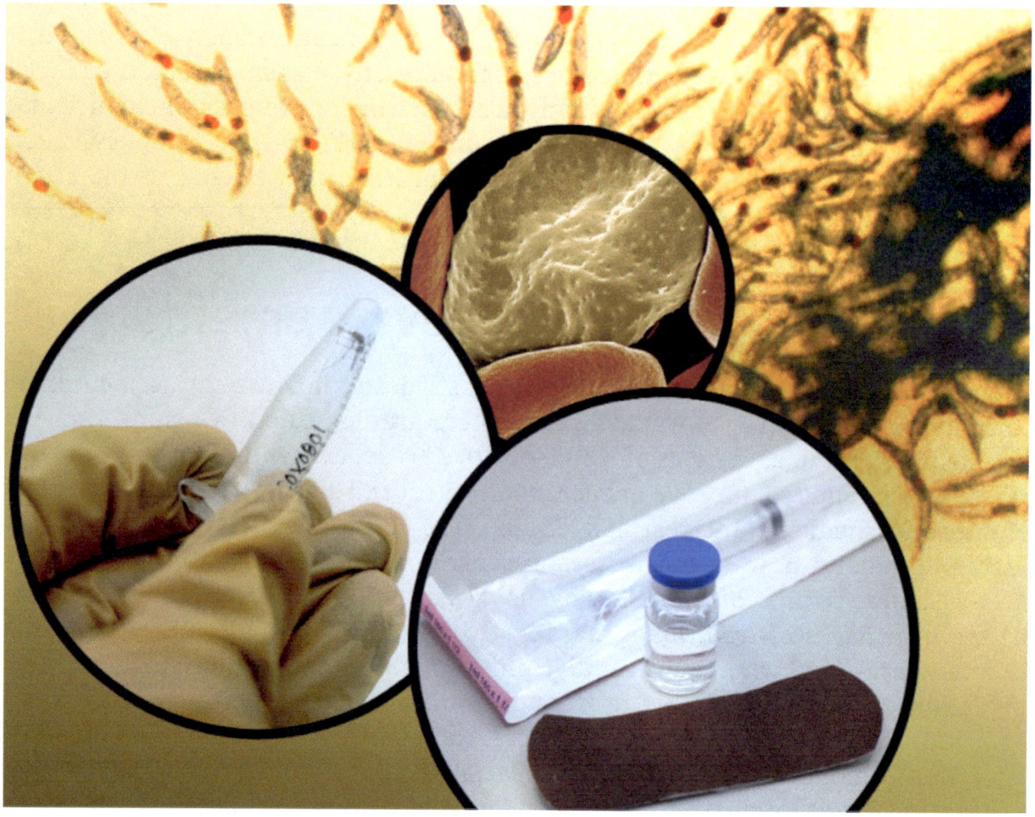

Figure 1.16. Current research and developments of malaria.

Source: National Institute of Allergy and Infectious Diseases. (n.d.). *Malaria Sporozoites and Image Circles.* https://www.niaid.nih.gov/sites/default/files/malaria-sporozoites-and-image-circles.jpg.

1.6.1. Advances in Malaria Vaccine Research

Malaria's devious character has caused scientists to be creative in their strategies, vaccines at the forefront, to contain the disease and, hopefully, eliminate it. Laboratories have been experimenting of late by integrating molecular tools with vaccine development, which gives much greater understanding of the parasite's working and behavior and how it interacts with its host. Whole-genome sequencing, for instance, has permitted scientists to examine the genetic variability of *Plasmodium falciparum* and enable them to focus on the antigen fragments needed to elicit a protective immune response. Such molecular mapping significantly heightens the challenge of developing vaccines that might outwit antigenic variation and work adequately in different endemic areas. Additionally, the capacity to identify hidden parasite pockets using advanced diagnostic equipment complements vaccine approaches by diminishing channels of transmission. In totality, all these elements are signaling a positive future direction toward malaria control measures in which vaccines have a role to play alongside other measures (Gavinho et al., 2019). There is also growing hype on extracellular vesicles (EVs) in vaccine development. EVs full of proteins, lipids, and nucleic acids, seem to be playing a role in the ping-pong between host and pathogen. Researchers who have been studying the vesicles that *Plasmodium*-infected cells release have, in most cases, discovered new leads for promising vaccine targets—pieces of the puzzle that might trigger the hoped-for immune response.

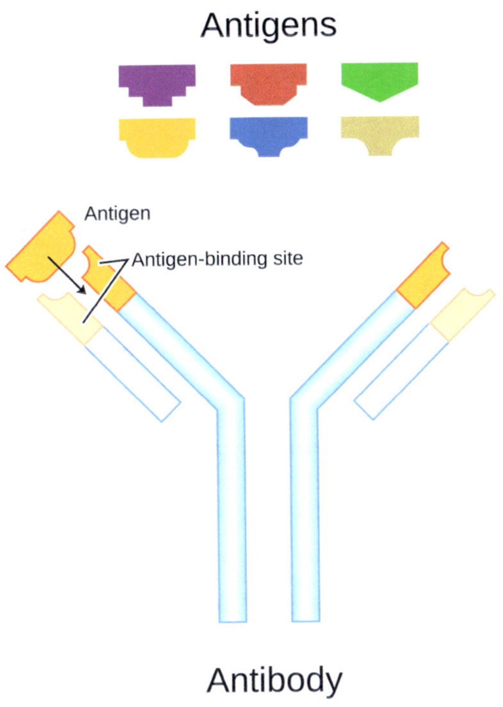

Figure 1.17. Advances in malaria vaccine research.

Source: By Fvasconcellos 19:03, 6 May 2007 (UTC) - Color version of Image:Antibody.png, originally a Work of the United States Government, Public Domain, https://commons.wikimedia.org/w/index.php?curid=2067564

It so occurs that EVs would either help the parasite to escape or even induce immunity; essentially, this is opening new ways to improve vaccine-induced immunity by targeting ways older approaches did not even target. This avenue, which brings cell biology expertise together with antigen delivery adjustments, is opening a new avenue to build vaccines that provide a better and longer-lasting defense against malaria (Gavinho et al., 2019). Field research combining molecular monitoring with vaccine studies has been an important breakthrough in bringing laboratory advances to tangible effect. Whole organism malaria vaccine reports from recent endemic countries have depended on genome-wide sieve analyses, which in most cases helps to anchor genes linked to immune protection. These indications have driven the development of next-generation vaccines aimed at the parasite stages most dominant in particular regions. In addition, the use of handheld molecular analysis tools in the field – sometimes with some on-the-spot adjusting – increases our ability to monitor vaccine efficacy. Such tools can detect hidden parasite populations that are not in plain sight of immune cells or that are avoiding standard tests. In all, the merging of these strategies not only maximizes vaccine formulations but also constitutes adaptive, locally adaptive malaria control interventions, leading us progressively toward global elimination goals (Stabler et al., 2024) (Figure 1.17).

1.6.2. Innovations in Treatment Methods

Natural remedies have traditionally been a significant portion of malaria treatment, and now that legacy is being put in a new twist. Before, drugs like quinine and artemisinin directly from the plant, a clear sign that nature centuries ago already had the formula to fight the disease. Nowadays, with more recent scientific breakthroughs, researchers are scouring the globe for lesser-known compounds that offer chemical characteristics you don't find much in lab-made libraries. Naturally, there are hurdles along the way, like the need for quick, efficient bioassays and extraction methods that can deliver at scale. Interdisciplinary collaborations and uniting historical ethnobotanical knowledge with contemporary pharmacology are now essential. In all, this combination of old and new technology seems poised to deliver new medicines that may even overcome the resistance issues plaguing some treatments of the present day (Chaachouay & Zidane, 2024). Artificial intelligence is meanwhile quietly revolutionizing the way we conduct malaria research and treatment. Machine learning computer algorithms, powered by data mountains, now aid in the discovery of possible drug targets and optimizing treatment with predictive models.

This can drive the entire drug discovery process much faster, getting therapies to patients more rapidly and, in most instances, at a lower cost. Even AI software is enabling more personalized medicine—customizing treatments to the individual patient, enhancing efficacy while minimizing side effects. Yet, pitfalls like data privacy matters, algorithmic bias and the imperative for human judgment surface along the way. Generally, in spite of these hiccups, AI is a trend-setting force that thrusts us beyond the traditional ways of fighting malaria (Alowais et al., 2023). Novel ideas in drug design and delivery are also changing the malaria game. Take into account such as delivering in nanoparticles or creating controlled-release systems, they make the drug travel more directly to where it is needed, which can improve outcomes and even decrease toxicity and frequency of dosing. By providing effective drug levels constantly, such plans also keep the parasite at bay, so resistance is less likely to develop. In addition, when new drugs are used alongside the known ones, it offers a multi-front attack that seems to reduce the chances of further developing resistance. Ongoing research into new delivery systems and combination therapy remains at the forefront of meeting the current challenges, supporting global control plans and even eradication in the long term. Conjointly, these advances herald the shift toward more precise, effective, and sustainable malaria treatments (Alowais et al., 2023; Chaachouay & Zidane, 2024) (Figure 1.18).

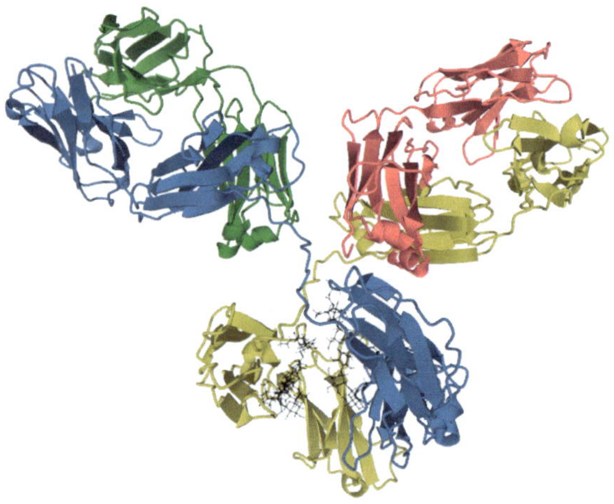

Figure 1.18. Innovations in treatment methods in malaria vaccine.

Source: By Tokenzero - Own work, CC BY-SA 4.0, https://commons.wikimedia.org/w/index.php?curid=95724189

1.6.3. Ongoing Studies on Transmission Reduction

Chipping away at malaria transmission strategies focused on innovative insecticide strategies—indoor residual spraying (IRS), for instance, with new chemical mixtures. In Côte d'Ivoire, clothianidin-based IRS was rolled out in previously untreated zones, and the drop in malaria was hard to overlook. Decades of health facility trends show that within months of the 2021 campaign, malaria cases dropped by an astounding 37.9%, a reduction of thousands of infections averted. Even after adjustment for seasonal trends and environmental variation, these declines were strong. The control sites without IRS did not see this same decline, indicating clothianidin's capacity, especially when in combination with pyrethroid-treated nets, to repress transmission. As a whole, the outcomes here suggest that IRS with new neonicotinoid insecticides is truly promising towards lowering malaria's burden (Hilton et al., 2024). Further research considered the performance of clothianidin, either alone or in combination with deltamethrin, in comparison to conventional ones like pirimiphos-methyl. In northern Benin, teams of human landing catches and mosquito collections identified that while clothianidin-based products persisted for most of the transmission season, their efficacy in lowering mosquito bites and inoculation rates was less than that of pirimiphos-methyl. Still, both strategies helped to decrease the amount of *Anopheles gambiae s.l.* indoors, a high priority given that these mosquitoes are the major culprits in malaria transmission. At the same time, researchers noticed that rates of feeding on blood were relatively stable, which implies that while decreasing mosquito numbers, some other behavioral or physiological mechanisms may be altering transmission dynamics. Mostly, the results highlight the need to carefully select insecticides to ensure that vector control efficacy can be successfully improved (Odjo et al., 2024). Control of malaria remains a priority in global health, and a multi-intervention combination seems a sensible way forward. The combination of LLINs and IRS provides a kind of layered protection; by targeting the mosquito at various points and sites, the combined approach provides added protection. Figures from periods when simultaneous mass net distributions and IRS were used show that layering can be associated with very significant decreases in both mosquito levels and actual malaria cases. Of course, altering levels of resistance among insects and levels of effectiveness in the field over time means we've had to constantly adapt our methods. It is indeed important to monitor ecological and mosquito behavior patterns to guide policy and remain on track. Generally, though progress is seen, it is still important to adapt various interventions to the local context if we are eventually going to eliminate malaria (Hilton et al., 2024; Odjo et al., 2024).

CLOSER LOOK

MOSQUITO BREEDING

Mosquito breeding is the biological process through which mosquitoes breed and reproduce, primarily in stagnant or slowly flowing water. Understanding this process is necessary because mosquitoes are not only nuisance insects but also dangerous disease-carriers for diseases such as malaria, dengue, chikungunya, Zika virus, and yellow fever. Mosquito has a four-stage life cycle: egg, larva, pupa, and adult, with complete metamorphosis. Female mosquitoes, after they have a blood meal, in most cases, from animals or humans, lay eggs in or on water bodies. The water bodies could be natural, e.g., ponds, marshes, and tree holes, or artificial, e.g., flowerpots, used tires, buckets, and clogged drains. Eggs are laid individually or in groups called rafts depending on the mosquito species. Eggs hatch within 24 to 48 hours into larvae, also referred to as "wrigglers" since they wriggle about on water. Larvae live on water and feed on organic matter and bacteria. Larvae tend to rise to the water's surface to breathe through a very small air tube. Larvae eventually mold several times before developing into pupae, or "tumblers," a non-feeding phase while preparing for adulthood. Within 1 to 3 days, the emergent adult mosquito will exit the pupal skin and will remain floating on the water surface until it is capable of flight.

Different species have different breeding behaviors. For example, *Aedes aegypti*, the primary vector of dengue and Zika, prefers clean, stagnant water commonly found in cities, whereas *Anopheles* mosquitoes responsible for transmitting malaria are capable of breeding in relatively cleaner, rural water bodies. The ability of mosquito eggs to survive dry conditions for weeks or even months is responsible for their persistence and international dissemination. Due to their short breeding cycle, requiring as little as one week to reach full development, populations of mosquitoes can grow quickly if left unchecked. Mosquito breeding can be controlled most effectively by removing or reducing breeding sites. Draining, covering, or treating containers holding water, clearing clogged drains and gutters, and good water storage practices will achieve this. Larvicides and biological control methods, such as the introduction of fish that feed on larvae in ponds, are also used in most areas. Participation and education among the people are important in developing consistent and large-scale mosquito control operations. In endemic regions, public health agencies may carry out fogging and insecticide spraying as a preventive or in an emergency situation. However, these should be incorporated into an integrated broader mosquito management plan that targets environmental sanitation and sustainable utilization. In conclusion, mosquito breeding is dynamic and speedy, and it largely plays a role in passing on the majority of infectious diseases. Mosquito breeding is controllable by individual and community intervention with the support of health authorities and environmental regulation in order to reduce the population of mosquitoes and achieve public health successfully.

SUMMARY

Malaria is not cured by some magic trick. It takes a patchwork solution that combines new ways of diagnosing it, better treatments, and getting members of the community to care about prevention. For example, if drug shops start using RDTs, this means that local businesses can help by making sure drugs like the artemisinin combinations are being used appropriately. Naturally, making such ideas work on a large scale requires you to have good rules, regular check-ups, and all on board. Uganda's experience in its own right, where community teams and local health workers led the word spreading—is that talking to people directly builds trust and, in the end, leads to better care, even if record keeping and referrals continue to catch you out (Mbonye et al., 2015). Money matters a great deal in all this too. Health programs have trouble breaking even on cost and benefit where things like ITNs, indoor spraying, and even the potential introduction of malaria vaccines are concerned. With budgets always tight and so many programs relying on outside funding, planners are forced to double-check all expenditures. Supporting the capacity to crunch numbers and requiring policymakers to collaborate on funding translates into money being able to be expended both on treating and preventing the disease from spreading in the first place. All things considered, this means long-term, stable funding is not just a nicety, it is a requirement (Mtui & Osoro, 2011). In summary, combating malaria means combining sage clinical measures, social moments of truth, and prudent budgeting. While innovations like RDTs represent a great step forward, they only find their footing when the entire system, including community support, has been in place. You just can't skip over the money side of things, without solid money and careful budgeting, even the best ideas will crumble. By merging healthcare professionals', policymakers', and everyday people's work, one can ease the malaria burden and enhance total community health, proving that an integrated strategy is key to lasting success (Mtui & Osoro, 2011; Mbonye et al., 2015).

Malaria under control has increased some very remarkable achievements in different regions of the country, all due to national initiatives made available to address needs at the local level. In Suriname, for example, the Medical Mission Malaria Program (MM-MP) implemented a set of mixed strategies, dispensing long-lasting ITNs, residual insecticide sprays, enhanced case detection, as well as even tackling rising case of the local health system. The numbers dived dramatically, malaria infections declined and vector groups broke down in fact, so the transmission threat was shifted from settled village conditions to more transient gold mines at the margins (Hiwat et al., 2012). The whole episode illustrates how bringing together community specific measures with a solid health infrastructure can sustain progress but always entails the need to sharpen interventions as new challenges emerge. Bhutan offers another interesting example of dealing with malaria when resources are tight and geography is not on your side. Over about a decade, the Bhutan Vector-Borne Disease Control Program increased access to diagnosis and treatment, rolled out ACTs for *Plasmodium falciparum*, and upped its game with IRS and ITNs. Thanks partly to broader socioeconomic improvements and better healthcare access, confirmed malaria cases dropped by nearly 99%! However, imported cases, , specifically from the Indian bordering states of Bhutan, present a difficult challenge to saying goodbye to malaria for good. Bhutan's efforts to screen at borders and focus surveillance efforts on risk groups highlight that you need to address both local transmission and cross-border disease if you are to maintain those improvements (Dev et al., 2012). Together, these cases highlight just how complex malaria control can become. It so turns out interventions have to be specialized, whether that is intense vector control, hands-on care management, or surveillance for migrant and moving populations that keep the disease in play. Developing health systems, sustaining pressure on behavioral change, and investing in surveillance are at the core of long-term success, though the transmission patterns keep evolving. In general, malaria eradication needs a bird's-eye view approach that brings together scientific professionalism, grassroot operations, and policy actions with genuine grassroots participation and local support (Hiwat et al., 2012; Dev et al., 2012).

KEY TERMS FROM THIS CHAPTER

Plasmodium	Anopheles Mosquito	Vector
Parasite Lifecycle	Sporozoites	Merozoites
Gametocytes	Erythrocytic Cycle	Exoerythrocytic Cycle
Insecticide-treated Nets	Indoor Residual Spraying	Antimalarial Drugs
Chloroquine Resistance	Intermittent Preventive Treatment	Malaria Endemicity
Fever and Chills	Hemolysis	Cerebral Malaria
Malaria Eradication		

References

1. Accoti, A., Damiani, C., Nunzi, E., Cappelli, A., Iacomelli, G., Monacchia, G., Turco, A., D'Alò, F., Peirce, M. J., Favia, G., & Spaccapelo, R. (2023). Anopheline mosquito saliva contains bacteria that are transferred to a mammalian host through blood feeding. *Frontiers in microbiology, 14*, 1157613. https://doi.org/10.3389/fmicb.2023.1157613(accessed on 13 May 2025).

2. Aderoyeje, T. G., & Erhuanga, O. G. (2024). A review on the exploration of genomic approaches to malaria prevention and treatment in Nigeria. A Review on the Exploration of Genomic Approaches to Malaria Prevention and Treatment in Nigeria. J. Appl. Sci. Environ. Manage. 28 (9) 2937-2941(accessed on 13 May 2025).

3. Alowais, S. A., Alghamdi, S. S., Alsuhebany, N., Alqahtani, T., Alshaya, A., Almohareb, S. N., Aldairem, A., et al. (2023). Revolutionizing healthcare: The role of artificial intelligence in clinical practice. *BMC Medical Education, 23*. https://doi.org/10.1186/s12909-023-04698-z.

4. Rolland, E., Checchi, F., Pinoges, L., Balkan, S., Guthmann, J. P., & Guerin, P. J. (2006). Operational response to malaria epidemics: are rapid diagnostic tests cost-effective?. *Tropical medicine & international health : TM & IH, 11*(4), 398–408. https://doi.org/10.1111/j.1365-3156.2006.01580.x (accessed on 13 May 2025).

5. Andrean, M., & Assafah, A. F. (2025). Rare malaria case in Jakarta: Diagnostic challenges and treatment strategies for general practitioners in non-endemic area. *Asian Journal of Social and Humanities*. https://doi.org/10.59888/ajosh.v3i6.539(accessed on 13 May 2025).

6. Atah, F. P., Longdoh, N. A., Thumamo, B. P., & Akoachere, J. F. (2023). Knowledge, Attitudes and Practices Among Adult Malaria Patients Co-Infected with Opportunistic Intestinal Coccidian Parasites in Fundong Health District, Northwest, Cameroon: A Cross Section Study Design. *European Journal of Theoretical and Applied Sciences, 1*(4), 1121-1140. https://doi.org/10.59324/ejtas.2023.1(4).105(accessed on 13 May 2025).

7. Ruberto, I., Camara, S., Banek, K., & Loua, M. K. (2014). Knowledge, attitudes and practices of malaria control among communities from the health district of Forécariah in the Republic of Guinea, West Africa. *Journal of vector borne diseases, 51*(2), 119–127. (accessed on 13 May 2025).

8. Briët, O. J., & Chitnis, N. (2013). Effects of changing mosquito host searching behaviour on the cost effectiveness of a mass distribution of long-lasting, insecticidal nets: a modelling study. *Malaria journal, 12*, 215. https://doi.org/10.1186/1475-2875-12-215 (accessed on 13 May 2025).

9. Hiwat, H., Hardjopawiro, L. S., Takken, W., & Villegas, L. (2012). Novel strategies lead to pre-elimination of malaria in previously high-risk areas in Suriname, South America. *Malaria journal, 11*, 10. https://doi.org/10.1186/1475-2875-11-10

10. Casamitjana, N., & Clotet, B. (2020). Use of antiviral drugs to reduce COVID-19 transmission. *The Lancet Global Health, 8*, e639–e640. https://doi.org/10.1016/s2214-109x(20)30114-5.

11. Chaachouay, N., & Zidane, L. (2024). Plant-derived natural products: A source for drug discovery and development. *Drugs and Drug Candidates, 3*, 184–207. https://doi.org/10.3390/ddc3010011.

12. https://core.ac.uk/download/42634679.pdf Mbonye, A. K., Clarke, S. E., Lal, S., Chandler, C. I., Hutchinson, E., Hansen, K. S., & Magnussen, P. (2015). Introducing rapid diagnostic tests for

malaria into registered drug shops in Uganda: lessons learned and policy implications. *Malaria journal, 14*, 448. https://doi.org/10.1186/s12936-015-0979-6 (accessed on 13 May 2025).

13. Chukwuocha, U., Okereke, U., Bosede, A. O., & Ogboeze, J. C. (2024). Prospect of social marketing in enhancing the acquisition and utilization of insecticide-treated nets (ITNs) for the prevention of malaria in a rural area of Imo State, South-Eastern Nigeria. *Social Marketing Quarterly*. https://www.semanticscholar.org/paper/7781cb3e8b48aa37fe607b88ba7990da1ff8f64f (accessed on 13 May 2025).
14. Sicuri, E., Vieta, A., Lindner, L., Constenla, D., & Sauboin, C. (2013). The economic costs of malaria in children in three sub-Saharan countries: Ghana, Tanzania and Kenya. *Malaria journal, 12*, 307. https://doi.org/10.1186/1475-2875-12-307 (accessed on 13 May 2025).
15. Crowley, B., O'Brien, É., & Kabota, S. (2024). The state of malaria in a rural-mission hospital in Nkhoma, Malawi. *UCC Student Medical Journal*. https://www.semanticscholar.org/paper/36d13aed3f83eec46e027a40c146d8e261adf88e (accessed on 13 May 2025).
16. de Young, T., & Raju, J. (2024). Histories intertwined: Tracing the evolution of the South African Astronomical Observatory Library and Information Service within the historical development of astronomy in South Africa. *Journal of Astronomical History and Heritage*. https://doi.org/10.3724/SP.J.1440-2807.2024.03.11(accessed on 13 May 2025).
17. Dev, V., Galappaththy, G. N. L., Gosling, R., Gueye, C. S., et al. (2012). Malaria control in Bhutan: Case study of a country embarking on elimination. https://core.ac.uk/download/pdf/8681713.pdf.
18. Fekri Jaski S, Khosravani M, Boutsika K, Ghadarjani S, Raeisi A, et al. The First Case Series of Malaria Overlapped with COVID-19 in Iran.J Adv Immunopharmacol.2023;3(1):e136527. https://doi.org/10.5812/tms-136527.(accessed on 13 May 2025).
19. Ngowo, H. S., Kaindoa, E. W., Matthiopoulos, J., Ferguson, H. M., & Okumu, F. O. (2017). Variations in household microclimate affect outdoor-biting behaviour of malaria vectors. *Wellcome open research, 2*, 102. https://doi.org/10.12688/wellcomeopenres.12928.1
20. Gavinho, B., Rossi, I. V., Evans-Osses, I., Inal, J., & Ramirez, M. I. (2018). A new landscape of host-protozoa interactions involving the extracellular vesicles world. *Parasitology, 145*(12), 1521–1530. https://doi.org/10.1017/S0031182018001105 (accessed on 13 May 2025).
21. Gubernatorova, E. O., Горшкова, E. A., Polinova, A. I., & Drutskaya, M. S. (2020). IL-6: Relevance for immunopathology of SARS-CoV-2. *Cytokine & Growth Factor Reviews, 53*, 13–24. https://doi.org/10.1016/j.cytogfr.2020.05.009.
22. Gyaase , Philip, Emmanuel Boateng Acheampong, David Ben Sampson, and Richard Owusu. 2023. "Factors Influencing the Utilization of Insecticide Treated Bed Nets in the Prevention of Malaria in the Berekum East Municipality, Ghana". *Asian Journal of Research in Infectious Diseases* 13 (2):1-14. https://doi.org/10.9734/ajrid/2023/v13i2259.
23. Hilton, E. R., Gning-Cisse, N., Assi, A., Eyakou, M., Koffi, J., Gnakou, B., Kouassi, B., Flatley, C., Chabi, J., Gbalegba, C., Alex Aimain, S., Yah Kokrasset, C., Antoine Tanoh, M., N'Gotta, S., Yao, O., Egou Assi, H., Konan, P., Davis, K., Constant, E., Belemvire, A., ... Burnett, S. (2024). Reduction of malaria case incidence following the introduction of clothianidin-based indoor residual spraying in previously unsprayed districts: an observational analysis using health facility register data from Côte d'Ivoire, 2018-2022. *BMJ global health, 9*(3), e013324. https://doi.org/10.1136/bmjgh-2023-013324(accessed on 13 May 2025).

24. Hu, B., Guo, H., Zhou, P., & Shi, Z. L. (2020). Characteristics of SARS-CoV-2 and COVID-19. *Nature Reviews Microbiology, 19*, 141–154. https://doi.org/10.1038/s41579-020-00459-7.

25. Kabore, K. K., & Guel, D. (2024). Addressing challenges in data quality and model generalization for malaria detection. *ArXiv, abs/2501.00464*. arXiv:2501.00464

26. https://www.semanticscholar.org/paper/d4e962ad61ea0bfe6888e275add0a922eec7a060 (accessed on 13 May 2025).

27. Kamnoi, J. (2024). Adapting Through Belief: The Persistent Rituals of Phuket's Jia Cai Festival. Humanities and Social Sciences, 12(6), 236-245. https://doi.org/10.11648/j.hss.20241206.18(accessed on 13 May 2025).

28. Amosi Kikwata G.H., Bofoe Lokango S., Badjoko Eya F., Bene Amisa A., Pami Kakunda L. Katanda Fundi J., Saliki Lifita M., Tagoto Tepungipamea A., Basandja Longembe E. and Panda Kitronza J. (2024). SOCIOENVIRONMENTAL DETERMINANTS OF MALARIA TRANSMISSION IN URBAN AREAS: A CASE STUDY FROM KISANGANI, DRC, International Journal of Applied Science and Engineering Review (IJASER) 5 (5): 44-60 Article No. 209 Sub Id 320 (accessed on 13 May 2025).

29. Kruk, M. E., Gage, A., Arsenault, C., Jordan, K., Leslie, H. H., Roder-DeWan, S., Adeyi, O., et al. (2018). High-quality health systems in the Sustainable Development Goals era: Time for a revolution. *The Lancet Global Health, 6*, e1196–e1252. https://doi.org/10.1016/s2214-109x(18)30386-3.

30. Lewis, S. M., Williams, A., & Eisenbarth, S. C. (2019). Structure and function of the immune system in the spleen. *Science Immunology, 4*. https://doi.org/10.1126/sciimmunol.aau6085.

31. Livingston, G., Huntley, J., Sommerlad, A., Ames, D., Ballard, C., Banerjee, S., Brayne, C., et al. (2020). Dementia prevention, intervention, and care: 2020 report of the Lancet Commission. *The Lancet, 396*, 413–446. https://doi.org/10.1016/s0140-6736(20)30367-6.

32. Lopci, E., Hicks, R., Dimitrakopoulou-Strauss, A., Dercle, L., Iravani, A., Seban, R., Sachpekidis, C., et al. (2022). Joint EANM/SNMMI/ANZSNM practice guidelines/procedure standards on recommended use of [18F]FDG PET/CT imaging during immunomodulatory treatments in patients with solid tumors version 1.0. *European Journal of Nuclear Medicine and Molecular Imaging, 49*, 2323–2341. https://www.semanticscholar.org/paper/b062e34802e78c69c42f97e6006cca9835667617 (accessed on 13 May 2025).

33. Mahajan, R., & Tyagi, A. K. (2025). Evaluation of MAL Card rapid test versus microscopic methods for malaria diagnosis in resource-limited rural settings of India. *International Journal for Multidisciplinary Research*. https://doi.org/10.36948/ijfmr.2025.v07i02.38406

34. (accessed on 13 May 2025).

35. Maina Mwaura F. (2024). Interplay Between Infant Nutrition and Malaria Susceptibility in West Africa: Socioeconomic, Environmental, and Cultural Perspectives. IDOSR JOURNAL OF APPLIED SCIENCES 9(2):48-53. https://doi.org/10.59298/IDOSRJAS/2024/9.2.485300(accessed on 13 May 2025).

36. Mhelembe, T., Ramroop, S., & Habyarimana, F. (2025). Assessing the influence of socioeconomic and environmental variables on malaria risk in Nigerian children under 5 years: a GLMM

approach. *Malaria journal, 24*(1), 55. https://doi.org/10.1186/s12936-025-05289-7(accessed on 13 May 2025).

37. Mtui, J., & Osoro, O. (2011). Aggregate cost implications of selected cost-drivers in the Tanzanian health sector. Final Report 12/1/2011. Commissioned by: Ministry of Health and Social Welfare. https://core.ac.uk/download/pdf/11307328.pdf (accessed on 13 May 2025).
38. Murray, C. J. L., Ikuta, K. S., Sharara, F., Swetschinski, L. R., Robles Aguilar, G., Gray, A. P., Han, C., et al. (2022). Global burden of bacterial antimicrobial resistance in 2019: A systematic analysis. *The Lancet, 399*, 629–655. https://doi.org/10.1016/S0140-6736(21)02724-0.
39. Mwandama, D., Gutman, J., Wolkon, A., Luka, M., Jafali, J., Ali, D., Mathanga, D. P., & Skarbinski, J. (2015). The use of intermittent preventive treatment in pregnancy and insecticide-treated bed nets for malaria prevention by women of child-bearing age in eight districts in Malawi. *Malaria journal, 14*, 316. https://doi.org/10.1186/s12936-015-0840-y(accessed on 13 May 2025).
40. Chandler, C. I., Webb, E. L., Maiteki-Sebuguzi, C., Nayiga, S., Nabirye, C., DiLiberto, D. D., Ssemmondo, E., Dorsey, G., Kamya, M. R., & Staedke, S. G. (2017). The impact of an intervention to introduce malaria rapid diagnostic tests on fever case management in a high transmission setting in Uganda: A mixed-methods cluster-randomized trial (PRIME). *PloS one, 12*(3), e0170998. https://doi.org/10.1371/journal.pone.0170998 (accessed on 13 May 2025).
41. Ndayishimiye Havyarimana P. (2024). Challenges in Malaria Control and Prevention in East Africa. NEWPORT INTERNATIONAL JOURNAL OF BIOLOGICAL AND APPLIED SCIENCES, 5(2):24-27. https://doi.org/10.59298/NIJBAS/2024/5.2.24271(accessed on 13 May 2025).
42. Ng'ang'a, P. N., Aduogo, P., & Mutero, C. M. (2021). Strengthening community and stakeholder participation in the implementation of integrated vector management for malaria control in western Kenya: A case study. *Malaria Journal, 20*. https://doi.org/10.1186/s12936-021-03692-4.
43. Odjo, E.M., Akpodji, C.S.T., Djènontin, A. *et al.* Did the prolonged residual efficacy of clothianidin products lead to a greater reduction in vector populations and subsequent malaria transmission compared to the shorter residual efficacy of pirimiphos-methyl?. *Malar J* **23**, 119 (2024). https://doi.org/10.1186/s12936-024-04949-4(accessed on 13 May 2025).
44. OECD. (2018). *Stemming the Superbug Tide* (OECD Health Policy Studies). https://doi.org/10.1787/9789264307599-en.
45. Ogunsakin, R., Babalola, B., Olusola, J., Joshua, A. O., & Okpeku, M. (2024). GIS-based spatiotemporal mapping of malaria prevalence and exploration of environmental inequalities. *Parasitology Research, 123*. https://www.semanticscholar.org/paper/f86da593f11cd84eec6aa4c6d49dab6783d8eb04 (accessed on 13 May 2025).
46. Omale U. I. (2024). A qualitative study on determinants of the use of malaria rapid diagnostic test and anti-malarial drug prescription practices by primary healthcare workers in Ebonyi state, Nigeria. *Malaria journal, 23*(1), 120. https://doi.org/10.1186/s12936-024-04958-3(accessed on 13 May 2025).
47. Puszko, A. K., Batista, F. A., Ejjoummany, A., Bouillon, A., Maurel, M., Adler, P., Legru, A., Martinez, M., Ortega Varga, L., Hadjadj, M., Alzari, P. M., Blondel, A., Haouz, A., Barale, J. C., & Hernandez, J. F. (2025). Towards Improved Peptidic α-Ketoamide Inhibitors of the Plasmodial Subtilisin-Like SUB1: Exploration of N-Terminal Extensions and Cyclic Constraints. *ChemMedChem, 20*(8), e202400924. https://doi.org/10.1002/cmdc.202400924(accessed on 13 May 2025).

48. Rajneesh, Tiwari, R., Singh, V. K., Kumar, A., Gupta, R. P., Singh, A. K., Gautam, V., & Kumar, R. (2023). Advancements and Challenges in Developing Malaria Vaccines: Targeting Multiple Stages of the Parasite Life Cycle. *ACS infectious diseases*, *9*(10), 1795–1814. https://doi.org/10.1021/acsinfecdis.3c00332(accessed on 13 May 2025).

49. Riaz, A., Kinwan, M., Mustafa, K. M., Rauf, M. S., Shah, A., Ahmad, M., Hussain, W., et al. (2024). Exploring Gaucher disease: A pediatric case of severe dyslipidemia and unique symptoms. *World Journal of Advanced Research and Reviews*. https://www.semanticscholar.org/paper/f0da506197a600186cb1abcc430d6ff28b433c0f (accessed on 13 May 2025).

50. Roth, G. A., Abate, D., Abate, K. H., Abay, S. M., Abbafati, C., Abbasi, N., Abbastabar, H., et al. (2018). Global, regional, and national age-sex-specific mortality for 282 causes of death in 195 countries and territories, 1980–2017: A systematic analysis for the Global Burden of Disease Study 2017. *The Lancet, 392*, 1736–1788. https://doi.org/10.1016/s0140-6736(18)32203-7.

51. Sallum, M. A. M., Obando, R. G., Carrejo, N., & Wilkerson, R. C. (2020). Identification keys to the *Anopheles* mosquitoes of South America (Diptera: Culicidae). I. Introduction. *Parasites & Vectors, 13*. https://doi.org/10.1186/s13071-020-04298-6.

52. Sambo, Elkanah, Deborah, Otoikhian, Cyril S.O, Bosah, Bernadette Obiageli, Elkanah Obadiah Sambo, Odozie, Esther Uche, and Oyegoke, Paul Ifeleke. 2024. "A Cross-Sectional Study of the Prevalence and Risk Factors Associated With Malaria Transmission Among Sickle Cell Anaemia Patients in Urban Communities of Taraba Northeastern Nigeria". *International Journal of TROPICAL DISEASE & Health* 45 (8):27-35. https://doi.org/10.9734/ijtdh/2024/v45i81579.

53. Sammons, S., Van Swearingen, A. E. D., Noteware, L., Bagegni, N., Moulton, K., Threatt, S., Jaggers, D., et al. (2024). Abstract PO5-20-02: Secondary brain metastases prevention after isolated intracranial progression on trastuzumab/pertuzumab or T-DM1 in patients with advanced HER2+ breast cancer with addition of tucatinib (BRIDGET). *Cancer Research*. https://www.semanticscholar.org/paper/56374cdbf7b096cfda10d5f58e2d0f254b4f79b9 (accessed on 13 May 2025).

54. Shooraj M, Mahdavi S A. A Review on the Clinical Symptoms and Treatment Methods of Human Hookworm Infections. Tabari Biomed Stu Res J 2022; 4 (3) : 39 URL: http://tbsrj.mazums.ac.ir/article-1-3763-en.html(accessed on 13 May 2025).

55. Stabler, T. C. (2024). Using whole *Plasmodium falciparum* genomes for monitoring of escape from diagnosis, drug treatment and vaccine-induced immunity in Central-West Africa. https://core.ac.uk/download/636766095.pdf (accessed on 13 May 2025).

56. Subaneg S, Sitdhibutr R, Pornpanom P, Lertwatcharasarakul P, Ploypan R, Kiewpong A, Chatkaewchai B, To-adithep N, Kasorndorkbua C. Molecular Prevalence and Haematological Assessments of Avian Malaria in Wild Raptors of Thailand. *Birds*. 2024; 5(3):428-439. https://doi.org/10.3390/birds5030029(accessed on 13 May 2025).

57. United Nations. (2016). *Millennium Development Goals Report*. https://doi.org/10.18356/98544aa9-en.

58. Volkan E, Karanis P. Current Risks and Prevention Strategies Against Vector-Borne Diseases in Cyprus. *Microorganisms*. 2025; 13(4):726. https://doi.org/10.3390/microorganisms13040726(accessed on 13 May 2025).

59.

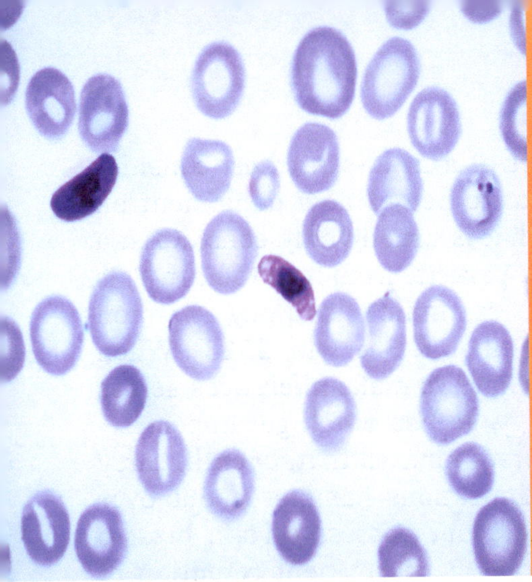

Chapter 2

BIOLOGY OF PLASMODIUM PARASITES

Contents

Introduction

Parasites and hosts engage in this odd, almost random relationship that has fascinated biologists for centuries, especially when it involves things that do impact our health. Take Plasmodium, for example; this particular genus is infamous for being responsible for malaria in people. It's pretty clear that understanding how Plasmodium does what it does is the number one concern when learning about its life cycle, adaptability, and pathogenicity. If one traces back to where everything began, there is an evolutionary tale that spans thousands of years, diverging from other eukaryotes; you have many characteristics—some old, some strangely unique—existing to allow it to survive. In most cases, such a long history shines not just on its clever survival strategies, but also on possible new therapy approaches, and that is precisely why stripping away these details so far down is so significant (Tobin et al., 2012). Stripping away somewhat further, rumor even surrounds Plasmodium having evolved from a photosynthetic ancestor. Even some scientists hazard that it's possibly some form of decayed algae, demonstrating just how much can occur in a time. It's sort of a head-scratcher: consider organisms once built to live independently, slowly becoming parasite beings now dependent on unlikely hosts like mosquitoes. Interestingly enough, a mosquito that is usually only considered a small pollinator winds up being significant because it transports the parasite from host to host. This role reversal is evidence of how loose and untidy evolution can be, reminding us to pay attention to how pressures in the environment drive such unique changes (Gillen & Sherwin, 2013). When you go and attempt to make sense out of Plasmodium biology, you have to make inferences across different domains—molecular biology, evolutionary biology, ecology, and so on all get hopelessly entwined. Consider its kinome, for instance: it is a jumble of protein kinases that, overall, carry signatures of both ancient eukaryotic origins and of unique optimizations hammered out over millions of years. These kinases belong to well-established clusters but possess certain bizarre features as a result of isolated, long-term evolution. This chimera—the permanent retention of ancient systems alongside the development of new specialized activities—enables the parasite to change gear as it chugs along between hosts and residences. Researchers studying these molecular features not only make progress in our foundational biological understanding but also inform the development of targeted antimalarial strategies, hence making research on this parasite increasingly important (Tobin et al., 2012) (Figure 2.1).

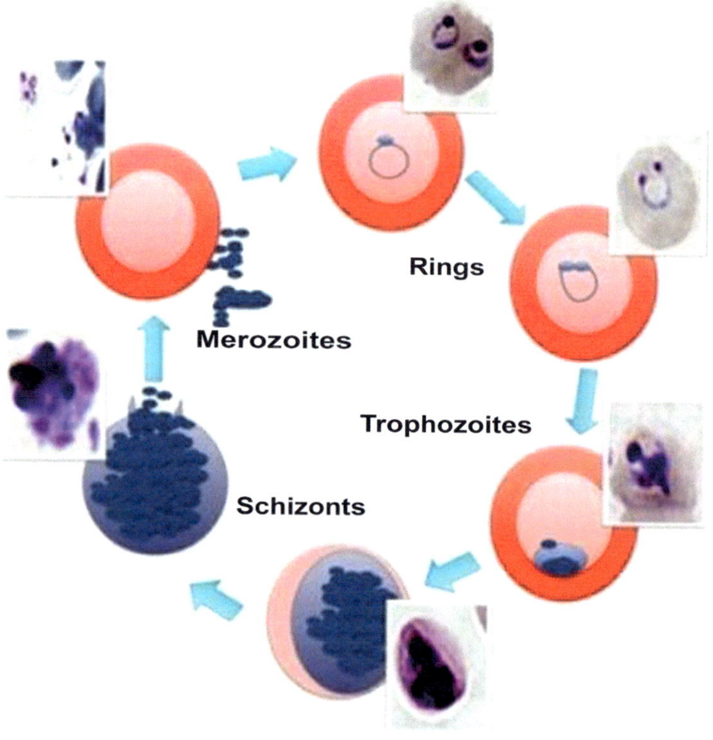

Figure 2.1. Biology of Plasmodium parasites.

Source: Shahinas, Dea, Asongna Folefoc, and Dylan R. Pillai. 2013. "Targeting Plasmodium falciparum Hsp90: Towards Reversing Antimalarial Resistance" *Pathogens* 2, no. 1: 33-54. https://doi.org/10.3390/pathogens2010033

Definition of Plasmodium Parasites

Eukaryotic microbes vary in shape and size, and most of the small organisms are implicated when large health issues across the globe are concerned. Take the Plasmodium parasites, for instance, tiny single-celled insects that cause malaria, a disease infamous for being pricey in terms of both disease and death. They belong to the group known as Apicomplexa, essentially meaning they have a special cell tip to use for infiltrating host cells. Their life cycle is quite complicated; they hop between vertebrate hosts and invertebrate vectors, showing just how well-adapted they have gotten over time. For the most part, it's been newer technology such as molecular phylogenetics that has unraveled their taxonomy, suggesting a combination of genetic anomalies and ecological niches that sustain malaria (Adl et al., 2018). All of this sets the stage for exploring the biological deceptions these parasites employ to survive, reproduce, and interact with hosts. The Plasmodium parasites are interesting in a taxonomic sense alone—they have the distinction of needing to live inside cells. They infect human red blood cells (RBCs) and are transmitted by female Anopheles mosquitoes. There are a small number of species within this group, but two of them, Plasmodium falciparum and Plasmodium vivax—are the major perpetrators of human disease. These parasites cause intermittent fevers and anemia by invading RBCs, multiplying, and bursting the cells open, releasing new, infective forms. Their life cycle has many stages, including sporozoites, merozoites, and gametocytes, each adapted to live either in the mosquito or human body. This rather unpredictable process makes malaria persist even with our immune systems, so it is a real headache for treatment and elimination (Shretta et al., 2017). Beyond their unusual biology, Plasmodium parasites are a major force behind global public health and disease control efforts. In spite of all our medical progress and population control measures for the mosquitoes, the parasites manage to adapt and resist medicines and immune attacks as well. For example, in most cases P. falciparum has even started resisting artemisinin derivatives, thereby making treatment procedures more difficult and necessitating regular observation and fresh ideas in therapy (Shretta et al., 2017). For the most part, having some familiarity with their general biology, for example, their genetic diversity, transmission dynamics, and interactions with the host—is what it takes to design effective vaccines and medicines. All of this knowledge essentially goes into broad strategies that integrate vector control, early diagnosis, and treatment to push malaria towards elimination. In general, keeping Plasmodium in mind in both biologic and public health perspectives remains relevant to our ongoing battle with one of the oldest parasitic foes of humankind (Figure 2.2).

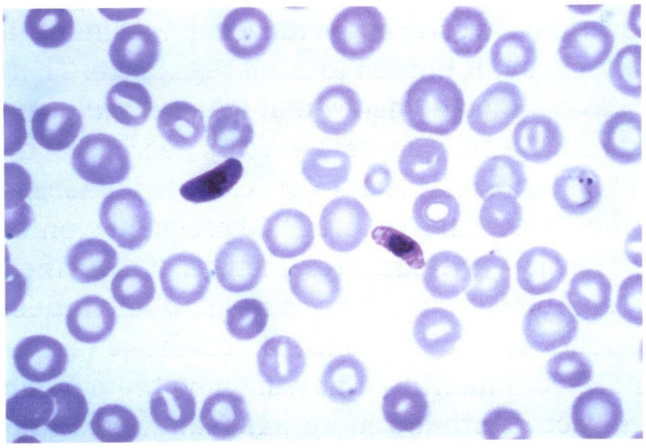

Figure 2.2. Plasmodium parasites.

Source: By Photo Credit:Content Providers(s): CDC/Dr. Mae MelvinTranswiki approved by: w:en:User:Dmcdevit - This media comes from the Centers for Disease Control and Prevention's Public Health Image Library (PHIL), with identification number #2704.Note: Not all PHIL images are public domain; be sure to check copyright status and credit authors and content providers. | Deutsch | English | македонски | slovenščina | +/−, Public Domain, https://commons.wikimedia.org/w/index.php?curid=2740653

Importance of Studying Plasmodium

Plasmodium biology is complicated and has an extensive effect on health worldwide, especially where the disease is endemic, and malaria is no different. The fact that the parasite can evade frontline medications like artemisinin is a great worry. Researchers have looked into genetic alterations, such as those in pfatp6 and pfmdr1 genes—to determine how it develops after treatments are given. These mutations can undermine how well our current treatments work, so it is important to keep a close eye on the parasite. It means that a combination of molecular surveillance with clinical data can allow us to control artemisinin resistance better (Pillai et al., 2012). Looking at Plasmodium on a deep, molecular level is the key to creating smarter, more effective treatments that protect the advances in the fight against malaria. Additionally, the importance of Plasmodium biology is not limited to drug resistance. There is strong good evidence that widespread use of insecticide-treated nets (ITNs) decreases the transmission of malaria, especially in vulnerable groups like young children and pregnant women. But because the parasite's method of movement is complex, protection overall does indeed depend on having enough coverage across entire communities. Knowing how the parasite interacts with both humans and mosquito vectors helps scientists and policymakers shape these interventions. In a way, achieving the right levels of ITN coverage and going into the lifecycle of the parasite shows that such research is intertwined with more efficient preventative measures and longer-term decreases in malaria incidence (Killeen et al., 2007). In the meantime, an investigation of Plasmodium gives valuable information regarding the way that parasites and hosts interact, and that's significant for charting new diagnostic assays and therapeutic agents. Its life cycle, which swings back and forth between mosquito and human hosts, holds many dangers and possibilities. Knowing exactly how the parasite outsmarts the immune system or commandeers its host's resources can spark vaccine breakthroughs and designer drug targeting, often in unexpected ways. Furthermore, tracking genetic differences between strains helps refine outbreak surveillance and projections of disease spread. In all, a closer examination of Plasmodium not only drives biomedical research forward but also strengthens our general capacity to counter malaria's evolving menace.

2.1. Taxonomy and Classification

Plasmodium parasites have eukaryotic ancestry that is far from simple. They split relatively early from the broad mass of eukaryotic life, and their long, independent history has given rise to some very distinctive biological characteristics. Their kinome—a heterogeneous group of protein kinases containing clades like AGC, CMGC, TKL, CaMK, and CK1—tethers them to yeast, plants, and mammals in surprising ways. In spite of their parasitic specialization, these organisms still share molecular features signaling an early origin. A shift from photosynthetic ancestors to a parasitic lifestyle seemed to have initiated the appearance of new, taxon-specific kinase and some notably aberrant enzyme features. Overall, this integration of ancient and modern clues is required in an effort to understand both their genetic relationships as well as how they may function (Tobin et al., 2012). Given the way Plasmodium parasites are separated out, it must be more than where they split off on the evolutionary tree. There is a complex overlay of molecular and functional differences that renders them different from closely related apicomplexans. Take piroplasmid parasites, for example, they share alveolate ancestry with Plasmodium but evolve into genetic and parasitic traits that lead us to consider different groupings. Babesia and Theileria species, just to mention a few, infect hosts of diverse types and are, in general, divided into roughly six or so lineages based on molecular phylogenetics. Notably, protein family diversification, for example, the C1A cysteine-proteinases in some lineages—reflects specialized adaptations on the basis of life cycle details and host affiliation. This molecular data adds further strata to the taxonomy, disclosing significant evolutionary and ecological distinctions even within parasites on the same niches (Ascencio et al., 2018).

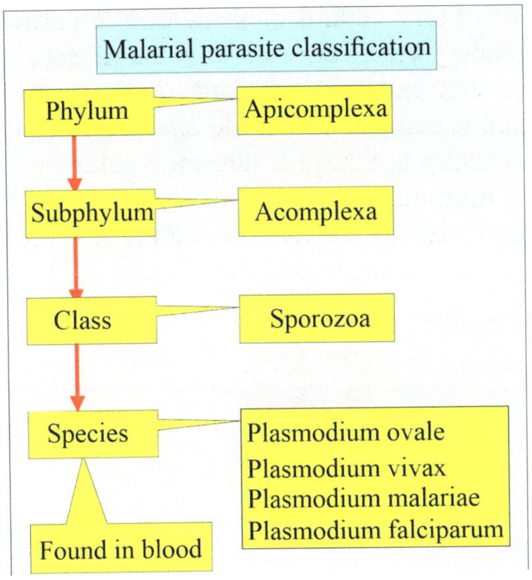

Figure 2.3. Taxonomy and classification of Plasmodium parasites.

Source: Labpedia.net. (2020). Malaria Classification and Plasmodium Life Cycle.

A further pathway for the refinement of Plasmodium taxonomy is examining gene family expansions underpinning key biological traits and host specialism. Phylogenetic analysis generally uncovers gene duplication events and expansions that define lineages, most frequently correlating such changes with more advanced phases of their life cycle, such as the schizont. Such molecular markers, it appears, are markers of vertebrate and invertebrate host pressures as well as transmission variation. For instance, differences in cysteine-proteinase paralogs between some piroplasmid parasites point to a molecular explanation for their alternative phenotypes and ecological niches. It is in the majority of cases that these ongoing evolutionary stresses underscore the requirement to integrate molecular, phylogenetic, and functional data when classifying Plasmodium and relatives (Ascencio et al., 2018) (Figure 2.3).

2.1.1. Overview of the Plasmodium Genus

Scientists have long been fascinated by the complex associations that bind Plasmodium parasites to the animals they infect. These insects don't just plague humans—also found in birds, reptiles, and other vertebrates—so it's clear that the Plasmodium genus, a collection of fairly diverse species, has much more behind it than it initially seems. Each species has its uniqueness and host preferences, which betray a long, winding evolutionary past. Take Plasmodium falciparum and Plasmodium vivax, for instance, while they tend to excel as the main perpetrators of human malaria, how they are distributed across the globe and what symptoms they cause can be very different. Overall, there is ubiquitous evidence supporting non-human primates as the main reservoirs for these parasites, especially when one considers the extent to which P. vivax is similar to the strains known to infect African great apes. Such data, in most cases, points to malaria parasites having made multiple jumps between hosts over human history, highlighting how highly adaptable they are (Gilabert et al., 2018). New genome tools have completely transformed the game, offering us entry-level access to high-resolution windows into Plasmodium biology we could never have dreamed about. Instead of merely taking it on faith that all that is in the genome behaves similarly, researchers found that while the core genetic areas—those parts that remain pretty much unchanged and even line up nicely in the P. vivax and its ape-infesting relatives—are there are families of genes that evolve at far higher, lineage-specific rates. For example, the genes responsible for the synthesis of reticulocyte-binding proteins (utilized by the parasite for infecting RBCs) show substantial modification, a kind of divergence in conformity with the process of the parasite adapting to infect human beings. Besides that, there are other genes that seem to be under positive selection pressure, indicating molecular transitions that would enable these organisms to escape our immune systems as well as acclimatize to mosquito species having a preference for feeding on human blood. In most cases, these genome hints not only explain parts of the evolutionary past but also determine potential targets that could affect how infectious and virulent the pathogen could be (Gilabert et al., 2018). There is a lot of genomic and post-genomic data these days that has given new and integrative ways to examine Plasmodium biology on many levels. Instead of keeping current isolates in isolation, researchers now assemble full biological spaces from the genetic blueprints of P. falciparum and its closest relatives; doing this allows them to forecast key novel drug targets and map metabolic pathways essential to the parasites' survival. This systems-wide, panoply view relies on dense data sets from protein sequence alignments through phylogenetic trees that expose important shared pathways as well as unique features that are unique to Plasmodium. When you assemble chemical libraries, you can discover and design lead antimalarial molecules using techniques like molecular docking and structure-based design. Further, these bioinformatics methods have become essential weapons in the fight against malaria, wonderfully illustrating the interplay between genomic insight and chemoinformatics as necessary for gains in preventing Plasmodium infections (Figure 2.4).

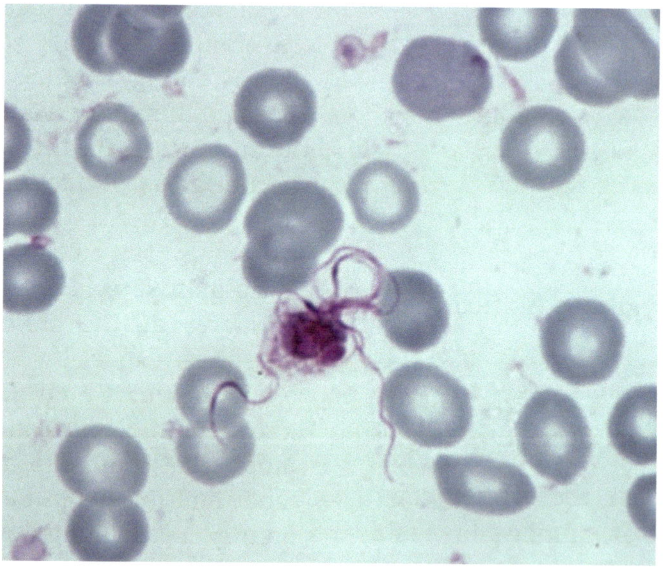

Figure 2.4. Overview of the Plasmodium genus.

Source: Flickr. (n.d.). Photograph of a Landscape. https://external-content.duckduckgo.com/iu/?u=https%3A%2F%2Flive.staticflickr.com%2F1795%2F41943814710_894b5d4ce7_w.jpg&f=1&nofb=1&ipt=fa603dccb2e32d403289df571893692fa6008641b329316503070a6d129831bf.

2.1.2. Different Species of Plasmodium

Malaria parasites have a boggling life cycle, and that's evident in the range of Plasmodium species that infect everything from man to great apes. Plasmodium vivax, for example, is being discussed a great deal in the news—it's common outside Africa and is directly linked to similar strains occurring in African apes. Such transfer reflects that the parasite has shifted hosts a number of times over the passage of time. As scientists dig deeper into the genomes, they can see that although the central sections match up well between vivax and its ape-adapted relative, finer details diverge them into other clades; this inconsistency reflects the complex, gradual process of host evolution and adaptation (Gilabert et al., 2018). But it is not only about P. vivax. The Plasmodium species also include others like P. falciparum, P. ovale, P. malariae, and even the recently discovered P. knowlesi. Each of them has its own specificities regarding biology and disease presentation, with P. falciparum tending to be the most lethal and causing most of the deaths due to malaria worldwide. Deciphering these subtleties involves deciphering a host-parasite labyrinth, a task that now has the benefit of modern-day genomic technologies and systems biology strategies. Scientists, with the aid of high-throughput sequencing and other -omics approaches, are piecing together the molecular mysteries these parasites use to cause infection, resist drugs, and resist the immune system, all of which could get us closer to better treatments and vaccines (Swann et al., 2015). It is even more interesting when one considers how evolutionary divergence is seen in specific genes, specifically the ones that allow the parasite to invade red blood cells (RBCs). Comparative genome studies reveal gene family members, like the reticulocyte-binding proteins—have been shaped by species-specific selective pressures infecting humans to increase their invasion and multiplication efficiency. In most cases, some of these positively selected P. vivax genes seem to follow evolutionary paths that are shared with those of P. falciparum; overlap indicates co-functional pathways required for parasite survival in human hosts as well as even within their insect vectors. All this suggests possible targets for therapies that one day could shut down crucial steps in the infection process (Gilabert et al., 2018) (Figure 2.5).

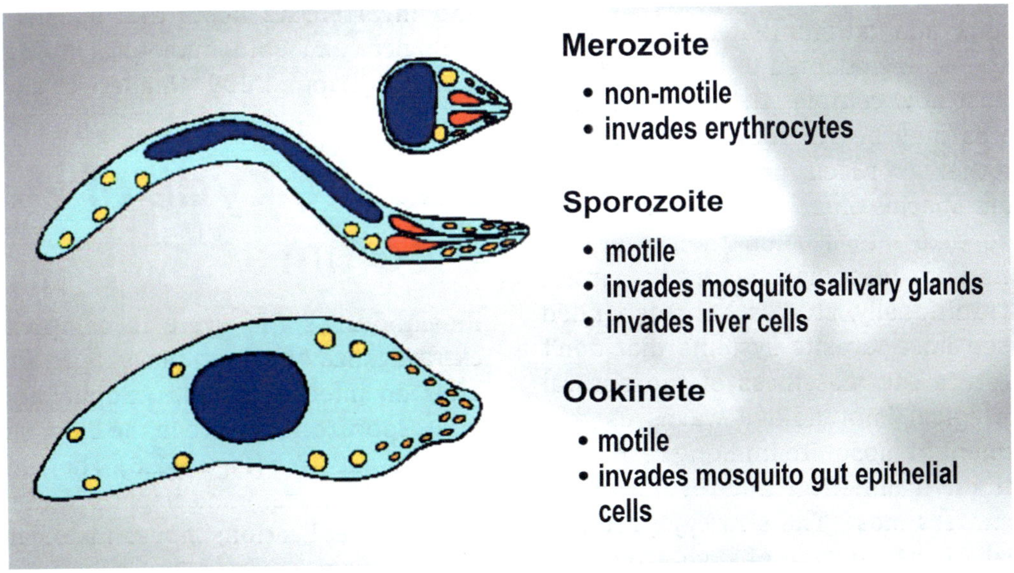

Figure 2.5. Different species of Plasmodium.

Source: Biology Notes Online. (n.d.). Diagram of Biological Concept. https://external-content.duckduckgo.com/iu/?u=https%3A%2F%2Fbiologynotesonline.com%2Fwp-content%2Fuploads%2F2024%2F04%2Fimage-1301.png&f=1&nofb=1&ipt=c8b37f029d30946453d9ef7967aa65934dc986752e4544dca7452fc4040da8ae.

2.1.3. Evolutionary Relationships Among Species

Following the history of Plasmodium gives us an idea of how these parasites developed into such experts at infecting not just one, but a whole array of hosts , including humans. Finding a Plasmodium vivax-like parasite in African great apes, for example, gave us an unexpected clue about where human P. vivax might have come from. Recent analyses using both long- and short-read sequencing in general exhibited an astounding similarity between the genome of P. vivax and that of its ape counterpart, even though they still belong to distinct groups. This implies that the jump to human infection was not a singular occurrence but rather happened on several occasions throughout the long evolution of the Homo lineage. For the most part, you will notice that lineage-specific changes – like gene family alterations that are accountable for invading RBCs – have the mark of evolutionary pressure on strains infecting humans. Detecting genes under positive selection that are also found in P. falciparum once more pinpoints the molecular adaptations that allowed these parasites to become adapted to humans, and it shows us just how complex their evolutionary relationships may be (Gilabert et al., 2018). Taking another approach, understanding how Plasmodium species emerged also means that we need to take into account their everyday interactions with mosquito vectors in natural settings. Traditionally, studies have depended on lab-based host-parasite systems that don't exactly capture the messiness of the natural world. Ecological immunology warns us that the assessment of mosquito immune responses in natural environmental and evolutionary contexts matters most. The strategy promises a more realistic assessment of such aspects as parasite virulence, immune defense diversity, and transmission dynamics. By focusing on natural population structures and the push-pull of coevolutionary pressures, scientists are able to more clearly track the selective drivers of Plasmodium diversification and its ability to infect specific hosts. Such insights, in a broader sense, are invaluable in attempting to tease apart the evolutionary trajectories that influence the spread of malaria and its effect on control measures (Tripet, 2009). The larger picture is even more complex when you add in the ways that parasite adaptations mix with host-vector coevolution. Not only do genetic divergences mirror host shifts, but they also mirror how factors like vector immune responses and environmental pressures influence evolutionary trajectories. Merging genomic data with evolutionary ecology gives an insight into why certain traits endure in certain parasite lineages. For instance, the evolutionary dynamics of reticulocyte-binding proteins in P. vivax reveal that expansions or contractions in gene families can be consistent with the level of ecological specialization and host invasion effectiveness. Collectively, these evolutionary findings sketch a mosaic of parasite diversification , shaped by successive host transfers and coevolutionary reciprocal selection between vertebrate and invertebrate hosts that speaks to broad biological and epidemiological frameworks of malaria (Tripet, 2009; Gilabert et al., 2018).

2.2. Life Cycle of Plasmodium

Plasmodium's life cycle is complex—a true extravaganza of evolutionary ingenuity. Shortly after an infected female Anopheles mosquito bites, sporozoites arrive in the bloodstream and travel to the liver (Figure 2.6). They invade liver cells (hepatocytes) and begin a kind of stealth, but vital, replication; thousands of merozoites emerge from these cells. Generally, this liver stage, though clinically quiescent, initiates the whole infection. Because the parasite is so prolific, it has to keep its gene activity under control in very heterogeneous environments. mRNA-binding protein studies reveal that, instead of extensive transcriptional refinement, Plasmodium falciparum is highly reliant upon post-transcriptional regulation— stabilizing and controlling its mRNA is crucial for uneventful development (Bunnik et al., 2016). That is, behind the apparent randomness is an undertow order that controls all of these processes. Once the merozoites leave the liver, they release into the blood and are inside RBCs. There, the parasite doesn't cooperate by the script—it goes through a ring stage, then a trophozoite, subsequently a schizont stage leading to schizogony, which results in more merozoites ready to infect new cells. This unstable phase in the blood not only sets up the cyclical fevers and all the symptoms of malaria but also enables the parasite to thrive in a relatively hostile setting. And don't forget, some merozoites even develop into gametocytes—the sexual stages that ensure the cycle is repeated when some other mosquito bites. Again, gene expression here is regulated mostly post-transcriptionally, with several RNA-binding proteins fine-tuning protein synthesis to meet the conditions (Bunnik et al., 2016).

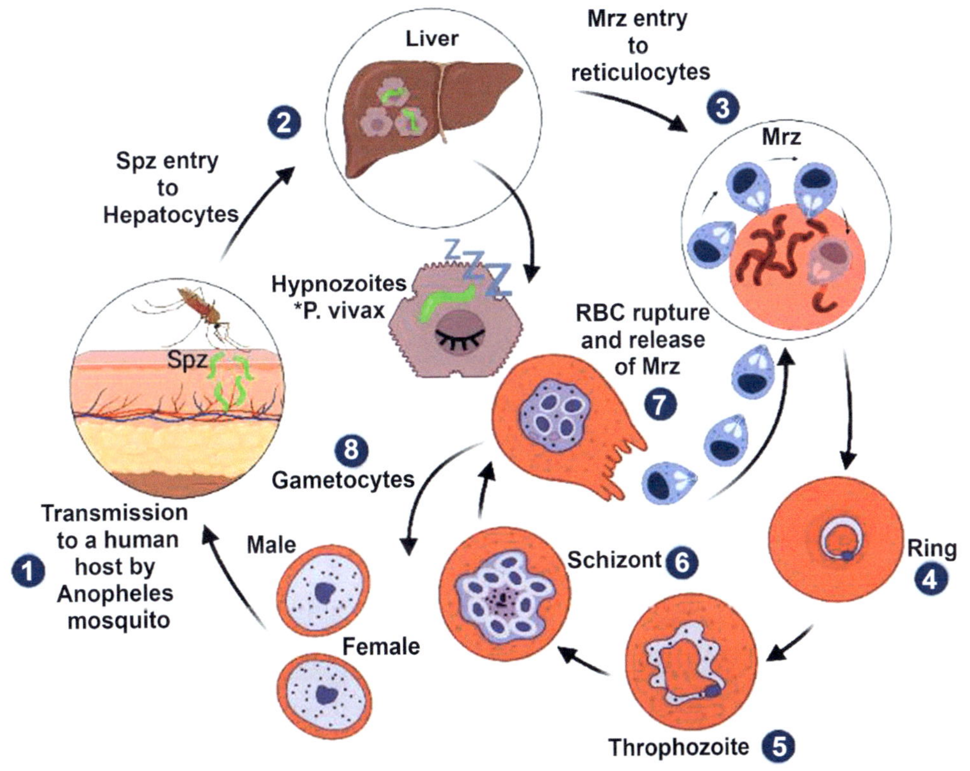

Figure 2.6. Plasmodium malariae life cycle.

Source: García, L. B., Tena, G., & Solano, R. (2022). MAP kinase signaling in plants: New insights into the last pieces of the puzzle. International Journal of Molecular Sciences, 23(22), 14528.

Such a blood stage, with all its twists, is meanwhile crucial not only for disease transmission but also for survival. Subsequently, in the mosquito gut, another surprise in store. Internalized gametocytes develop and form male and female gametes to become zygotes, which soon develop into speedy ookinetes. The ookinetes penetrate the gut wall and insert themselves as oocysts;

afterward, the oocysts develop and release sporozoites which migrate onto the salivary gland of the mosquito, until the next meal. New advances in genomic and systems biology have further informed our knowledge of these host-parasite interactions, uncovering a fairly complex network of mechanisms governing development and transmission. Generally, studying Plasmodium's complete life cycle demonstrates real hope: by attacking these molecular processes at the heart, we might unlock the door to smarter therapies and, hopefully, eventually send malaria packing.

2.2.1. Stages of the Life Cycle

Plasmodium parasites are rather capable of getting around, switching between habitats in stepwise ways that are not just the ordinary steps but advanced moves for survival and commuting from humans to mosquitoes.

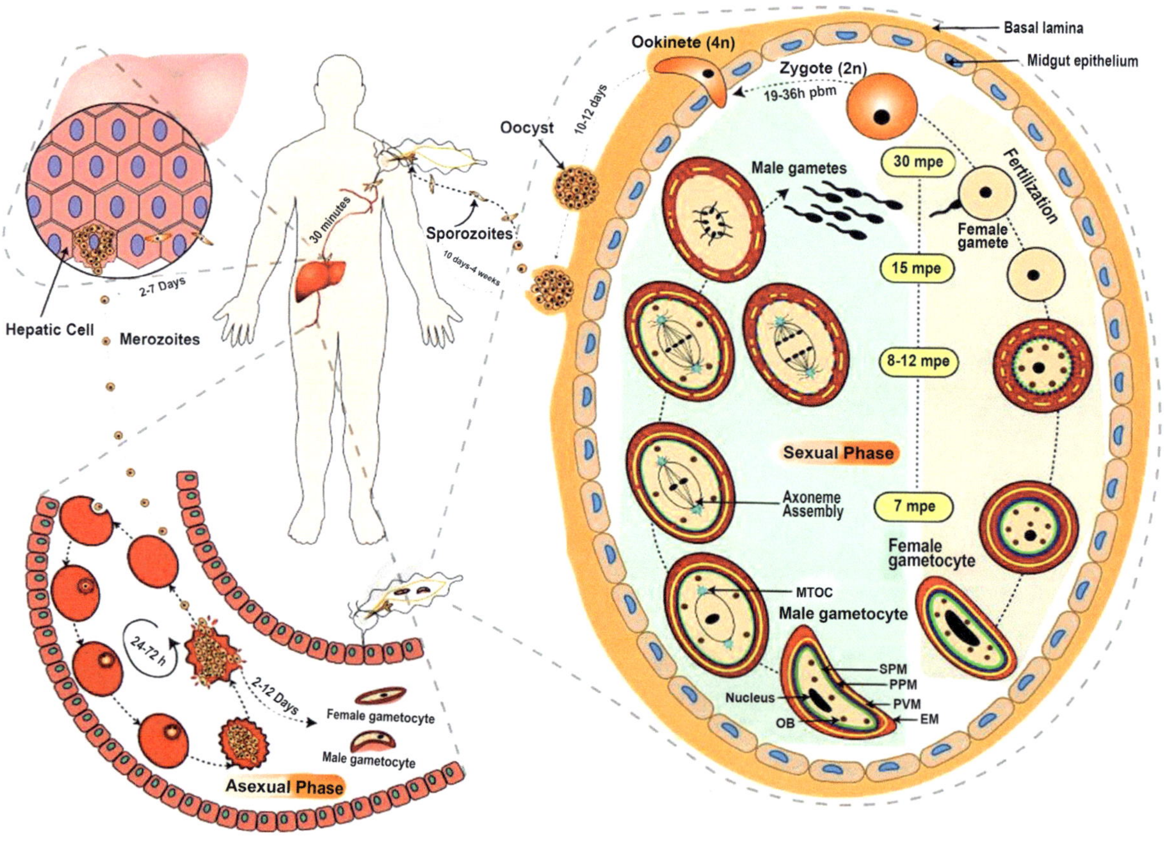

Figure 2.7. Consider the given stages in the life cycle of Plasmodium.

Source: Dash M, Sachdeva S, Bansal A and Sinha A (2022) Gametogenesis in Plasmodium: Delving Deeper to Connect the Dots. Front. Cell. Infect. Microbiol. 12:877907. doi: 10.3389/fcimb.2022.877907

When the parasite first invades the human blood, it quickly starts dividing inside RBCs, a process that, in most cases, is immediately related to malaria's manifestation. Then, out of the blue like a light switch, the parasite goes into high gear and begins producing gametocytes, a type of sexual differentiation crucial to riding inside a mosquito. Recent single-cell transcriptomics studies have begun to unveil this transformation, pointing out certain genetic markers that diverge from the general metabolic flows, all aimed at readying the parasite for its impending adventure (Brancucci et al., 2018). If you want to understand Plasmodium, you have to look at the whole host-parasite conversation. Each phase, from the sporozoites that infect the liver to the merozoites that infect RBCs—seems to have its own bag of tricks for immune evasion and replication boost. Genomic and systems biology studies have even mapped comparatively complex networks that manipulate the parasite's genes as it makes its way through its cycle. For the most part, this sweeping strategy is simply how the parasite faces the different stresses of the environment; it even allows scientists to pinpoint where certain treatments might be effective. It is a dynamic, complex association that shows just how clever and advanced these parasites are (Swann et al., 2015). Recent advances in molecular and genetic technologies have shifted the focus toward disrupting the cycle of the parasite as a means to fight malaria. Targeting that all-important phase of sexual differentiation— the period the parasite gets ready to move from human to mosquito—seems like a pretty solid move. By investigating the highly specific markers and signals that drive this phase, scientists are not just adding to our basic knowledge about parasite biology but are setting the stage for developing drugs and vaccines that would cut off transmission. This approach is a move away from simply treating symptoms and toward strangling the parasite's ability to propagate and thrive. Continued investigation of every twist and turn in the Plasmodium life cycle gives hope that more effective control, and even elimination of malaria is within sight (Swann et al., 2015; Brancucci et al., 2018) (Figure 2.7).

2.2.2. Role of the Mosquito Vector

Plasmodium parasites and mosquito vectors share a rich relationship that drives malaria transmission. Anopheles mosquitoes, for instance, are the major culprits in helping the parasite develop and jump onto humans—a fact that recent surveys conducted in the Greater Mekong Subregion have brought to light by finding a varied group of Anopheles species with Plasmodium infections. In our collections within the field, Anopheles sinensis would be found in large numbers, with high parasite burdens; this suggests in most cases that its role might be more important than in the known vectors like Anopheles dirus and Anopheles minimus. It seems that several vector species play a role in the transmission of malaria, which quite complicates things if one is to attempt to target one form. Having knowledge about which local species are present, and how heavily infected as well as what their behavior is, continues to be valuable in coming up with responsive control measures within the complicated epidemiological landscape of endemic regions (Zhang et al., 2022). Mosquito biology itself plays a determining role in how effectively Plasmodium can grow and spread. Neurochemical mechanisms within such insects, specifically those employing serotonin (5-hydroxytryptamine or 5-HT)—overall regulate types of behaviors that are significant to malaria dangers. Some experiments have indicated that when mosquitoes take a blood meal that has malaria-related levels of 5-HT, they undergo a shift in flight speed and host-seeking behavior such that they are more inclined to make multiple fast blood feeds. This change may improve transmission chances because the mosquito is essentially interacting with multiple hosts within a short time period. Furthermore, 5-HT levels appear to influence the susceptibility of mosquitoes to infection with

Plasmodium, proposing an intimate neurophysiological connection between parasite development and behavior. These discoveries in mosquito neurobiology offer intriguing avenues to disrupt malaria transmission through manipulating selected vector signaling pathways (Briggs et al., 2022). The developmental phase of a mosquito also plays a part in determining the feeding behavior of such mosquitoes, ultimately affecting transmission dynamics. When, for example, midgut oocysts exist, then the mosquitoes will moderate blood-feeding to some extent—potentially bringing the spread to an end. But when sporozoites have formed in the salivary glands, feeding levels rise dramatically to enable the parasite to jump onto new hosts with greater ease.

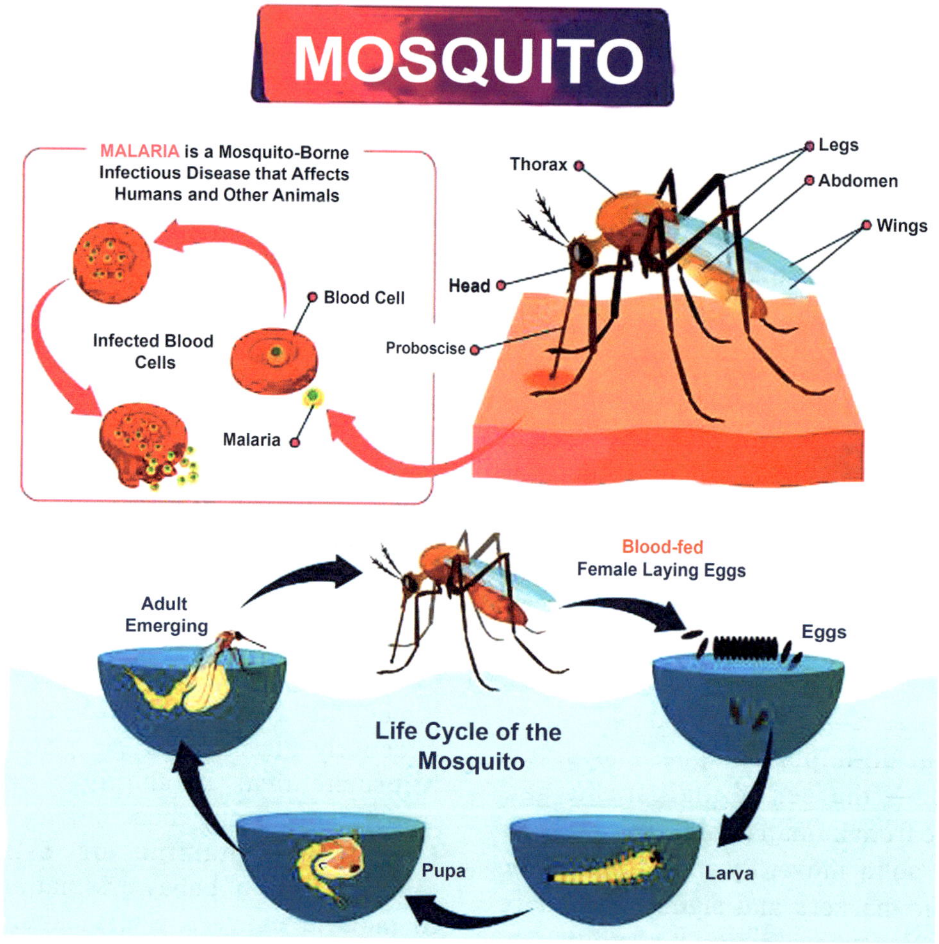

Figure 2.8. Mosquito vector.

Source: Freepik. (n.d.). Mosquito Vector. https://external-content.duckduckgo.com/iu/?u=https%3A%2F%2Fas2.ftcdn.net%2Fv2%2Fjpg%2F02%2F80%2F99%2F93%2F1000_F_280999363_O3eV9JPfITJ2GkHE4i7yrfi3Rc1Y4NXJ.jpg&f=1&nofb=1&ipt=0c098ba3e36f552c805eca9845bd2251f38f86e046baff9a8d0893a21f1f4243.

This interaction among feeding behavior, environmental stimulus, and such variables as 5-HT modulation weaves a complex tapestry of mosquito efficacy as parasitic carriers. Oftentimes, the discovery of such interrelated factors indicates why it is positively crucial to pair behavioral studies with molecular ones. Certain interventions that either block or disrupt a mosquito's capacity to feed could possibly go a long way toward ending the cycle of malaria (Briggs et al., 2022) (Figure 2.8).

2.2.3. Transmission to Humans

The Plasmodium parasites and their hosts have a complicated interaction that makes transmission of malaria short of simple. In the host human, the parasites mature into gametocytes that drift in the blood for amazingly extended periods of time, sometimes even weeks—until the timing is right when a hungry Anopheles mosquito comes by. Meanwhile, their immature forms persist in tissues like the bone marrow, in effect evading immune detection and serving as a standby reserve. This fusion of asexual development and its shift to sexual stages, for most cases, enables the parasite to balance its dual life in mosquitoes and humans. This type of dynamic, if you observe closely, not only facilitates ongoing transmission but also indicates crucial points for intervention (van der Watt et al., 2022). When a female Anopheles mosquito feeds, the parasite is introduced to an entirely new world that requires immediate accommodation. In the mosquito midgut's hiding places, its proteins and the insect's receptors associate in a molecular ballet—a dynamic interaction honed through the centuries, as if both have learned to coexist. Overall, interfering with these subtle interactions can potentially pave the way for novel interventions like targeted medication or vaccines that are designed to inhibit parasite development in the mosquito. However, challenges ensue since the parasite can move into discrete biological niches that are significantly divergent from those encountered during human infection, and thus the research approach has to be as agile (Keleta et al., 2021). If real advances in reducing malaria are the goal, then descending deep into the process of transmission, mosquito bite to infection in humans, is well and truly necessary. Current therapies bring together older therapies that target the parasite in the blood and liver and newer strategies that target the sexual stages on which mosquitoes feed. Researchers persist in refining focus on gametocyte behavior and molecular nuances within mosquito intestines, all in an effort to identify the exact parasite molecules at play for transmission. Briefly, stopping the chain of infection comes down to an interdisciplinary endeavor, one that balances historical therapies with novel, scientifically driven treatments based on a thorough understanding of Plasmodium's transmission tactic (Keleta et al., 2021; van der Watt et al., 2022).

2.3. Pathogenesis and Symptoms

Plasmodium falciparum causes havoc in quite a hidden way in the human body – infected RBCs are responsible (Figure 2.9). As soon as the RBCs are infected by the parasite, their surface is altered immediately by exposing their PfEMP1 proteins in a manner that sticks to the walls of blood vessels. This attahcment, known as sequestration, keeps the body from clearing out these infected cells, yet also causes problems like plugged up small vessels and inflammation. Interestingly, the parasite seems to use many different forms of PfEMP1, allowing it to attach to many different endothelial receptors; this variation influences how severe the disease will be. The latest transcriptomic research, in general, shows that the most severe malaria cases usually possess PfEMP1 variants with binding to the endothelial protein C receptor, whereas less severe cases express proteins with a tendency to bind to CD36 (Wichers-Misterek et al., 2021). For those suffering from the first infection, a poor immune response may allow the parasite to survive for a longer time, and thus, it will further enhance the pathogenesis and symptoms of malaria. The symptoms, in part, arise from the capacity of P. falciparum to adhere to host tissues. A classical sign of severe malaria is when the brain is involved : infected cells adhere to the microvessels of the brain, causing endothelial activation and inflammation in a not-so-direct fashion. This intimate interaction serves to disrupt the blood-brain barrier, both by physically blocking it and through cytokine-mediated damage to the endothelial cells. In the vast majority of cases, recent work using three-dimensional blood-brain barrier models has shown that the parasite invades brain endothelial cells only if it can bind via both ICAM-1 and EPCR. This double binding causes the barrier to swell and break, which is associated with brain edema and neurological symptoms that are usually seen with cerebral malaria (Adams et al., 2021). These results, while quite roundabout in explanation, do link the tiny adhesion events at the molecular level to the big picture of neurological complications. Advancing from a benign infection to a life-threatening case of malaria, to a large extent, depends on these same processes of adhesion, which then determine a wide variety of symptoms. Beyond the brain, when the parasite seizes other organs, it is capable of inducing multisystem complications – think acute respiratory distress or even renal failure. Parasites carrying EPCR-binding PfEMP1 variants are typically found to induce more severe inflammatory responses and vascular issues. Also, the general immune status of the individual; in a person experiencing malaria for the first time, the lack of pre-existing immunity can result in a more intense, and at times excessively severe, immunopathological response that enhances the development of a more virulent parasite form. Together, this array of parasite virulence, the specific receptors they bind to, and the host immune status weaves the complex clinical tapestry of malaria – from uncomplicated fever and anemia to lethal organ damage (Adams et al., 2021; Wichers-Misterek et al., 2021).

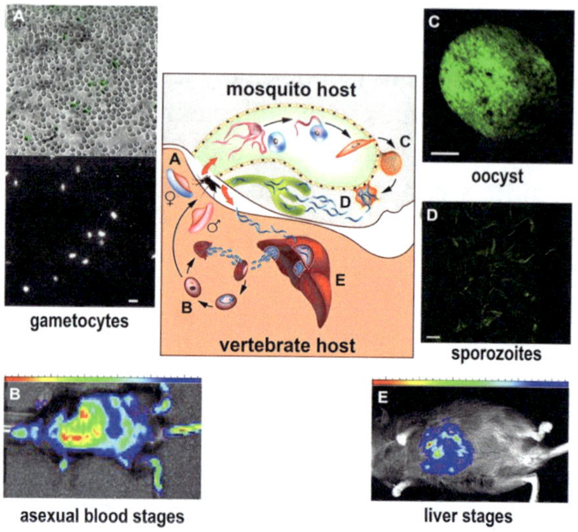

Figure 2.9. Pathogenesis and symptoms of Plasmodium falciparum.

Source: Siciliano G and Alano P (2015) Enlightening the malaria parasite life cycle: bioluminescent Plasmodium in fundamental and applied research. Front. Microbiol. 6:391. doi: 10.3389/fmicb.2015.00391

2.3.1. Mechanism of Infection in Humans

When the infected mosquito ingests blood, sporozoites, tiny infiltrators concealed in its salivary glands, find entry into human skin. They settle mostly in the dermis subsequently start to travel about, migrating off towards nearby blood vessels. Not many of these sporozoites penetrate the skin barrier, which seems to be an actual site of weakness for the parasite. Once within the bloodstream, they stream to the liver, infecting liver cells where they silently develop and multiply, even before we notice any symptoms. In the majority of cases, this silent amassing eventually leads to the release of merozoites infecting RBCs, which initiates the sequence of processes that ends in malaria (Waide et al., 2020). Upon reaching the liver, they dive into quite a complex cycle of exoerythrocytic schizogony. Inside liver cells, they become transformed from the sporozoites into so-called schizonts, with each of these harboring thousands of merozoites as a result of successive nuclear division cycles, without dividing up turn by turn. Most often, this quick reproduction goes unnoticed, not stimulating much immune reaction, and the body overlooks the first warning signals. The liver stage ends with the rupture of infected cells, liberating the merozoites into the blood; a crucial step in initiating the blood stage that ultimately causes symptoms.

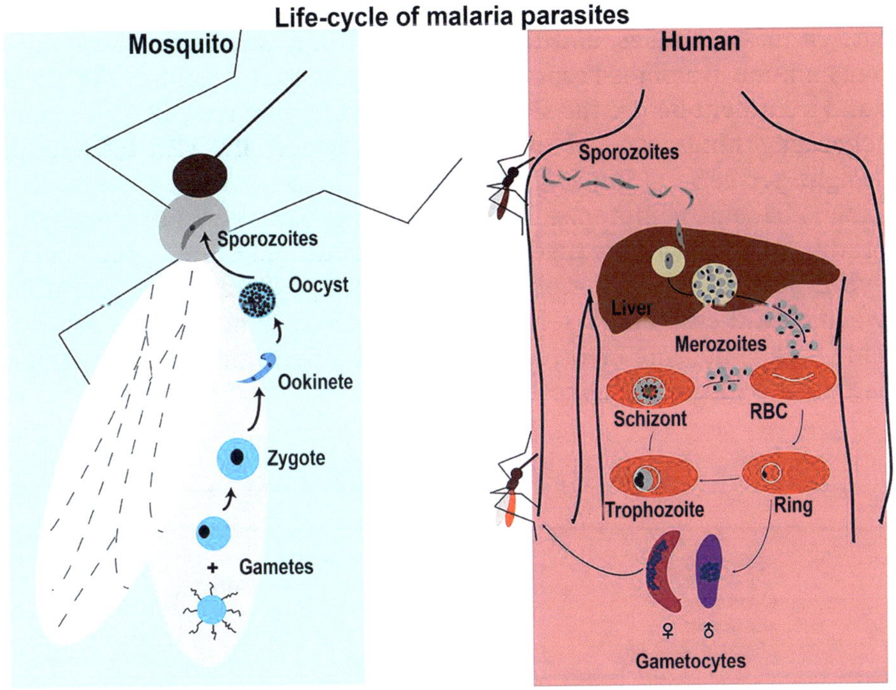

Figure 2.10. Mechanism of infection in humans of Plasmodium falciparum.

Source: Su X-z, Zhang C and Joy DA (2020) Host-Malaria Parasite Interactions and Impacts on Mutual Evolution. Front. Cell. Infect. Microbiol. 10:587933. doi: 10.3389/fcimb.2020.587933

Perhaps not coincidentally, processes like the gut microbiota may infrequently alter immune reactions, having a gentle adjustment of parasite numbers and host antibody production (Waide et al., 2020). When they escape liver cells, merozoites spring immediately into RBCs, starting the blood stage that gets noticed. In these cells, parasites asexually multiply, consuming hemoglobin until the red cell is no longer able to cling and bursts wide open—this, in turn, releases even more merozoites to infect additional cells. This oscillating invasion and lysis of the red cells is the foundation for most of the typical presentations of malaria, including fever, anemia, and generalized inflammation. Of note is that certain of the parasites change to another form, the gametocytes, which are the ones responsible for the cycle to restart entry into mosquitoes with new bites. For most cases, the seamless progression from that first bite to gametocyte production is controlled by the way the host immune system responds and by a number of variable bottlenecks that finally regulate the parasite's general infectious ability and malaria transmission (Graumans et al., 2020) (Figure 2.10).

2.3.2. Common Symptoms of Malaria

Malaria emerges when Plasmodium parasites make their way through the body—first infecting the liver, subsequently spreading to RBCs. The whole ordeal is not quick; it takes a while, and the wait varies based on which type of Plasmodium is present. Fever, chills, and bouts of sweating set in a short while around the time infected blood cells burst, dumping merozoites and some very nasty toxins into the bloodstream. These bouts of fever normally coincide with the parasite undergoing its cycle of replication, typically with headache, aching muscles, and general "off" feeling. This is generally the pattern in most cases, and the pattern not only shows the parasites are increasing but also that your immune system is responding, a response that amplifies the signs and demands rapid diagnosis and treatment before the situation worsening (Laurens, 2019). If malaria is allowed to progress unchecked, things can get extremely bad, especially with Plasmodium falciparum infections. You might get serious impacts like extreme anemia or even cerebral malaria, where confusion or seizures become symptoms. In the meantime, parasitized cells can stick to the blood vessel lining, creating small blockages that worsen the condition. Even a spectacular splenomegaly can happen as your body is trying a more effortful attempt at removing the infected cells. The distinction between a mild case and a serious one typically lies in the intensity of the symptoms and whether many organs become involved, which in turn determines the treatment strategy and what to anticipate in the future (Talapko et al., 2019).

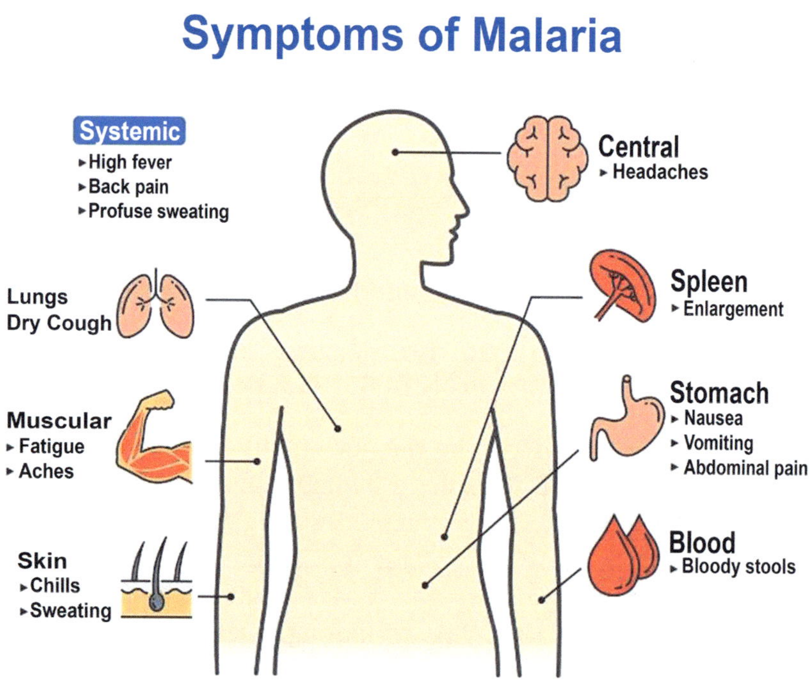

Figure 2.11. Common symptoms of malaria.

Source: Cambridge Independent. (n.d.). Image of a Plant Défense Mechanism. https://external-content.duckduckgo.com/iu/?u=https%3A%2F%2Fwww.cambridgeindependent.co.uk%2F_media%2Fimg%2F0YY38TZV2RQVHQMEKV3W.jpg&f=1&nofb=1&ipt=59a40bf20d8b5ae452de40ebb70641375b747d4a5eb32964d0b91fd423d15afd.

In areas where malaria is prevalent, the signs and symptoms don't always come in a pre-scripted form—they change based on the immune history of the host and how many times he or she has been exposed. People who have some immunity will have milder or even somewhat atypical symptom, which can complicate a simple diagnosis.

While this is happening, tourists or immune individuals tend to acquire a sudden onset of hectic fever, chills, pulsating headache, and gastrointestinal disturbance like nausea and vomiting. Since the initial symptoms are so nonspecific that they are shared with other etiologies of fever, clinical acumen alone is not enough; laboratory tests become an absolute requirement to make the diagnosis. This pairing of presentations emphasizes why understanding the local infection pattern and more specific diagnostic tools remains essential in attempts to fight malaria worldwide (Laurens, 2019; Talapko et al., 2019) (Figure 2.11).

2.3.3. Complications Arising from Plasmodium Infection

Plasmodium parasites wreak havoc in the human body after the initial infection. They don't just nest; they conduct a stealth operation, evading our immune system by sending small packages in the form of extracellular vesicles (EVs). These EVs, packages containing proteins, lipids, and even strands of nucleic acid—can trick surrounding cells to change their behavior, which, in most cases, leaves our immune system rather baffled. When subjected to stress or when the disease turns virulent, this ongoing dripping of vesicles seems to propagate malaria's effect throughout the body. While our immune cells are thrown out of kilter by such hidden messages, inflammation builds up and can lead to serious problems like cerebral malaria, extreme anemia, or even multi-organ failure (Gavinho et al., 2019).

Dissecting how these vesicles work gives us new, albeit somewhat vague, information about how the host and parasite constantly exchange blows. Heart and muscle tissue are not immune to it either, cardiac or skeletal muscles alike are in the crosshairs. It is one of the tendencies in most protozoan infections: the parasite triggers an inflammatory cascade that not only provokes oxidative stress but also triggers a rise in pro-inflammatory cytokines. The outcome? Widespread muscle cell destruction can take the form of arrhythmias (irregular heartbeats) or even myocarditis, along with general muscle weakness that does little but add to the patient's discomfort. When normal muscle function spirals out of control, malaria's cumulative disrupting effects worsen, disturbing the body's natural balance (Marrelli et al., 2020). Such additional complications beyond the bloodstream demonstrate clearly that the parasite's influence penetrates deep, leading us to consider treatments that address inflammation as well as infection. Meanwhile, these complex complications present enormous challenges for treatment.

The EV strategy of the parasite not only worsens the disease but also poses challenges to vaccine and drug development. Additionally, muscle and heart injury necessitate therapies to play a double function, killing parasites while reducing inflammatory damage. Early data suggest that antioxidant and anti-inflammatory therapies might limit tissue damage, but their testing in clinical settings is required. Finally, a greater understanding of these biological processes is the foundation for designing targeted therapies and public health initiatives that may reduce the global burden of malaria (Gavinho et al., 2019; Marrelli et al., 2020) (Figure 2.12).

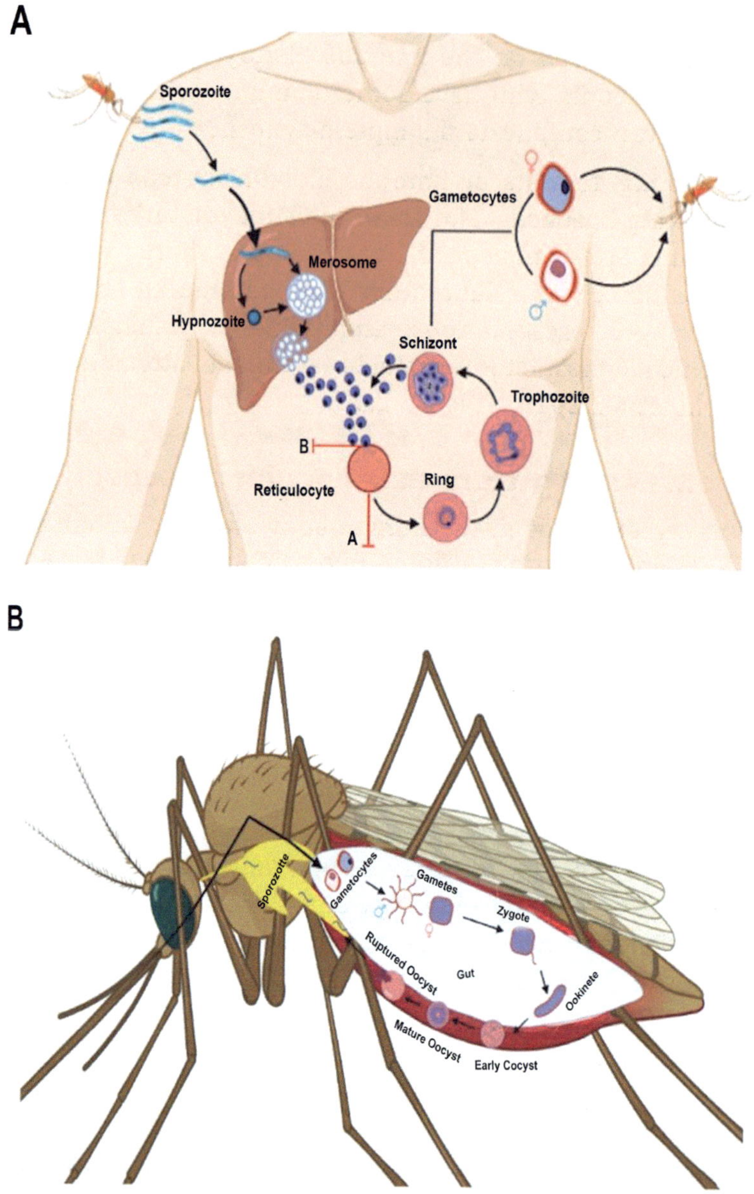

Figure 2.12. Complications arising from mosquitoes.

Source: Kumari S and Sinha A (2023) Culture and transfection: Two major bottlenecks in understanding Plasmodium vivax biology. Front. Microbiol. 14:1144453. doi: 10.3389/fmicb.2023.1144453

2.4. Immune Response to Plasmodium

Plasmodium parasites and our immune system are playing an insidious association that indeed determines the progression of the disease. At the onset of the parasite, the body takes off—macrophages and dendritic cells roll into action, releasing bursts of inflammatory cytokines that, in an attempt to slow parasite, spread, tend to cause fever and shivering. However Plasmodium falciparum has some tricks of its own for avoiding detection, so that even while these early defenses become established, the parasite mysteriously persists. Adaptive responses try to catch up but take a while to develop and maybe fall behind, leaving us with a persistent global health challenge. Scientists are also studying these avoidance methods and creating vaccines that may provoke greater, longer-lasting immunity (Bonam et al., 2021).

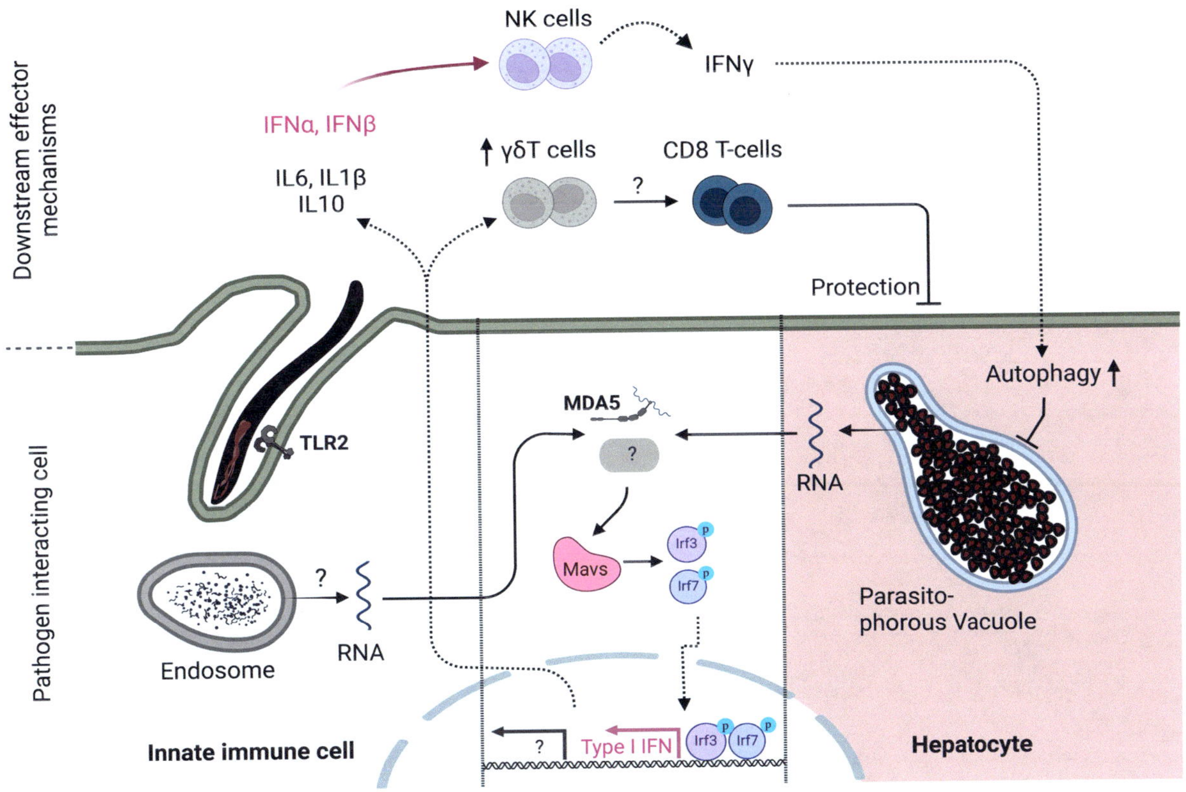

Figure 2.13. Immune response to Plasmodium.

Source: Pohl K and Cockburn IA (2022) Innate immunity to malaria: The good, the bad and the unknown. Front. Immunol. 13:914598. doi: 10.3389/fimmu.2022.914598

Humoral immunity, though, is the seeming game changer for eradicating Plasmodium infections. We learn that our gut microbiota, bacteria that we most often take for granted, play a surprising role in controlling our antibody responses. Experiments in mice, for example, have shown that mice with a gut microbiota skewed towards lower parasite loads develop a more active germinal center in the spleen. This leads to an expansion of B cells and higher titers of parasite-specific antibodies that not only seem to work better but are likely to be different in quality, giving better protection. Very clearly, however, the microenvironment of the gut does have an opinion regarding the building of immunity, and that injecting gut bacteria into the body may represent a convenient extra strategy to boost humoral immunity and vaccine efficacy (Waide et al., 2020). Apart from such antibody-driven defenses, the ability of the body to memorize earlier infections is also a prime consideration. Good immunological memory hinges significantly on strong germinal center responses that produce high-affinity memory B cells and long-term plasma cells, ready to pounce if the parasite returns. For good measure, a couple of vaccine adjuvants, by stimulating these germinal centers that little bit harder, offer promising new ways to boost malaria vaccines. Because the parasite can shift antigens and avoid our defenses, means of augmenting and extending the protective immune response are crucial to the point of being absolute. In most cases, the integration of insights from immunology and parasitology remains our best hope for meeting the obstinate challenge of malaria control (Waide et al., 2020; Bonam et al., 2021) (Figure 2.13).

2.4.1. Human Immune Response Mechanisms

Plasmodium parasites and human bodies are locked in a filthy, constant struggle. When dropped by a mosquito, the parasite, the sporozoites race quickly into liver cells and start rubbing shoulders with the body's indigenous immune system. Liver macrophages, uncontrolled Kupffer cells, are an initial stumbling block but often get bypassed; sometimes the parasite literally forces them into apoptosis, which affects their ability to engulf intruders.

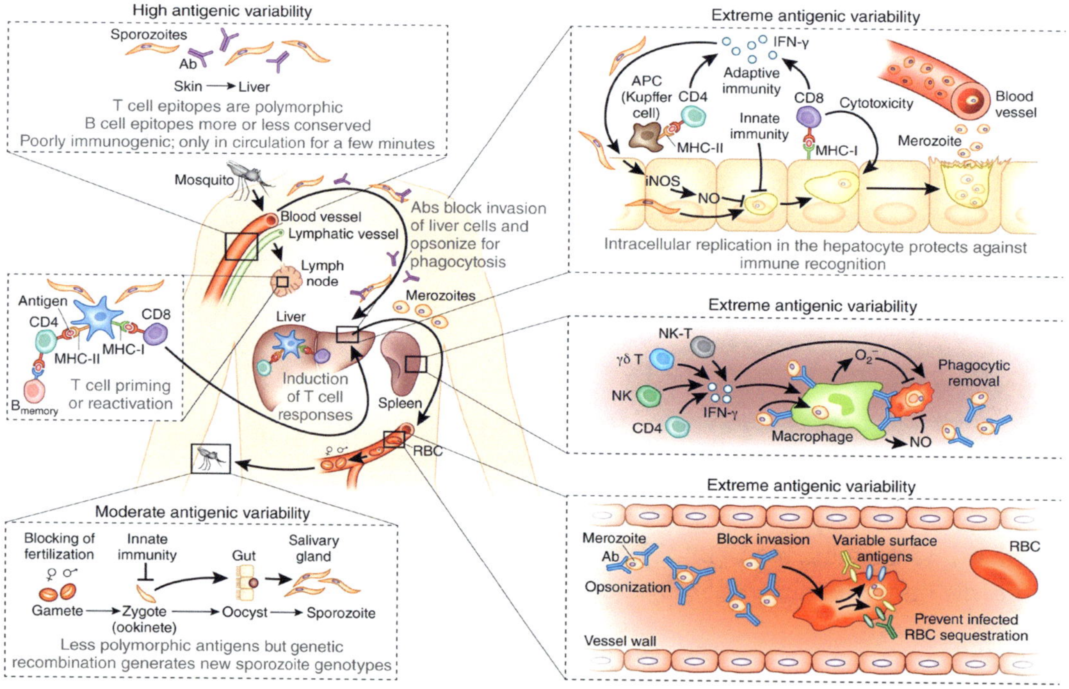

Figure 2.14. Human immune response mechanisms.

Source: Riley, E. M., & Stewart, V. A. (2013). Immune mechanisms in malaria: New insights in vaccine development. Nature Medicine, 19(2), 168–178.

The parasite also downregulates the expression of major histocompatibility complex-I on the infected RBCs, so cytotoxic CD8+ T cells won't likely detect the threat. In the majority of cases, these mechanisms operate synergistically to enable the parasite to slip through the cracks, and it becomes challenging to get rid of the infection (Belachew, 2018). Recognition has a significant role on the adaptive side, but when working with Plasmodium falciparum, it becomes complicated. This parasite is notorious for regularly changing its surface proteins so the host's capability to establish a long-term immune response gets out of balance. For the most part, this constant reshuffling, including both epigenetic modifications and odd transcriptional switching, undermines the body's immunological memory. Thus, the infection continues and the parasite gains more chances of spreading. This perpetual shift is a typical illustration of Plasmodium's tendency to evade innate as well as adaptive immunity, posing true challenges in the production of vaccines (Deitsch et al., 2017). And here is the bizarre episode of the complement system. The parasite even succeeds in recruiting host complement proteins into its cause. For instance, they use these proteins to shield extracellular gametes from complement lysis in the mosquito midgut, so that they can return into the mosquito with ease. Meanwhile, once in humans, the parasite hides away inside RBCs, which, having no major histocompatibility complex markers, properly camouflage the threat from cytotoxic lymphocytes. Interestingly, on some occasions, these complement proteins help the parasite sneak into erythrocytes, showing a form of ironic twist in host defense. All of this goes to emphasize the significance of learning about receptor-ligand interactions at various stages of parasites with the hope of envisioning vaccines that could potentially cut these evasive maneuvers (Belachew, 2018) (Figure 2.14).

2.4.2. Evasion Strategies Employed by Plasmodium

Plasmodium can persist inside its hostile host in large measure because it employs many shrewd evasive action. One major means is the ejection of small parcels called EVs – these little packages, which are packed with proteins, lipids, and nucleic acids, have the power to change the activity of surrounding cells. Under stress or as things become worse, the parasite seems to boost EV play, communicating with host cells in a way that masks its presence. Overall, releasing EVs helps Plasmodium tip the balance toward it along the trajectory of an infection, which makes it hard for the immune system to attack it (Gavinho et al., 2019). This type of immune manipulation, though a bit unconventional, prolongs the parasite's stay in the game. Another ingenious trick is antigenic variation, where the parasite continuously modifies the proteins on the surface of infected RBCs. It has been discovered in studies conducted on Plasmodium knowlesi and Plasmodium falciparum that proteins like SICA and PfEMP1 continue to change in order to avoid the antibodies of the body. This incessant toggling—owing to huge multigene families—results in the spleen's screening process struggling to keep up. The majority of the time, the resulting confusion not only allows the parasite to cling to the host but also makes it more difficult to create potent vaccines (Galinski etal., 2018). It is somewhat like the parasite having its closet perpetually updated to remain in immune shadows. Besides that, Plasmodium exploits sequestration to make a further escape from immune clearance. Sequestered red blood cells are attached to the endothelial surfaces of organs such as the brain and placenta and therefore escape the regular sweep of the spleen. Essentially, parasite proteins on the cell surface are binding with host cell receptors in novel configurations, which has the effect of making these cells drop below the immunological radar. This form of localized protection is not just reducing exposure to immune detection to a low level but is also creating refugia where the parasite can grow. Include other mechanisms like molecular mimicry and subtle immunomodulation and you have a whole arsenal of explanations as to how Plasmodium long survives in a very hostile environment. All these interconnected strategies show the complex nature of Plasmodium's deceptions and the challenge they pose to drug targeting (Figure 2.15).

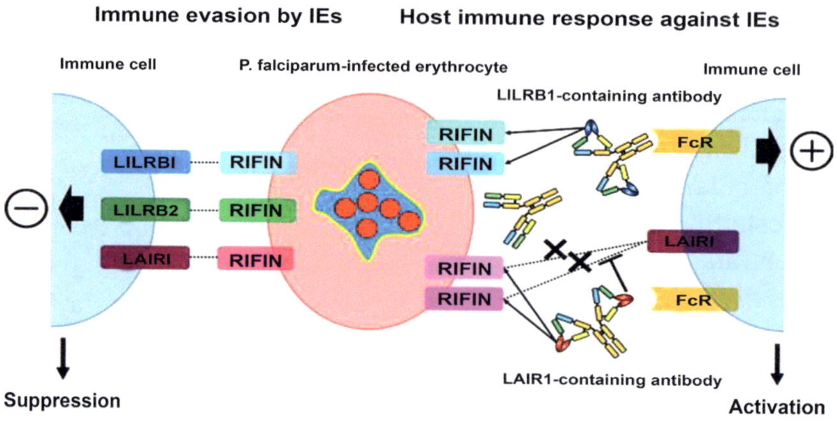

Figure 2.15. Evasion strategies employed by Plasmodium.

Source: Sakoguchi, A., & Arase, H. (2022). The immunosuppressive functions of RIFINs towards host immunity and the host immune response against RIFINs. In A. Sakoguchi & H. Arase, Mechanisms for host immune evasion mediated by Plasmodium falciparum-infected erythrocyte surface antigens. Frontiers in Immunology, 13, Article 901864.

2.4.3. Role of Vaccines in Immunity

Plasmodium parasites are recalcitrant biology, deciphering the details is necessary to develop effective vaccines that can protect us against malaria. These insects travel through a number of different stages within human beings and mosquitoes, and that complex life cycle offers many points where a vaccine might hit them. Vaccines should train our immune system to see and destroy the parasite pieces before they can gain a solid foothold or become actual disease. But it is even more sinister when you factor in that the parasite is able to change its antigen presentation based on such factors as available current nutrients present or interaction with its host. Researchers have found that laboratory culturing of the parasite alters its gene function, especially those concerning how lethal it can be. Hence, what we learn from watching parasites under real-life conditions (in vivo) becomes very applicable for choosing vaccine targets that induce strong, persistent immunity (Brown et al., 2020). Vaccine immunity depends on attacking specific proteins of the parasite, usually those that help the parasite gain entry into host cells and interfere with the immune system. An example would be that studies on Plasmodium vivax have pointed out the Reticulocyte-Binding Protein (PvRBP) family as pivotal in breaking through reticulocytes—the very cells the parasite seems to have a special affinity for invading. One protein, PvRBP2b, is rather skilled at binding to reticulocytes by itself and this has researchers thinking it might be a prime candidate for vaccines. Fascinatingly, natural responses, such as responses of IgG1 and IgG3 antibodies to proteins such as PvRBP2b and PvRBP1a, have been linked, in most cases, with a lower risk of infection of malaria in endemic areas. Practically speaking, through inhibition of the proteins that form the core of the parasite's entry, vaccines are able to retard its ability to slip into RBCs, restraining replication and the resulting disease; such an idea underscores the need for vaccine targets that have been confirmed through extensive molecular research (França et al., 2016). Other than selecting the right antigen, whether a vaccine for malaria will work is a question of give-and-take between our immune system and the parasite's own cleverness. Plasmodium has acquired a variety of tricks—changing its appearance by antigenic variation or sticking to cells through something called cytoadherence—to allow it to get away from us. Even external factors like a fever or the stress of circulating blood can re-tune its gene expression, like for proteins like PfEMP1, presumably lowering the overall effectiveness of a vaccine if such modifications are not factored in. Adding to that is the fact that lab-cultured parasites might not entirely reflect those in a living body, which is why studies into genuine host-derived samples are so important. In total, a deep and integrated understanding of the way the parasite develops and communicates with our immune systems is, on the whole, essential in creating vaccine strategies conferring a broad, enduring protection from malaria (Brown et al., 2020) (Figure 2.16).

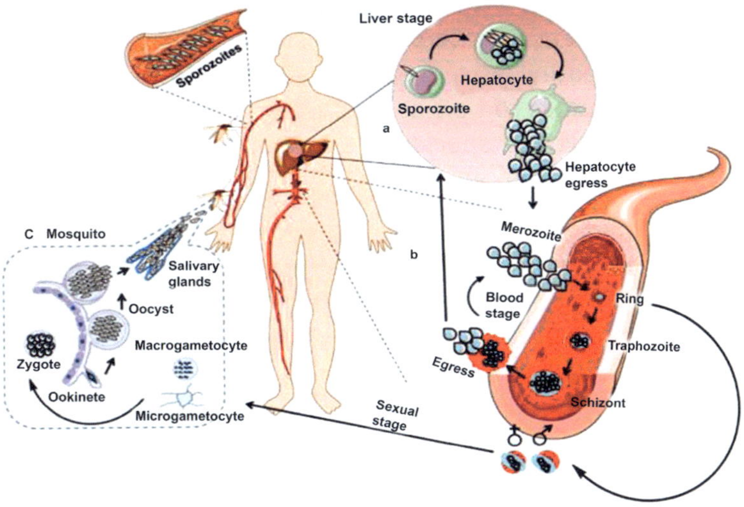

Figure 2.16. Plasmodium falciparum malaria vaccines and vaccine adjuvants.

Source: Bonam SR, Rénia L, Tadepalli G, Bayry J, Kumar HMS. Plasmodium falciparum Malaria Vaccines and Vaccine Adjuvants. *Vaccines*. 2021; 9(10):1072. https://doi.org/10.3390/vaccines9101072

2.5. Diagnosis of Plasmodium Infections

Diagnosis of malaria is still the backbone of our overall activities to cure and manage the disease (Figure 2.17). Traditional microscopy, once the gold standard, enables us to see Plasmodium parasites within RBCs; however, with low parasitemia or if several species mix together, its usefulness decreases quite quickly. Relying solely on microscopy might shortchange the actual numbers for some species like Plasmodium vivax and Plasmodium malariae, which prefer to live at lower densities or lie dormant in areas outside the standard blood sample. In most cases, new approaches filled in the picture more clearly by picking up even those stealthy, asymptomatic carriers through techniques such as polymerase chain reaction (PCR). An accurate, and detailed, diagnosis is critical; not only does it direct treatment decisions, but it is also the foundation of the kind of epidemiological tracking that public health initiatives depend upon. P. vivax is especially troublesome; in that it has some peculiarities. For one, it can live in the liver in a latent phase known as hypnozoites—phases that standard blood tests simply don't pick up on, leaving room for relapses long after the blood seems clear. This hidden pool of parasites undoubtedly makes diagnosis and treatment more complex, requiring specially tailored tests and longer, more complex treatment that targets both the blood and liver phases. There is even newer data indicating that P. vivax can sequester in other body compartments, once more avoiding our usual detection methods and emphasizing just how clandestine it can be. All of this, in a general sense, is to state that we might have to alter our approach and rethink diagnostic methods to be able to detect these stubborn forms (Baird, 2021). On the other hand, chasing after Plasmodium malariae can also be challenging. Its low blood presence, added to being mixed with a more common species like P. falciparum, sometimes leads to diagnosis errors and the following underreporting. This, in turn, leaves us with an unclear picture of exactly how big a role P. malariae malaria contributes to the overall burden of the disease, especially in regions like sub-Saharan Africa. Typical tests simply lack the sensitivity necessary for large-scale, routine detection of this insidious parasite. But recent progress in next-generation sequencing and genomic surveillance is starting to fill some of these gaps, allowing its transmission pathways to be more readily traced and genetic modifications that may herald emerging drug resistance to be watched. Lastly, bringing our diagnostic capabilities up to speed on more poorly characterized species like P. malariae seems required if we are to stand any hope of a generalized strategy for all forms of human-infecting malaria eradication (Oriero et al., 2021).

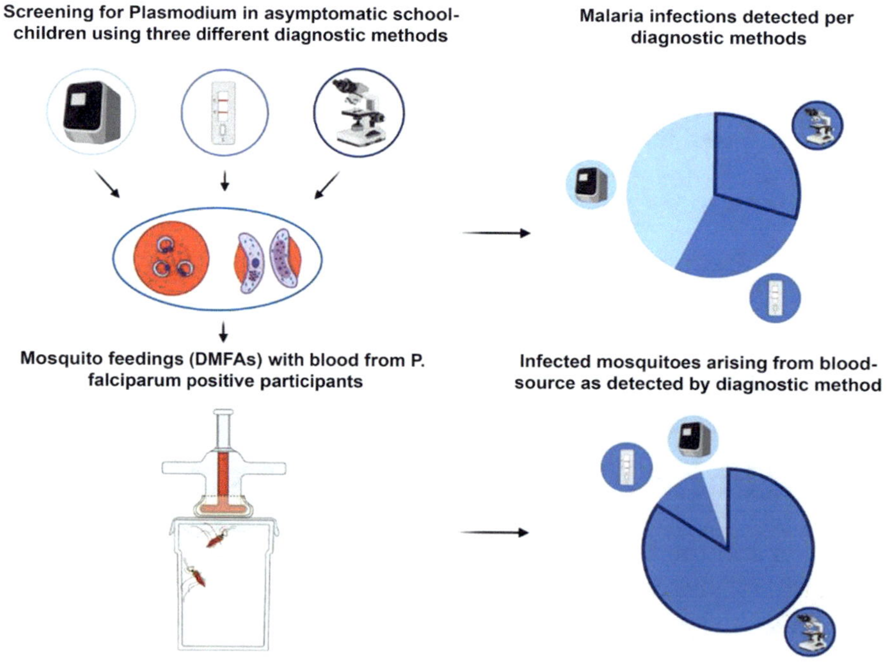

Figure 2.17. Diagnosis of Plasmodium infections.

Source: Hofer, L. M., et al. (2024). Additional blood meals increase sporozoite infection in Anopheles mosquitoes but not Plasmodium falciparum genetic diversity. Scientific Reports, 14, Article 17467.

2.5.1. Common Diagnostic Methods

Diagnosis of Plasmodium infection is tasked with keeping malaria in check—a disease notorious for having a multifaceted biology. Labs generally start by examining stained blood smears microscopically; this old-school method reveals the parasite in RBCs at different stages. Although it is a labor-intensive process, it allows you to see the parasites firsthand and even indicate the species by its shape.

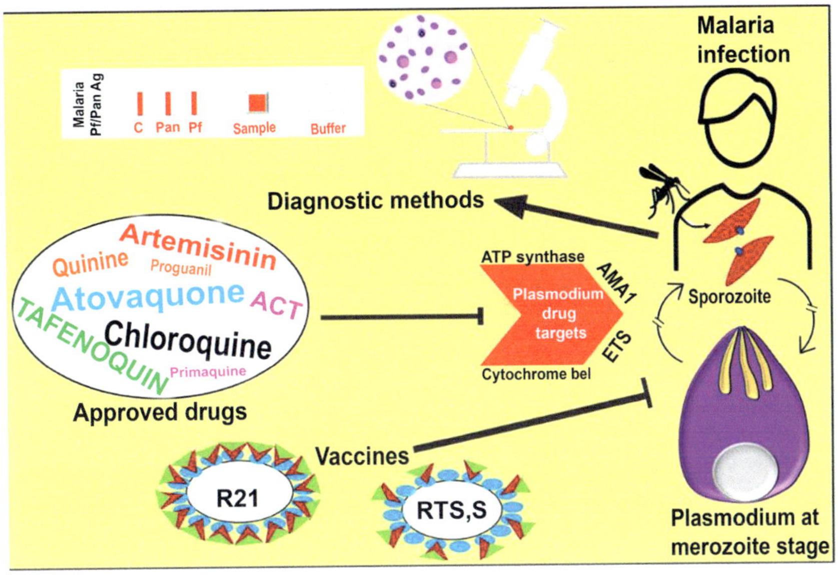

Figure 2.18. Common diagnostic methods.

Source: Tripathi, H., et al. (2023). Life cycle of malaria parasite. In Malaria therapeutics: are we close enough? Parasites & Vectors, 16(1), Article 130.

However, the technique is dependent largely on the competence of the operator and fails where parasite levels are very low or where more than one species is present together. PCR, i.e., Polymerase Chain Reaction, was designed to circumvent these limitations. In general terms, PCR works on particular pieces of parasite DNA, giving absolute sensitivity and specificity. It can also identify infections too slight to be identified under a microscope—making it especially valuable for asymptomatic illness detection and informing initial treatment, critical because of the devious lifecycle and adaptation methods of the parasite. Immunological tests have instead become a second major tool for diagnosing malaria. Rapid diagnostic tests (RDTs) are aimed at parasite proteins—take histidine-rich protein II (HRP2) or lactate dehydrogenase (LDH), and they travel rapidly even when you are operating without a high-tech laboratory. They are simple to use, but occasionally the outcomes are not consistent because different Plasmodium species can express these proteins differently. In some cases, gene deletions can even result in false negatives, and therefore interpreting the results is not always straightforward. These tests are in line with our overall impression of the parasite since they identify proteins that are present during major phases of the parasite's life, pointing to its metabolic state. Still, especially in low transmission and low parasite-load cases, a cautious approach to treating RDT results is advisable. In the meantime, fresh investigations into the parasite's molecular markers are opening up encouraging new paths for diagnosis. Scientists currently explore proteins related to parasite development and reproduction that may also serve as warning signs. For instance, recent studies highlighted the activation of specific kinases in sexual differentiation (Reininger et al., 2012), a procedure that can be employed to label parasite populations prone to transmission. Apart from this, knowledge of biological mechanisms such as telomere control (essential to parasite survival and cell division) is uncovering new targets at the protein and genetic levels (Religa et al., 2014). Integration of these molecular signals within diagnostic platforms may not only improve sensitivity and specificity but offer a more sophisticated answer to the control of malaria overall (Figure 2.18).

2.5.2. Advances in Diagnostic Technology

Malaria, caused by Plasmodium parasites, has been fought for centuries by dashing to identify the culprit. In the majority of cases, it usually is earlier diagnosis using such techniques as conventional microscopy or antigen rapid tests that falls short, especially when parasite loads collapse or mixed infections occur. Progress has recently shifted the tide, though, in separating unique genetic signatures of these parasites. Scientists now use techniques to identify short nucleic acid sequences with velocity and accuracy.

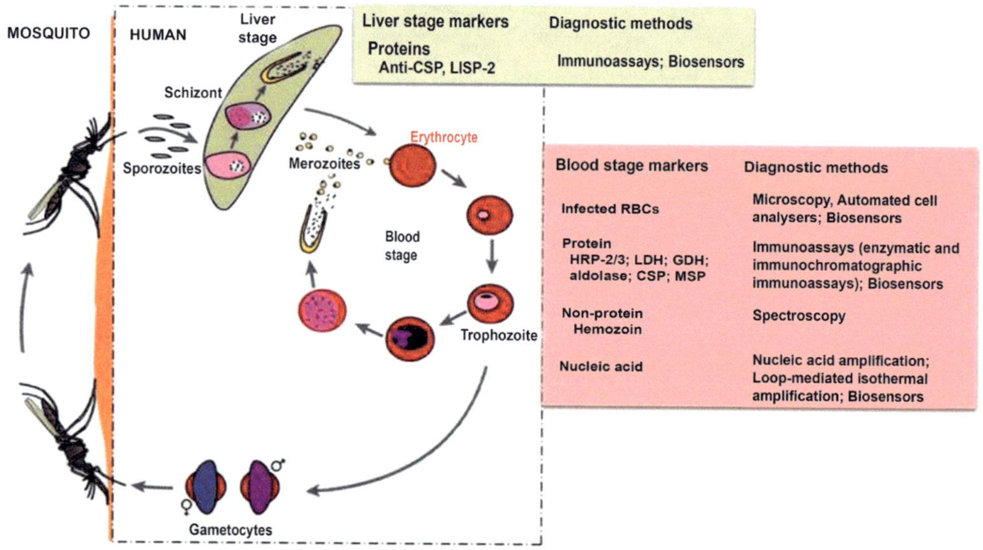

Figure 2.19. Advances in diagnostic technology of malaria.

Source: Krampa FD, Aniweh Y, Kanyong P, Awandare GA. Recent Advances in the Development of Biosensors for Malaria Diagnosis. *Sensors*. 2020; 20(3):799. https://doi.org/10.3390/s20030799

For instance, CRISPR-based tools, especially CRISPR-Cas13, which edits RNA without making permanent changes—offer a new window not only for identifying Plasmodium but also for exploring its RNA messages. Overall, these advancements help to inform malaria control efforts while opening up further inquiry into the parasite's nature (Quansah et al., 2023). By contrast, immunological methods are no longer static; developments come along as sensor technology is brought into antibody tests. A prime example is how tests for the search for proteins like lactate dehydrogenase (PfLDH) are currently married with systems like inductively coupled plasma mass spectrometry. Together, thanks in part to gold nanoparticle-conjugated monoclonal antibodies, the sensitivity of detection is brought to picogram levels, which is rather impressive. The resultant ability to accurately quantify parasitemia throughout various stages of the parasites, even among asymptomatic carriers, provides a more comprehensive understanding of the transmission of malaria and steers public health interventions in the right direction (Mu et al., 2021). On another front, genomic editors are redefining research approaches and clinical usefulness while working with Plasmodium. In most cases, the parasite's nonfunctional natural RNA interference mechanism earlier stalled RNA-editing strategies, but CRISPR-Cas13 sidesteps that issue by targeting RNA transcripts directly. This technique, with its transient and scarless edits, is considered safer and more universal by many. Through the integration of CRISPR-Cas13 with other molecular techniques, researchers are now able to visualize parasite gene expression in real time, gradually peeling away layers of the parasite's complex life cycle and pushing the boundaries of diagnostic innovation (Quansah et al., 2023) (Figure 2.19).

2.5.3. Challenges in Accurate Diagnosis

Diagnosing malaria is less straightforward than one might desire. The fight begins with parasites that wildly vary in number and activity, a headache to test because they need a moving target. Sometimes, a patient will have little more than a handful of parasites—fewer than 200 asexual parasites per microliter—so the test can simply miss them, leading to false negatives. Fever, or even a complete lack of fever, is added to the equation; as a rule, fever does increase detection but a lack of it can bias results. In most community settings, this inconsistency in sensitivity and specificity makes it very hard to handle cases. But where lab facilities are scarce, the RDTs truly shine, minimizing wastage of treatment for what is not needed by trying to separate parasitic fevers from other illnesses (Ishengoma et al., 2011). In pregnancy-associated malaria (PAM), however, the issue is even more complex. The whole process is inextricably linked with the unique ways pregnancy affects immune function, and, quite frankly, sometimes the traditional methods just do not cut it. Standard microscopy, a.k.a. the gold standard, is prone to underestimating infections since it performs poorly with low-level parasitemia and parasites invading the placenta. Although rapid tests sometimes show enhanced sensitivity compared to microscopes, inconsistencies continue to emerge when compared to more advanced techniques like PCR. Such microscopic infections slip through regular screenings in the majority of cases, compromising mothers and infants. PAM diagnostic methods, therefore, have to balance between simplicity and the detection of as many cases as can be detected, especially where active case management is increasingly being considered as an option as opposed to prevention treatment (Minja et al., 2012). To make matters worse, the performance of these diagnostic instruments is not consistent across all areas. Where malaria is declining, test results can become seriously obscure, altering the positive predictive values of RDTs. Variation in parasite antigen expression, host immunity variability, and even co-infection can obfuscate diagnostic reliability. For example, malaria antigens can persist when parasites are no longer present—causing false positives, and genetic variability in target proteins can decrease the sensitivity of a test. Also, the extent to which healthcare providers follow treatment protocols by these results can make a difference in overall malaria management outcomes. In spite of suboptimal specificity and sensitivity, integrating RDT with microscopy and a pinch of clinical judgment still remains the best, most practical choice in resource-limited settings, informing treatment decisions and preventing drug abuse (Ishengoma et al., 2011).

2.6. Treatment and Prevention

Recent advancements in the battle against malaria have been trying to stay ahead of drug resistance by focusing on other areas of the Plasmodium lifecycle , not quite the simplest of tasks. ACT, or artemisinin-based combination therapies (ACTs), have been the standard for targeting blood-stage parasites for centuries, but when ACT-resistant strains started to emerge, researchers were forced to adopt a new strategy. They are now working on ways of inhibiting certain of the enzymes the parasite needs to develop and invade. For example, new drugs aimed at aspartic proteases, such as Plasmepsin IX and X, with dual inhibitors such as WM382, seem to interfere with liver and blood stages, effectively preventing the parasite from escaping and spreading. Overall, this protease inhibitory method illustrates a type of multi-layered protection against the parasite that offers one potential route for future generations of antimalarial drugs (Favuzza et al., 2020). The complex Plasmodium biology adds extra complicating issues, especially for relapsing malaria caused by Plasmodium vivax. As opposed to P. falciparum, though, P. vivax can withdraw in the liver as hypnozoites - dormant forms that can result in a relapse even if the blood parasites are apparently cleared. Overall, differentiating a relapse from recrudescence or reinfection is a headache as each case calls for a different action. New probabilistic models that integrate genetic leads with clinical data have improved how we determine the cause of relapsing infections. For instance, in the absence of a radical cure using primaquine, relapses can occur in approximately 75% of patients; while, if a high dose primaquine is effectively administered, relapse diminishes to approximately 3% (Taylor et al., 2019). Prevention remains central to the fight against malaria. Day-to-day practices like the use of ITNs and indoor residual spraying (IRS) complement treatments by cutting down opportunities for transmission. Of course, making these effective treatments available and used consistently – especially in settings where malaria is common , remains important to avoiding drug resistance and relapses. In the majority of cases, new antimalarial agents that attack multiple life stages of the parasite, when used in combination with more acute diagnostic tools to distinguish recurrences, would entirely transform how we treat malaria. Lastly, marrying deep biological knowledge with new treatment and prevention advances paints an extremely optimistic scenario for long-term eradication measures against malaria.

2.6.1. Antimalarial Medications

Malaria treatment has been a zag-and-zig history spanning decades—its history is closely entwined with the unpredictability of Plasmodium parasites that just keep adapting to us. Such pesky parasites seem to adapt so fast that doctors have had to constantly adapt drug regimens to attack other phases of the parasite's lifecycle. Much of the development initially came from nature; many innovations started life as plant chemicals. Think about quinine, for instance, obtained from cinchona bark, it was one of the first medicines to provide hope and even spur the creation of its synthetic relatives. While chemically created medicines have progressed considerably, natural substances still offer a collection of chemical forms that can drive Plasmodium's clever biology. More generally, the real task is getting these leads to function effectively but still be sustainable and cost-effective, using cutting-edge high-throughput methods to find new candidates

(Chaachouay & Zidane, 2024). Medicine is not just a matter of messing around with chemicals, though. Increasingly, drug research has spread out of the domain of drugs into other areas, such as stopping the mosquitoes that spread malaria. Gene drive techniques, applied to re-engineer Anopheles mosquitoes (the primary vectors of transmission), are in the testing stages with a view to lowering the risk of getting infected by lowering the transmission of the parasite. It is promisingly named for controlling malaria in the long term, potentially alongside drug therapies.

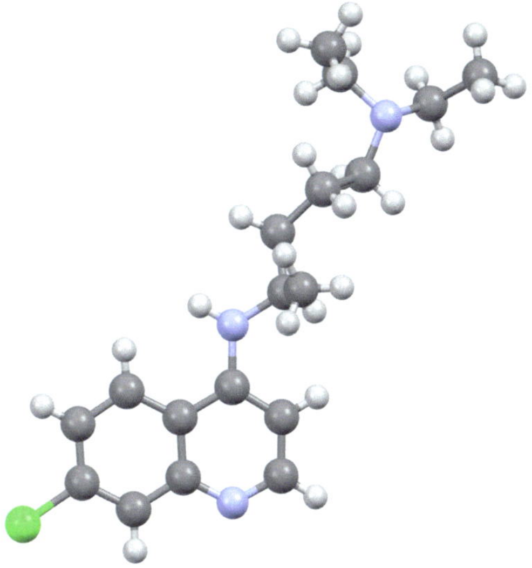

Source: By Ben Mills - Own work, Public Domain, https://commons.wikimedia.org/w/index.php?curid=89995618

But manipulating mosquito genes is a serious issue, with real regulatory and ethical problems, so there need to be strict safety and social acceptability trials. In general, the debate between drug refinement and vector control itself shows how complicated the battle against malaria is (James et al., 2018). With all of this, however, drug resistance in Plasmodium is still a nagging problem, undermining the effectiveness of our current interventions. This resistance not only makes treatment regimens difficult but also puts pressure on researchers to keep on the lookout for new drug targets hidden in the parasite's quixotic metabolic features. Combination therapies, like those that act on artemisinin—are a buffer, relying on overlapping activity to kill the parasite more thoroughly. However, long-term solutions need sustained support in drug development research which marries natural product studies, parasite genetic research, and contemporary molecular methodologies. In essence, through these hybrid and occasionally confusing efforts, the scientific community can hope to stay one step ahead of Plasmodium, ensuring our therapies are robust in the global fight against malaria (James et al., 2018; Chaachouay & Zidane, 2024).

2.6.2. Preventive Measures and Strategies

The global toll of malaria shows just how difficult it is to keep the Plasmodium parasites at bay. Treated nets and indoor spraying are used by people in numerous areas, but the traditional methods have worked only so far—the persistent Anopheles mosquitoes just keep adapting. The parasite itself also mutates rapidly and resists most drugs, so we usually have to think outside the box. Modern work in immunology and molecular biology has led us to vaccines that try to stop an infection at its very beginning. As an example, the RTS,S vaccine targets the stage before the parasite settles down in the human host and is now being recommended for use in children in high-risk regions (Mariano et al., 2023). Even with RTS,S available, a vaccine that confers wide, long-lasting protection is still elusive because the parasite's life cycle is very complex. Researchers now prefer a combination strategy that targets more than one developmental stage at a time. Some are working on transmission-blocking vaccines, which try to stop the sexual stages of the parasite in mosquitoes—a tactic that would break the transmission cycle. A Transmission-blocking and pre-erythrocytic combination could effectively cut down the parasite's ability to transmit and replicate. Nevertheless, in most cases, building immunity that is long-term and works well in diverse settings is a tough nut to crack; ongoing research continues in a bid to plug these loopholes and augment existing measures (Mariano et al., 2023). Apart from vaccines, malaria also comes with other problems like anemia, which call for a more integrated approach. Anemia, common with malaria infections, is the result of a multiplicity of factors, malnutrition, chronic inflammation, and even genetic blood disorders, all of which make the control of the disease very complex. Effective control programs must take into account nutritional status enhancement, reduction of infection, and control of the other health burdens found in most low- and middle-income countries. In large part, identifying the many etiologies of anemia that are linked to malaria can help to target public health efforts to the specific needs of the population, so that fighting the parasite also reduces other related health emergencies, like morbidity and mortality.

2.6.3. Global Efforts to Combat Malaria

Malaria remains such a gigantic problem that afflicts so many people, and people worldwide are now competing to find a means of finally defeating it. Different solutions are put on the table – experts and health establishments are investigating the unyielding character of the parasite as well as testing local environments and seeking to upgrade community health centers. In other places, as simple as an insecticide-treated bed net has been a matter of life and death, though medications for treatment and prevention sometimes meet resistance. This tangle of thinking means that malaria is not just a matter of an insect; it also intersects with social, political, and geographical puzzles, especially in far-flung, underserved populations. Take Cambodia, for example, mediocre healthcare makes it even more difficult to control malaria, and worldwide collaborations all the more important to assist these susceptible groups and fight recalcitrant, resistant strains (DeHart et al., 2020). New research is also making waves on vaccines designed to teach our bodies how to identify and fight the Plasmodium parasite. The idea is to give our immune systems a bit of practice so they can react more swiftly and successfully, reducing how often or badly people get sick. All right, vaccines have eradicated diseases like smallpox and polio, but malaria is a harder one to crack because the parasite's lifecycle keeps changing and it has so many different disguises. Despite this, the partial success of some candidate vaccines promises an era in which they help to decrease transmission and limit the burden of disease, supplementing nets, medication, and other methods. In most cases, this partnership of high-tech science and ground-level strategies is a crucial step forward in the fight against malaria (Tonna, 2006). Nevertheless, despite these positive measures, the battle against malaria is ever wound up under slanted social and environmental circumstances. In some remote, inhospitable regions where health care is, well, sort of iffy, it is absolutely critical to have a constant supply of reliable tests, treatment, and prevention technology. International agencies tend to stress local expertise development and spreading basic information about how to identify and protect against symptoms – reconciling advanced surveillance with good old-fashioned neighborhood contact. Such systems allow the monitoring of nuisance resistance patterns and behavioral changes in the parasite so that productive stopgaps can be put in place when needed. Overall, coordinating scientific breakthroughs with suitably corresponding public health policy illustrates the way forward toward malaria eradication is not a straight one – it is a complex, ongoing undertaking involving many sectors and taking some jurisdictions across the board (Tonna, 2006; DeHart et al., 2020).

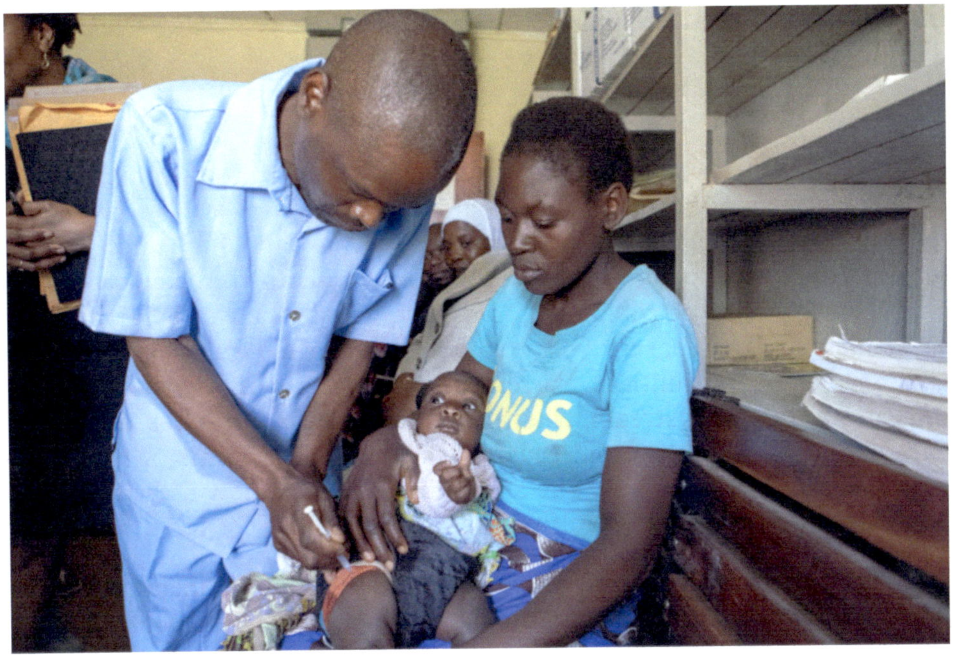

Source: The Global Fund. (n.d.). Malaria Vaccine. https://external-content.duckduckgo.com/iu/?u=https%3A%2F%2Fwww.theglobalfund.org%2Fmedia%2F11941%2Fmalaria-vaccine.jpg&f=1&nofb=1&ipt=45dab557f282fd2e681c6fe58cc9b8c6f6cead3338fb301741e557ed7162f7ed.

CLOSER LOOK

PLASMODIUM VIVAX

Plasmodium vivax is among the five *Plasmodium* species of malaria parasites that infect humans and is the most widespread outside the sub-Saharan region of Africa. The protozoan parasite is spread through the bite of an infected female *Anopheles* mosquito that injects the parasite into the human bloodstream. Once inside the body, *P. vivax* travels to the liver, where it infects liver cells and undergoes a dormant phase known as the hypnozoite phase. This phase is unique to *P. vivax* and *P. ovale* and allows the parasite to remain in the liver for weeks, months, or years before becoming active once again and initiating a relapse of malaria symptoms. After this liver phase, the parasite migrates to the bloodstream, where it invades RBCs, multiplies, and eventually causes the cells to burst, releasing parasites and causing the classic symptoms of malaria—fever, chills, sweating, headache, nausea, and fatigue. The symptoms usually follow a cyclical pattern every 48 hours, which coincides with the lifecycle of the parasite in RBCs.

Plasmodium vivax also differs from *P. falciparum*, the most lethal malaria parasite, in several important aspects. While less virulent in general, *P. vivax* can cause severe illness, especially in vulnerable groups such as children, pregnant women, and individuals with weak immune systems. One of the main issues with *P. vivax* is that it can relapse from hypnozoites and requires a different treatment approach. In addition to blood-stage antimalarials like chloroquine or ACTs, a liver-stage drug like primaquine or tafenoquine has to be part of the treatment to eliminate hypnozoites and prevent relapse. These drugs do, nevertheless, pose a risk to those with G6PD (glucose-6-phosphate dehydrogenase) deficiency, an inherited condition that can lead to severe anemia when exposed to certain medications, so testing and careful monitoring are necessary.

Geographically, *P. vivax* occurs in Asia, Latin America, and parts of the Middle East and Oceania. It can survive in temperate climates and at higher altitudes than *P. falciparum*, which is most successful in tropical and subtropical climates. This broader ecological tolerance makes *P. vivax* a deeply rooted public health issue. In addition, the parasite can also infect young RBCs (reticulocytes), which are fewer in number, thus limiting parasite density in the blood but also making detection more difficult and infections more likely to be undervalued. Diagnosis of *P. vivax* is routinely done through microscopy of blood smears or RDTs, while molecular methods like PCR are more precise.

Although historically viewed as a "benign" malaria species, *P. vivax* is now recognized to contribute to significant morbidity, have the potential for life-threatening complications, and play an important role in sustaining malaria transmission. Its management and eventual eradication require multifaceted approaches using improved diagnostics, access to effective and complete treatment, vector control, and public education. In conclusion, *Plasmodium vivax* poses unique challenges to the control of malaria due to its biological features of dormancy and relapse, its wide geographic range, and its capacity to cause repeated illness, indicating the need for targeted interventions and global health engagement.

SUMMARY

The Plasmodium parasites do possess some very complex cell mechanisms that serve to emphasize both the advanced biology of these parasites and how vulnerable they may be in certain areas. Recent published studies on protein kinase CK2, which is, PfCK2, established that you just can't manage without its catalytic subunit or its regulatory subunit when the parasite is in the asexual blood stage. In RBCs, these subunits function hand in glove to keep the cell alive and sustain it for replication. It is intriguing that PfCK2 is not just floating around in the outer part of the cell but also tucked away within the nucleus, which indicates that it might be serving more than a single purpose, especially with the arrangement of chromatin. Relating this to chromatin assembly, and that it triggers phosphorylation of nucleosome assembly proteins, histones, and even Alba family members, in fact implies quite strongly that it does influence gene activity and organize the genome. Combined, these discoveries add depth to our knowledge of Plasmodium's inner life and provide new, compelling targets for treatment, which generally has a lot to do with why kinase research is a large undertaking in the fight to understand and treat malaria (Dastidar et al., 2012). Apart from mere molecular details, combating Plasmodium infection is all the more complicated since effective vaccines are on the horizon as yet and drug resistance keeps piling up. With next-generation sequencing and vast genomic databases entering the scene, research into the relationship between parasites and hosts took a not-so-unexpected turn; scientists are piecing together multi-omics data to find complex, complex webs that sustain the parasite's vitality and virulence. With this broader canvas, researchers have the toolkit they need to crack the code of the parasite's unique biology, find new drug targets, and drive the emergence of new antiparasitic treatments. In most cases, systems biology not only extends our basic knowledge regarding the mechanism of the parasite but also lays out a strategic plan to circumvent the bottlenecks that we currently face in controlling and even eradicating malaria (Swann et al., 2015). In conclusion, the combination of intimate molecular examinations with the larger context constitutes a kind of guidebook for future investigation and intervention strategies against malaria. The central role of PfCK2 in orchestrating cell processes shows just how much the parasite relies on those very particular biochemical networks, networks we can potentially turn on to our own benefit. In the meantime, merging high-throughput data with traditional research promises to shed some light on hidden weak links within the parasite lifecycle. This two-pronged strategy—investigating individual molecular hacks while keeping an eye on the global biological system—bodes valuable potential for malaria biology and treatment progress. Interdisciplinary future research, combining approaches like reverse genetics, proteomics, and systems biology, will be key to meeting the world malaria challenge and lessening the socioeconomic impact of this disastrous disease (Dastidar et al., 2012; Swann et al., 2015).

Plasmodium parasites have a surprisingly complex life, they cycle between vertebrate hosts such as humans and invertebrates such as mosquitoes. Their life cycle is not a straightforward tale; instead, it wriggles between different stages, sometimes asexually multiplying numerous times inside RBCs and at other times undergoing sexual reproduction within the mosquito. It is this incessant toggling that allows them to survive and thrive, making them quite skilled at causing disease. Recently, a series of papers have pointed out that apoptosis or programmed cell death is feasible even in such single-celled life, which in a general sense goes against the old premise that survival is just reproduction. To one extent or another, realizing how apoptosis is part of their plan of attack not only enables us to observe their population control tricks but also suggests targets for therapy to disrupt their life cycle and cut malaria transmission (Pollitt et al., 2010). If we delve into their evolutionary past, it just becomes more complex. It is suggested by some researchers that Plasmodium might have evolved from non-parasitic ancestors, perhaps even from some alga-like organisms, subsequently evolved to parasitic life, while mosquitoes increasingly took on the role of a vector instead of having some pivotal ecological function. Such a concept creates a picture of evolution as an active, chaotic process where role adjustments are the rule. By weighing mainstream evolutionary explanations against more off-the-beaten-path ones, and even some creationist theories that come into the mix, scholars explore all kinds of theories about how malaria and its notoriously deadly perpetrator came into being. It is a useful reminder that malaria science is not one dedicated discipline in itself; it is all about molecular details, ecological observations, and even historical methods (Gillen & Sherwin, 2013). To summarize, studying Plasmodium parasites interweaves the complex themes of biology everything from the most minute cellular functions like apoptosis to the greater, more disorderly web of host and vector interactions. Their capacity for adjusting phases of the life cycle for different hosts allows them to persist, which makes them that much harder to eliminate. Investigating these parameters offers potential areas of intervention, i.e., possibly blocking the apoptotic mechanisms in order to decrease the number of parasites and decrease transmission. Also, embracing several viewpoints—be they evolution-based, alternative theories, or yet even more unconventional hypotheses—offers further dimensions to the argument and enriches a deeper research approach. Lastly, the Plasmodium story informs us about how cellular processes, adaptation of the organism, and prolonged evolutionary shifts all come together in the battle against infectious disease (Pollitt et al., 2010; Gillen & Sherwin, 2013).

KEY TERMS FROM THIS CHAPTER

- Plasmodium falciparum
- Plasmodium vivax
- Plasmodium malariae
- Plasmodium ovale
- Plasmodium knowlesi
- Definitive Host (Mosquito)
- Intermediate Host (Human)
- Sporozoite Stage
- Merozoite Stage
- Trophozoite Stage
- Schizont Stage
- Hypnozoites
- Gametocytes
- Erythrocytic Cycle
- Antigenic Variation
- Cytoadherence
- Immune Evasion

References

1. Adams, Y., Olsen, R. W., Bengtsson, A., Dalgaard, N., Zdioruk, M., Satpathi, S., Behera, P. K., et al. (2021). Plasmodium falciparum erythrocyte membrane protein 1 variants induce cell swelling and disrupt the blood–brain barrier in cerebral malaria. The Journal of Experimental Medicine, 218(7), e20201266. https://doi.org/10.1084/jem.20201266.
2. Adl, S. M., Bass, D., Lane, C. E., Lukeš, J., Schoch, C. L., Смирнов, A. B., Agatha, S., et al. (2018). Revisions to the classification, nomenclature, and diversity of eukaryotes. Journal of Eukaryotic Microbiology, 66(1), 4–119. https://doi.org/10.1111/jeu.12691.
3. Gilabert, A., Otto, T. D., Rutledge, G. G., Franzon, B., Ollomo, B., Arnathau, C., Durand, P., Moukodoum, N. D., Okouga, A. P., Ngoubangoye, B., Makanga, B., Boundenga, L., Paupy, C., Renaud, F., Prugnolle, F., & Rougeron, V. (2018). Plasmodium vivax-like genome sequences shed new insights into Plasmodium vivax biology and evolution. PLoS biology, 16(8), e2006035. https://doi.org/10.1371/journal.pbio.2006035 (accessed on 13 May 2025).
4. Ascencio, M. E., Florin-Christensen, M., Mamoun, C. B., Weir, W., Shiels, B., & Schnittger, L. (2018). Cysteine Proteinase C1A Paralog Profiles Correspond with Phylogenetic Lineages of Pathogenic Piroplasmids. Veterinary sciences, 5(2), 41. https://doi.org/10.3390/vetsci5020041 (accessed on 13 May 2025).
5. Galinski, M. R., Lapp, S. A., Peterson, M. S., Ay, F., Joyner, C. J., LE Roch, K. G., Fonseca, L. L., Voit, E. O., & MAHPIC CONSORTIUM (2018). Plasmodium knowlesi: a superb in vivo nonhuman primate model of antigenic variation in malaria. Parasitology, 145(1), 85–100. https://doi.org/10.1017/S0031182017001135
6. Baird, J. K. (2021). Basic research of Plasmodium vivax biology enabling its management as a clinical and public health problem. Frontiers in Cellular and Infection Microbiology, 11, 696598. https://doi.org/10.3389/fcimb.2021.696598.
7. Birkholtz, L. M., Bastien, O., Wells, G., Grando, D., Joubert, F., Kasam, V., Zimmermann, M., Ortet, P., Jacq, N., Saïdani, N., Roy, S., Hofmann-Apitius, M., Breton, V., Louw, A. I., & Maréchal, E. (2006). Integration and mining of malaria molecular, functional and pharmacological data: how far are we from a chemogenomic knowledge space?. Malaria journal, 5, 110. https://doi.org/10.1186/1475-2875-5-110
8. Bunnik, E. M., Batugedara, G., Saraf, A., Prudhomme, J., Florens, L., & Le Roch, K. G. (2016). The mRNA-bound proteome of the human malaria parasite Plasmodium falciparum. Genome biology, 17(1), 147. https://doi.org/10.1186/s13059-016-1014-0
9. Belachew, E. B. (2018). Immune response and evasion mechanisms of Plasmodium falciparum parasites. Journal of Immunology Research, 2018, 6529681. https://doi.org/10.1155/2018/6529681.
10. Marrelli, M., Fiedler, M., Biguetti, C., & Brotto, M. (2020). Detrimental effects of malaria, toxoplasmosis, leishmaniosis and Chagas disease on cardiac and skeletal muscles. Medical Research Archives, 8(9). https://doi.org/10.18103/mra.v8i9.2218
11. https://core.ac.uk/download/161865555.pdf Brancucci, N. M. B., De Niz, M., Straub, T. J., Ravel, D., Sollelis, L., Birren, B. W., Voss, T. S., Neafsey, D. E., & Marti, M. (2018). Probing Plasmodium falciparum sexual commitment at the single-cell level. Wellcome open research, 3, 70. https://doi.org/10.12688/wellcomeopenres.14645.4 (accessed on 12 May 2025).

12. Bonam, S. R., Rénia, L., Tadepalli, G., Bayry, J., & Kumar, H. M. S. (2021). Plasmodium falciparum malaria vaccines and vaccine adjuvants. Vaccines, 9(10), 1072. https://doi.org/10.3390/vaccines9101072.
13. Briggs, A. M., Hambly, M. G., Simão-Gurge, R. M., Garrison, S. M., Khaku, Z., Van Susteren, G., Lewis, E. E., et al. (2022). Anopheles stephensi feeding, flight behavior, and infection with malaria parasites are altered by ingestion of serotonin. Frontiers in Physiology, 13, 911097. https://doi.org/10.3389/fphys.2022.911097.
14. Brown, A. C., & Güler, J. L. (2020). From circulation to cultivation: Plasmodium in vivo versus in vitro. Trends in Parasitology, 36(11), 914–926. https://doi.org/10.1016/j.pt.2020.08.008.
15. Chaachouay, N., & Zidane, L. (2024). Plant-derived natural products: A source for drug discovery and development. Drugs and Drug Candidates, 3(1), 184–207. https://doi.org/10.3390/ddc3010011.
16. Chaparro, C. M., & Suchdev, P. S. (2019). Anemia epidemiology, pathophysiology, and etiology in low- and middle-income countries. Annals of the New York Academy of Sciences, 1450(1), 15–31. https://doi.org/10.1111/nyas.14092.
17. Dastidar, E. G., Dayer, G., Holland, Z. M., Dorin-Semblat, D., Claes, A., Chêne, A., Sharma, A., Hamelin, R., Moniatte, M., Lopez-Rubio, J. J., Scherf, A., & Doerig, C. (2012). Involvement of Plasmodium falciparum protein kinase CK2 in the chromatin assembly pathway. BMC biology, 10, 5. https://doi.org/10.1186/1741-7007-10-5 (accessed on 13 May 2025).
18. Pollitt, L. C., Colegrave, N., Khan, S. M., Sajid, M., & Reece, S. E. (2010). Investigating the evolution of apoptosis in malaria parasites: the importance of ecology. Parasites & vectors, 3, 105. https://doi.org/10.1186/1756-3305-3-105 (accessed on 13 May 2025).
19. DeHart, Ciera, "Health Concerns in Cambodia Compounded by Historical and Rural Setbacks" (2020). *Senior Honors Theses*. 967. https://digitalcommons.liberty.edu/honors/967 (accessed on 13 May 2025).
20. Deitsch, K., & Dzikowski, R. (2017). Variant gene expression and antigenic variation by malaria parasites. Annual Review of Microbiology, 71, 625–641. https://doi.org/10.1146/annurev-micro-090816-093841.
21. Ishengoma, D. S., Francis, F., Mmbando, B. P., Lusingu, J. P., Magistrado, P., Alifrangis, M., Theander, T. G., Bygbjerg, I. C., & Lemnge, M. M. (2011). Accuracy of malaria rapid diagnostic tests in community studies and their impact on treatment of malaria in an area with declining malaria burden in north-eastern Tanzania. Malaria journal, 10, 176. https://doi.org/10.1186/1475-2875-10-176 (accessed on 13 May 2025).
22. Favuzza, P., de Lera Ruiz, M., Thompson, J. K., Triglia, T., Ngo, A., Steel, R. W. J., Vavrek, M., et al. (2020). Dual plasmepsin-targeting antimalarial agents disrupt multiple stages of the malaria parasite life cycle. Cell Host & Microbe, 27(4), 642–658.e12. https://doi.org/10.1016/j.chom.2020.02.005.
23. França, C. T., He, W., Gruszczyk, J., Lim, N. T. Y., Lin, E., Kiniboro, B., Siba, P. M., et al. (2016). Plasmodium vivax reticulocyte binding proteins are key targets of naturally acquired immunity in young Papua New Guinean children. PLoS Neglected Tropical Diseases, 10(5), e0005014. https://doi.org/10.1371/journal.pntd.0005014.
24. Gavinho, B., Rossi, I. V., Evans-Osses, I., Inal, J., & Ramirez, M. I. (2018). A new landscape of

host-protozoa interactions involving the extracellular vesicles world. Parasitology, 145(12), 1521–1530. https://doi.org/10.1017/S0031182018001105 (accessed on 12 May 2025).

25. Gillen, Alan L. and Sherwin, Frank, “The Genesis of Malaria: The Origin of Mosquitoes and Their Protistan Cargo, Plasmodium falciparum” (2013). Faculty Publications and Presentations. 136. https://digitalcommons.liberty.edu/bio_chem_fac_pubs/136 (accessed on 13 May 2025).

26. Graumans, W., Jacobs, E., Bousema, T., & Sinnis, P. (2020). When is a Plasmodium-infected mosquito an infectious mosquito? Trends in Parasitology, 36, 705–716. https://doi.org/10.1016/j.pt.2020.05.011.

27. James, S. L., Collins, F. H., Welkhoff, P. A., Emerson, C., Charles, H., Gottlieb, M., Greenwood, B., et al. (2018). Pathway to deployment of gene drive mosquitoes as a potential biocontrol tool for elimination of malaria in sub-Saharan Africa: Recommendations of a scientific working group. American Journal of Tropical Medicine and Hygiene, 98(Supplement), 1–49. https://doi.org/10.4269/ajtmh.18-0083.

28. Swann, J., Jamshidi, N., Lewis, N. E., & Winzeler, E. A. (2015). Systems analysis of host-parasite interactions. Wiley interdisciplinary reviews. Systems biology and medicine, 7(6), 381–400. https://doi.org/10.1002/wsbm.1311

29. Religa AA, Ramesar J, Janse CJ, Scherf A, Waters AP (2014) *P. berghei* Telomerase Subunit TERT is Essential for Parasite Survival. PLoS ONE 9(10): e108930. https://doi.org/10.1371/journal.pone.0108930 (accessed on 13 May 2025).

30. Keleta, Y., Ramelow, J., Cui, L., & Li, J. (2021). Molecular interactions between parasite and mosquito during midgut invasion as targets to block malaria transmission. npj Vaccines, 6, Article 128. https://doi.org/10.1038/s41541-021-00401-9.

31. Pillai, D. R., Lau, R., Khairnar, K., Lepore, R., Via, A., Staines, H. M., & Krishna, S. (2012). Artemether resistance in vitro is linked to mutations in PfATP6 that also interact with mutations in PfMDR1 in travellers returning with Plasmodium falciparum infections. Malaria journal, 11, 131. https://doi.org/10.1186/1475-2875-11-131 (accessed on 13 May 2025).

32. Laurens, M. B. (2019). RTS,S/AS01 vaccine (Mosquirix™): An overview. Human Vaccines & Immunotherapeutics, 16(3), 480–489. https://doi.org/10.1080/21645515.2019.1669415.

33. Killeen, G. F., Smith, T. A., Ferguson, H. M., Mshinda, H., Abdulla, S., Lengeler, C., & Kachur, S. P. (2007). Preventing childhood malaria in Africa by protecting adults from mosquitoes with insecticide-treated nets. PLoS medicine, 4(7), e229. https://doi.org/10.1371/journal.pmed.0040229

34. Reininger, L., Garcia, M., Tomlins, A., Müller, S., & Doerig, C. (2012). The Plasmodium falciparum, Nima-related kinase Pfnek-4: a marker for asexual parasites committed to sexual differentiation. Malaria journal, 11, 250. https://doi.org/10.1186/1475-2875-11-250(accessed on 13 May 2025).

35. Mariano, R. M. S., Gonçalves, A. A. M., de Oliveira, D. S., Ribeiro, H. S., Pereira, D. F. S., Santos, I. S., Lair, D. F., et al. (2023). A review of major patents on potential malaria vaccine targets. Pathogens, 12(2), 247. https://doi.org/10.3390/pathogens12020247.

36. Minja, D. T., Schmiegelow, C., Oesterholt, M., Magistrado, P. A., Boström, S., John, D., Pehrson, C., Andersen, D., Deloron, P., Salanti, A., Lemnge, M., Luty, A. J., Alifrangis, M., Theander, T., & Lusingu, J. P. (2012). Reliability of rapid diagnostic tests in diagnosing pregnancy-associated

malaria in north-eastern Tanzania. Malaria journal, 11, 211. https://doi.org/10.1186/1475-2875-11-211 (accessed on 13 May 2025).

37. Mu, J., Yu, L. L., & Wellems, T. E. (2021). Sensitive immunoassay detection of Plasmodium lactate dehydrogenase by inductively coupled plasma mass spectrometry. Frontiers in Cellular and Infection Microbiology, 10, 620419. https://doi.org/10.3389/fcimb.2020.620419.

38. Oriero, E., Amenga–Etego, L., Ishengoma, D. S., & Amambua-Ngwa, A. (2021). Plasmodium malariae, current knowledge and future research opportunities on a neglected malaria parasite species. Critical Reviews in Microbiology, 47(1), 44–56. https://doi.org/10.1080/1040841x.2020.1838440.

39. Quansah, E., Chen, Y., Yang, S., Wang, J., Sun, D., Zhao, Y., Chen, M., et al. (2023). CRISPR-Cas13 in malaria parasite: Diagnosis and prospective gene function identification. Frontiers in Microbiology, 14, 1076947. https://doi.org/10.3389/fmicb.2023.1076947.

40. Shretta, R., Liu, J., Cotter, C., Cohen, J. M., Dolenz, C., Makomva, K., Newby, G., et al. (2017). Malaria elimination and eradication. In Disease Control Priorities (3rd ed.). The World Bank. https://doi.org/10.1596/978-1-4648-0524-0_ch12.

41. Talapko, J., Škrlec, I., Alebić, T., Jukić, M., & Včev, A. (2019). Malaria: The past and the present. Microorganisms, 7(6), 179. https://doi.org/10.3390/microorganisms7060179.

42. Taylor, A. R., Watson, J. A., Chu, C. S., Puaprasert, K., Duanguppama, J., Day, N., Nosten, F., et al. (2019). Resolving the cause of recurrent Plasmodium vivax malaria probabilistically. Nature Communications, 10, Article 5599. https://doi.org/10.1038/s41467-019-13412-x.

43. Tobin, A. B., Carvalho, T. G., Doerig, C., Talevich, E., Kannan, N., Wells, T. N., & Wilson, R. J. (2012). An evolutionary perspective on the kinome of malaria parasites. https://core.ac.uk/download/9649485.pdf (accessed on 13 May 2025).

44. Tonna, I. (2006). Is vaccination the only option for possible global malaria eradication? Malta Medical Journal Volume 18 Issue 02 July 2006. https://core.ac.uk/download/46602052.pdf

45. Tripet F. (2009). Ecological immunology of mosquito-malaria interactions: Of non-natural versus natural model systems and their inferences. Parasitology, 136(14), 1935–1942. https://doi.org/10.1017/S0031182009006234van der Watt, M., Reader, J., & Birkholtz, L. M. (2022). Adapt or die: Targeting unique transmission-stage biology for malaria elimination. Frontiers in Cellular and Infection Microbiology, 12, 901971. https://doi.org/10.3389/fcimb.2022.901971.

46. Waide, M. L., Polidoro, R. B., Powell, W., Denny, J. E., Kos, J. T., Tieri, D., Watson, C. T., et al. (2020). Gut microbiota composition modulates the magnitude and quality of germinal centers during Plasmodium infections. Cell Reports, 33(9), 108503. https://doi.org/10.1016/j.celrep.2020.108503.

47. Wichers-Misterek, J. S., Tonkin-Hill, G., Thye, T., Krumkamp, R., Kreuels, B., Strauss, J., von Thien, H., et al. (2021). Common virulence gene expression in adult first-time infected malaria patients and severe cases. eLife, 10, e69040. https://doi.org/10.7554/eLife.69040.

48. Zhang, C., Yang, R., Wu, L., Luo, C., Yang, Y., Deng, Y., Wu, J., et al. (2022). Survey of malaria vectors on the Cambodia, Thailand and China-Laos borders. Malaria Journal, 21, Article 241. https://doi.org/10.1186/s12936-022-04418-w.

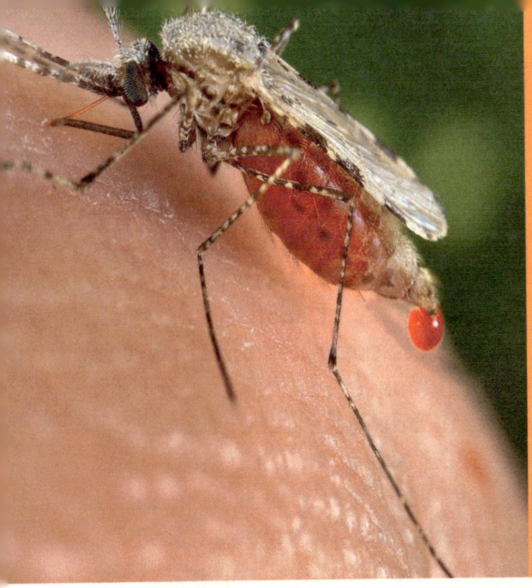

Chapter 3

VECTOR BIOLOGY OF MOSQUITOES

Contents

Introduction

Scientists have been fascinated with mosquitoes , these tiny pests have a knack for spreading terrible diseases. They don't just spread malaria; they're busy spreading arboviruses like dengue, Zika, and chikungunya, making a right mess of global public health. It is interesting to think about how information, either at the finest microscopic scale or at larger ecological levels, comes into play in how these insects' spread disease. Their population dynamics, which are fueled by environmental features and genetic adaptation, seem to alter their ability to spread disease and resist control methods. Overall, teasing out these levels contains the key to developing new methods of protecting communities from increasing health and economic issues caused by these pests. Looking more deeply into the ways that mosquitoes transmit disease, many influences, such as genetic mutations, variations in enzyme activity, and even features of behavior—can alter their interactions with pathogens. Some recent research has raised red flags about insecticide resistance. For example, elevated levels of P450 monooxygenases, enzymes that break down chemicals, are making known solutions like pyrethroids obsolete. Research on Zanzibari populations of *Anopheles arabiensis* even revealed widespread resistance due partly to such enzymatic changes (Jones et al., 2013). If you break it down at the molecular and the more population-level, information on such patterns of resistance becomes critical to devising vector control initiatives that can bypass or overcome the impact of resistance, with the perspective of attaining something sustainable in disease control. Subsequently there is the puzzling role of vertebrate hosts in the life cycle of mosquito-borne arboviruses. Initially, scientists had assumed that vertebrates were simply transporting viruses in nature. But more recent findings call that idea into question, and we ought to be thinking about arbovirus ecology differently. This lack of knowledge makes it increasingly difficult to model transmission accurately and formulate control measures that target both the insects and their vertebrate counterparts (Kuno et al., 2017). It seems we need to get to the bottom of these interactions if we are to cut off the transmission cycle at several points and break the cascade effects of these mosquito-borne diseases (Figure 3.1).

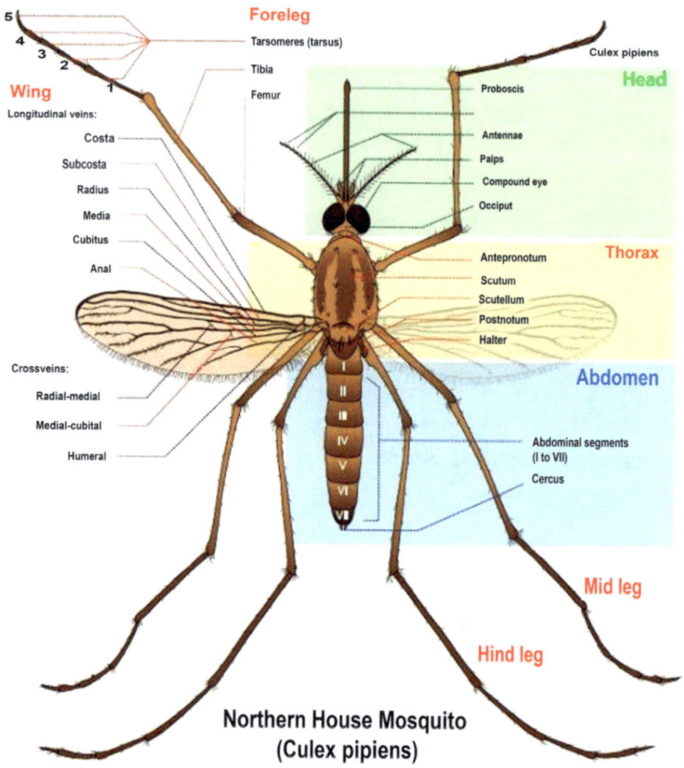

Figure 3.1. Vector biology of mosquitoes.

Source: Central Massachusetts Mosquito Control Project. (n.d.). *Culex Mosquito Anatomy*. https://www.cmmcp.org/sites/g/files/vyhlif2966/f/imce/culex_anatomy.jpg.

Definition of Vector Biology

Understanding how disease jumps from animals to people is key to trying to keep epidemics at bay. Pathogens like mosquitoes are not just messengers, they circulate microbes back and forth among hosts, and that's why learning about their existence is so vital. Vector biology reveals all facets of these little animals: their life cycle, behavior, the places where they are likely to amass, and how they deal with pathogens as well as hosts. Scientists typically look for those all-important moments when you can interrupt the chain of infection, and what they discover is that these animals are not quite so relaxed, these are dynamic players in disease transmission. This active role sets the stage for formulating strategies against diseases such as dengue fever and malaria. Looking closer at this realm, it must be said regarding the day-to-day lives of these vectors. Generally speaking, what and when they are fed usually immediately sets the state on how diseases are spread. Consider the *Anopheles* mosquito, for instance; it has a keen appetite for biting humans indoors at night. A number of surveys of concurrent human and mosquito activity in various regions of Africa, have confirmed that most human exposure to bites is within homes at night (Huho et al., 2013). Such a practice directly dictates how interventions, like indoor spraying or ITNs, function to lower infection risk. Monitoring these daily movements is at the heart of refining current control schemes and even creating new, adaptable approaches. Yet, the science of vector biology is not merely the tracking of transmission—it also involves assessing risk whenever these insects infest new areas or trigger outbreaks. An example is the study of *Ochlerotatus camptorhynchus* in New Zealand, exemplifying how observations in the field can support surveillance and improve biosecurity protocols (de Wet et al., 2005). By investigating the mosquito's biology and natural environment, scientists can create models that predict the emergence of diseases and guide control measures early on. In most cases, the insights gained here build a broader framework, one that can be wedded to strategies for tackling other vectors globally, ultimately serving as a crucial tool in shaping public health policy.

Importance of Mosquitoes as Vectors

Mosquitoes camouflage themselves in a manner that ends up altering the method of disease transmission to humans. Human alterations, sprawl, global warming, and so on, mean such pests are finding new places to hide to survive, and sometimes they even inhabit areas they never occupied previously. All this generally means is natural landscapes are changing so more mosquitoes are around human beings. Invasive species like Aedes albopictus and Aedes aegypti, for instance, have started appearing in regions with fewer competitors that are native and plenty of urban spaces perfect for reproduction. They are specifically well-adapted to spread viruses like dengue, chikungunya, and Zika because of their behavior, which includes feeding patterns and where they lay eggs, making experts closely watch them under vector control programs (Giunti et al., 2023). How they spread these diseases is intertwined with the nature of the mosquitoes. Different species step into the limelight depending on where you are—you may be in a jungle or a city, for example. In Africa, you'll find it familiar to hear names like *Ae. furcifer*, *Ae. luteocephalus*, and *Ae. taylori* keeping dengue thriving in woodlands, while cities have to deal with *Ae. aegypti* and *Ae. albopictus* doing most of the contribution. This twinning setting makes control efforts very challenging because the insects respond so differently in the wild versus the urban setting. Overall, understanding factors like vertical transmission and the nature of mosquitoes and pathogens is crucial in formulating interventions. The recent upsurge in dengue cases clearly demonstrates the need for strengthened targeted surveillance and tailored control interventions (Diallo et al., 2022). Mosquitoes not only contribute to the spread of infections; they also inform large-scale policy regarding health across the world. Ongoing research into the activity of these insects has led to interventions intended to break the cycle of disease. Control measures proposed by organizations such as the WHO

Vector Control Advisory Group, for example, aim at lowering mosquito numbers and limiting the contact between mosquitoes and humans. Most effective sustainable strategies typically involve merging ecological knowledge with community involvement. Such an integrated vision, demonstrated by One Health, reminds us, most of the time, that human, animal, and ecosystem health are interconnected. In short, even though mosquitoes are small, their impact on disease dynamics and public health policy is colossal (Giunti et al., 2023) (Figure 3.2).

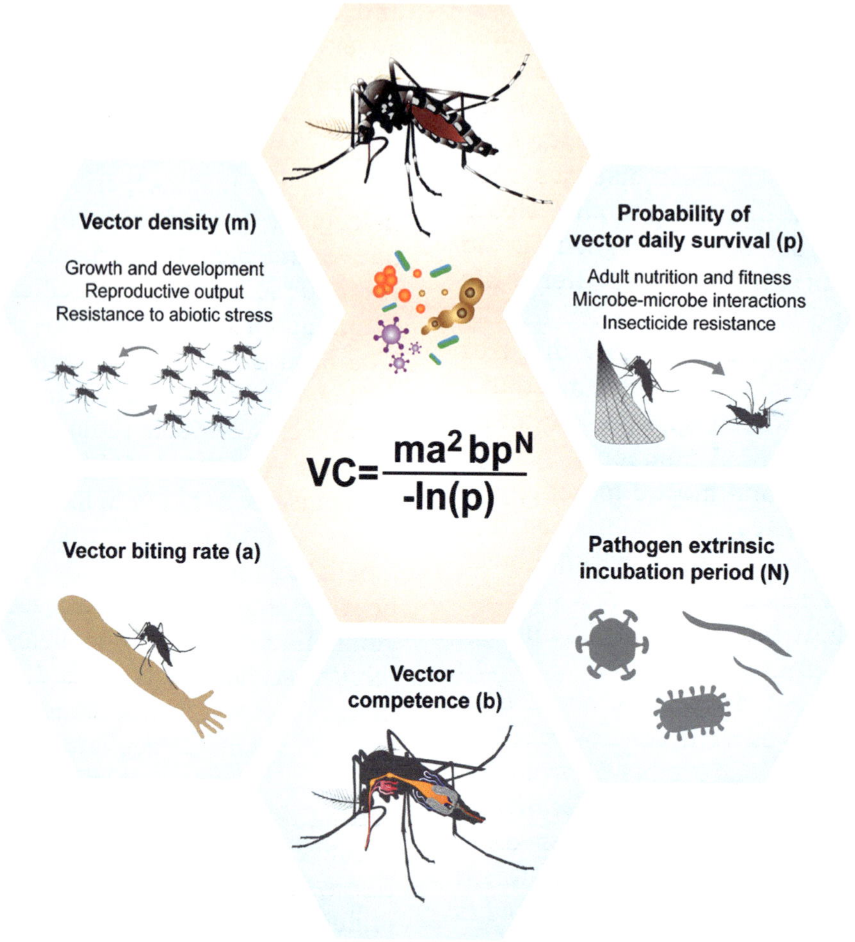

Figure 3.2. Mosquitoes as vectors.

Source: Cansado-Utrilla, C., Zhao, S. Y., McCall, P. J., Coon, K. L., & Hughes, G. L. (2021). The microbiome and mosquito vectorial capacity: Rich potential for discovery and translation. *Microbiome, 9*, Article 111.

3.1. Mosquito Anatomy and Physiology

Mosquitoes use a keen sense of smell to home in on hosts with incredible accuracy. Both their antennae and the small maxillary palps are covered with microscopic, hair-like features called sensilla—small sacs that hold olfactory receptor neurons (ORNs). These neurons pick up many chemicals floating in the air, including the odors humans and animals give off. Essentially, this peripheral odor-smelling system relays information on odor type and strength to the brain, particularly to regions such as the glomeruli of the antennal lobe, where things are processed in a rather complicated way. Even small variations in the receptors suggest that some mosquitoes are simply better adapted to particular environments or host types. Single sensillum recordings have uncovered how these neurons work, with a range of types that are particularly sensitive to detecting key human skin chemicals like heptanal and nonanal (Ghaninia et al., 2007). Beneath this sensory equipment, the general anatomy of the mosquito is adapted to lead a double life—drinking nectar some of the time and, at other times, harvesting blood. Their mouthparts are oddly adapted to pierce the skin and suck blood, a necessity for egg development in the females. The proboscis is not one unit; it is made up of parts like the labium, mandibles, and maxillae that function together in unexpected combinations to slip under the skin while keeping things as unobtrusive as possible. Their digestive system, for instance, is quickly set up to process blood meals using enzymes that glean the nutrients required for reproduction. Both the respiratory and circulatory systems are maximized to provide the high energy demands of flight and host seeking. All of these traits somehow come together to guarantee that mosquitoes not only survive but accomplish a remarkably efficient task as disease vectors. Thinking about how these complex characteristics evolved leads to all manner of interesting ideas about mosquito evolution and their roles in nature. Some individuals suggest that mosquitoes, and their relationships with *parasites* like *Plasmodium*—may originally have had roles that were completely unrelated to disease transmission at all, possibly even helping to pollinate (Gillen & Sherwin, 2013). In most cases, it seems their complex systems got reassigned along the line as they evolved into the parasite vectors, we know today. Whatever their original function, their modern anatomy and physiology reveal a design perfectly suited to harboring and propagating *parasites*. Exploring these varied perspectives not only deepens our knowledge of mosquito biology but also points to new possibilities for managing disease through targeting the very vulnerabilities in their design (Figure 3.3).

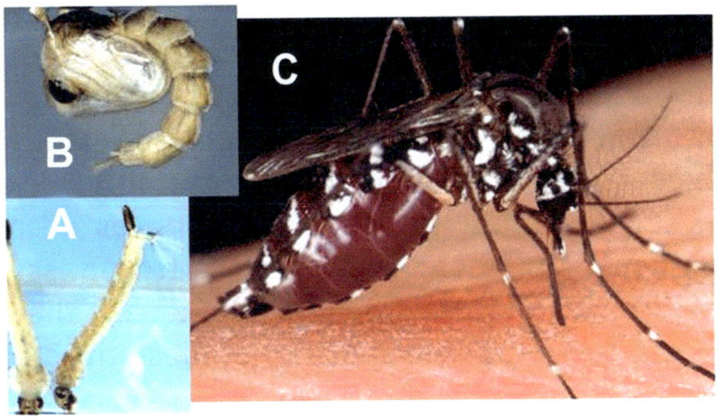

Figure 3.3. Anatomy of a mosquito.

Source: Dahmana H, Mediannikov O. Mosquito-Borne Diseases Emergence/Resurgence and How to Effectively Control It Biologically. *Pathogens*. 2020; 9(4):310. https://doi.org/10.3390/pathogens9040310

3.1.1. Key Anatomical Features of Mosquitoes

Mosquito bodies are remarkably complex and fuel their ability to spread disease. They survive on many sensor pieces distributed around the body that pick up on subtle hints from the environment. For example, ORNs hidden in antennae and maxillary palps allow them to pick up on hints like body odors and carbon dioxide. Interestingly, these neurons don't work alone – the adjacent ones seem to communicate via lateral inhibition, which serves to sharpen the signals somewhat. This kind of neural communication, likely combined to ephaptic coupling rather than to traditional synapses, enables them to filter out useful signals from background noise. To a large extent, a grasp of these sensory adaptations is key to an understanding of mosquitoes' host-seeking behavior and can even stimulate novel directions in vector control strategies (Carlson et al., 2012). Apart from this internalized sensing game, external features are equally critical in their role as vectors of disease. Their proboscis is a very specialized feeding structure that not only pierces the skin but also works via an orchestrated choreography of several needle-like structures to draw blood , a necessary function for females needing blood meals for egg development. The mosquito's body, which is covered in scales and setae, might also tip the scales when it comes to flying effectively and managing heat. It is amusing how, despite molecular methods becoming increasingly clever, checking characteristics such as wing patterns and body size is still the preferred way of species identification in the field (Carlson et al., 2012). Things are just as fascinating indoors. The midgut is not only where blood digestion takes place, it is also an early checkpoint where pathogens have to survive in order to establish an infection. Lined with a special epithelial layer, it battles on the fly unwelcome travelers like malaria *parasites* or arboviruses. Meanwhile, the salivary glands have their own essential task to perform; pathogens infect and multiply there before hitching a ride during the next blood meal. Likewise, the combination of sensory input with motor responses keeps the mosquito on its toes while targeting a host, condensing detection and disease transmission. Generally, this close relationship between inner design and disease-spreading ability is the reason why it is so critical in vector biology to be aware of the minute specifics of mosquito anatomy (Bharti et al., 2020) (Figure 3.4).

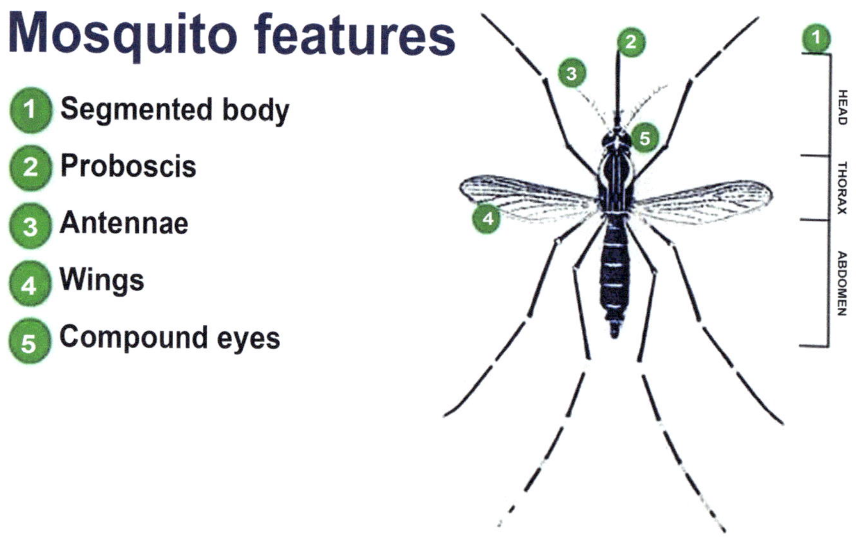

Figure 3.4. Key anatomical features of mosquitoes.

Source: Terminix. (2025). *Mosquito Features Chart.*

3.1.2. Physiological Processes Relevant to Vector Biology

Unraveling how a disease is transmitted often boils down to deconstructing the internal life of mosquito biology. These small animals don't just passively carry disease—their digestive cycles, energy balancing, and immune cues all have gargantuan significance in whether or not they catch, hold, subsequently convey infection. In the majority of cases, how parasite development crosses over with a mosquito's natural defenses dictates what we call vector competence, essentially the innate ability a mosquito population has to transmit disease. Researchers have been building these structured maps of insect biology recently—relating processes such as metabolism and immune signals—to help integrate information into smarter ways of controlling disease outbreaks (Topalis et al., 2011). Drilling deeper, transcriptomic studies have revealed spectacular shifts in a mosquito body at pivotal moments in time. Take the case of *Anopheles gambiae*, the notorious African malaria vector; after a blood meal, it sees high gene expression changes that are vital to digestion, support for the immune system, and regulating parasite interactions. These alterations, recorded in single tissues and phases of life, indicate how mosquitoes respond to infections and sometimes develop resistance to insecticides. Frequently, in the majority of cases, this more detailed knowledge of gene activity not only sheds light on how they resist infection but also identifies new ways of interrupting the parasite life cycle and improving devices like ITNs (Domingos et al., 2017). Along with these changes inside, mosquitoes also alter their behavior and metabolism to increase their chances of finding hosts and staying active under adverse conditions. They are adjusting how they can sense the world and decide how to use their energy—behavior that is very important for sensing a good blood meal and eventually for sensing pathogens. In addition, the mechanisms they use to break down insecticides, through metabolic detoxification processes, are able to alter their sensitivity to chemical controls. Synthesizing all these ideas—gene regulation and immunity and behavior and metabolism—gives a more comprehensive picture of vector competence, unveiling new, innovative ways to counteract vector-borne diseases (Topalis et al., 2011; Domingos et al., 2017) (Figure 3.5).

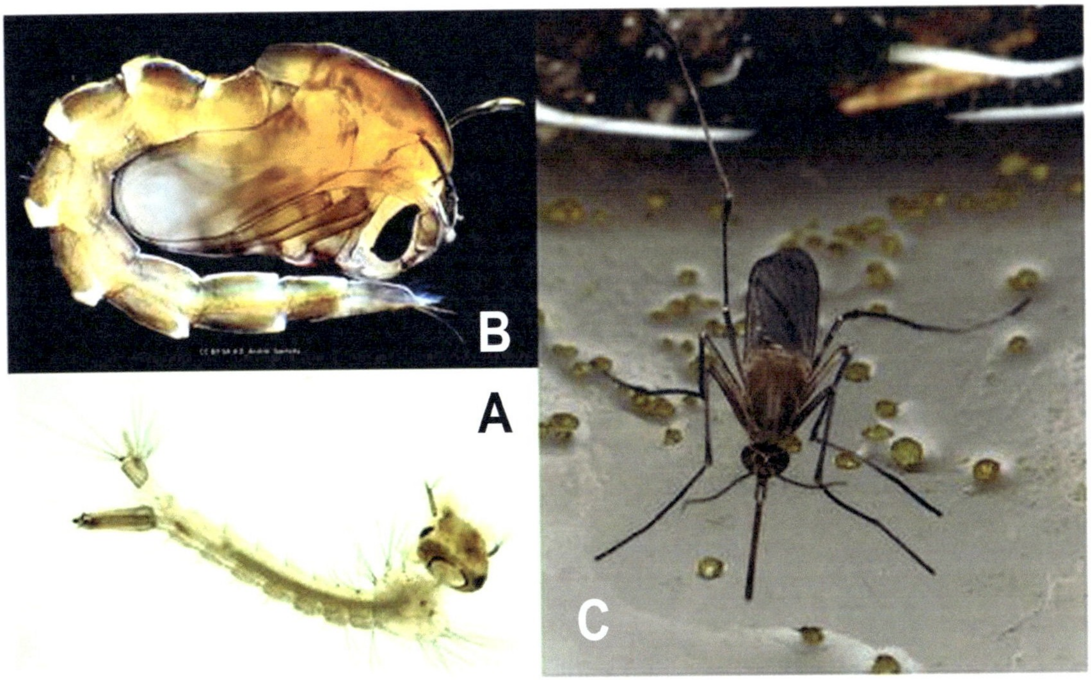

Figure 3.5. Physiological processes relevant to vector biology of mosquitoes.

Source: Dahmana H, Mediannikov O. Mosquito-Borne Diseases Emergence/Resurgence and How to Effectively Control It Biologically. *Pathogens*. 2020; 9(4):310. https://doi.org/10.3390/pathogens9040310

3.1.3. Adaptations for Blood-Feeding

Mosquitoes rely on blood capture to exist and keep on reproducing and thus have had to become very clever at doing it. They do not just pick a host at random—different species have different preferences that can modify their potentiality as disease vectors. Take, for example, *Anopheles gambiae* s.s.; this major malaria mosquito feeds almost exclusively on humans, which is believed by many to give it a survival advantage. However, experiments have shown that when these pathogens are fed a single blood meal, they live longer on human or cow blood compared to dog or bird blood. For most, this is where the blood type comes into play, though using just human blood repeatedly does not necessarily yield more benefits than mixing it, a testament to the fact that their feeding pattern is indeed complex for real (Lyimo et al., 2012). It is equally intriguing within the mosquito. Other than what they engage in outdoors, immune defenses and midgut handle the task of managing blood meals while at the same time dealing with invading pathogens. After the mosquito ingests a blood meal, *parasites* like *Plasmodium* have to fight through a form of living barrier, the midgut lining, which is not just a physical hindrance but also poses immune challenges. Overall, protein family signals like protein kinase C (PKC) control this barrier, affecting both the potential of the mosquito to fight off infections and the capacity of the parasite to grow. For instance, a spike of different PKC isoforms in the midgut shortly after feeding is seen for most Anopheles species, indicating their function in the preservation of lining integrity and immune response modulation. Interestingly, decreasing PKC activity has also been shown to make the barrier stronger and block parasite growth, which is a nice illustration of how these pathways balance immunity, blood digestion, and disease transmission (Camp et al., 2013). Getting a full meal is not entirely about internal defenses, however—bodies are built for it too. Mosquitoes have evolved some very impressive mouthparts, such as long, narrow proboscises with infinitesimally small, serrated tips that are capable of piercing skin almost undetected. They also secrete saliva that contains anticoagulants and even mild anesthetic compounds, which discourage the blood from clotting and prevent the host from feeling what is occurring. Further, their sensory organs, which pick up on cues like body heat and carbon dioxide, work in a kind of loosely coordinated fashion to find hosts. To summarize, these different adaptations demonstrate a subtle, almost elegant trade-off between finding a meal and staying hidden that makes mosquitoes such successful disease vectors even though, sometimes, their behavior can seem rather capricious (Figure 3.6).

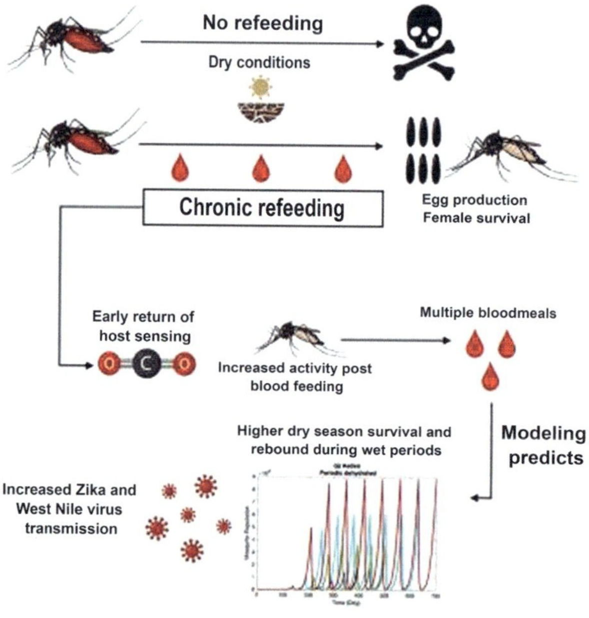

Figure 3.6. Multiple blood feeding bouts in mosquitoes.

Source: Holmes, C. J., Chakraborty, S., Ajayi, O. M., Uhran, M. R., Frigard, R., Stacey, C. L., et al. (2025). Multiple blood feeding bouts in mosquitoes allow for prolonged survival and are predicted to increase viral transmission during dry periods. *iScience, 28*(2), 111760.

3.2. Life Cycle of Mosquitoes

Mosquito growth is a unique cycle that begins when eggs are laid right on or by standing water—this watery location is not just any old location but a prerequisite stage for what is yet to be. After hatching, the larvae plunge into life as tiny water inhabitants, feasting on organic matter and small microorganisms that allow them to develop through a series of stages. Except for the most unusual cases, the larval stage is totally key; this is where their bodies reorganize themselves in a manner that makes way for pupation. Water chemistry, availability of nutrients, and other local factors govern their survival chances.

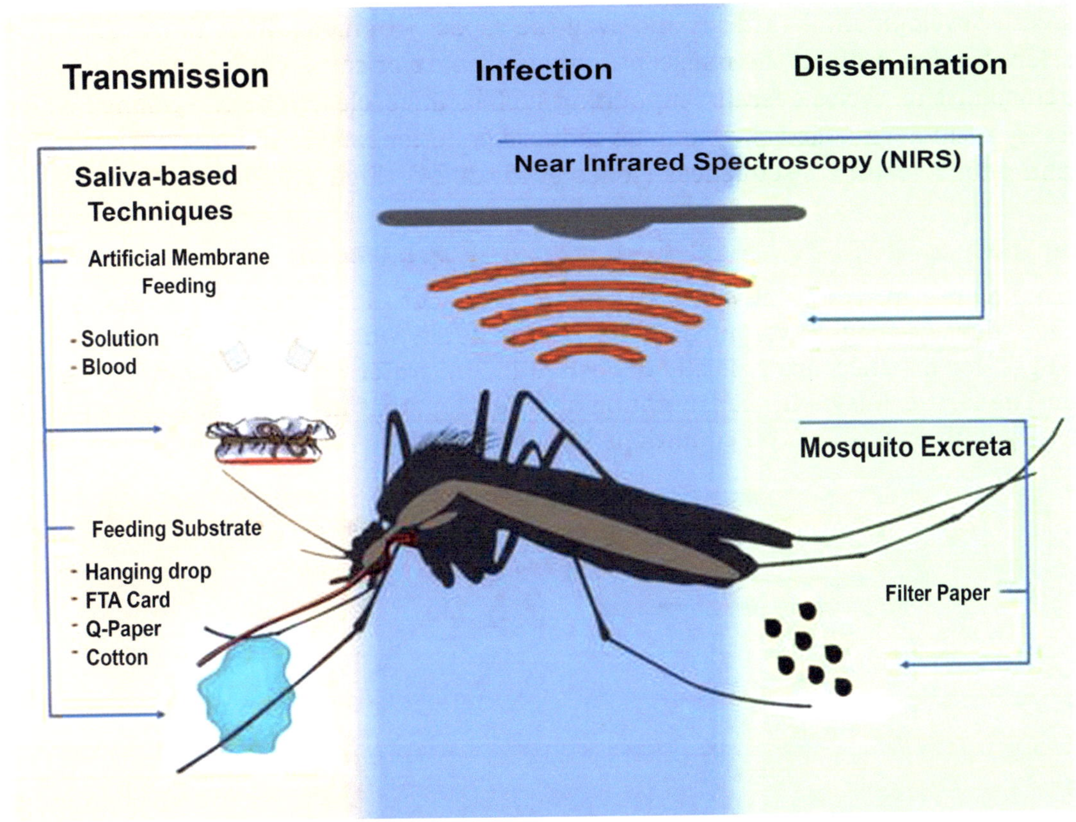

Figure 3.7. Mosquito life cycle.

Source: Meireles ACA, Rios FGF, Feitoza LHM, da Silva LR, Julião GR. Nondestructive Methods of Pathogen Detection: Importance of Mosquito Integrity in Studies of Disease Transmission and Control. *Pathogens*. 2023; 12(6):816. https://doi.org/10.3390/pathogens12060816

As it happens, the environment is less like the static backdrop and more like an active partner, with areas of potential to strike at the mosquito life cycle's proper vulnerabilities. Delving deeper at the molecular level reveals even more surprises. Researchers have found that microRNAs (miRNAs) unexpectedly take center stage during the larval stage. Mostly, these small RNA molecules help regulate molting, metamorphosis, and even cell differentiation by modulating which genes get expressed. That is, they prepare the doors for the immature mosquitoes to eventually become completely adult-ready mosquitoes that are fertile and can spread diseases. At times, the identical molecules also force modifications in feeding behavior, which further shapes the capability of mosquitoes to act as disease vectors. Such observations, in most cases, trace the true worth of basic biological research, implying that a greater understanding of these molecular details may open new avenues for innovative intervention strategies designed to disrupt their development (Shaalan et al., 2024). Subsequently there is the added twist of microplastic contamination contaminating the waters. One might overlook small plastic pieces in water breeding grounds at first, but witness accounts from other aquatic organisms indicate that such pollutants have the potential to induce stress as well as interfere with immune processes. Although data more directly involving microplastics in the biology of mosquitoes is still relatively scant, it is quite reasonable that such pollutants can interfere with developmental patterns and even the capacity of mosquitoes to transmit pathogens. This interference may redirect their susceptibility to disease or cause shifts in population balances, affecting transmission cycles overall. Pinpointing such lacunae, clearly, better-planned experiments are necessary to untangle exactly how human-induced pollution may be indirectly affecting mosquito vectors and public health consequences (Jones et al., 2024) (Figure 3.7).

3.2.1. Stages of Development: Egg, Larva, Pupa, Adult

Comprehending the growth of mosquitoes is not as clear-cut as it appears. Mosquitoes go through a four-stage journey—egg, larva, pupa, subsequently adult, which is full of rapid, transformative changes. Eggs, for instance, are typically deposited in still water, where they emerge as larvae not long after. The larvae, busy with consumption and development in water, undergo a growth spurt that can vary with environmental conditions like temperature.

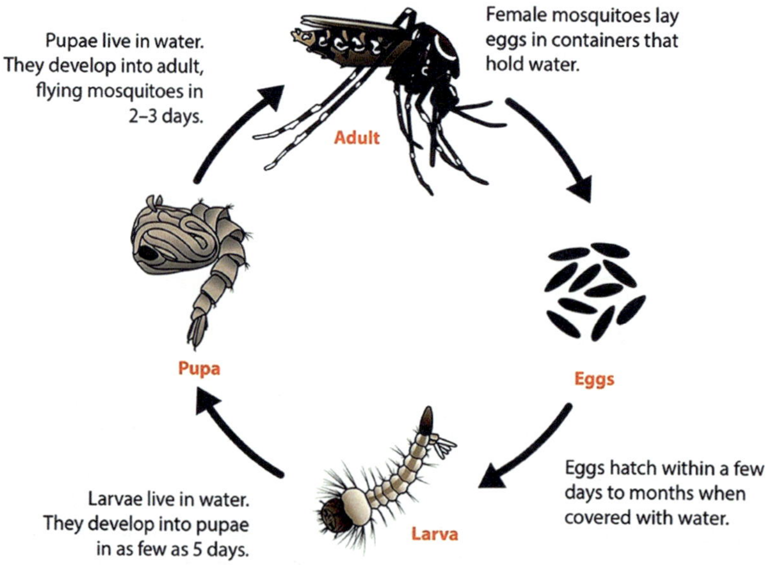

Figure 3.8. Stages of development of mosquitoes.

Source: Centers for Disease Control and Prevention. (n.d.). *Aedes Mosquito Life Cycle*. https://www.cdc.gov/mosquitoes/images/Aedes-life-cycle.jpg.

Each stage possesses its uniqueness, and those uniquenesses are avenues of stopping the mosquito's life cycle, sometimes halting their rise as disease disseminators. Passing from the larva to the pupa is a majestic, almost abrupt change. Generally speaking, it is like the push of a reset button, the mosquito stops eating and remakes itself, developing wings, legs, and other features specific to adults. Temperature is generally the culprit here in most cases; cold weather tends to extend such periods, and occasionally even keeps adults from emerging well, since some investigation throughout Culex species in colder areas has shown (Grech et al., 2023). This sort of data, though in a way somewhat complex in its manner of occurring, does a great deal to inform whether and how population control would ideally be applied. Once it has finally burst out of its juvenile state and into adulthood, the mosquito can now breed and, sadly, also transmit diseases. Research on *Anopheles funestus* has shown that gene expression of microRNAs varies dramatically throughout its life stages. Extremely fascinatingly, many microRNAs are expressed specifically over certain durations, indicating their role in controlling growth and differentiation. Normally, it ought to be manageable to alter with these microRNAs and create a new method of disrupting mosquito development and inhibiting their growth (Keller et al., 2016). Altogether, seeing these four pieces of development gives us a broad sketch of mosquito biology and promises directions to slice disease transmission—although not necessarily along a gleaming direct or tidy trajectory (Figure 3.8).

3.2.2. Environmental Factors Influencing Life Cycle

Environmental pressures and mosquito populations intersect in ways that have an impact, especially when you're dealing with things like *Aedes albopictus* species that appear to just keep popping up in new places. Urbanization and the resulting changes due to human development create spaces that are perfect for mosquitoes, even the random pockets of green around the city can suddenly become high-use breeding grounds. In a study conducted in Rome, scientists noted how even a small city park seemed to enhance the mosquito population subsequently consider the additional factor of late summer rains triggering a second influx of adult mosquitoes. Temperature, rain, and the like all play a part in every step: from eggs first starting to hatch, through larva development, all the way up to those pesky adult stages (Manica et al., 2016). It seems to be logical that being aware of even these microscale habits about environments is crucial if we are to establish effective ways of restricting their spread in our cities. Weather is not just a question of where mosquitoes end up, it also seems to be linked to how diseases these insects transmit end up spreading. In East Africa's highlands, shifting weather has been linked to the changing areas where malaria-carrying mosquitoes occur. Now, while some continue to dispute exactly how much global warming is the culprit, there's more than enough evidence that warmer temperatures and altered rain patterns weaken nature's ecosystems, making it easy for mosquitoes to thrive. Okay, blaming it all on the weather might be simplifying things too much; land use changes, human migration, and even mosquito adaptation all mix into this complex situation. Schmalhausen's law, for example, describes that when nature is stressed to start with, even small changes will have more significant impacts, producing more unstable mosquito levels and heightening disease threats. Often, it takes many many variables—more than climate—into which we need to feed our models if we are to ever get in front of vector-borne diseases (Chaves & & Koenraadt, 2010). Local circumstances, like the way a landscape becomes fragmentary or the volume of water that persists around, may be as influential as weather or urban growth in shaping the life of a mosquito. Whether in terms of the selection of egg-laying places or the nature of larval habitats, all these micro-scale differences directly affect the number of adult mosquitoes. However, in break-up city landscapes where water-holding containers suddenly materialize, such as *Aedes albopictus*, they can achieve seasonal population peaks with alarming speed. Temperature seems to expedite the development process too speeding up life cycles so that mosquitoes can achieve more generations in a season, which maximizes their potential for disease transmission. All these little and grand things illustrate how the mosquito populations respond quite dramatically to the larger picture as well as the details of their life. Viewing things integratively, in how eco-climatic and human factors come together, serves well in understanding mosquito behavior and designing wise control strategies (Figure 3.9).

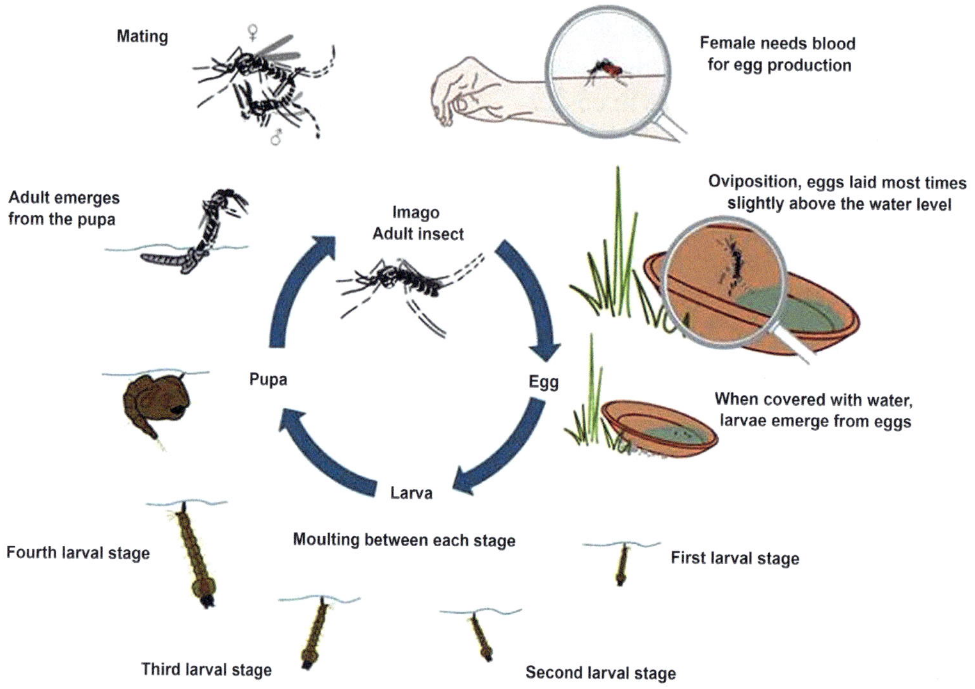

Figure 3.9. Environmental factors influencing life cycle of mosquitoes.

Source: Biogents. (n.d.). *Life Cycle of Aedes Aegypti (Yellow Fever Mosquito).* https://us.biogents.com/wp-content/uploads/life-cycle-aedes-aegypti-yellow-fever-mosquito-en-768x549.jpg.

3.2.3. Duration of Each Life Stage

Mosquitoes' development timing isn't nice to have—it governs how populations grow and disease spreads. These are pathogens that go through an entire cycle—eggs, larvae, pupae, adults—in cycles that each seem especially sensitive to temperature. When it is warmer, eggs hatch sooner and the larval stage rushes along; this rapid turnover is what allows new generations to emerge soon. Still, in the majority of cases, not all phases react the same way: a pinch of extra heat can lower death risks in one stage and anomalously raise them in another because of some crafty, nonlinear mechanisms. All these ambiguities make our predictions more complicated, although the awareness of these subtleties still continues to be important for estimating risks and planning interventions (Ewing et al., 2016). As a whole, having a precise measure of each phase's duration is important in mapping vector dynamics. It is not just the temperature alone; the environment has a hand in the action by reacting with the mosquito's microbiota. That is, the small microbes lying around in their tissues and gut can shift the balance where nutrition, immune systems, and even disease resistance come into play—all of which, as a result, affect how long each phase of life lasts. Microbes, for example, might add extra amino acids and vitamins that fast-forward larvae development, cutting down the overall time taken for development. On the other hand, these microbes, however, fortify the immune system of the mosquito and help them weather those pivotal moments when infection takes hold. This mixing of biological factors and environmental stress presents a complex picture that reflects just how intertwining these forces are (Douglas, 2014). Overall, understanding these microbe-host interactions is key to understanding how mosquitoes live out their short lives. Mixing stage-specific length of life into solid population models requires accounting for temperature fluctuations throughout the year, and even those infinitesimal biotic particulars. Scientists tend to use temperature-based delay-differential equations to simulate how things such as diapause and mortality rates change with the weather, providing more earthy insight into seasonal mosquito highs. In general, warmer temperatures push peak counts higher by speeding growth through more stages, giving a broader window for the spread of disease. It is not always easy, though, as parts of their life move quicker on the swing with warmth, but others might see greater mortality when extremes happen—giving a perpetually shifting balance (Ewing et al., 2016). Add microbial forces to the mix, and the situation becomes even more complex. These additional thoughts indicate maybe; by targeting the microbes, we could throw a monkey wrench into the usual timeline and mitigate the risks of vector-borne diseases. In most cases, judicious consideration of each stage in the face of both environmental and biological challenges is extremely critical to effective vector control measures.

3.3. Mosquito Behavior

Mosquito behavior matters, a close look at the way these insects act can turn the tide when it comes to stopping the spread of disease. What they eat, for example, depends on all sorts of things from mercurial weather to what people happen to be doing in the general vicinity. Different species, and even the same ones at different times, can differ in when or where they bite, sometimes because of things like ITNs or indoor spraying. This complex mix of variables makes it tough to interrupt the cycle of transmission, and generally, as we push harder to eliminate malaria, mosquitoes seem to change their ways. Increasingly, they are biting outdoors or earlier in the day than you would anticipate them to while humans are resting, so our traditional inside repairs aren't constantly effective (Lyimo et al., 2012). Things get even more involved when you look at the larval end of the equation. Larvae contribute a lot to the number of mosquitoes that end up flying around, and sometimes they even end up feeding on one another, especially in the case of species like *Aedes albopictus*. Experiments have shown that crowding, food levels, and the configuration of a breeding site all contribute to how often one larva will cannibalize another. In the vast majority of cases, the simple geometry of a larval habitat—its shape, size, and spatial irregularities—alters the frequency of these interactions, adding a new dimension to the regulation of numbers in a population. This sort of behavior implies extreme competition for resources and survival strategies that over time move the balance in suppressing or enhancing mosquito populations in temporary aggregates of water (Mastrantonio et al., 2018). If you look at the big picture, when you step back and see it, it's clear that fighting mosquitoes is a matter of keeping up with their wily adaptations with an adaptive, multi-pronged strategy. Even having many indoor safety measures in place, there is always persisting transmission remaining; mosquitoes are just too resistant at times. As they start biting outdoors and earlier in the evenings, finding out what their habits are outdoors takes precedence. Therefore, instead of simply relying on standard interior means, control measures must reach out to cover spaces in which the insects find themselves resting outside and adjust to new feeding patterns. For the most part, reconsidering mosquito reactions to different stresses, either environmental shifts or our efforts at controlling them—opens up a broader plan that does not merely stay ahead of these insects but leads the way to elimination (Lyimo et al., 2012) (Figure 3.10).

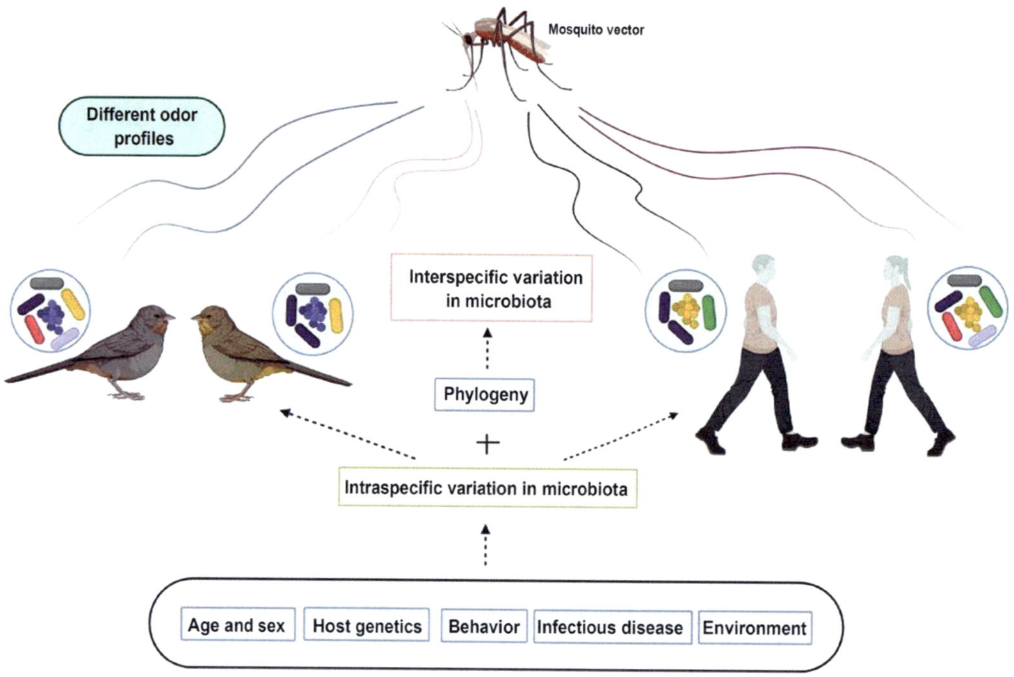

Figure 3.10. Mosquito behavior.

Source: Ruiz-López, M. J. (2020). Mosquito behavior and vertebrate microbiota interaction: Implications for pathogen transmission. *Frontiers in Microbiology, 11,* Article 573371. https://www.frontiersin.org/files/Articles/573371/fmicb-11-573371-HTML/image_m/fmicb-11-573371-g001.jpg.

3.3.1. Feeding Habits and Preferences

Seeing how the mosquitoes feed tells us a great deal about how they spread disease. They are not all the same protocol followers, some feed almost exclusively of human blood, whereas others seem to sample the blood of every warm-blooded creature they find themselves around. In the majority of cases, the key malaria vectors prefer human blood, a feature which not only enhances their disease transmission potential but also renders them susceptible to control measures like ITNs, and even indoor residual spraying (IRS); paradoxically though, certain species manage to deceive it by taking outdoor bites or by feeding on animal hosts, more or less dodging the conventional indoor treatments. This kind of flexibility implies that disease transmission can stubbornly maintain itself even when the most vulnerable types are contained to a large degree. Feeding changes appear to typically occur after changes in which species are present or simply due to natural plasticity in host searching rather than due to genetic resistance. Therefore, observing these feeding patterns is quite significant if we are to improve our vector control activities (Govella et al., 2013).

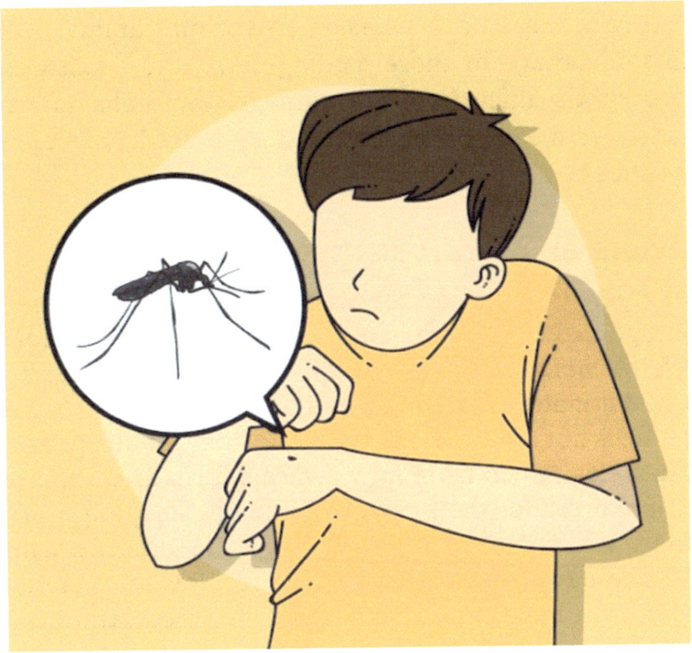

Figure 3.11. Mosquito feeding behavior.

Source: Freepik. (n.d.). *Hand Drawn Composition of Mosquito Bite.* https://external-content.duckduckgo.com/iu/?u=https%3A%2F%2Fimg.freepik.com%2Ffree-vector%2Fhand-drawn-composition-mosquito-bite_23-2147929510.jpg%3Fsemt%3Dais_hybrid&f=1&nofb=1&ipt=27c32ef65a2c6b2b7b6e1cf0df23a8067ad380cf035f5fd9e3eaf90169e234dc.

Apart from whom they bite, where and when mosquitoes choose to take their meal also plays a major role in how diseases are transmitted. For the most part, most of these pathogens show up at dawn, dusk, or even stay awake throughout the night—times that generally overlap with when hosts are available but also shun further environmental dangers. These timing-of-feeding changes occasionally disrupt control measures that depend on the protection of humans when they sleep. Besides, some species are not satisfied with being found at a single place; they switch between outdoors and indoors depending on the facility with which a host can be reached and the level of insecticide pressure. Such strategies are more characteristic of a persistence behavior than complete resistance, and as such, they present a strong case for integrated vector management (IVM) that cuts across a range of ecological environments. A better knowledge of these habits can help frame interventions to break mosquito-human interaction in different environments (Govella et al., 2013). Looking back, the interaction between feeding behavior in mosquitoes and our control measures has significantly changed, especially as our insecticide materials and biological insights have evolved. Much of the control was early based on insecticides, but as soon as resistance started to emerge in some species of mosquitoes, we realized that we had to think about how these insects feed. For instance, those mosquitoes that occur around livestock possess a different host choice system that alters both their potential for transmission and response to control. While the arrival of effective insecticides at one time looked like a genuine breakthrough, the intersection of trends toward resistance and changes in feeding behavior continues to throw curveballs to sustainable control. New methods, like releasing sterile males or de-worming animals with endectocides—offer promising ways of taking advantage of these feeding behaviors against the mosquitoes. On the whole, a balanced, rather subtle analysis of mosquito feeding behavior remains at the heart of conceiving innovative, effective means of managing these pests in our constantly evolving public health landscape (Figure 3.11).

3.3.2. Mating Behaviors and Reproductive Strategies

Mosquito breeding also largely depends on the way these pathogens come at mating—a process, over the course of time, optimized to allow genes to travel and populations to thrive in different contexts. In the *Anopheles gambiae* complex, mosquitoes' group in swarms, a formation that not only makes it easier to find a mate but also naturally drives them to stick together. It does occur, however, that this swarming is not always along the same lines for all species; regional idiosyncrasy and behavior tend to cause deviations from how swarms form and function. *An. coluzzii* females, for example, are strongly preferred for their conspecific males, keeping hybridization to an absolute minimum even when there is a composite of several species present, while *An. quadriannulatus* appears rather less picky. These sorts of differences are a result of an evolutionary trade-off between gene mixing and keeping narrow mate choice, something that affects traits like how good a mosquito is at causing disease. In most contexts, being able to gain control over such mating preferences is rather core to population structure planning and intervention design for minimizing disease transmission (Bolton et al., 2015). In control measure strategy, the mating choice of mosquitoes fits perfectly into strategies using the deployment of new genetic tools. The releasing insects with a dominant lethal gene (RIDL) release through to gene drives and CRISPR-based adjustments takes advantage of the idea of breaking up natural mating systems in order to eliminate or replace entire populations. Generally, their achievement relies on a plunge into the details of mosquito breeding—how preferences in mating rearrange gene movement, for instance. Looking at these processes from an evolutionary lens helps researchers to forecast whether resistance will occur or not, thus idea creation for mixed or combinatorial approaches to circumvent that challenge. It is a bit akin to controlling antibiotic resistance elsewhere, which highlights the need to bring together behavioral ecology knowledge and technical genetic intervention (Tippelt et al., 2018). Some other methods even try to disrupt the usual reproductive signals or use RNA interference to impose limitations on fertility directly. By investigating details like sperm competition, mating frequency, and the highs and lows of insemination success among different mosquito species, researchers are refining biocontrol methods to function more effectively with less off-target ecological spill. Experiments that demonstrate variability in mating success and cross-pairing demonstrate how complex mosquito reproduction can be—creating challenges as well as new prospects for innovative control approaches. Generally speaking, the application of such reproductive nuances enhances the accuracy of vector control measures as much as it facilitates the evolution of sustainable management programs that respect conservation agendas in sensitive ecosystems under threat from vector-borne diseases (Bolton et al., 2015; Tippelt et al., 2018) (Figure 3.12).

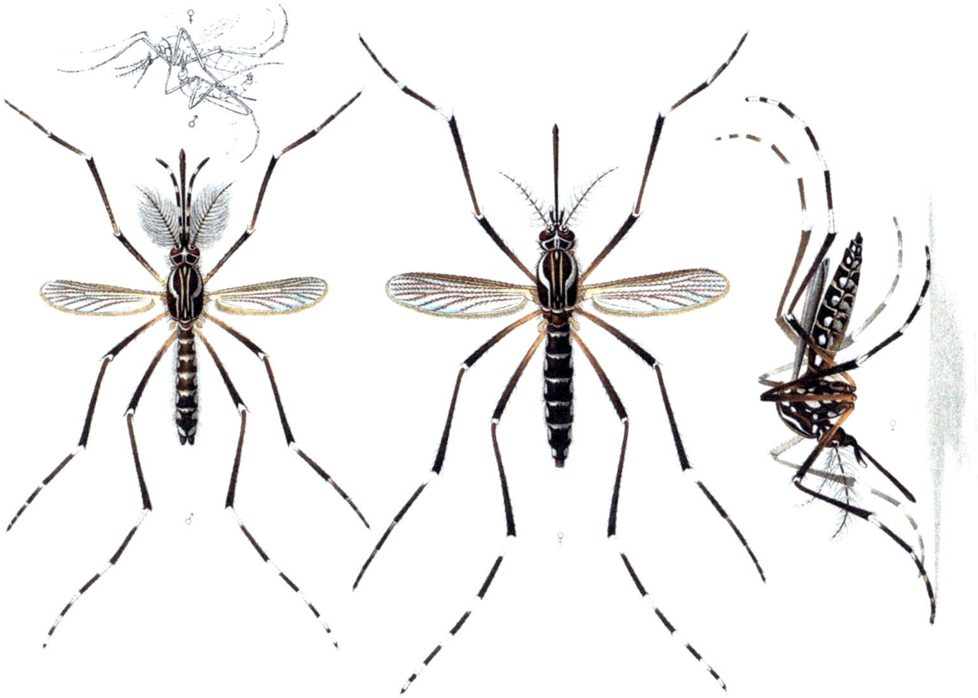

Figure 3.12. Mosquito mating.

Source: By Own scan, slightly modified. Original by Emil August Goeldi (1859 - 1917). - E. A. Goeldi (1905) Os Mosquitos no Pará. Memorias do Museu Goeldi. Pará, Brazil. Figures 3 (left) 1 (middle) and 2 (right) of Plate 1 in the Appendix., Public Domain, https://commons.wikimedia.org/w/index.php?curid=5469706

3.3.3. Host-Seeking Mechanisms

Mosquitoes must find a host to live, propagate, and spread disease. They depend on an arsenal of sensory gear, primarily their antennae and maxillary palps, which come equipped with small structures known as sensilla. Each and every one of these small areas contains ORNs that are responsible for sensing specific chemical signals from other animals. Overall, these neurons notice the strength and nature of odors, reporting that data back to the central nervous system to guide the zigzag flight of the mosquito toward prey. Experiments on species like *Anopheles gambiae* and *Aedes aegypti* have even mapped areas of their antennal lobes, and it is shown that ORN signals are spatially sorted with different clusters responding to chemicals like heptanal and nonanal, compounds routinely found in human odors. This increased sense shows how mosquitoes can pick the right host (Ghaninia et al., 2007). The environment also has a say on how these insects travel. Distribution of such resources as breeding areas and blood hosts ultimately has them decide where the mosquitoes will go and in what quantity, which, in turn, has them decide about their chances of encountering humans and causing disease. Scientists using multi-patch mathematical models discovered that when scented molecules cluster or disperse, mosquitoes locate them- and themselves-exhibiting in different ways-they might, for instance, cover longer distances searching for a host. In most cases but a couple of exceptions, the use of spatial repellents throws a wrench in these movements, reducing mobility as well as host encounter rates and hence reducing transmission rates for disease. In general, having this spatial and behavioral feature information is a win big time for engineering better vector control methods in heterogeneous real-world environments (Lutambi et al., 2012). The integration of chemical signals with spatial information gives additional depth to the way mosquitoes find hosts. Their ORNs pick up many volatile compounds from the skin of humans, and interestingly, the mixture can differ by body region such as feet or underarms, suggesting a very subtle level of discrimination. These chemical signals, along with variables such as patchiness in the resource and even the repellents, are among the factors that factor into making the mosquito an expert at targeting a host. Advances in techniques like single sensillum recording have allowed scientists to distinguish different ORN types and their specific stimuli, expanding our window into how these tiny sensors translate odor molecules into action. Collectively, these results open the door to targeted strategies that fragment the sensory inputs mosquitoes rely on, potentially diminishing their role as disease vectors (Ghaninia et al., 2007; Lutambi et al., 2012) (Figure 3.13).

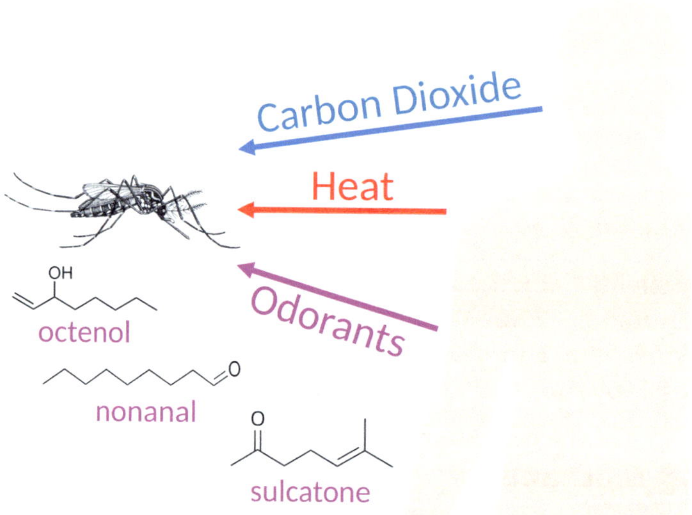

Figure 3.13. Mosquito host-seeking mechanisms.

Source: By Chiswick Chap - Own work; embedded images File:Human body silhouette.svg and File:Stegomyia fasciata.jpg, CC BY-SA 4.0, https://commons.wikimedia.org/w/index.php?curid=142120692

3.4. Role of Mosquitoes in Disease Transmission

Mosquito-borne illnesses result from an interconnected mix of the insects' inherent nature and what they do in interaction with their surroundings. Take *Aedes aegypti* as an instance, such insects breed rapidly and seem to acclimatize rapidly to differences in temperature fluctuations. They can adapt at will to heat and climate differences that can make all the difference in disease transmission. In most cases, attributes that encompass thermal tolerance and even the adaptable nature of the mosquitoes themselves ultimately decide where and when such outbreaks like dengue take place. You stated that models that run on such climate adaptation data give a better picture of public health threats in general (Couper et al., 2021).

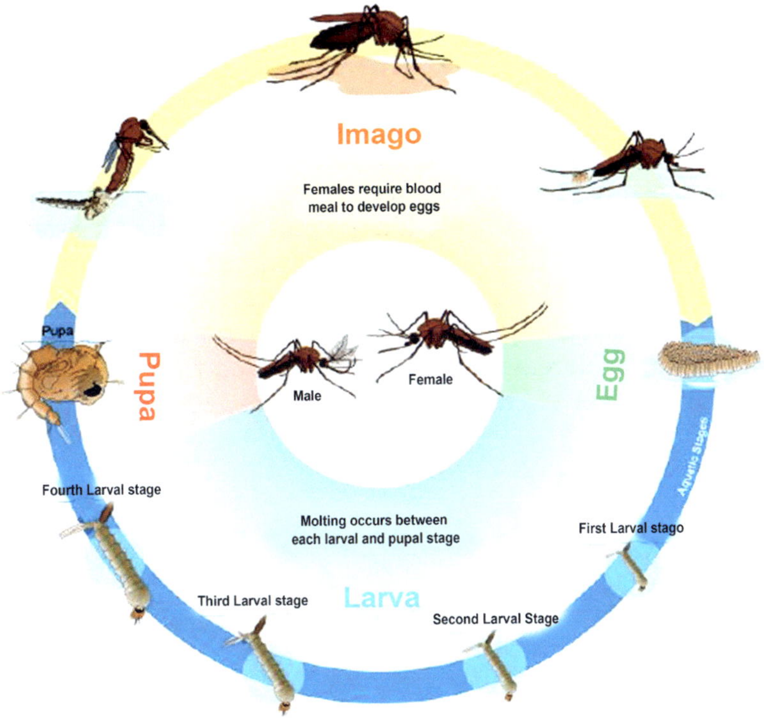

Figure 3.14. Role of mosquitoes in disease transmission.

Source: https://en.m.wikipedia.org/wiki/File:Culex_mosquito_life_cycle_en.svg

Generally speaking, their natural features make it hard to control disease and fight them. These microbes, for example, *Plasmodium* spp., travel within mosquitoes through a series of challenges that either pass or fail an infection. After a mosquito has sucked in infected blood, the *parasites* get to work by starting sexual reproduction subsequently moving through stages—gametocytes, zygotes, ookinetes, and oocysts—before they finally end up as sporozoites. It is a rough ride from the midgut to the salivary glands, and only a minority of those *parasites* make it through round two. These bottlenecks, where so many *parasites* just do not survive, contribute significantly to how well an illness propagates. Factors like parasite load, the immune state of the mosquito itself, and even the way molecules interact at the level of the salivary glands all work together to dictate malaria transmission, with the possibility for additional interventions (Graumans et al., 2020). And for the terminal jump—the actual deposition of sporozoites into a mammalian host—the story is even more intriguing. When an infected mosquito feeds and probes, it deposits sporozoites directly into tissue just under the skin. There, those *parasites* fight the host immune system before they travel to the liver. How many is transmitted depends on the particular design of the mosquito salivary glands and on the extremely specific way sporozoites adhere. Furthermore, how long these sporozoites exist in the mosquito and how they are released out during feeding periods also play a significant role in the infectivity of the insect. All this environmental variability that regulates mosquito behavior only adds to the overall complexity. Indeed, it is crucial to master these details if we are to be able to create precision control initiatives that may decimate the global incidence of mosquito-borne diseases (Graumans et al., 2020) (Figure 3.14)..

3.4.1. Overview of Diseases Transmitted by Mosquitoes

Mosquitoes don't just bite—diseases spread by them have, in many cases, changed world public health. Zika virus, chikungunya, dengue fever, and yellow fever, to mention a few, are on the rise; much of this rise can be explained by the unexpected adaptability of pathogens like *Aedes aegypti* and *Aedes albopictus*. In spite of research plodding along and constant attempts at intervention, making effective vaccines continues to be challenging, and our reliance on keeping the insects at bay has not yet been enough to keep outbreaks at bay. These endemic viruses demonstrate how complicated it is to deal with mosquito populations that thrive in densely populated cities and their underserved borderlands, the underemphasized areas, and, on the whole, transmitting insecticide resistance only adds another layer of challenge (Achee et al., 2019).

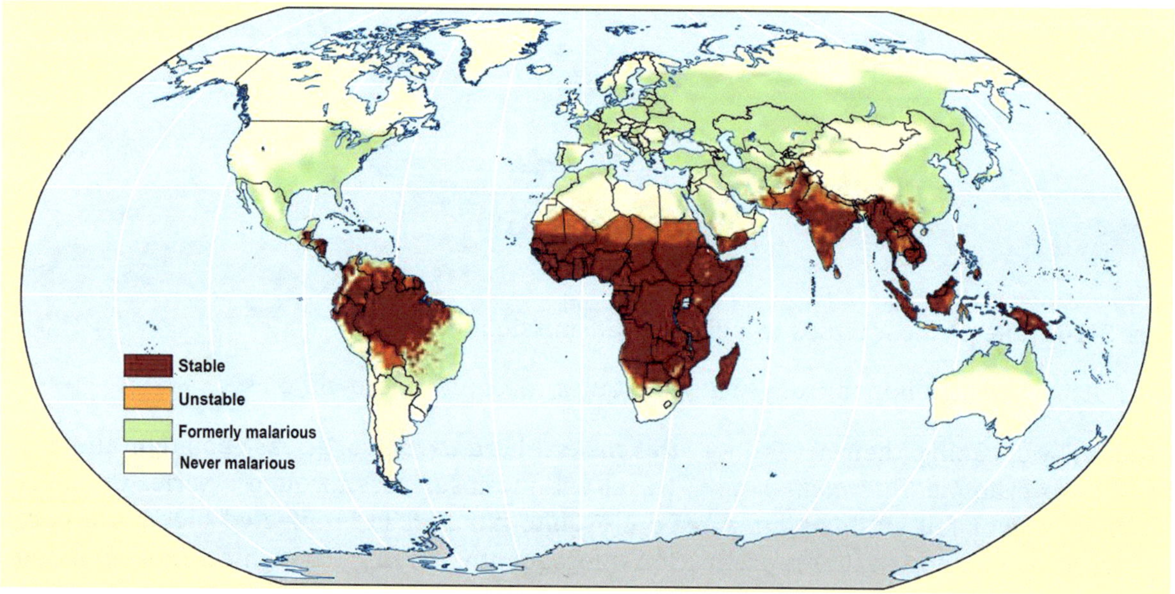

Figure 3.15. Diseases transmitted by mosquitoes.

Source: By World Development Report (2009)5 - https://ourworldindata.org/health-meta, CC BY 4.0, https://commons.wikimedia.org/w/index.php?curid=82822311

Briefly stated, attaining a solid grasp of mosquito biology is the foundation for creating long-lasting solutions that can finally halt virus transmission and decrease the global disease burden. Apart from these arboviral problems, malaria is another intractable menace, spread by *Anopheles* mosquitoes nearly exclusively. The *Plasmodium parasites* responsible for malaria are accompanied by an envelope of biological features that make them difficult to eradicate well into the decades of control attempts. Early measures like ITNs and indoor spraying have increasingly given way to more holistic, integrated strategies—ones that now combine surveillance, drug therapies, and even changes to the environment—to combat the disease. Overall, the momentum behind these efforts closely mirrors the ambitious goals initiated by organizations like the World Health Organization (WHO) through its Global Technical Strategy. Yet the ever-changing habits of malaria vectors, coupled with growing drug and insecticide resistance, emphasize the need for fresh research and fresh control strategies. All this frenzied scientific activity lies at the very center of moving us closer to eliminating malaria once and for all (Rabinovich et al., 2017). Besides these old-familiar diseases, mosquitoes also transmit agents that cause other debilitating diseases like lymphatic filariasis and West Nile virus infection. Lymphatic filariasis, spread predominantly by Culex mosquitoes with the help of small filarial worms, often leads to permanent disability and even social exclusion in impacted communities. West Nile virus, spread through complex bird–mosquito cycles, is a prime example of how zoonotic pathogens can suddenly switch to human populations and create havoc. Together, these diseases highlight the astounding diversity of pathogens transmitted by mosquitoes, so that a subtle understanding of their ecology and host association is of such significance. One that combines epidemiological insights with ecological data is finally necessary to develop targeted public health interventions for these complex threats (Rabinovich et al., 2017; Achee et al., 2019) (Figure 3.15).

3.4.2. Mechanisms of Pathogen Transmission

Understanding how mosquitoes deal with the microbes they transmit isn't as simple as it may appear (Figure 3.16). To get a grip on things, one must delve into all the small steps that allow a pathogen to travel from host to host. It begins when a mosquito feeds on someone who is already infected bringing the microbe along for the ride. Then the disease must work its way past the natural defenses of the mosquito, multiply in places like the midgut and salivary glands, subsequently be present in its saliva when the mosquito bites once more. Those leaps and hurdles play a big part in whether that microbe ever reaches a new person. In recent times, scientists have been experimenting with genetic alterations and other methods of dealing with mosquitoes in an effort to break this chain in the hope of slowing disease transmission (Kohl et al., 2016). The features of mosquitoes themselves help bring about this dynamic mélange. Their habits, when and where they feed, how long they live, even where they prefer to congregate—can make it that much more likely for a microbe to be transmitted. Take Aedes mosquitoes. Both *Aedes albopictus* and *Aedes aegypti* have this capacity to bite in the daytime and stick around human habitations, which, in large part, makes them near-perfect virus vectors like dengue and chikungunya. And it is not just behavior in action, small differences in their genes, the way their immune systems react, or even the bacteria they're attached to inside their bodies can slow down or speed up viral copying. All these naturally hybridized characteristics give us clues about why certain diseases occur and sometimes recur around (Boyer et al., 2012). But it is not all that happens inside a mosquito; the world they inhabit matters a lot, as well. The temperature fluctuates, humidity rates, even the season cycle could affect how fast mosquitoes reproduce or how fast a virus replicates once swallowed. For instance, if it is warmer, the time for a pathogen to prepare for transmission can be shortened, and reproductive and survival chances for a mosquito can be enhanced. At the same time, if human beings change their environments through urbanization or land use modification, breeding sites become randomly variable and the rate of mosquitoes coming across novel hosts varies. New techniques, including using Wolbachia-mediated biocontrol or even genetically modified mosquitoes, are trying to take advantage of these ecological weaknesses. More than likely, these integrated measures rely on our growing, if sometimes uncontrolled, sophisticated understanding of how pathogens ride their lifecycle through mosquito vectors (Kohl et al., 2016).

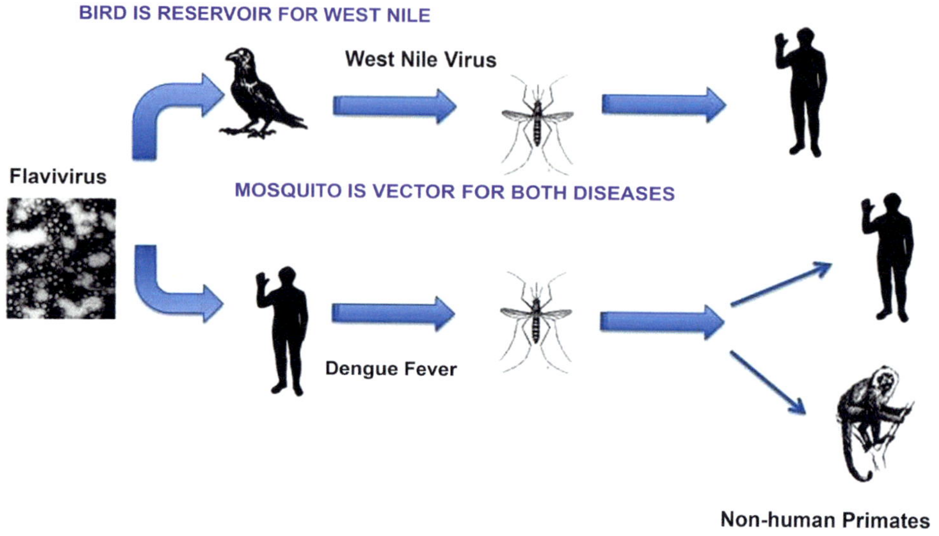

Figure 3.16. The schematic diagram of pathogen transmission by the mosquito.

Source: By Kwasnyje - Own work, CC BY-SA 4.0, https://commons.wikimedia.org/w/index.php?curid=49676794

3.4.3. Impact of Mosquito-Borne Diseases on Public Health

Mosquitoes are spreading their wings across the globe in manners that public health systems simply hadn't seen before. *Aedes aegypti* and *Anopheles stephensi* are a couple of the species that are particularly adept at wriggling their way into new territories, due to weather cycles and, naturally, climate change. They move into areas where people have not been exposed to diseases like dengue, malaria, chikungunya, and Zika, which used to limit themselves to tropical or subtropical areas. For the most part, the WHO feels that climate change will heighten the burden of such diseases, pushing morbidity and mortality rates even higher (George et al., 2023). In nearly all low-resource settings, the infrastructure for detection, treatment, and prevention of these diseases is already overburdened, and outbreaks tend to erode labor productivity and overwhelm health systems, all of which strongly advocate for IVM strategies. The complex interaction between mosquito vectors and the environment is complicated; it is a complex web that interrupts disease transmission. You see, everything ranging from what these insects prefer to eat, where they prefer to breed, and even the coming and going of the seasons come into play when talking about the transmission of disease. For instance, feeding behaviors of *Culex pipiens* species, like *Cx. pipiens pipiens* and *Cx. pipiens molestus*, have been found to influence West Nile virus transmission risk by changing the rate at which they feed on birds, which amplifies the virus, versus humans, who typically do not pass it on again (Ferraguti et al., 2023). Epidemiological models frequently suggest that small changes in local mosquito behavior can modify invasion risks and shape outbreak patterns. Most importantly, it is coming to an understanding of these specific ecological and behavioral traits that are key if we are to target surveillance and control measures. Human movement and travel are also thrown into this complex equation. Rapid urbanization and heightened global travel have made it easier than ever for invasive mosquito species, and the diseases they carry—to surface in new areas, which only boosts epidemic potential. In urban areas with high population density, discarded items that hold water, for example, can turn into perfect makeshift nurseries for vectors like *Aedes aegypti*, which further elevates the prospect of dengue and Zika outbreaks (George et al., 2023). Moreover, the socio-economic situation, whereby large parts of the population have limited access to proper vector control and healthcare facilities, largely dictates how these diseases play out, especially in the developing world. In total, the prevention of mosquito-borne disease needs to involve a marriage of vector biology science with an emphasis on social and behavioral determinants so that we can build public health interventions that truly succeed over the long haul.

3.5. Mosquito Control Strategies

Mosquitoes simply will not give us a break, they just continue to spread diseases and send us on an endless quest for better control. Humans have utilized chemical insecticides for ages to kill adult mosquitoes and baby mosquitoes, but over time the chemicals lose their potency because the pests learn to shrugged them off, and this normally hurts the environment and our health as well. In a sort of mixed strategy, farmers and public health authorities have resorted to programs that mix chemicals with other strategies, such as biological and even mechanical methods—to slow down that resistance factor. It is interesting how even less common Anopheles species like *Anopheles squamosus*, which can circumvent the usual sprays, remind us there is still much we do not completely understand about these pests (Nguyen et al., 2025). Even newer, greener approaches are being developed that aim to minimize the negatives of chemical pesticides. Many researchers are now looking at genetic control measures, releasing sterile insects or even using CRISPR/Cas9 gene editing, to directly modify or shrink mosquito populations. And nature also has some clever tricks up its sleeve. Bacteria such as *Bacillus thuringiensis* subsp., for instance, *israelensis* (Bti) and *Lysinibacillus sphaericus* (Ls) are toxins that kill larvae of mosquitoes, and they seem to do this without disrupting other organisms.

These biologics have at least in the field passed the test of time, showing little to no resistance signs, and they are a very significant part of green mosquito control (Miranda et al., 2024). However, for all our newer gimmicks and better technology, all is not settled. Globalization and a changing climate—warmer temperatures, more rainfall, and ease of travel—are spreading mosquito habitats and enabling the pests to move into new areas, bringing an entire new dimension of difficulty to their control. Control in most circumstances now requires a patchwork strategy that combines new and old ideas with sensitivity to local ecosystems and disease trends. Continued monitoring, community participation, and measures like habitat manipulation are all seemingly among the methods for keeping resistance at bay while tackling the problem forcefully. In short, coupling the old tools with the new, innovative approaches, and continued study of mosquito behavior, remains at the heart of fighting these diseases globally (Miranda et al., 2024; Nguyen et al., 2025) (Figure 3.17).

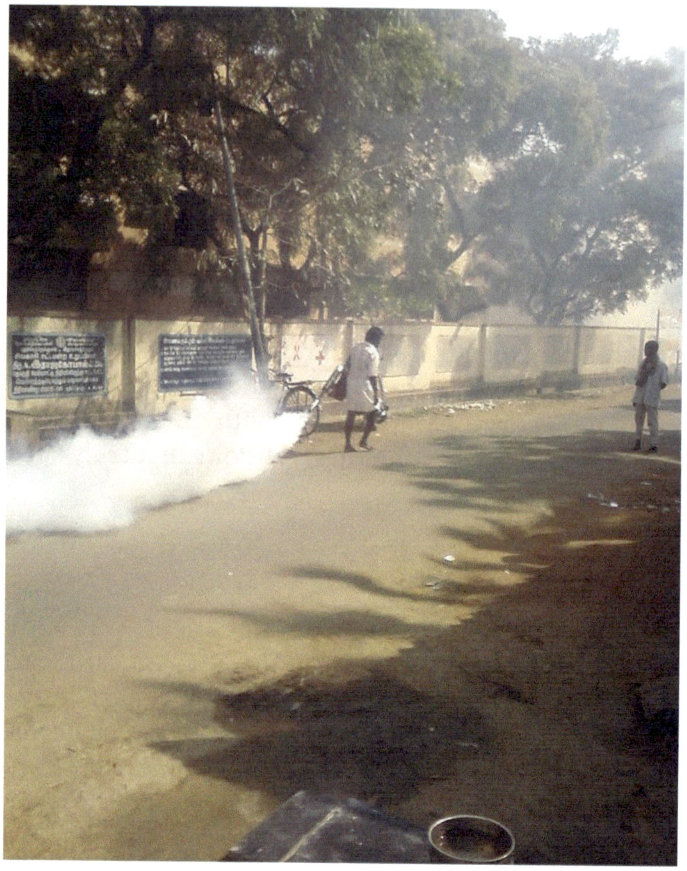

Figure 3.17. Mosquito control.

Source: By Srithern - Own work, CC BY-SA 3.0, https://commons.wikimedia.org/w/index.php?curid=23524718

3.5.1. Chemical Control Methods

Mosquito-borne diseases have been a nuisance lately and have led us to try out different ways of fighting the disease-ridden pests. Chemicals have been attempted and employed for a long time now as an instant measure, spraying adult pests and larvae to interfere with their cycle and slow down the multiplication. Sometimes this approach is quite instant, but it is not snag-free. Mosquitoes can build up resistance over time, and there is that risk of chemicals damaging the environment or even striking off-target baddies we'd prefer to leave alone. In spite of these deterrents, chemical solutions keep reappearing as a one-size-fits-all answer in epidemic situations due to their speed and ability to be scaled up when needed, though they definitely need to be optimized as part of an overall strategy (Aguilar-Durán et al., 2024). Examining more closely chemical control within urban environments—particularly in locations that often struggle with dengue—the outcomes can be a bit of a mixed bag. Some research within affluent urban centers indicates that insecticides and larvicides are able to significantly reduce the number of Aedes. Strangely, however, lower numbers of mosquitoes do not always translate to lower incidences of disease. Mosquito behavior, human behavior, and the environmental conditions of the area seem to mix together and form a puzzle that can't be fully solved by simple spraying alone. Overall, this means that reducing the number of mosquitoes is key, but it's not the whole story; incorporating practices like enhanced environmental control and biological controls may be the missing spark needed (Durrance-Bagale et al., 2024). Combining chemical methods with newer strategies offers a promising, if not always linear, way forward. To date, for instance, the use of traps, such as autocidal gravid ovitraps, to be used in combination with larvicidal and adulticidal sprays has resulted in spectacular reduction in the populations of *Aedes aegypti*, but only where adequate traps and chemicals reach saturation. The combined strategies are based on mosquito behavior in innovative ways, seeking more targeted impact and possibly slowing down resistance development. But on closer inspection, it appears that the magic bullet is wide coverage and real community participation; in the absence of a lot of traps or frequent chemical spraying, populations of mosquitoes can recover at once, undermining early successes. Chemical treatments in most cases should instead be viewed not as singletons but as useful supporting pieces inserted into locally modified vector management plans (Aguilar-Durán et al., 2024).

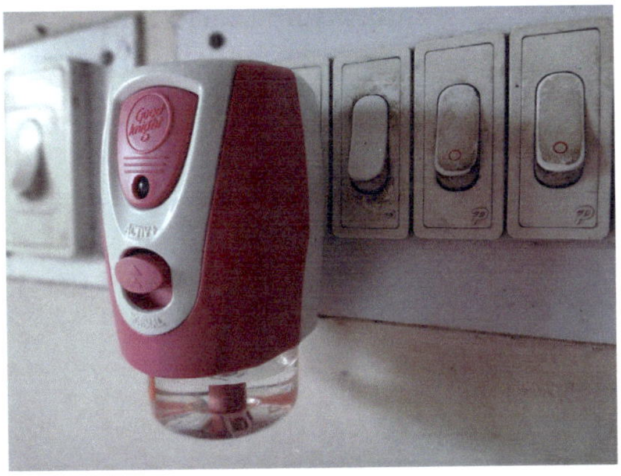

Source: By Gausanchennai - Own work, CC BY-SA 4.0, https://commons.wikimedia.org/w/index.php?curid=75802178

3.5.2. Biological Control Methods

Mosquito control has become an interesting turn these days as people opt more into biological practices for sustainability and a lighter environmental impact. Adult resting collections, for example, allow us to have a glimpse into the behavior of mosquitoes and even into the ways of their physiology—information that could give rise to more targeted interventions. Researchers have tried sampling designs concentrating on the resting behavior of primary and secondary vectors to deconvolute disease dynamics; however, even quite thorough efforts on species like *Aedes triseriatus* and its invasive relatives, some resting site collections end up with just too few catches. This combination of outcomes, though not entirely unexpected—suggests that ecological systems have limitations, and it often underscores the need to alter our methods of sampling to better augment vector behaviors and environments so that ultimately, there can be more efficient means of control (Nordgulen et al., 2024). One of the most interesting features of biological control is that it is carried out through the use of symbiotic friendly bacteria like Wolbachia. This tiny bacterium has been in the spotlight for its power to regulate mosquito reproduction and disease transmission. Techniques such as the sterile insect technique (SIT) and the incompatible insect technique (IIT) take advantage of the reproductive-disrupting capacity of Wolbachia, which generally yields fewer mosquitoes. These techniques have proven useful not only against a number of insect pest species but also, most importantly, against Aedes mosquitoes—the unwanted arboviral disease vectors. Outside vector control, Wolbachia can even be involved in managing agribusiness pests, proposing a multi-functional, nature-sourced means. With modern molecular tools helping to bridge the gap between SIT and IIT, there is an entirely new generation of sustainable vector control that seeks to find an equilibrium between raw efficacy and environmental sensitivity (Hyder et al., 2024). How effective these Wolbachia-based methods are ultimately depends on figuring out the challenging dynamics between mosquitoes and their bacterial symbionts. The bacterium works in all sorts of modes, sometimes as a beneficial mutualist and sometimes more akin to a pest in itself—impacting everything from reproductive biology to the efficiency with which a mosquito can spread disease. New research, integrating multi-omics data with functional tests of genes, is slowly unspooling these complex interactions, which in turn enables researchers to engineer Wolbachia strains for very specific control applications. However, there remain challenges, ecological threats, moral concerns, and an ongoing need for proper risk evaluations to occur along the way. In most cases, going forward means developing interdisciplinary collaborations and remaining open to furthering these biological methods so they are responsibly integrated into more holistic vector control programs aimed at reducing the prevalence of mosquito-borne illness over the long term (Hyder et al., 2024) (Figure 3.18).

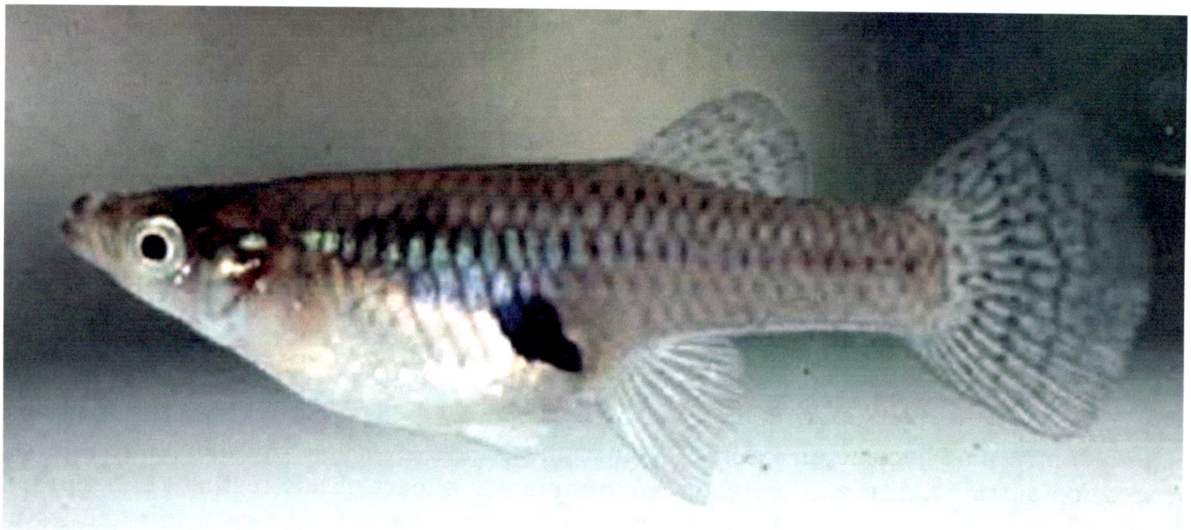

Figure 3.18. Biological control methods.

Source: Public Domain, https://commons.wikimedia.org/w/index.php?curid=1616904

3.5.3. Integrated Pest Management (IPM) Approaches

Mosquito populations are a nasty, complex lot, and since these little insects spread disease, we have to use a whole arsenal of strategies short of spraying pesticides. Integrated pest management (IPM) combines biological, chemical, environmental, and even genetic methods to cut their numbers down without decimating nature. Humans track how many there are and where they breed, taking action only when things get way out of hand. In Thailand and other nations where local environments vary, the use of GIS and land-use maps has refined these efforts (Overgaard et al., 2025). By integrating spatial data with information on mosquito behavior, the approach enables us to cut back on large-scale use of insecticides and averts the build-up of resistance. This balanced, dynamic method shows that we need to adjust our strategies to protect nature as well as public health. Advances in genetic and molecular technology have in fact opened the playbook of mosquito control in recent years. Techniques like SIT, RIDL, and gene drive systems disrupt the reproduction of mosquitoes as well as their genetic composition. These approaches in the majority of cases draw ideas from evolution to prevent undesirable side effects, like resistance—in a collaborative endeavor by joining many steps. There are also RNAi and CRISPR-based approaches that appear to be good for adjusting mosquito biology at the very minute level. When these newer techniques are integrated with the core IPM operations, we are seeing a boost in effectiveness and long-term duration that also decreases environmental harm (Bolton et al., 2015). This multi-layered approach takes us into a future for vector control that gets down to the nasty business of disease transmission. Even with all of these new concepts, IPM is not without its problems. Natural variability in the ecosystem, cumulative community reactions, and occasional off-target hit on non-target organisms guarantee that the problems never cease. Effective programs must be regularly checked and fine-tuned as mosquito populations and environmental variables fluctuate. Occasionally, the integration of the introduction of the addition of such measures as habitat manipulation or water management adjustments along with genetic and chemical interventions could prove to augment control while leaving ecosystems relatively unscathed (Overgaard et al., 2025). Education and gaining public support are no less crucial ensuring that local customs and cultures are preserved and that the effort continues. Controlling disease-transmitting vectors ultimately boils down to cooperation, remaining up to date with research, and achieving a balance between human health and an honest regard for nature, a refrain repeated in modern conservation and public health policy (Bolton et al., 2015).

3.6. Current Research in Vector Biology

Technology's sudden bounds are now disrupting how scientists monitor mosquitoes, and this change is providing us with a new perspective on vector biology. The traditional methods—those clunky, hands-on approaches—are usually restrictive, giving us a limited view and too much tunnel vision, making it difficult to get the complete ecological picture. Recently, the marriage of computer vision with deep learning has provided a clean, continuous way of monitoring insects over sunny days and seasons of change. Insect monitoring systems outdoors and in laboratories, for instance, now automatically gather mountains of data about the numbers, size, and kind of mosquitoes with unimagined levels of accuracy before. These digital methods even enable researchers to capture minor changes in behavior and physical features, repeatedly going over and over their focus on central details. Yet there is more to be done – like demanding better image-based taxonomic checks, robust training collections, and balanced reference databases – all of which are crucial if we are to augment sensor-based surveillance for vector research and disease management schemes (Høye et al., 2021). Mosquito-borne diseases seem to be making quite the return in our fast-moving world, which is driving us to integrate evolutionary biology and biomedical knowledge. It seems that the early enthusiasm of outwitting infectious diseases has paled a little before the harsh reality of drug-resistant diseases and mosquitos (yes, occasionally with a single 's' surprisingly) spreading their wings in the context of, for instance, malaria and dengue. Generally, new research calls us to wonder how pathogens learn to adapt and how resistance to insecticides finds its way in. It's no longer Band-Aids, no; it's a long-haul, adaptive strategy for health, and one that evolutionary ecology can guide us toward. Observing the challenging, interconnected connections of mosquitoes, their disease vectors, and the world in general gives us opportunities that can lead to the prevention of resistance and the shelf life of our control measures.

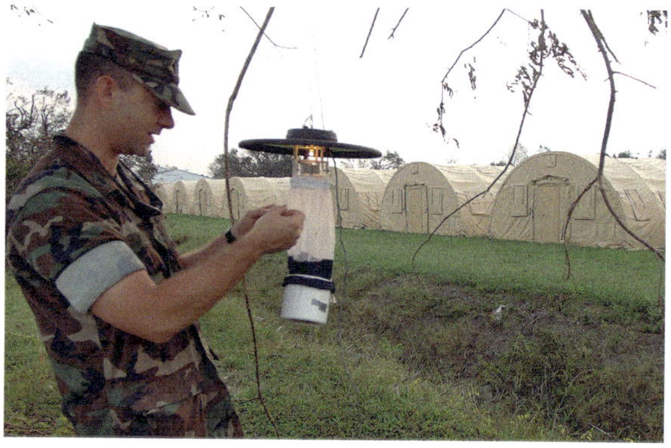

Source: By U.S. Navy photo - This image was released by the United States Navy with the ID 050910-N-2653P-132 (next).https://commons.wikimedia.org/w/index.php?curid=8215246

For most cases, these ideas align with greater sustainable health goals as we are also confronted with issues necessitated by climate change and urbanization (Echaubard et al., 2018). There is also mounting literature that is putting a spotlight on the mosquito disease transmission evolutionary association. Researchers are currently unlayering unsuspecting trade-offs in mosquito genetics and environmental pressure - conditions that regulate such traits as parasite survival inside the insect as well as how the life strategy of the mosquito can shift, especially in the face of such instruments as ITNs. From time to time, these kinds of computational models, which combine reasonable evolutionary principles with real data, propose means by which changing our strategy can minimize resistance risk and maximize overall control success. Primarily, through enabling evolutionary ideas to inform our investigations and public health policy—a reasoning that occasionally stumbles into vernacular words somewhere along the line—we could perhaps finally make headway to stay one jump ahead of the mosquito-pathogen race, prolonging our disease management programs further and better (Echaubard et al., 2018).

3.6.1. Advances in Genetic Modification of Mosquitoes

Molecular biology has recently literally turned our understanding of mosquito genetics on its head, especially for those pestiferous species that transmit malaria. New genetic tools enable scientists to observe and even alter with the *Anopheles* genome, yielding eye-opening revelations into how these pathogens defend themselves, produce more of themselves, and behave. Oftener than not, these novel findings engender ideas for particular treatments that may suppress mosquitoes or make them less effective at carrying diseases. New-edge transgenic methods now hold the promise of breaking free from the conventional chemical chemicals to a more targeted, genetic strategy (Catteruccia et al., 2009). In a way, it is a potential turning point in the fight against mosquito-borne disease through targeting the very makeup of the insect. One of the giant strides in this regard is engineering mosquito genes to induce sterility—a shift that could revolutionize population management. Traditionally, programs utilize the SIT where males are sterilized using radiation and compete with wild ones, but radiation sometimes renders these mosquitoes vulnerable, thus lowering overall effectiveness. Genetic modification circumvents that issue by making sterile males through non-irradiation, a condition that in most cases enhances their competitiveness and allows population control more effectively. Strategies employed with insects like *Drosophila* tend to be rough blueprints for adapting the same methods for use with *Anopheles* mosquitoes. In general, the idea of genetically breeding mosquitoes to be sterile is a significant step toward more effective, sustainable means of controlling vectors (Catteruccia et al., 2009)—once more illustrating the growing marriage of molecular genetics and public health. The study is also more than just inducing sterility. Researchers are also tampering with mosquito genes in order to block transmission of pathogens altogether. They're employing vectors to deliver genes that can make the mosquitoes resistant to malaria *parasites*, shorten their lifespans, or even alter their feeding patterns, something that could bring the disease cycle to a standstill.

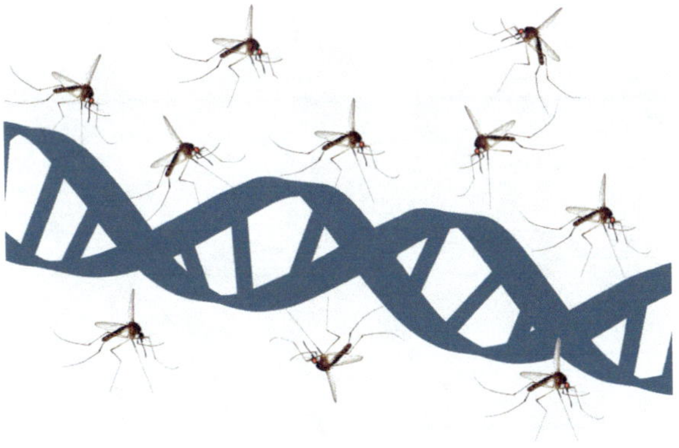

Source: National Institutes of Health. (2015). Gene drive research takes aim at malaria. *NIH Director's Blog*. https://directorsblog.nih.gov/wp-content/uploads/2015/11/mosquito-and-dna1.jpg.

The rapidity of gene editing—thanks to CRISPR-Cas technology—is now enabling researchers to design mosquito strains with very specific traits almost in real-time. Initial laboratory and half-field experiments show that these genetically modified mosquitoes withstand real-world conditions, making the possibility of future field trials imminent. However, the ecological and ethical risks involved in releasing genetically modified mosquitoes need to be carefully weighed. In most cases, merging molecular biologists, ecologists, and policymakers is essential to ensure that such innovations are introduced safely (Catteruccia et al., 2009; Catteruccia et al., 2009).

3.6.2. Studies on Mosquito Ecology and Behavior

Mosquito larvae that associate in breeding locations control their population in far more complicated patterns than simple association. Cannibalism, for instance, is an essential force that modulates personal fitness as well as the overall constitution of the population. This is not some random behavior at all—it tends to be a matter of local circumstances such as how densely packed the region is, how rich the resources are, and even the shape of the breeding habitats. A combination of laboratory tests and simulation studies on *Aedes albopictus* suggests that spatial arrangements of aquatic conditions can have the effect of getting predators and potential victims to meet each other at certain frequencies. In the majority of cases, natural heterogeneity in breeding sites not only modulates encounter rates but also determines the conditions for the presence of cannibalism, and this increases the level of insight into mosquito larval ecology and vector control programs (Mastrantonio et al., 2018). Reading through the details of mosquito resistance and its battle with malaria *parasites* reminds us that the natural environment is worth a great deal. Traditional lab models have long given us some clues about mosquito–*Plasmodium* interactions, but they often disregard the details of the field. Ecological immunology, in most instances, examines how environmental pressures, for example, variations in host density, parasite diversity, and shifting environments—cause immune responses to vary. This way of thinking values that evolutionary pressures and population dynamics influence both immune function and pathogen virulence, so fieldwork is key to understanding transmission dynamics. This is a critical form of strategy in informing malaria control via mechanisms that are ecologically sound and evolutionary sensible (Tripet, 2009). Integration of ecological and behavioral studies also provides an understanding of how populations of mosquitoes rapidly adapt to their environments, which also informs disease risk. Behavioral elements—whether looking at larval interactions, where they mate, or feeding behavior—have their roots in some interaction between genetic makeup and external pressures. The unique features of breeding sites, for example, can affect larval survival through cannibalism but also affect adult emergence rates and overall vector potential. It needs a complete integration of laboratory experiments, computer simulations, and field measurements to account for all the aspects of ecological processes. Information regarding these various layers is utilized to develop enhanced predictive models for the population of mosquitoes and makes control measures based on natural knowledge to disrupt mosquito life cycles more accurately (Figure 3.19).

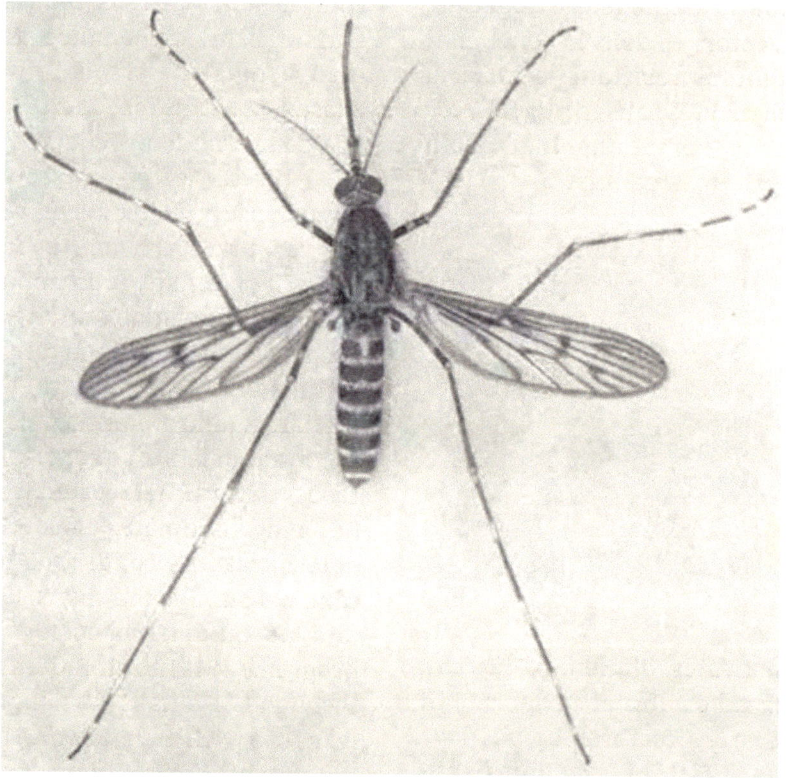

Figure 3.19. Ecology of mosquitoes.

Source: By John Frederick Marshall, 5. 8. 1875 - 5. 12. 1949John Frederick Marshall, British Entomologist, born 5 September 1874, died 5 December 1949 - J. F. Marshall (1938) The British Mosquitoes. Plate XIII., Public Domain, https://commons.wikimedia.org/w/index.php?curid=8968177.

3.6.3. Innovations in Disease Prevention and Control

Vaccine research has come a long way in fighting mosquito-borne illnesses, malaria, for instance, being one of the strongest contenders. One idea that is picking up steam is the use of genetically attenuated parasites (GAP) to suppress their own development in the liver, a process which in most cases prevents the *parasites* from ever making it to the blood stage where symptoms and signs are expressed. This illusion not only decreases the potential for infection but also seems to lead the immune system to create some kind of sterile, long-term protection. Take, for example, the *P. berghei* Δb9Δslarp GAP; it not only fully prevents liver-stage growth and even causes immunity in other mouse models with quite low doses of parasites. These focused vaccine approaches portend live vaccines that combine safety and efficacy, a gradual but transformative pathway toward preemptive disease control within regions where such diseases are prevalent (Kaindoa et al., 2013). Addressing mosquito population control, there have been a few forward-thinking developments in recent years. Genetic tools like gene drive technologies are now used to make changes in mosquitoes by introducing traits that either render them incapable of transmitting diseases or stop them from propagating—a green solution to the majority of conventional insecticides which, in all honesty, have issues with resistance and environmental toxicity. apart from that, advances in mapping the spatial location of breeding places of mosquitoes currently pinpoint high-risk areas more effectively, which facilitates planning interventions better aligned with reality. In most but a few cases, integrating these tools enables public health teams to achieve more with their resources and interrupt disease transmission in a way that tackles a broader image of mosquito biology as well as control interventions (London School of Hygiene & Tropical Medicine, 2013). On a separate front, developments in surveillance and diagnostic technologies are making early detection of outbreaks easier. Molecular diagnostics combined with handheld devices enable scientists to quickly identify pathogens in mosquitoes—a vital asset for coping with diseases like dengue, Zika, and chikungunya. Data platforms, however, help to form a world view of outbreak patterns, giving public health officials a critical edge when epidemics begin. This forward-looking thinking is a tidy synthesis of molecular biology wisdom, entomology's attention to detail, and information technology know-how, all combining new and interesting ways. Overall, when you combine these novel vaccine strategies, genetic adjustments, and speedy diagnostic advances, you get a multilayered system that contemporary disease prevention relies on, despite the occasional glitch in delivery.

CLOSER LOOK

CHIKUNGUNYA

Chikungunya is a viral disease transmitted by the Chikungunya virus (CHIKV), transmitted predominantly by the bite of an infected female *Aedes aegypti* or *Aedes albopictus* mosquito, as with dengue and Zika viruses. First discovered in Tanzania in 1952, chikungunya has since caused numerous outbreaks in Africa, Asia, Europe, and the Americas. The title "chikungunya" is from the Makonde language and translates as "to become contorted," depicting patients' stooping posture resulting from severe joint pain, one of the typical symptoms of the disease. After being bitten by an infected mosquito, the virus stays in the human body for 3 to 7 days before it manifests as symptoms. Chikungunya typically begins with an acute onset of high fever, accompanied by severe pain in the joints, particularly the hands, feet, wrists, and ankles. Muscle ache, headache, fatigue, nausea, vomiting, and rash are also typically present. The acute symptoms usually last for a duration of about a week; however, pain in the joints may continue to weeks or even months in some individuals, especially older adults, or those with previous joint disease, to produce chronic arthritis-like signs.

Though chikungunya is never lethal, it is a very disabling and uncomfortable disease, which has social as well as economic consequences in the endemic regions. Most of the patients recover, but there are occasional complications such as neurological syndromes, myocarditis, ophthalmic disease, or aggravation of pre-existing diseases. The disease is clinically diagnosed and later supported by laboratory studies such as RT-PCR, which detects the viral RNA, or serological studies such as ELISA, which identifies specific antibodies (IgM and IgG) against the virus. There is no known specific antiviral drug for the treatment of chikungunya till date; treatment is symptomatic and supportive with rest, fluids, and analgesic medication such as paracetamol. Non-steroidal anti-inflammatory drugs (NSAIDs) must be given with caution, particularly in case of suspected co-infection with dengue, to prevent the danger of bleeding disorders.

Prevention of chikungunya relies mostly on the control of mosquitoes and avoidance measures. They include destroying mosquito breeding sites by drainage of standing water in containers, use of insect repellents, use of long-sleeved clothing, and screening windows and doors. Control of outbreaks and public health education also play significant roles at the community level in the control of mosquitoes and limiting the virus transmission. While there is no vaccine commercially available for chikungunya as of this writing, research and testing are ongoing, with some vaccine candidates showing promise. Chikungunya continues to pose a threat to public health, particularly in subtropical and tropical regions where the Aedes mosquito is prevalent. Urbanization, climate change, and increasing international travel have facilitated the virus's spread to new regions. In conclusion, chikungunya is a debilitating but generally non-lethal viral illness causing intense joint pain and swelling. Mosquito population control, public awareness, and vaccine development are essential to managing and ultimately preventing chikungunya within populations globally.

SUMMARY

Mosquito activity is a complex mix of circumstances. Weather isn't just scenery—sudden temperature fluctuations, unexpected humidity changes, and even an unexpected shower or sprinkle will guide their actions in ways you can't always predict. You'll notice that each type will react in its own way, and factors like these will drive population highs and lows in specific seasons as well as modulate their potential to be vectors of disease. And behold, the entire process is rather complex: these environmental signals are combinable with the internal processes of every mosquito, such that there can be no doubt that it is imperative to know such strange responses to craft a good control regimen. When researchers synthesize real-world information and field observations, they acquire wisdom such that they can forecast outbreaks and perfectly time interventions (Baril et al., 2023). Even when weather provides the backdrop, what is happening inside the mosquito is also important. Generally speaking, feeding habits and reproductive features play a large role in deciding how they are going to function as disease agents. Studies suggest that mating is not necessarily going to alter a mosquito's first blood meal but will affect feedings down the road and eventually egg laying. A finer inspection of sugar intake and dieting factors makes it even more complex, and laboratory experiments will supposedly have to try to mimic such natural conditions as precisely as possible (League et al., 2021). It tends to make it a lot more complicated when it comes to internal processes vs. external factors, which adds yet another essential detail to our information on how such insects operate. In summary, marrying insight into nature's sudden signals with mosquito inner life gives us a richer, if more frantic, image for public health. In the majority of cases, effective control measures can't be complete; they need to match local weather features and the pests' unique life rhythms to effectively hold disease transmission in check. Simplified, when you combine ecology with internal physiological processes like feeding and mating, you realize that each turn of the tale matters. Ongoing, cross-disciplinary research activities that integrate ecology, physiology, and epidemiology remain necessary to enhance the control of mosquitoes and reduce the global health burden of vector-borne diseases (League et al., 2021; Baril et al., 2023).

Effective public health depends to a very large degree on our comprehension of how vector biology is engaged with disease transmission. In earlier times, controlling these insects meant a plunge into local environmental details – subsequently insecticides became the center of attention. That revolution, however, sometimes overlooked the nasty, capricious character of mosquitoes and the delicate sensitivities of the diseases they carry; resistance to insecticides ensued. More recently, experts are calling for the integration of experiential ecological understanding with technical entomological skills. In most cases, integrating a variety of control methods—each altered to the uniqueness of a specific mosquito species and its habitat—can improve the quality and the longevity of interventions. These principles remind us that adaptation to fluctuate environmental cues and vector change is paramount, and that chemicals by themselves are not enough; we need to look for non-insecticidal avenues as well to keep disease cycles in check (Wilson et al., 2020). Recent research on vector biology has unearthed novel biocontrol methods that present a most welcome alternative to conventional insecticides. Take, for instance, the release of Wolbachia-infected mosquitos—most famously the wAlbB strain within *Aedes aegypti*, which tends to work by biological interference to cut back on dengue virus transmission. Field trials, held within many urban settings, have established that Wolbachia can stably get a foothold within mosquito populations while causing disruption to the usual process of pathogen transmission; most crucially, these trials even saw an overall decrease in human cases of dengue. Moreover, the heat tolerance of the wAlbB strain, in the majority of cases, surpasses that of past Wolbachia strains and thus it is an option for use in warmer climates where dengue is prevalent. All this signifies a paradigm shift in vector control, with pathogen blocking and gene modification of mosquitoes being given priority as a path toward long-term disease control (Nazni et al., 2019). In summary, the bottom line is that preventing mosquito-borne disease requires a multifaceted approach with solid evidence. While insecticides previously provided answers in the short term, now they need to be buttressed by ecological insight and novel biological tools to fight resistance and ecological changes. The addition of Wolbachia-based strategies presents innovative potential and very well complements the traditional methods, a reflection of the dynamic nature of vector biology science. Continued, diligent dedication to these mixed programs—integrating native ecological knowledge with modern technology—appears imperative for keeping cycles of disease at bay. Ultimately, sustainable mosquito control is about putting local ecology first, utilizing a wide array of intervention tools, and keeping a vigilant eye for improvement to address the global burden of the diseases (Nazni et al., 2019; Wilson et al., 2020).

KEY TERMS FROM THIS CHAPTER

Anopheles	Aedes	Culex
Vector Competence	Vector Capacity	Host Preference
Anthropophilic	Zoophilic	Endophagic
Exophagic	Endophilic	Exophilic
Larval Habitat	Breeding Sites	Gonotrophic Cycle
Sporogonic Cycle	Vectorial Efficiency	Insecticide Resistance
Entomological Inoculation Rate	Parous Rate	

References

1. Kohl, A., Pondeville, E., Schnettler, E., Crisanti, A., Supparo, C., Christophides, G. K., Kersey, P. J., Maslen, G. L., Takken, W., Koenraadt, C. J., Oliva, C. F., Busquets, N., Abad, F. X., Failloux, A. B., Levashina, E. A., Wilson, A. J., Veronesi, E., Pichard, M., Arnaud Marsh, S., Simard, F., ... Vernick, K. D. (2016). Advancing vector biology research: a community survey for future directions, research applications and infrastructure requirements. *Pathogens and global health*, *110*(4-5), 164–172. https://doi.org/10.1080/20477724.2016.1211475 (accessed on 13 May 2025).
2. Huho, B., Briët, O., Seyoum, A., Sikaala, C., Bayoh, N., Gimnig, J., Okumu, F., Diallo, D., Abdulla, S., Smith, T., & Killeen, G. (2013). Consistently high estimates for the proportion of human exposure to malaria vector populations occurring indoors in rural Africa. *International journal of epidemiology*, *42*(1), 235–247. https://doi.org/10.1093/ije/dys214 (accessed on 13 May 2025).
3. Achee, N. L., Grieco, J. P., Vatandoost, H., Seixas, G., Pinto, J., Ching-NG, L., Martins, A. J., et al. (2019). Alternative strategies for mosquito-borne arbovirus control. *PLoS Neglected Tropical Diseases, 13*, e0006822. https://doi.org/10.1371/journal.pntd.0006822.
4. Aguilar-Durán, J. A., Hamer, G. L., Reyes-Villanueva, F., Fernández-Santos, N. A., Uriegas-Camargo, S., Rodríguez-Martínez, L. M., Estrada-Franco, J. G., & Rodríguez-Pérez, M. A. (2024). Effectiveness of mass trapping interventions using autocidal gravid ovitraps (AGO) for the control of the dengue vector, Aedes (Stegomyia) aegypti, in Northern Mexico. *Parasites & vectors*, *17*(1), 344. https://doi.org/10.1186/s13071-024-06361-y(accessed on 13 May 2025).
5. Jones, C. M., Haji, K. A., Khatib, B. O., Bagi, J., Mcha, J., Devine, G. J., Daley, M., Kabula, B., Ali, A. S., Majambere, S., & Ranson, H. (2013). The dynamics of pyrethroid resistance in Anopheles arabiensis from Zanzibar and an assessment of the underlying genetic basis. *Parasites & vectors*, *6*, 343. https://doi.org/10.1186/1756-3305-6-343 (accessed on 13 May 2025).
6. Grech, M. G., Miserendino, M. L., & Almirón, W. R. (2023). The role of temperature in shaping *Culex acharistus* mosquitoes life history traits in its southern limit of distribution (Patagonia-Argentina). *Heliyon*, *9*(2), e13696. https://doi.org/10.1016/j.heliyon.2023.e13696 (accessed on 13 May 2025).
7. Lutambi, A. M., Penny, M. A., Smith, T., & Chitnis, N. (2013). Mathematical modelling of mosquito dispersal in a heterogeneous environment. *Mathematical biosciences*, *241*(2), 198–216. https://doi.org/10.1016/j.mbs.2012.11.013 (accessed on 13 May 2025).
8. Baril, C., Pilling, B. G., Mikkelsen, M. J., Sparrow, J. M., Duncan, C. A. M., Koloski, C. W., LaZerte, S., et al. (2023). The influence of weather on the population dynamics of common mosquito vector species in the Canadian Prairies. *Parasites & Vectors, 16*, Article 183. https://doi.org/10.1186/s13071-023-05760-x.
9. Bellini, R., Crasta, G., Mastrantonio, V., Porretta, D., et al. (2018). Cannibalism in temporary waters: Simulations and laboratory experiments revealed the role of spatial shape in the mosquito *Aedes albopictus*. https://core.ac.uk/download/158822477.pdf Mastrantonio, V., Crasta, G., Puggioli, A., Bellini, R., Urbanelli, S., & Porretta, D. (2018). Cannibalism in temporary waters: Simulations and laboratory experiments revealed the role of spatial shape in the mosquito Aedes albopictus. *PloS one*, *13*(5), e0198194. https://doi.org/10.1371/journal.pone.0198194 (accessed on 13 May 2025).

10. Catteruccia, F., Crisanti, A. & Wimmer, E.A. Transgenic technologies to induce sterility. *Malar J* **8** (Suppl 2), S7 (2009). https://doi.org/10.1186/1475-2875-8-S2-S7
11. Bharti, P., Carney, R. M., Chellappan, S., McClinton III, D., et al. (2020). Automating the surveillance of mosquito vectors from trapped specimens using computer vision techniques. http://arxiv.org/abs/2005.12188 (accessed on 13 May 2025).
12. Bolton, M., Chapman, T., & Leftwich, P. (2015). Evolutionary biology and genetic techniques for insect control. https://core.ac.uk/download/41991375.pdf (accessed on 13 May 2025).
13. Boyer, S., Dehecq, J. S., Delatte, H., Fontenille, D., et al. (2012). Life traits of Aedes mosquitoes as factors of arboviruses emergence: S1304TU01. Medical and Veterinary Entomology. http://agritrop.cirad.fr/568193/1/document_568193.pdf (accessed on 13 May 2025).
14. Camp, L., Luckhart, S., Nadler, S. A., Pakpour, N., et al. (2013). Protein kinase C-dependent signaling controls the midgut epithelial barrier to malaria parasite infection in anopheline mosquitoes. https://core.ac.uk/download/323068952.pdf.
15. Manica, M., Filipponi, F., D'Alessandro, A., Screti, A., Neteler, M., Rosà, R., Solimini, A., Della Torre, A., & Caputo, B. (2016). Spatial and Temporal Hot Spots of Aedes albopictus Abundance inside and outside a South European Metropolitan Area. *PLoS neglected tropical diseases, 10*(6), e0004758. https://doi.org/10.1371/journal.pntd.0004758 (accessed on 13 May 2025).
16. Carlson, J. R., Menuz, K., Reisert, J., Su, C. Y., et al. (2012). Non-synaptic inhibition between grouped neurons in an olfactory circuit. https://core.ac.uk/download/323066407.pdf.
17. Chaves, L. F., & Koenraadt, C. J. M. (2010). Climate change and highland malaria: Fresh air for a hot debate. https://core.ac.uk/download/pdf/29238217.pdf (accessed on 13 May 2025).
18. Couper, L., Farner, J. E., Caldwell, J. M., Childs, M. L., Harris, M., Kirk, D., Nova, N., et al. (2021). How will mosquitoes adapt to climate warming? *eLife, 10*, e69630. https://doi.org/10.7554/elife.69630.
19. Domingos, A., Pinheiro-Silva, R., Couto, J., do Rosário, V., & de la Fuente, J. (2017). The Anopheles gambiae transcriptome - a turning point for malaria control. *Insect molecular biology, 26*(2), 140–151. https://doi.org/10.1111/imb.12289(accessed on 13 May 2025).
20. de Wet, N., Hales, S., Slaney, D., Warrick, R., et al. (2005). Hotspots: Modelling capacity for vector-borne disease risk analysis in New Zealand: A case study of *Ochlerotatus camptorhynchus* incursions. https://core.ac.uk/download/29194963.pdf (accessed on 13 May 2025).
21. Diallo, D., Diouf, B., Gaye, A., Ndiaye, E. H., Sene, N. M., Dia, I., & Diallo, M. (2022). Dengue vectors in Africa: A review. *Heliyon, 8*, e09459. https://doi.org/10.1016/j.heliyon.2022.e09459.
22. Douglas, A. E. (2014). Multiorganismal insects: Diversity and function of resident microorganisms. *Annual Review of Entomology, 60*, 17–34. https://doi.org/10.1146/annurev-ento-010814-020822.
23. Durrance-Bagale, A., Hoe, N., Lai, J., Liew, J., Clapham, H., & Howard, N. (2024). Dengue vector control in high-income, city settings: A scoping review of approaches and methods. *PLOS Neglected Tropical Diseases, 18*. https://www.semanticscholar.org/paper/a9117fdc2de531d46c34a1df1076d4da9c73e3cf (accessed on 13 May 2025).
24. Echaubard, P., Rudge, J. W., & Léfèvre, T. (2018). Evolutionary perspectives on human infectious diseases: Challenges, advances, and promises. *Evolutionary Applications, 11*, 383–393. https://doi.org/10.1111/eva.12586.

25. Ewing, D. A., Cobbold, C. A., Purse, B. V., Nunn, M. A., & White, S. M. (2016). Modelling the effect of temperature on the seasonal population dynamics of temperate mosquitoes. *Journal of Theoretical Biology, 400*, 65–79. https://doi.org/10.1016/j.jtbi.2016.04.008.

26. Lyimo, I. N., Keegan, S. P., Ranford-Cartwright, L. C., & Ferguson, H. M. (2012). The impact of uniform and mixed species blood meals on the fitness of the mosquito vector Anopheles gambiae s.s: does a specialist pay for diversifying its host species diet?. *Journal of evolutionary biology*, *25*(3), 452–460. https://doi.org/10.1111/j.1420-9101.2011.02442.x (accessed on 13 May 2025).

27. Govella, N. J., & Ferguson, H. (2012). Why Use of Interventions Targeting Outdoor Biting Mosquitoes will be Necessary to Achieve Malaria Elimination. *Frontiers in physiology*, *3*, 199. https://doi.org/10.3389/fphys.2012.00199(accessed on 13 May 2025).

28. Ferraguti, M., Martins, A. D., & Artzy-Randrup, Y. (2023). Quantifying the invasion risk of West Nile virus: Insights from a multi-vector and multi-host SEIR model. *One Health, 17*, 100638. https://doi.org/10.1016/j.onehlt.2023.100638.

29. George, A. M., Ansumana, R., de Souza, D. K., Niyas, V. K. M., Zumla, A., & Bockarie, M. J. (2023). Climate change and the rising incidence of vector-borne diseases globally. *International Journal of Infectious Diseases, 139*, 143–145. https://doi.org/10.1016/j.ijid.2023.12.004.

30. Ghaninia, M. (2007). Olfaction in mosquitoes. https://core.ac.uk/download/11695204.pdf (accessed on 13 May 2025).

31. Gillen, Alan L. and Sherwin, Frank, "The Genesis of Malaria: The Origin of Mosquitoes and Their Protistan Cargo, Plasmodium falciparum" (2013). Faculty Publications and Presentations. 136. https://digitalcommons.liberty.edu/bio_chem_fac_pubs/136 (accessed on 13 May 2025).

32. Giunti, G., Becker, N., & Benelli, G. (2023). Invasive mosquito vectors in Europe: From bioecology to surveillance and management. *Acta Tropica, 239*, 106832. https://doi.org/10.1016/j.actatropica.2023.106832.

33. Kuno, G., Mackenzie, J. S., Junglen, S., Hubálek, Z., Plyusnin, A., & Gubler, D. J. (2017). Vertebrate Reservoirs of Arboviruses: Myth, Synonym of Amplifier, or Reality?. *Viruses*, *9*(7), 185. https://doi.org/10.3390/v9070185 (accessed on 13 May 2025).

34. Govella, N.J., Chaki, P.P. & Killeen, G.F. Entomological surveillance of behavioural resilience and resistance in residual malaria vector populations. *Malar J* **12**, 124 (2013). https://doi.org/10.1186/1475-2875-12-124 (accessed on 13 May 2025).

35. Høye, T. T., Ärje, J., Bjerge, K., Hansen, O. L. P., Iosifidis, A., Leese, F., Mann, H. M. R., et al. (2021). Deep learning and computer vision will transform entomology. *Proceedings of the National Academy of Sciences, 118*, e2002545117. https://doi.org/10.1073/pnas.2002545117.

36. Hyder, M., Lodhi, A. M., Wang, Z., Bukero, A., Gao, J., & Mao, R. (2024). *Wolbachia* interactions with diverse insect hosts: From reproductive modulations to sustainable pest management strategies. *Biology, 13*. https://www.semanticscholar.org/paper/3e14fcaa16ece553accfbebde704b47c8a39d38b (accessed on 13 May 2025).

37. Jones, C. M., Hughes, G. L., Coleman, S., Fellows, R., & Quilliam, R. S. (2024). A perspective on the impacts of microplastics on mosquito biology and their vectorial capacity. *Medical and Veterinary Entomology, 38*, 138–147. https://doi.org/10.1111/mve.12652.

38. Okumu, F. O., Sumaye, R. D., Matowo, N. S., Mwangungulu, S. P., Kaindoa, E. W., Moshi, I. R.,

Madumla, E. P., & Lwetoijera, D. W. (2013). Outdoor mosquito control using odour-baited devices: development and evaluation of a potential new strategy to complement indoor malaria prevention methods. *MalariaWorld journal, 4*, 8. https://doi.org/10.5281/zenodo.10894810

39. Keller, A., Kiszewski, A., Kozomara, A., Marco, A., Nikaki, A., Oshlack, A., Teleman, A. A., et al. (2016). Identification and characterization of microRNAs expressed in the African malaria vector *Anopheles* funestus life stages using high throughput sequencing. https://core.ac.uk/download/80548975.pdf (accessed on 13 May 2025).

40. Knipling, E. F., & Lindquist, A. W. (1957). Recent advances in veterinary entomology. https://doi.org/10.1146/annurev.en.02.010157.001145 https://core.ac.uk/download/323061734.pdf (accessed on 13 May 2025).

41. League, G. P., Degner, E. C., Pitcher, S. A., Hafezi, Y., Tennant, E., Cruz, P. C., Krishnan, R. S., et al. (2021). The impact of mating and sugar feeding on blood-feeding physiology and behavior in the arbovirus vector mosquito *Aedes aegypti. PLOS Neglected Tropical Diseases, 15*, e0009815. https://doi.org/10.1371/journal.pntd.0009815.

42. London School of Hygiene & Tropical Medicine. (2013). *Annual Report 2013*. https://core.ac.uk/download/19452766.pdf (accessed on 13 May 2025).

43. Topalis, P., Dialynas, E., Mitraka, E., Deligianni, E., Siden-Kiamos, I., & Louis, C. (2011). A set of ontologies to drive tools for the control of vector-borne diseases. *Journal of biomedical informatics, 44*(1), 42–47. https://doi.org/10.1016/j.jbi.2010.03.012 (accessed on 13 May 2025).

44. Miranda, L. S., Rudd, S. R., Mena, O., Hudspeth, P. E., Barboza-Corona, J. E., Park, H. W., & Bideshi, D. K. (2024). The Perpetual Vector Mosquito Threat and Its Eco-Friendly Nemeses. *Biology, 13*(3), 182. https://doi.org/10.3390/biology13030182(accessed on 13 May 2025).

45. Nguyen, V. T., Dryden, D. S., Broder, B. A., Tadimari, A., Tanachaiwiwat, P., Mathias, D. K., Thongsripong, P., et al. (2025). A comprehensive review: Biology of *Anopheles squamosus*, an understudied malaria vector in Africa. *Insects, 16*. https://www.semanticscholar.org/paper/d837b9aca018d3da27766dd0a6815279d8a59b99 (accessed on 13 May 2025).

46. Nordgulen, M., Lewandowski, K., Burkett-Cadena, N., Mathias, D., & Byrd, B. D. (2024). LA CROSSE VIRUS VECTOR RESTING BEHAVIORS - FIELD STUDIES WITH PROKOPAK AND RESTING SHELTER COLLECTIONS PROVIDE LOW YIELD. *Journal of the American Mosquito Control Association, 40*(3), 141–144. https://doi.org/10.2987/23-7161(accessed on 13 May 2025).

47. Overgaard, H. (2025). Malaria mosquito resistance to agricultural insecticides: Risk area mapping in Thailand. https://core.ac.uk/download/pdf/6405173.pdf (accessed on 13 May 2025).

48. Rabinovich, R. N., Drakeley, C., Djimdé, A., Hall, B., Hay, S. I., Hemingway, J., Kaslow, D. C., et al. (2017). malERA: An updated research agenda for malaria elimination and eradication. *PLoS Medicine, 14*, e1002456. https://doi.org/10.1371/journal.pmed.1002456.

49. Shaalan, M. G., et al. (2024). A highly efficient computational strategy for unraveling microRNA profiles in the aquatic larvae of the mosquito disease vector *Culex quinquefasciatus. Egyptian Journal of Aquatic Biology and Fisheries*. https://www.semanticscholar.org/paper/75a07eb908521079c0b18255f503e49ee2ecf566 (accessed on 13 May 2025).

50. Tippelt, S. (2018). *Assortative Mating in the Anopheles gambiae Species Complex*. https://core.ac.uk/download/159487594.pdf (accessed on 13 May 2025).

51. Tripet F. (2009). Ecological immunology of mosquito-malaria interactions: Of non-natural versus natural model systems and their inferences. *Parasitology, 136*(14), 1935–1942. https://doi.org/10.1017/S0031182009006234W A Nazni, Hoffmann, A. A., Ahmad, N. A., Cheong, Y. L., Mancini, M. V., Golding, N., Kamarul, G. M. R., et al. (2019). Establishment of *Wolbachia* strain wAlbB in Malaysian populations of *Aedes aegypti* for dengue control. *Current Biology, 29*, 4241–4248.e5. https://doi.org/10.1016/j.cub.2019.11.007.

52. Wilson, A. L., Courtenay, O., Kelly-Hope, L. A., Scott, T. W., Takken, W., Torr, S. J., & Lindsay, S. W. (2020). The importance of vector control for the control and elimination of vector-borne diseases. *PLOS Neglected Tropical Diseases, 14*, e0007831. https://doi.org/10.1371/journal.pntd.0007831.

53. Wouter Graumans, Jacobs, E., Bousema, T., & Sinnis, P. (2020). When is a *Plasmodium*-infected mosquito an infectious mosquito? *Trends in Parasitology, 36*, 705–716. https://doi.org/10.1016/j.pt.2020.05.011.

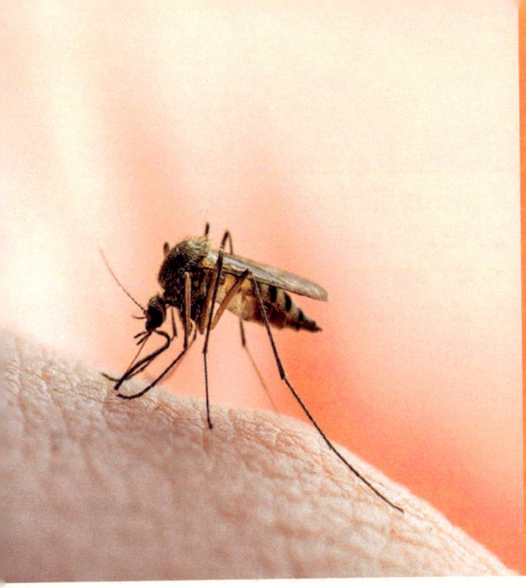

Chapter 4

PATHOPHYSIOLOGY OF MALARIA

Contents

Introduction

Malaria remains one of the globe's biggest health issues. It is caused primarily by *Plasmodium parasites* that somehow enter our system when an infected *Anopheles* mosquito bites us. Despite advances in medicine, areas with hot and humid conditions, where these insects thrive—remain the hardest hit. The parasite's winding journey, oscillating between human hosts and mosquitoes, only serves to make our efforts at control even more difficult. In general, comprehension of the way malaria distorts our normal body processes and elicits immune responses is the most crucial one since that forms the foundation of better treatments and prevention. The progression of disease is an intermixed mix between the infecting parasite and the host's own immune system. First, *Plasmodium* infects liver cells, silently growing before spilling over into the blood and starting to infect red blood cells (RBCs). As each red cell cycle is destroyed, individuals begin to experience fever, chills, and anemia. Meanwhile, our immune system, with the aid of macrophages, scrambles to the infection to fight a war, but those cells sometimes end up causing damage to the tissues along the way. These macrophages are not fixed in one state; they are there to toggle between a more active, pro-inflammatory state (M1) and a less active, anti-inflammatory state (M2) (Moghaddam et al., 2018). Where the balancing act fails, tissue damage becomes worse, pushing the disease toward more disastrous outcomes and showing how critical it is to have immune responses balanced. In recent times, scientists have been pointing out the fact that the effect of malaria extends way beyond the infection. Complications including cerebral malaria and multi-organ failure have also been seen to result—typically as a result of overcompensation by the body. Uncontrolled inflammatory response, along with infected red blood cells adhering to the walls of the vessels and clogging minute vessels, are some factors that lead to the severe complications. In the majority of cases, the surge of inflammation signals eventually leads to leaky blood vessels and interference with normal clotting, and this may lead to dangerous, even fatal, complications. Included as well is the observation that the economic and health cost of malaria commonly hits hardest at the most susceptible segments of the population, pregnant women and young children, due to their own already compromised immune and physical status (Blencowe et al., 2013). Overall, a comprehensive and advanced understanding of how malaria works is crucial to enhanced clinical control as well as public health policy formulation that aims to curb its propagation globally (Figure 4.1).

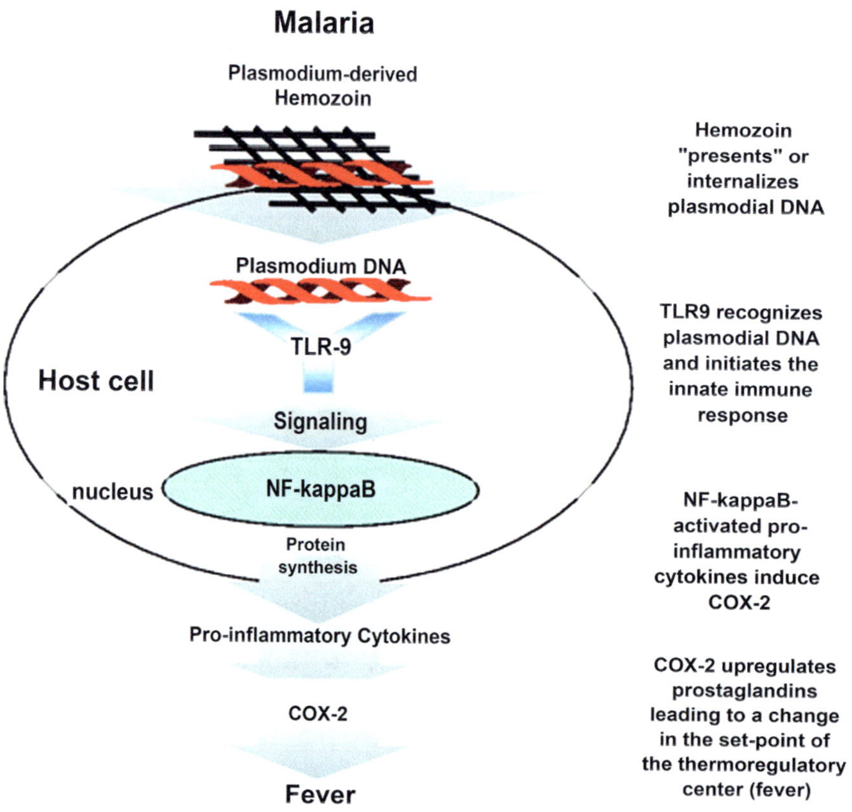

Figure 4.1. Pathophysiology of malaria.

Source: Srinivas. (2015). *Life Cycle of the Malaria Parasite.* https://i0.wp.com/www.malariasite.com/wp-content/uploads/2015/02/F1.medium.gif?resize=440%2C419&ssl=1.

Definition of Malaria

Malaria is a contagious illness that has been a persistent problem for the majority of communities. It starts with tiny *Plasmodium* group *parasites* entering one's blood after being bitten by an *Anopheles* female mosquito infected with malaria. Previously, this disease was seen as a monstrous world reversal, mostly because it still robs the body of its RBCs in a continuous cycle. That loss of cells triggers a storm of fever, chills, and even anemia, while our immune system and delicate control of blood vessel function all factor in to decide how bad the disease will get. In fact, to be aware of malaria is not just to recognize the parasite; it is also to be aware of the way that human genes, like when being sickle cell trait gives a bit of protection—interact with the parasite's own genetic features (Gibbs et al., 2022). Its clinical presentation can be all over the place. Other times the parasite exists without causing any visible issue, and sometimes the consequences swell into complications such as cerebral ones or even multi-organ failure. These are generally different depending on the response of the body triggered by the *parasites*, especially with *Plasmodium falciparum* usually being the cause of the worst. Infected RBCs aggregate in microvessels, interfering with normal tissue blood perfusion and initiating waves of inflammatory signals to intensify the severity. In areas where resources are scarce—most often in association with complications like severe anemia or shock—the overall effect becomes even more complex (Assies et al., 2022). In addition, how malaria develops neatly into an overarching story of genetic vulnerability, with host-pathogen interaction at the genetic level tipping scales of resistance against risk every so often. Current studies have emphasized the point that a number of genetic hotspots, either in hemoglobin modification or in immune system adjustments, decide exactly how badly one will fare. In summary, malaria isn't so much an issue of a parasite getting you ill; it is a challenging, complex association of genetics, immune systems, and environment that together control the disease as well as how we continue to fight it (Gibbs et al., 2022) (Figure 4.2).

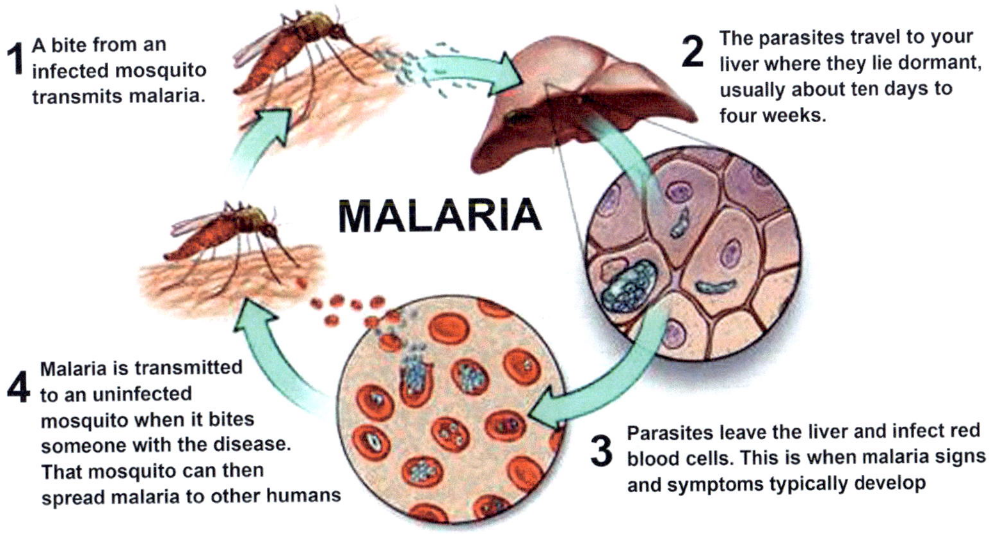

Figure 4.2. Malaria.

Source: Mayo Clinic. (2023). *Malaria Transmission Cycle.* https://www.mayoclinic.org/content/dam/media/en/images/2023/02/09/malaria-transmission-cycle.jpg.

Historical Context and Significance

The history of malaria begins many years ago, when the beginnings of tropical medicine research mixed bedside patient hints with new laboratory concepts. By the early 1900s, scientists were starting to recognize how insects communicated with our cells, and pioneers such as Carlos Chagas linked what we observed in patients to what was occurring under the microscope (Lidani et al., 2019). The leads at the time were scattered, sometimes just an observation here, a cellular hint there, but over time, scientists shifted from simply describing symptoms to digging into the parasite's journey through RBCs. This shift, not always smooth, eventually braided clinical symptoms and actions at the molecular level together, shaping our knowledge of how hosts and pathogens interact. It is noteworthy to mention that the impact of malaria goes well beyond its immediate symptoms. The advances in genetic and molecular medicine have come hand in hand with advances in other blood disorders. For instance, the path from the discovery of sickle cell anemia to the understanding of its inner workings (Williams et al., 2018) is comparable to the quest to understand the dynamics of malaria itself. The sickle cell trait—once thought to be nature's whim that happens to guard against malaria—is a kind of evolutionary tug-of-war between the parasite and our genes. For the most part, this tug-of-war blurs the line between a simple infection and a force that has driven human genetic diversity and even steered research into fields like immunology and hematology. Looking back at over a century, malaria research has been many triumphant advances and stubborn reverses. Early hopes for turning experimentally obtained molecular leads into solid therapies encountered difficulties somewhat similar to those we saw with sickle cell anemia (Williams et al., 2018). Especially in the tropical world, the disease's persistent burden led international groups to mix old knowledge with modern biology and even new drug approaches. Most frequently, these efforts resulted in new therapies and prevention methods that depend to a great extent on a detailed study of the disease mechanism. In general, the course of malaria knowledge is a twisted one where clinical observation, laboratory research, and public health incessantly influence one another, leaving an everlasting legacy in medicine and society.

4.1. Etiology of Malaria

Malaria begins with a complex interplay of factors. There is the parasite itself, mainly *Plasmodium falciparum* and *Plasmodium vivax* being passed on by the female *Anopheles* mosquito, subsequently there are the characteristics of the host itself. In the majority of cases, following the bite, the *parasites* infect the liver where they multiply silently before moving into red blood cells (RBCs), which is what eventually causes the symptoms. In many cases, the distribution of the disease is influenced by local climate and social conditions; tropical and subtropical regions, where mosquitoes thrive, experience more infections. Additionally, your body's natural immunity, genetic traits such as the sickle cell trait, and even your nutritional status have a part in determining the severity with which one may be affected. Overall, it is understanding these overlapping factors that hold the key to unlocking how malaria works and how to more effectively prevent and treat it. One of the more extreme consequences is the anemia that comes with malaria—not only from the parasite itself directly annihilating RBCs but also from our body's complex, sometimes overactive response. When the life cycle in the red cells is finished, they burst and release merozoites that continue to fuel infection and depletion of blood cells. This havoc, along with a decrease in the manufacture of new blood cells—partly because of bone marrow breakdown and those pesky inflammatory cytokines—leads to anemia of varying severity. Where malaria is common, nutritional problems like iron deficiency pile insult on injury, heightening dangers for worse outcomes (Chaparro & Suchdev, 2019). To compound the problem, ongoing infection or chronic inflammation can continue the anemia, which, admittedly, complicates treatment even further. In brief, this anemia isn't just a side effect—it disrupts oxygen transport and can set off a series of other problems. The other aspect manifests in pregnancy. *Plasmodium falciparum* sometimes implants itself in the placenta, and in doing so, interferes with the usual exchange of oxygen and nutrients between the fetus and mother. The interference usually ends up causing complications like fetal growth restriction, preterm births, and a higher possibility of perinatal death (Melamed et al., 2021). Here, the crosstalk between the maternal immune responses and the parasite's own mechanisms sets off pregnancy complications. Impaired placental vessel formation and alteration in cytokine levels also cloud the issue, worsening fetal outcomes. Overall, linking these events together makes it clear why it is so important to give priority to interventions in pregnant women, especially when managing malaria needs to be incorporated with overall maternal and fetal health measures (Figure 4.3).

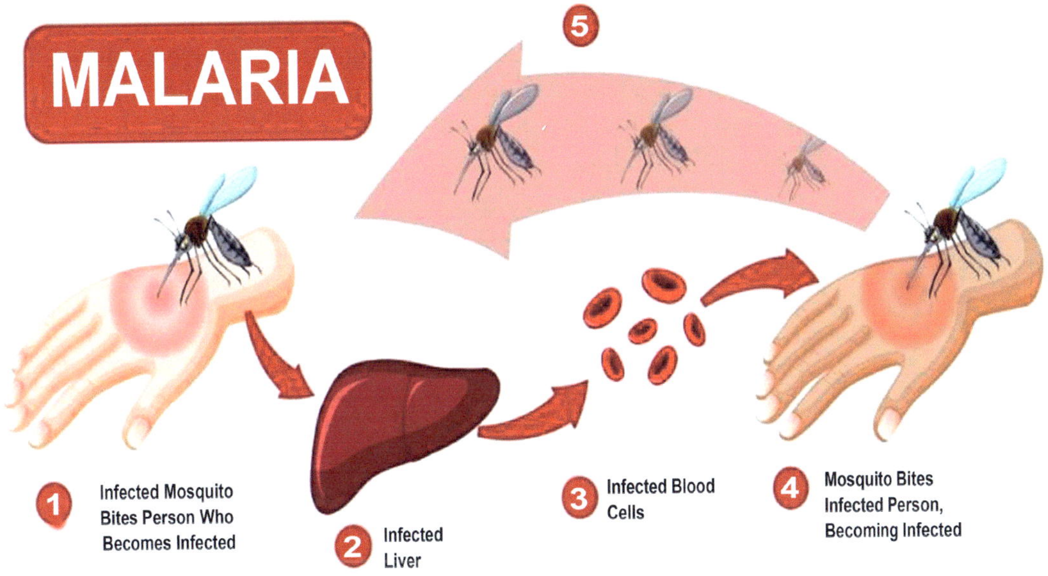

Figure 4.3. Etiology of malaria.

Source: Regency Medical Centre. (2021). *Malaria Causes, Symptoms, and Treatment.* https://external-content.duckduckgo.com/iu/?u=https%3A%2F%2Fwww.regencymedicalcentre.com%2Fwp-content%2Fuploads%2F2021%2F04%2Fcauses-malaria-1024x684.jpg&f=1&nofb=1&ipt=c60be2b3e53b58e42497291ab4d2d5ad9c2f623a91766bbd8fe534dae6d03fd5.

4.1.1. Causative Agents (Plasmodium Species)

Malaria is a deadly parasitic infection stemming from a complex interplay of human physiology and a very special kind of protozoan—*Plasmodium* species. It all begins when an infected female *Anopheles* mosquito bites a human being; the *parasites* then take a tortuous journey in the body. You have several key players here: *Plasmodium falciparum*, *P. vivax*, *P. ovale*, *P. malariae*, and more recently, *P. knowlesi*. Overall, *P. falciparum* has the worst reputation for producing the most severe symptoms and the highest number of deaths. After a short liver stage, these parasites slide into RBCs, a hidden maneuver that helps them evade detection by the immune system. For the most part, getting to know the individual life cycle and features of each of these *Plasmodium* types is central to knowing how malaria works and what that clinically means (Chopra et al., 2021). These parasite types are not only distinct by name, but their various behaviors, like parasite loads, relapse cycles, and tissues of choice—also impact how the disease progresses and responds to treatment. For instance, *P. vivax* and *P. ovale* can remain dormant in the form of liver stages, or hypnozoites, and cause relapses months or even years later; however, *P. falciparum* usually starts an acute and, all too often, fatal infection. Such latent activity impacts eradication efforts and, in most cases, suggests that different mechanisms are at work between species. Such subtleties highlight the need for research to dig into species-level differences so that more targeted and effective treatments can eventually be tailored (Chopra et al., 2021). The effects of a *Plasmodium* infection do not stop at disrupting RBCs, malaria can also cause large-scale inflammatory responses and even neurological issues. Cerebral malaria, mainly linked with *P. falciparum*, is a particularly serious disease in which neuroinflammation and blood-brain barrier problems lead to complex brain dysfunction. Recent studies have begun to elucidate how processes like the activation of glial cells, cytokine imbalance, and disrupted neurotransmitter signals can cause cognitive impairment as well as behavioral alterations. All these systemic effects illustrate that the damage is more than blood cell destruction alone and that malaria is a far more complex, multisystem disease than many might initially appreciate (Figure 4.4).

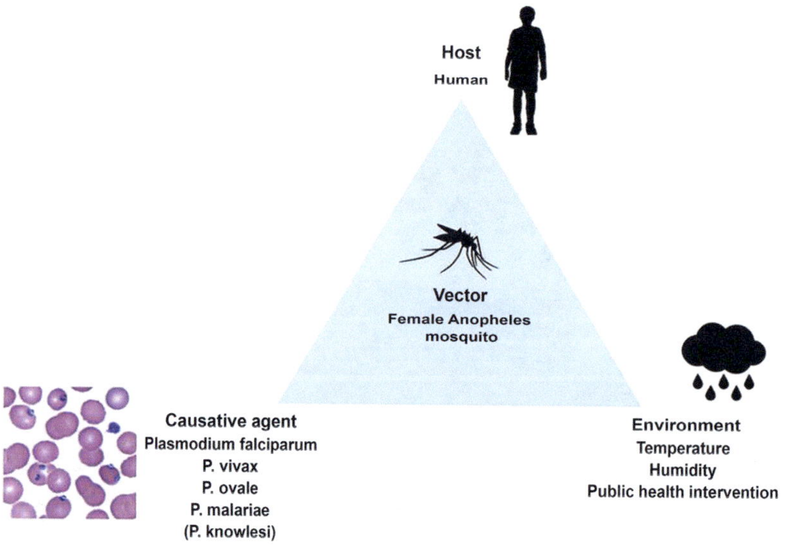

Figure 4.4. Causative agents.

Source: Wix.com. (n.d.). *Mosquito Life Cycle Diagram*. https://external-content.duckduckgo.com/iu/?u=https%3A%2F%2Fstatic.wixstatic.com%2Fmedia%2Fd05e83_a6e3d3dadd714fcaa503106ff6669aa0~mv2.png%2Fv1%2Ffill%2Fw_980%2Ch_637%2Cal_c%2Cq_90%2Cusm_0.66_1.00_0.01%2Cenc_auto%2Fd05e83_a6e3d3dadd714fcaa503106ff6669aa0~mv2.png&f=1&nofb=1&ipt=fe55604f540bc49322fbc0642c8c0838d8e0263c27e6ab3ba04e142f0287cd53.

4.1.2. Transmission Vectors (Anopheles Mosquitoes)

Malaria's spread amounts to an intertwined association between the minute *parasites* and the insects that carry them around. Malaria-carrying *Plasmodium parasites* are carried by *Anopheles* mosquitoes—those small insects that are found so abundantly in warm, humid areas. They thrive in tropical and subtropical areas where the climate simply happens to be apt for their survival and reproduction. You can see that in places like Sub-Saharan Africa, South Asia, and Central America, elevated mosquito infestation tends to coincide with regions that abound in malaria. Their potential to transmit the parasite relies on many factors, like how well they can support the pathogen, where and when they take their meal, and even simply for how long they live.

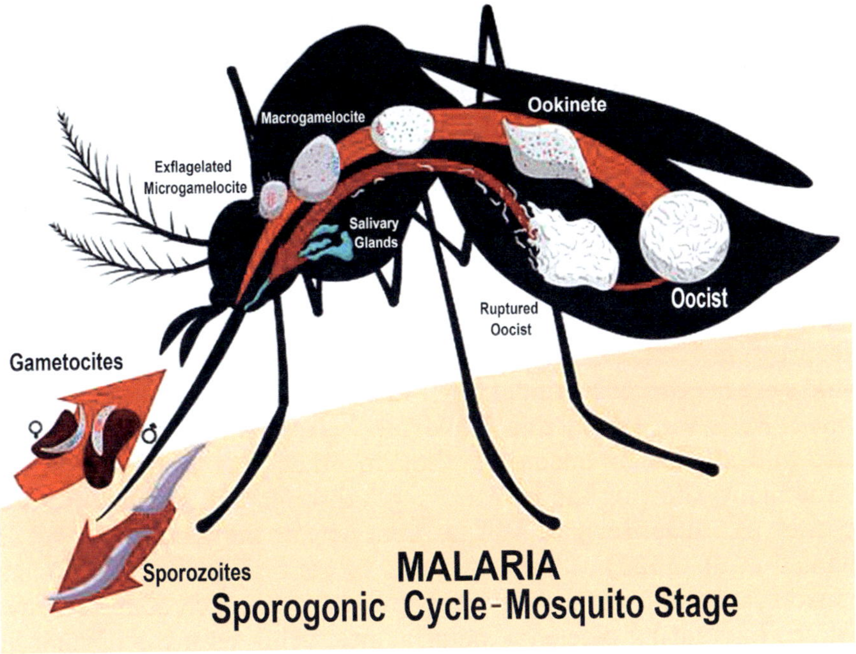

Figure 4.5. *Anopheles* mosquito.

Source: iStock. (n.d.). *Malaria Plasmodium Life Cycle Mosquito Infection Vector*. https://external-content.duckduckgo.com/iu/?u=https%3A%2F%2Fmedia.istockphoto.com%2Fvectors%2Fmalarian-*Plasmodium*-life-cycle-mosquito-infection-vector-id523625398%3Fk%3D6%26m%3D523625398%26s%3D612x612%26w%3D0%26h%3D6EMQS4bBR-qDVTRYWzN1JlXbDgkM2ag CYFDI8FgtIgs%3D&f=1&nofb=1&ipt=cee6d465de6310ba19804887b8577455fe87c4a4e6be7246f347b7edeae7f9ea.

All this contact maintains malaria chugging along in some parts of the world, while wealthier areas with lower populations of such insects have much lower rates of transmission (Bansal et al., 2023). When you look further into it, the whole transmission picture is even more complicated by the parasite itself and its insect vector's behavior. Take *Plasmodium vivax*, for instance; this is the group that shows us a set of peculiar traits that seem to influence its transmission. Traditionally, scientists have assumed that in regions such as sub-Saharan Africa, Duffy-negative RBCs meant that most were essentially immune. Yet with more recent studies, in most cases, things were not so simple – *vivax* somehow manages to infect locations such as the bone marrow and spleen, outside of the regular bloodstream cycle. This latent strategy can cause a low but steady parasite load, not merely making them hard to discover but continuing the transmission cycle even if the host has its usual defenses (Baird, 2022). Going further, the mosquito's own unique biology provides yet another complexity to how the disease takes hold in people. Their biting patterns—the timing, where on the skin they bite, and where gametocytes then find themselves in small blood vessels—can even tip the odds of parasite transmission. Compared to a controlled feeding situation using artificially fed blood samples, free-living mosquitos are more inclined to bite certain regions of the skin, almost as if following subtle parasite cues. This activity can make transmission rise even when blood testing indicates teeny-tiny parasite levels. Practically speaking, these temporary host-vector-parasite interactions help keep malaria in the picture where the mathematics just won't balance out. These nuances must be recognized when crafting clever control strategies that will break the transmission cycle without simply relying on blood test results (Baird, 2022; Bansal et al., 2023) (Figure 4.5).

4.1.3. Risk Factors for Infection

Risk from malaria is not a one-note story—it's the amalgamation of how people live, the functioning of nature, and even personal features. Mosquito bites, especially from *Anopheles*, start it all, and their spread is even very weather- and location- and population-habitation-dependent. Some populations, like pregnant women, infants, or HIV or malnourished individuals, possess more weakened immune systems that leave them open to extra vulnerability. Even a person's DNA, like variations in forms of RBCs, can modify this risk factor. Subsequently there are housing conditions—subpar healthcare and subpar or unsanitary housing that have a way of critically disrupting prevention and treatment, allowing the parasite to get through that much more easily. All of these, when mixed together in a disorderly sort of fashion, permit the parasite to get in, multiply, and sicken one (Melamed et al., 2021). Other infections or general health issues complicate matters sometimes. For instance, conditions that toy with the placenta, such as fetal growth restriction—end up looking much like during placental malaria, interfering with the normal flow of nutrients and immune signals, which can heighten infection risk (Melamed et al., 2021). Where malaria is endemic, individuals will experience repeated attacks of the disease; if it continues long enough, it can interrupt the balance of the immune system, rendering a person susceptible not only to further malaria but to other insects as well. In areas where resources and proper nutrition are scarce, like parts of sub-Saharan Africa or Asia, poor immunity only makes the situation worse. When there are conditions such as HIV or tuberculosis added to the mix, caring for the illness becomes an awful lot more complicated, and it highlights the importance of having a wide perspective of all of these risk factors (Rudd et al., 2020). It is not only a matter of being exposed or being sick with something else either—there are other indicators at work. Scientists observed that certain biomarkers, for instance, placental abnormal Doppler, could be an indicator that the organ is not functioning optimally, which would also imply a higher risk of placental malaria and could even lead to adverse outcomes for the baby (Melamed et al., 2021). Variation in the frequency with which these infections occur at the regional level also suggests that following local trends and combining that with targeted interventions for health, is vital. The large number of deaths due to sepsis and other infection-related factors in areas of ongoing malaria indeed underscores the need to detect and mitigate such risks. Overall, gaining control over these intersecting factors is important if we are to advance prevention and treatment efforts throughout the world (Rudd et al., 2020).

4.2. Life Cycle of Plasmodium

The two-step tango between *Plasmodium* and human host is at the heart of malaria's reach, a kind of smart, if not sinister, association by which the parasite can survive and reproduce. When an infected *Anopheles* mosquito bites its host, sporozoites invade the blood and march directly to the liver; there, they infect liver cells and start asexual reproduction. This brief liver phase subsequently overloads the blood with thousands of merozoites, beginning the stage at which symptoms become evident. In new transcript studies, even such earliest blood-stage *parasites* exhibit remnants of transitioning into a sexual form Adapa et al. (2019).

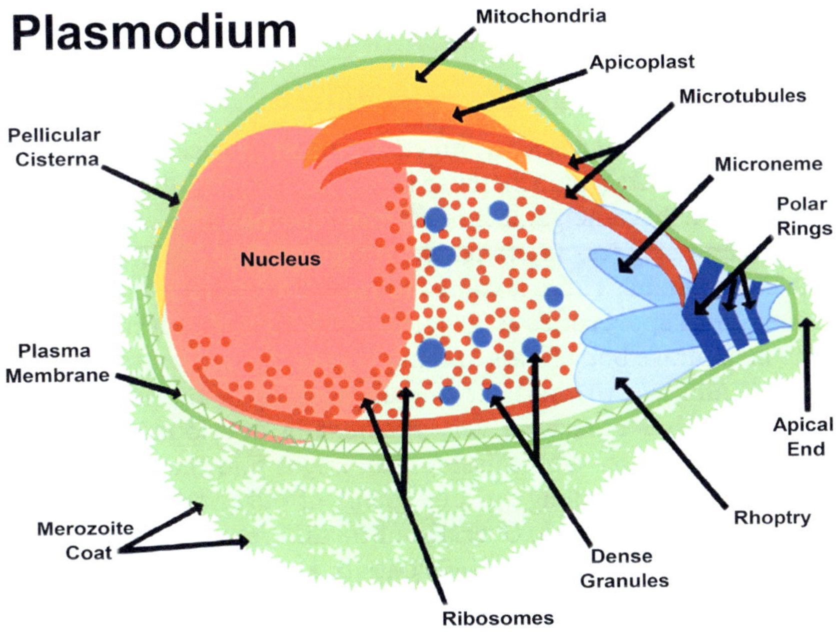

Figure 4.6. Life cycle of *Plasmodium*.

Source: By Jfbranch14 - Own work, CC BY-SA 3.0, https://commons.wikimedia.org/w/index.php?curid=19558260

By and large, this sexual head start disrupts traditional expectations of gametocyte production following multiple rounds of asexual replication, illustrating just how well-equipped *Plasmodium* is to balance survival in the host with readiness to leap to new mosquito vectors. Once those merozoites are released into the bloodstream, they immediately look for RBCs to live in, going through a process of stages referred to as ring, trophozoite, and schizont, each of which creates its own set of problems. The ongoing cycle of destruction of RBCs and a resultant new release of merozoites not only provoke inflammatory responses but also induce fever and anemia. In both cases, the parasite's metabolism during this active phase is amplified and depends heavily on the pentose phosphate pathway (PPP) to supply necessary nucleotides to support rapid growth and keep oxidative stress levels at a bare minimum (Stincone et al., 2014). The dual roles of the PPP—building blocks on the one hand, and defense against damage from reactive oxygen species on the other— demonstrate the metabolic sleight of hand the parasite employs to keep its lights on inside RBCs. It's not merely a question of rapid reproduction, however; the parasite also sets the stage for what comes next by entering into sexual forms, called gametocytes, which form within infected RBCs. As the mosquito feeds, these gametocytes develop further within its gut until they eventually mature into sporozoites. Other mathematical models even propose that a previous conversion to gametocyte output might speed up transmission and make control harder since infective stages may mature sooner than initially thought (Adapa et al., 2019). It is in almost all respects crucial to understand how *Plasmodium* progresses from asexual reproduction to gametocyte formation—both to ease the disease symptoms and to retard the spread of malaria. This complex life cycle, with all its overlapping stages, in effect serves as at once both the agent of the disease and a factor controlling its extensive spread (Figure 4.6).

4.2.1. Stages of the Parasite in the Mosquito

As the female *Anopheles* mosquito bites an infected person, it picks up the parasite in its sexual stage – the gametocytes. Inside its stomach, these forms do not just lie dormant; they rapidly change as the male and female cells become gametes and join together into a single zygote. That one-cell zygote then grows into an ookinete, an elongated structure that can creep along the lining of the midgut to locate the basal lamina. There it comes to rest and enters a phase called sporogony. Most of the time, an aggregate of sporozoites is generated inside the oocyst, and after maturing, they are excreted into the mosquito's body fluids and migrate to the salivary glands. The transformation cycle sets them up for jumping to the next human host upon the next bite (Al-Agroudi et al., 2017). *Plasmodium* species are otherwise very resilient in development in the mosquito, which indeed has implications for disease transmission. You might find that the timing and effectiveness of these stages are not identical among various forms of *parasites* – take *Plasmodium vivax*, for example, versus *Plasmodium falciparum*. Overall, subtle differences in biology and host preference lead to unique relationships with the vector. Scientists are yet to unravel how the *parasites* use their genetic plasticity and molecular sleight of hand – for instance, avoiding the immune system of the mosquito and using receptor–ligand binding – to find themselves a foothold within midgut cells and salivary glands. This survival tactic puts another twist in the evolutionary history of the parasite (Al-Agroudi et al., 2017). These features, in turn, make control all the more difficult and spur efforts toward finding more sophisticated means of targeting the parasite before it can incubate in the mosquito. How effectively the disease is transmitted ultimately hinges on the parasite's proficiency at mass-producing infectious sporozoites and depositing them in the salivary glands of the mosquito, where they can penetrate human skin and the liver. The whole process is a delicate balancing act because temperature and even interspecific differences in mosquitoes can influence the number of developing sporozoites and how infective they are. Astonishingly, even if human blood parasite numbers are virtually too low to measure, enough gametocytes may be consumed to induce transmission. This leads us to re-examine the typical relationship between observed parasitemia and risk; occasionally there are some in the form of hidden reservoirs of *parasites* in various tissues that contribute substantially (Bairt, 2022). The majority of the time, knowledge of these dynamics of the mosquito stage is of critical importance in developing interventions that could potentially break the malaria transmission cycle (Figure 4.7).

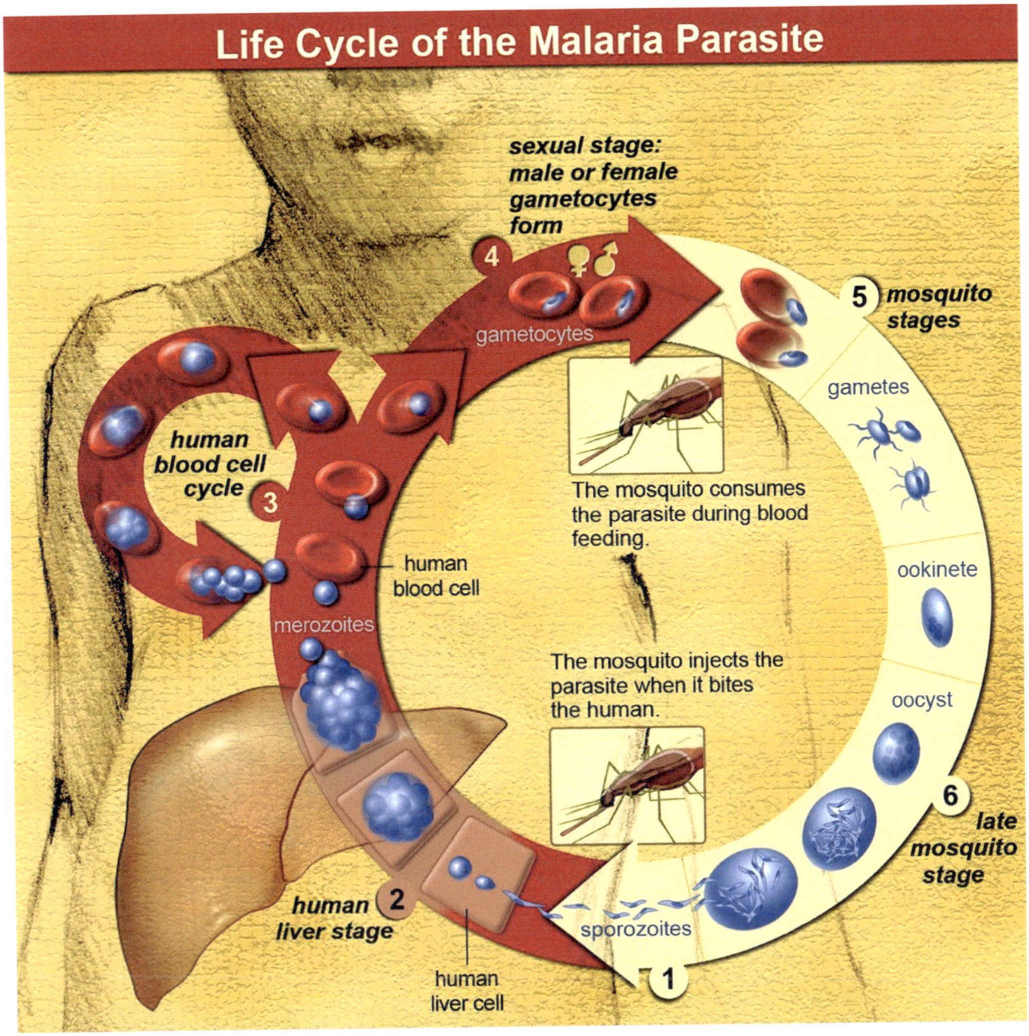

Figure 4.7. Stages of the parasite in the mosquito.

Source: By National Institutes of Health (NIH) - National Institutes of Health (NIH), Public Domain, https://commons.wikimedia.org/w/index.php?curid=29552307

4.2.2. Stages of the Parasite in the Human Host

Malaria starts with the bite of the mosquito that injects sporozoites into the blood. These tiny invaders go directly to the liver, infect liver cells, and start to divide under wraps. While in stealth mode, they form clusters known as schizonts that burst, releasing thousands of merozoites into the bloodstream. Upon entering the circulation, these merozoites infect RBCs, multiply, and kill cells, when symptoms like fever start appearing. The liver stage is imperceptible, yet in fact is an important preparation for the survival of the parasite in two essentially different environments, providing the basis for the complex course of the disease. In the blood stage, a rhythmicity appears. Merozoites invade RBCs and travel erratically in a sequence of recognizable shapes—the ring form, then the trophozoite, and finally the schizont stage—until the cell ruptures to form more *parasites*. This cycle sustains the classical chills and fever of malaria. Inexplicably, some of the *parasites* follow a different course: they transform into gametocytes that remain in the blood waiting to be engulfed by another mosquito. New evidence suggests that our own RBC microRNAs, like miR-92a-3p, shed off during infection, which seems to be accompanied by a rise in the virulence factor PfEMP1. The protein, in return, helps the parasite evade the immune system (Prabhu et al., 2023).

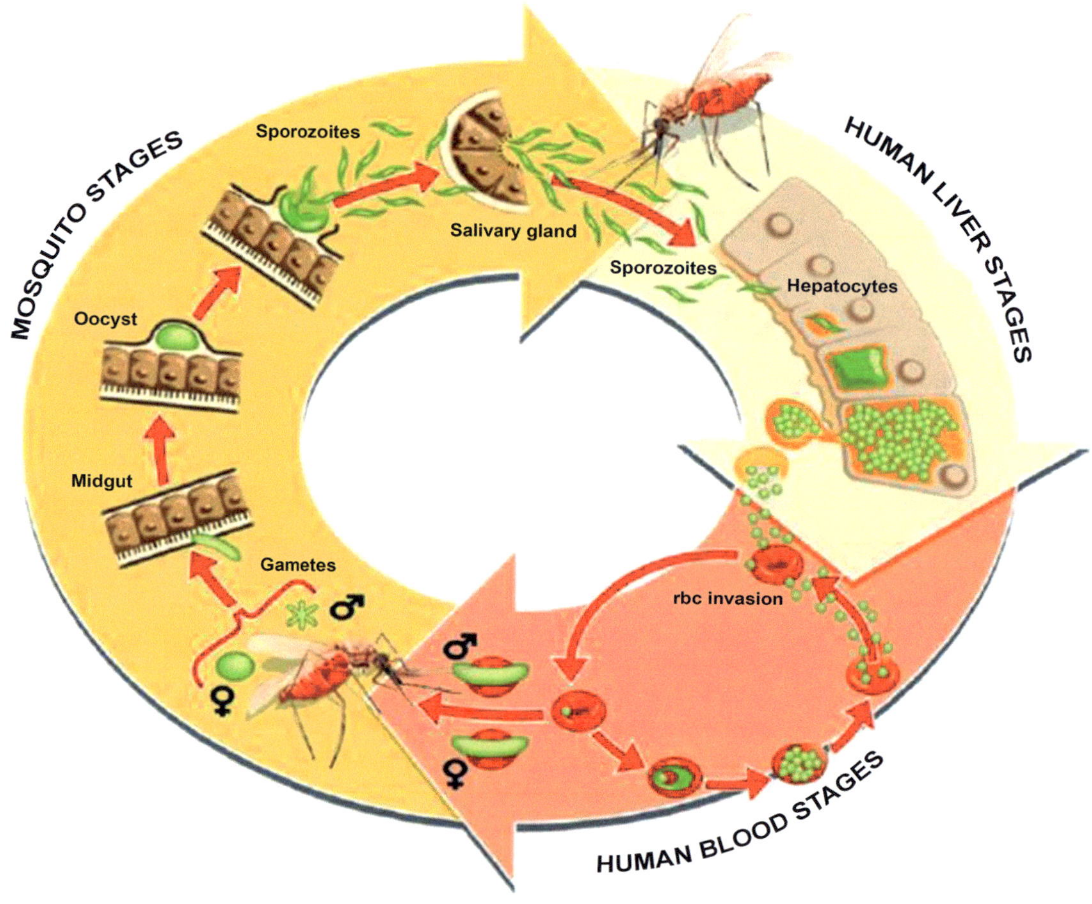

Figure 4.8. Parasite life cycle in the human host.

Source: Mota, M. M. (2010). *Parasite Life Cycle in the Human Host and Mosquito Vector.*

It is a neat example of how molecular interactions might be playing tricks with the survival methods of the parasite. Subsequently there is the issue with different *Plasmodium* species, with another layer of complexity. As an example, *Plasmodium vivax* prefers to feed exclusively on immature RBCs—reticulocytes, and its growth relies very much on the natural mechanism of maturation of the cells. Researchers trying to culture *P. vivax* in the lab have found it a real challenge to reproduce a true host environment, and this indicates how sensitive and picky the development of the parasite could be. This reliance on the cell state of the host could potentially be a weak point through which new treatments can be targeted. In general, this give-and-take between parasite and host reminds us how complicated malaria is, and it reminds us why potent interventions are so hard to achieve (Thomson-Luque et al., 2019) (Figure 4.8).

4.2.3. Duration and Phases of the Life Cycle

Malaria is a complex undertaking, at least in part because the life cycle of the parasite has phases that take place both in the mosquito and human bodies. Notice, however, that when an *Anopheles* mosquito bites, sporozoites immediately flood into the blood circulation and stream towards the liver, beginning what we call the hepatic phase – a period that usually lasts somewhere between 7 to 14 days. Meanwhile, they reproduce silently inside liver cells during that time and result in producing thousands of merozoites that burst out to re-enter the circulatory system. Then comes the invasion stage where RBCs are invaded; meanwhile, the parasite also reproduces and causes cell lysis in a sort of cyclic recurrence that defines how symptoms will appear. These stages, spurred by the level of the parasite's replication and by the immune response of the body, build layers into the overall clinical picture of malaria. This is not just a matter of the parasite simply moving from the liver to the blood stage—this also ramps up the body's immune system into overdrive. Generally speaking, while those sporozoites are busy getting themselves settled into liver cells, our immune systems take a brief vacation, and the parasite gets to enjoy its peaceful establishment in quiet contemplation. But once all of those merozoites flood the blood, the host takes the initiative to raise a tempestuous inflammatory response. Leukocytes, monocytes, lymphocytes, and more get activated and spill cytokines, chemokines, and cytoadhesion molecules of every description, and all contribute to that familiar bout of fever and chills. Generally, this sudden immune response highlights how the alteration stages of the parasite life are able to have direct effects on pathophysiological effects (Mavondo et al., 2019). Generally, the malarial parasite life cycle abounds with sly timing and physiological subtleties that are dependent on the parasite's own nature as well as the host state. While the overall time course is fairly uniform, the influence of other factors like nutrition or the external environment can push the parasite's behavior and shift the severity of the disease experienced. In fact, some high-resolution behavioral tracking experiments in other systems also show slight cyclical trends in body activity, trends which also seem to map overall health and disease state over time (Chiu et al., 2013). Similarly, if parasite phases are controlled by diet or immunological state, this can alter symptoms and recovery times. In general, having a complete understanding of how long each one lasts and what is happening within them is key to creating treatments that will, in most cases, disrupt the parasite's advancement in the host.

4.3. Immune Response to Malaria

Malaria's bite derives from the wild tango between our immune system and the parasite. As *Plasmodium* slides into the blood, the innate defenses are triggered with alacrity—dendritic cells and macrophages are activated to present fragments of the invader for the adaptive side to continue. Overall, a lot of rides on Toll-like receptors that sense generic signals in the parasite to induce pro-inflammatory cytokine bursts. But the parasite is clever; it alters parameters like endosomal pH and subtly interrupts TLR signaling in a way that it sometimes falls below the immune radar. Interestingly, antimalarial medications like hydroxychloroquine (HCQ) also disrupt endosomal acidification, which in turn impacts immune cell activation and cytokine release. In brief, the immune system's two-edged function—eliminating pathogens on one side but also dangerously overreacting on the other—is central to why infections of malaria end so differently (Nirk et al., 2020). Recent research has begun to demonstrate that additional infections can complicate the immune landscape in malaria. For example, in some rodent models, a latent viral infection persisting with *Plasmodium* induces a vigorous type I interferon response. This antiviral wave has the effect of depleting dendritic cell numbers and makes them less efficient at producing crucial signals like interleukin-12p70, which is critical for sufficient Th1 development. As the $CD4^+$ T cell response is dampened, cerebral malaria's dire consequences and even autoimmune problems are less severe. So, in some instances, the presence of another infection can—contrary to what one might expect—serve to alleviate the severity of malaria's impact. This result simply serves as a reminder that the combination of pathogens inhabiting the body has a large role to play in determining immune responses (Hassan et al., 2020). At the cellular level, the balance between the inflammatory fighters and the regulators dictates the final outcome of malaria. $CD4^+$ T cells, specifically the Th1 and Th17 subsets, are important in the clearance of the parasite by secreting cytokines, though if they are not controlled, they also trigger detrimental immune responses. In contrast, regulatory T cells function to limit excessive inflammation and tissue injury. Often, *Plasmodium* derails this delicate balance, pushing the body into overdrive. Researchers have also explored ways of manipulating intrinsic cell processes like autophagy and calcium signaling—by using immunomodulatory drugs that regulate TLR stimulation or calcium-dependent pathways—in order to restore balance. By trimming back overactive cytokine production and restoring T-cell ratio balance, these approaches illustrate how the pathology involved in malaria is revealed, even though the whole system sometimes appears a bit unbalanced (Nirk et al., 2020).

4.3.1. Innate Immune Response Mechanisms

Malaria triggers a kind of complex exchange between these *Plasmodium parasites* and our very initial defense line—the innate immune system. Upon invading the bloodstream, cells like macrophages and dendritic cells instantly recognize such invaders by sensing known molecular patterns using receptors like TLRs. A split second after, these cells start releasing pro-inflammatory cytokines—don't mind TNF-α, IL-6, and a load of interferons—attempting to hit the brakes to parasite multiplication and spread. You get TLR7 and TLR9, tucked away in endosomes, coming down hard on the nucleic acids of the parasite and triggering a chain reaction of signals crucial for that initial immune boost. When these signaling pathways ever get slightly off track, it can tip the scales toward more grievous disease outcomes because the host will lose its grip on controlling them. Observing how *Plasmodium* constituents interact with such receptors shines a light both on the initial defense mechanisms in malaria and on some potential areas for therapeutic realignments (Hu et al., 2021). Another component of our innate response is driven by the JAK/STAT signaling pathway. Essentially, this process translates extracellular cytokine signals into intracellular instructions that turn up pro-inflammatory genes and eliminator genes for invaders. When interferons and other immune messengers bind to their cytokine receptors, the JAK/STAT pathway is initiated, elevating the functions of macrophages to destroy microbes and initiating the production of reactive oxygen species that help in limiting parasite proliferation. This works well enough in most cases, but if the signaling does go wrong, it might either place the immune system in overdrive—risking tissue damage—or fail altogether in maintaining a lid on the parasite, demonstrating how delicate of an act even this pathway must attain. But overall, manipulating this cascade might be a desirable way to modulate immunity in malaria (Hu et al., 2021). Apart from such receptor cues, our body's own warriors also depend upon lysosomal mechanisms and autophagy-based techniques to kill the parasite within cells. Autophagy works quite similarly to a cellular recycling plant, helping eliminate infected RBCs or leftover plasmodial debris. But in a curious twist of fate, *Plasmodium* sometimes manages to outsmart such defenses, as if it were pledged to survival strategies that complicate the whole host-pathogen association. Small alterations in lysosomal pH and the activity of certain enzymes also play a very important role in antigen presentation and processing, and thereby in the immune response as a whole. Certain drugs employed in the treatment of malaria—extra credit, they also interfere with immune responses—seem to affect these mechanisms via altering cytokine release and the efficacy of parasite elimination. In general, knowledge of these within-cell defense strategies may potentially open new avenues for adjunct therapy targeting malaria (Nirk et al., 2020) (Figure 4.9).

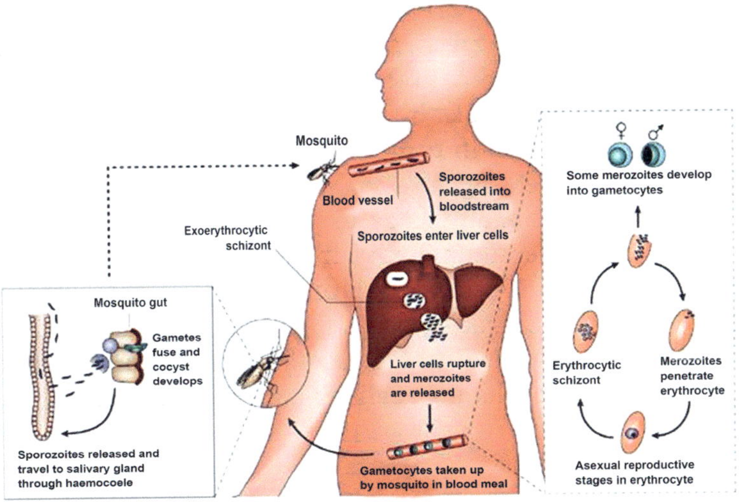

Figure 4.9. Immune response to malaria.

Source: Mota, M. M. (2010). *Parasite Life Cycle in the Human Host and Mosquito Vector.* https://media.springernature.com/full/springer-static/image/art%3A10.1038%2Fnri1311/MediaObjects/41577_2004_Article_BFnri1311_Fig1_HTML.jpg.

4.3.2. Adaptive Immune Response Mechanisms

The immune system's friend-or-foe discrimination is the most critical component of beating malaria. At the initial infection, our natal immunity, such as macrophages and dendritic cells—simply get to work, recognizing *Plasmodium* markers and transferring them to T cells that are in hiding in lymphoid tissues. The transfer triggers the adaptive response, with some T cells that start replicating to destroy infected liver and RBCs. T helper cells subsequently contribute by releasing chemical signals that activate macrophages into action and induce B cells into the production of antibodies that are specifically directed against the parasite. These antibodies help to counteract the attempts of the parasite to invade and remove infected RBCs. Of course, the parasite is not strictly sportsmanlike, its ability to change its surface properties (antigenic variation) acts to throw a spanner in the works. Drugs like HCQ, in the majority of cases, end up altering these immune pathways by interfering with endosome function and dampening pro-inflammatory signals (Nirk et al., 2020). Understanding these interplay dynamics is quite central to understanding how malaria works. The adaptability of macrophages plays a huge role in determining how our body combats malaria. At first, such cells will go into a pro-inflammatory M1 form, releasing cytokines like TNF-α and IL-12 which are used to trigger Th1 responses—all essential for parasite killing. But if that M1 form stays around for too long, it can cause tissue damage, so there is a need to switch over to an anti-inflammatory M2 form that releases IL-10 and TGF-β to calm everyone down and allow repair. This seesaw between M1 and M2 regulates the activation of T cells and the presentation of antigens to the immune system. In the clinical environment, malaria forces macrophages into switching states within different tissues, and this dynamic state can indeed govern both disease pathology as well as immune homeostasis. Some therapies are targeted toward regulating these macrophage moods to regain balance and maximize clinical response (Moghaddam et al., 2018). Overall, the chameleon function of macrophages bridges our initial defense to the later, more specific immune mechanisms of malaria. Permanent immunity to malaria depends on the concerted action of T and B lymphocytes whose specific responses maintain parasite populations low and reduce tissue damage. For example, in the liver stage, CD8+ T cells play a role in killing infected hepatocytes, while $CD4^+$ T helper cells assist by mobilizing B cells and increasing the macrophages' activity to remove the invaders. B cells, in turn, secrete high-affinity antibodies against the blood stage of *Plasmodium*, thereby preventing invasion of RBC and allowing opsonization. However, repeated exposure to malaria occasionally leads to problems like T cell exhaustion and skewed cytokine profiles, hence lowering overall immunity. In addition, pathways like the calcium pathway or alterations in the functioning of Toll-like receptors quietly control lymphocyte activation and differentiation, and some immunomodulatory drugs function by regulating these internal pathways (Nirk et al., 2020). Each of these adaptive strategies is not only essential for natural immunity but also serves as the foundation for developing realistic malaria vaccines.

4.3.3. Challenges in Developing Immunity

Malaria's stealthiness makes things tough for our immune system. The parasite messes up our RBCs, and that often leads to anemia—something that, by disrupting oxygen delivery and destabilizing cell environments, further complicates immune function. Anemia is not caused by a single factor alone; anemia is associated with nutrition issues, periods of inflammation, as well as some genetic defects, all of which tend to place additional burdens on how well the body can ward off an infection. In all but a few cases, however, the co-morbidity of other infections and inflammatory diseases in malarial areas only adds to the chaos, complicating the ability of the immune system to create the kind of long-term immunity that is at the core of a reduction in the health incidence of malaria (Chaparro & Suchdev, 2019). Then, of course, there is the whole question of macrophages, those cells that do a lot of contribution to our innate immune response. They tend to shift strategy depending on the situation—first, so-called M1 cells appear and release cytokines like TNF-α and IL-12 in an attempt to repel the parasite, but if they stay long enough, the excessive inflammation can damage tissues. On the other hand, M2 cells are involved in tissue repair and soothing inflammation but sometimes the overexpression of their activity paradoxically leads to the parasite escaping the immune response. This battle in macrophage function further complicates the matter in trying to stock up on a useful adaptive response to malaria (Moghaddam et al., 2018). To compound this, the parasite is a chameleon in itself. It constantly alters the proteins on its surface; a process known as antigenic variation—to pass through our antibodies, and that makes it hard for memory B cells to be able to do their job and makes it hard to develop effective vaccines. Repeated infection and persistent inflammation can even wear out the immune system and also lead to tolerance instead of the kind of protection that we would want. Alongside other issues like malnourishment and other diseases that also weaken immune defenses, all of these seem to spell trouble for achieving long-term immunity in regions that have experienced high levels of malaria infection.

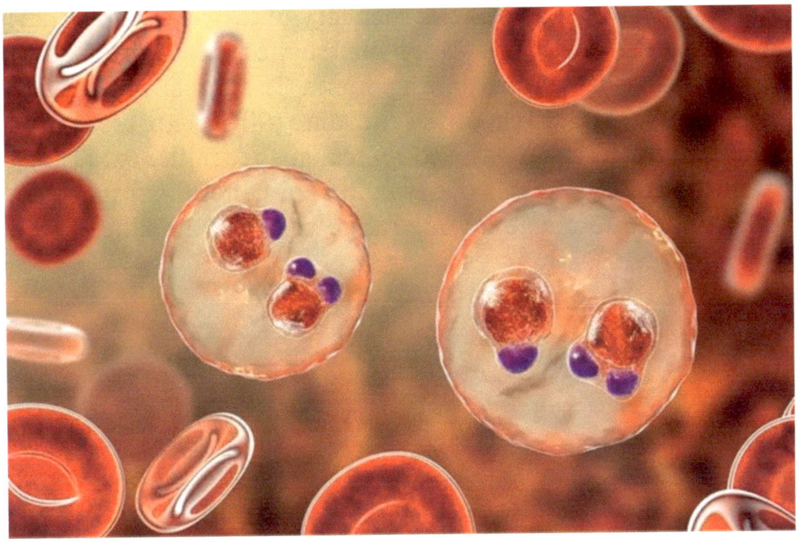

Source: Shutterstock. (2020). *Malaria Parasite Life Cycle and Transmission Vector Illustration*. https://d2jx2rerrg6sh3.cloudfront.net/image-handler/picture/2020/2/%40shutterstock_1521138356.jpg.

4.4. Pathophysiological Effects of Malaria

As soon as *Plasmodium* infects the human organism, a cascade of events quickly spirals out of control into a variety of medical issues. The parasite jumps into RBCs and kills them—this killing normally leads to anemia, one of the most important signs of malaria. Not only does loss of these cells decrease oxygen levels in the blood, but it also triggers a cytokine storm-type inflammatory process with very high levels of cytokines that cause fever and chills more intensely. Then, when these infected RBCs start clumping together in small blood vessels, they block blood flow, which interferes with tissue perfusion and can lead to organ complications, especially in the brain and kidneys. When those cells disintegrate and release parasitic components, the body responds with an aggressive immune reaction that can be beneficial and sometimes damaging. All of these jumbled processes form the basis for malaria's lethal effects, leading us to consider the host-pathogen association that has to be addressed in medicines. A huge concern with malaria is when it focuses on the brain, more frequently appearing as cerebral malaria. Here, things get very dangerous because blocked parasitized RBCs stick to the inner surfaces of capillaries within the brain, forming tiny clogs and clogging blood flow. This, in most cases, ruptures the blood-brain barrier and bumps up the pressure within the cranium, eventually leading to dire issues such as seizures, coma, or even death. Inflammatory mediators produced by the infection add additional stress to brain tissues and increase oxidative damage within the central nervous system. This type of stress is similar to that involved with other inflammatory diseases and has some molecular mechanisms in common with toxin- or viral infection-induced disease (Hahad et al., 2020; Petrakis et al., 2020). Generally, taking control of these processes is most important to writing treatments that counteract brain damage without totally compromising the resistance of the body. Malaria's reach does not stop at the brain—it also disrupts other vital organs like the lungs and kidneys, pushing the body in certain circumstances toward multi-organ failure. In the lung, increased capillary leak with inflammatory markers as well as aggregated infected RBCs may stimulate acute respiratory distress syndrome (ARDS), a complication that greatly worsens the recovery of the patient. Similarly, the kidneys may be influenced by the same kind of microvascular obstructions and direct cell damage, leading to acute kidney injury and further metabolic derangement. The nonspecific inflammatory response, better known as systemic inflammatory response syndrome (SIRS), expresses the damaging pathways of other life-threatening infections and points to typical suspects like oxidative stress and immune dysregulation (Hahad et al., 2020; Petrakis et al., 2020). In general, all these results highlight why severe malaria treatment needs to tackle a wide range of organ maladies rather than focusing on one causative factor (Figure 4.10).

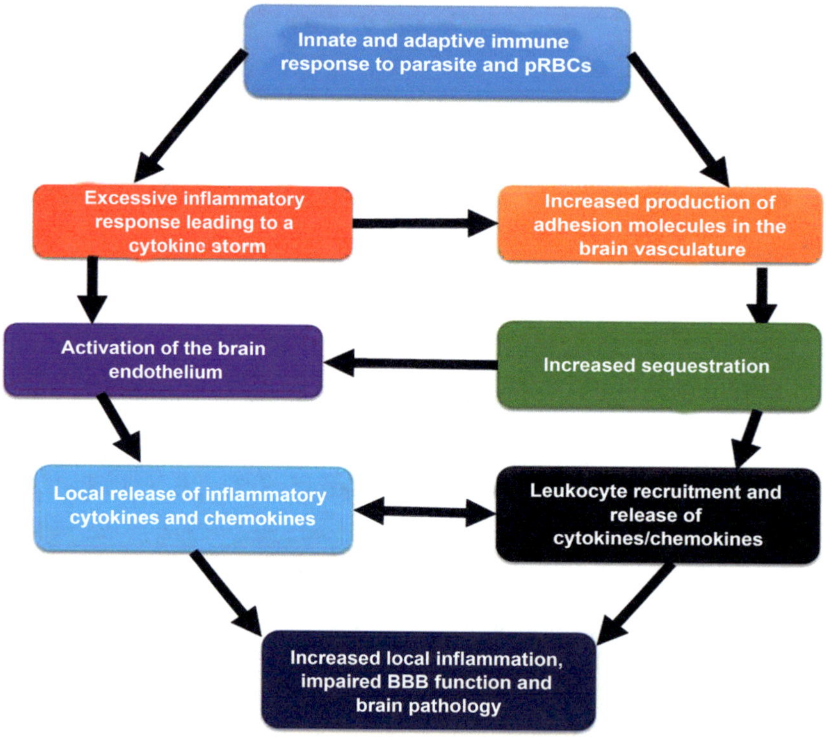

Figure 4.10. Pathophysiological effects of malaria.

Source: InTech. (n.d.). Image of plant defenses mechanisms. *In Plant defense Mechanisms and Secondary Metabolites.* https://cdnintech.com/media/chapter/68779/1512345123/media/F2.png.

4.4.1. Impact on Red Blood Cells (RBCs)

RBCs start to lose their usual resiliency as malaria becomes established. *Plasmodium*, especially *Plasmodium falciparum*, infects the blood and, to all intents and purposes suddenly, gets to work changing these cells both structurally and functionally. Infected cells become hard and sticky, sticking to one another in small blood vessels and interfering with the free flow of blood and supply of oxygen. The parasites manipulate membrane proteins such that the cells stick to vessel walls, a covert ruse to evade spleen clearance, which triggers a cascade: hemolysis, anemia, and turbulent microcirculation. In almost all cases, parasite-derived and host inflammatory mediators exacerbate mayhem, destabilizing the endothelium and providing an opening for systemic complications like metabolic acidosis and multi-organ failure (Sriboonvorakul et al., 2023). At the same time, the body's immune response isn't quite a good thing. When RBCs proudly display their altered surfaces, antibodies and splenic macrophages rush in for what is a clumsy cleanup job. This immune assault not only eliminates the infected cells but sometimes destroys healthy cells as well, aggravating the anemia. Concurrently, the JAK/STAT pathway, a key player in inflammatory signaling—is drawn into the situation by impacting RBC production and lifespan. Generally, if this pathway becomes slightly dysfunctional, it can further inhibit recovery from anemia. Essentially, the parasite's direct effect and these molecular signals become mated in a kind of complex relationship affecting the RBCs (Hu et al., 2021). When those damaged cells break down, the chain reactions go so much further than one might logically expect. When RBCs rupture, they also spill toxic heme and other by-products of the parasite into the blood, which have the potential to activate oxidative stress and get the lining of the blood vessel in overdrive, sometimes causing leakage of fluid and more inflammation. There is also some evidence that alterations in the gut microbiota, typically in the most severe forms of malaria, further drive the immune system out of equilibrium by permitting greater microbial translocation. All these factors, from the overt parasite blow to the host's reactive signals and even some microbial interference, all contribute to exacerbate metabolic acidosis and other complications. It is a complex, multi-faceted picture of disease far in excess of an uncomplicated invasion (Sriboonvorakul et al., 2023).

4.4.2. Effects on the Liver and Spleen

Malaria rattles the body up by triggering a whole series of reactions that impact major organs—mainly the liver and spleen. The liver leads the charge as it becomes the first stop for *Plasmodium parasites*, which need an important phase of their lifecycle there. In most cases, when such *parasites* settle in, they kill liver cells and initiate an inflammation that eventually disrupts metabolic activities and lays the ground for liver disease, usually marked by jaundice and raised levels of liver enzymes. Meanwhile, all of this is happening, the immune system responds in turn by nudging the hypothalamic-pituitary-adrenal axis, which in turn makes subtle changes in levels of glucocorticoids; these are the hormones that proceed to control the operation of blood vessels and immune responses, all part of the body's effort to contain the infection (Bosscher et al., 2019). So, glance over at the spleen, and it is only more fascinating and a little chaotic. Histologic examinations will typically show that the spleen does not stay normal but often ends up with degenerated white pulp, destroyed periarteriolar lymphoid sheaths, and even dilated sinusoids in the red pulp, which suggests that immune cells are piling up and tissue is being reorganized unexpectedly. Such reorganization impacts the spleen's role of eliminating infected erythrocytes efficiently, leading to most cases resulting in splenomegaly. It should also be noted that antimalarial drugs like chloroquine, Fansidar, and cotecxin can sometimes add insult to injury by causing additional histopathological changes and therefore slightly increasing the risk of splenic rupture or other derangements (Jimmy et al., 2014). All these effects on the liver and spleen are not merely direct consequences of the activity of the parasite—there is also an involvement of the immune mechanisms of the body and the drugs used during treatment. Broadly, the alteration in glucocorticoid levels during malaria may influence the extent of these organs' resilience, adding another level to the overall plan of the disease. While anti-malarial drugs still remain a requirement, there is a thin line involved: these drugs, as potent as they are, may sometimes induce hepatic jaundice or add further to spleen pathology. This integration of parasitic action, immune response, and drug action emphasizes the necessity of strict monitoring and regulation of treatment. All these interconnected elements enable us to realize just how complex malaria is in relation to impeding essential organ functions, and they point us in the direction of enhancing approaches to dealing with life-threatening complications (Bosscher et al., 2019; Jimmy et al., 2014) (Figure 4.11).

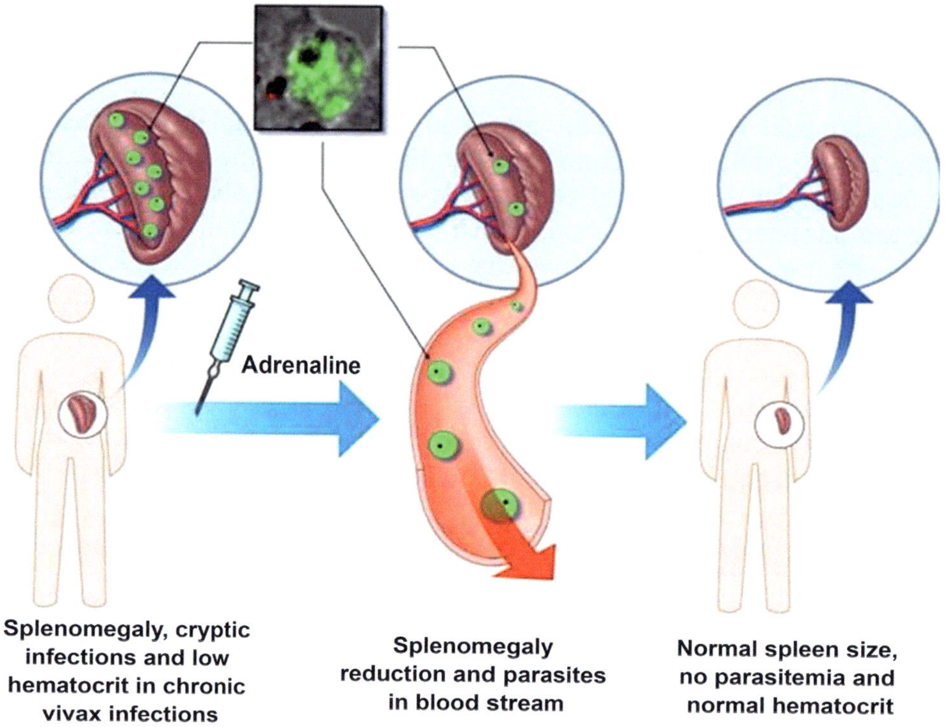

Figure 4.11. Effects of malaria on the liver and spleen.

Source: Monteiro, W., Brito-Sousa, J. D., Elizalde-Torrent, A., Bôtto-Menezes, C., Melo, G. C., Fernandez-Becerra, C., et al. (2020). Cryptic *Plasmodium* chronic infections: was *Maurizio Ascoli,* right? *Malaria Journal, 19*(1), 440.

4.4.3. Consequences for the Circulatory System

Malaria's assault on the circulatory system starts when the *parasites* infect RBCs, essentially breaking them apart and triggering a vague release of inflammatory signals. The breakdown (hemolysis) typically leads to anemia, so the blood's oxygen-carrying capacity is reduced and tissues become oxygen-deprived. In the meantime, the *parasites* wreak havoc on the flexibility of the cells—rigidifying them and making them unusually adhere to vessel walls. The sticking that is out of the ordinary, often called cytoadherence, has the impact of interfering with the free flow of blood through the tiny vessels and can even block them. The mechanical blockade and the activation of the vessel walls both initiate an inflammatory response that further worsens the dysfunction. These processes get complex and, in some cases, spin out into such disastrous complications as cerebral malaria, where impaired microcirculation causes neurological symptoms. Taken together, these processes illustrate the degree to which the impact of malaria on the blood system is multifactorial and capricious. Apart from causing mere blockage, malaria also triggers an inflammatory storm systemically that further undermines circulatory integrity. Overall, a surplus of cytokines, tumor necrosis factor-alpha, interleukins, etc., leads to generalized endothelial activation and makes the blood vessels leakier than normal.

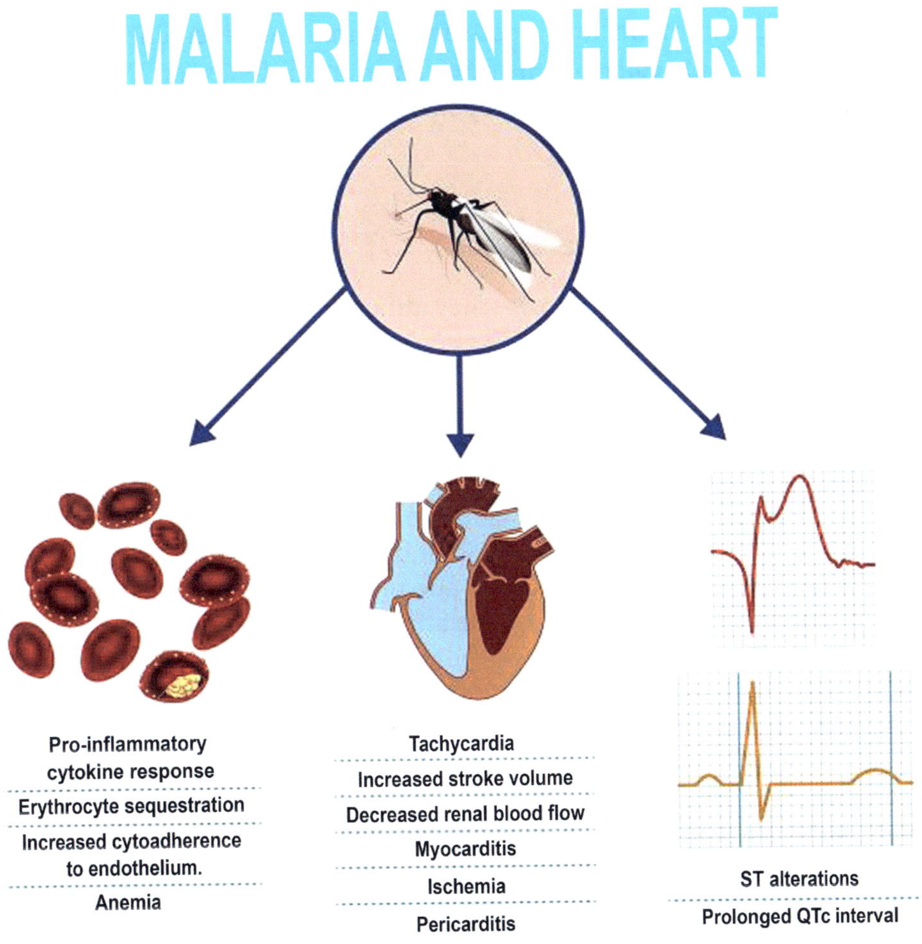

Figure 4.12. Consequences for the circulatory system.

Source: Elsevier. (n.d.). *Figure 2-02 from B9780323911221000039.* https://ars.els-cdn.com/content/image/3-s2.0-B9780323911221000039-f02-02-9780323911221.jpg.

The storm of inflammation may trigger capillary leakage, leading to a drop in blood volume and pressure, thereby hammering the heart with further stress. In addition, infection itself will drive the body into a hypercoagulable state, with the consequence that conditions like disseminated intravascular coagulation are more likely, with microclots forming and returning by feedback to further occlude small vessels. In the extreme, the additive effect of uncontrolled inflammation and circulatory failure can mimic the clinical appearance of septic shock—blurring boundaries between different cardiovascular emergencies (Gotts et al., 2016). If the malaria becomes severe enough, the circulatory system simply cannot cope at times, and more severe resuscitative measures are required. The European Resuscitation Council, for example, emphasizes that an immediate, detailed assessment and a rapid treatment designed to restore cardiovascular function is critical, especially if presentations resemble shock states (Perkins et al., 2021). Practically, stable blood pressure and good oxygen delivery generally mean fluid resuscitation at a very fast rate, with vasoactive support as needed. At the same time, however, one must also treat the underlying parasite with immediate antimalarial therapy, thereby interrupting the ongoing cascade of circulatory derangement. Even after initial stabilization, meticulous post-resuscitation management is accountable for the prevention of recurrent vascular collapse and allowance of full recovery. Together, understanding of these complex circulatory challenges posed by malaria is required to improve clinical outcomes in severely ill patients (Figure 4.12).

4.5. Clinical Manifestations of Malaria

The symptoms of malaria are fairly diverse—they differ not only with the type of *Plasmodium* involved but even with the intensity of an individual's immune response. At the onset, symptoms like chills, fever, sweats, headaches, and general malaise look almost identical to your run-of-the-mill fever, which makes early diagnosis an order of magnitude more difficult. Then, after the disease is established, you start to see more distinctive signs, in part because infected RBCs lyse and trigger a full-blown inflammatory response. You usually get a pattern of fever rhythm when these RBCs lyse synchronously, dumping merozoites and toxins into the bloodstream that, in turn, cause the release of pro-inflammatory cytokines. In more severe attacks, issues like severe anemia, hypoglycemia, and even metabolic acidosis occur due to cell lysis and inadequate organ perfusion, which is how both uncontrolled parasite proliferation and the body's own response shape the overall image of malaria (Phyo et al., 2022). Very young children and pregnant women, for instance, suffer most from severe malaria due to their compromised immune status. Anemia, particularly in children, is a serious issue, often fueled by chronic infections that cause both hemolysis and a type of bone marrow suppression. In pregnancy, *vivax* and *falciparum* infections tend to congest the placenta, disrupting the exchange of oxygen and nutrients and increasing risks like low birth weight, fetal loss, and severe maternal anemia. It now looks like vivax malaria, once thought to be benign, can hit hard, according to new evidence. And with the disease varying so extremely from one place—or even within the same place—to another, prognosis and treatment are an even more elusive target. This more subtle perspective demands personalized intervention for the most vulnerable while indicating persistent gaps in our knowledge (Phyo et al., 2022). Once malaria slips into its severe phase, the complications have the potential to strike several of the body's systems simultaneously due in part to the parasite's devious mechanisms for evading our defenses. Take cerebral malaria, for instance: it manifests as an altered state of consciousness and even seizures, the result of parasitized blood cells sticking firmly to the microvessels of the brain and causing enough inflammation to breech the blood-brain barrier. At the pulmonary end, ARDS can occur when the body's inflammatory response and the abnormal activity of endothelial cells combine to create leaky vessels and hypoxia. Kidneys can then become involved, and metabolic disturbances like acidosis add to the grim picture. In total, these complex difficulties are a muddled interaction between the *parasites*, the immune system, and small vessel disease. With such a wide range of these clinical presentations, early identification of the disease and institution of proper antimalarial treatment, rooted in a clear comprehension of these complex processes—remains of the utmost significance to better outcomes (Ohiagu et al., 2021) (Figure 4.13).

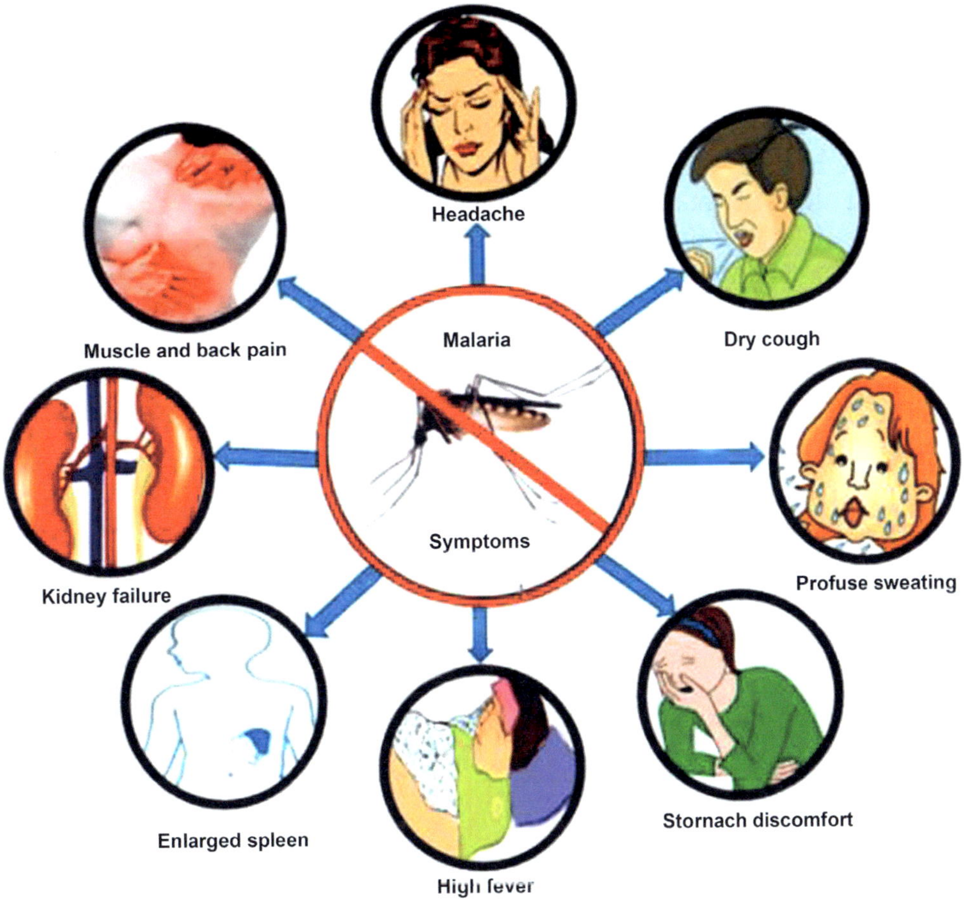

Figure 4.13. Clinical manifestations of malaria.

Source: Okello, D., & Kang, Y. (2019). Illustration of some common symptoms of malaria. In Exploring antimalarial herbal plants across communities in Uganda based on electronic data. *Evidence-based Complementary and Alternative Medicine.*

4.5.1. Symptoms of Uncomplicated Malaria

Malaria can start with very innocent-appearing symptoms that other feverish infections also display – rendering that initial diagnosis quite challenging. Victims of the uncomplicated form of this infection usually suffer recurring episodic fevers, sometimes with chills and shaking rigors that occur as the parasite lyses RBCs in a highly synchronous manner. The body, having been exposed to parts of this parasite, then releases some of the inflammation-causing chemicals (like TNF-α) that cause fever. You might also experience headache, overall feeling of sickness, muscle aches, and gastrointestinal upset like nausea or vomiting. All these symptoms display both the overall inflammatory response of the body and the more direct effects of chemicals this parasite secretes. Most often, such frequent fevers parallel the way *Plasmodium* develops in the blood cells, a common sign of its advanced in uncomplicated disease (Fikadu et al., 2023). Detection of such symptoms in the early stages is necessary so that treatment can be started in advance so as not to aggravate the disease. Taking a closer examination of what is happening inside, the symptoms have their origin in the way the parasite functions inside our RBCs and the ensuing immune resistance. Essentially, after entering the cells, the *parasites* start breeding—first becoming trophozoites, then shedding to become schizonts, before bursting the cells to release a flood of merozoites which go on to infect other cells. This constant cycle, which will eventually result in anemia, also triggers macrophage activity that attempts to clean up by engulfing the free *parasites* as well as the infected cells. The body's inflammation becomes more heightened with repeated exposure to these markers for *parasites*, hence why the fevers and that sickish feeling are so prevalent. While these symptoms are not unique to malaria, they are a critical juncture of intersection between the development of the parasite and immune response. In fact, some scientists suggest that sensing unique biochemical or molecular signals, like those involving how our blood vessel cells react—can potentially identify a more precise diagnosis (Gomes et al., 2023). And so, in a way, the big picture of all these symptoms shows how the parasite and our body are essentially always combined up. Despite all the excessive variation that is seen in how severe these symptoms can become; uncomplicated malaria does not usually endanger vital organs immediately. But that initial sign is important warning signs that encourage clinicians to start antimalarial drugs early before things turn for the worse. It is also significant that since these symptoms are very common in other febrile illnesses found in endemic areas, diagnosis of malaria based on clinical symptoms alone would be unreliable.

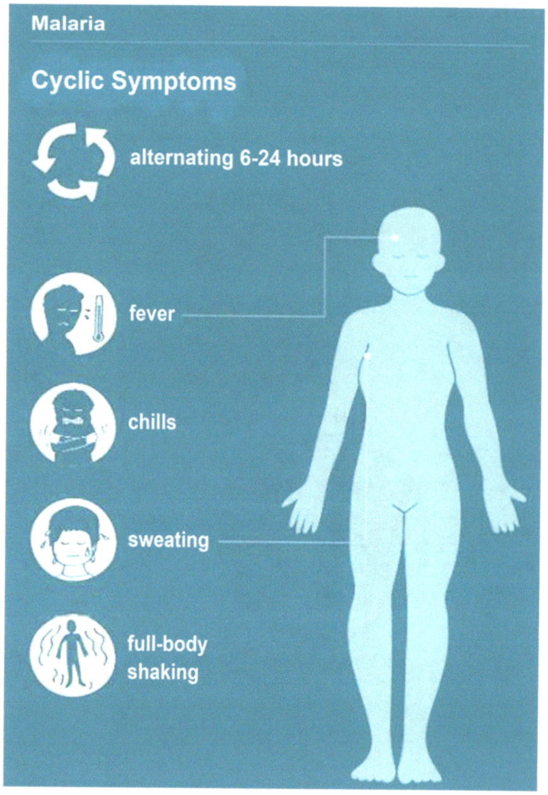

Figure 4.14. Symptoms of uncomplicated malaria.

Source: Verywell Health. (2018). *Symptoms of Malaria*. https://www.verywellhealth.com/thmb/HJLqJ-HM5eBb2TN33jP7vpOILGo=/1500x0/filters:no_upscale():max_bytes(150000):strip_icc()/malaria-symptoms-5ad7552c119fa8003660f7d0.png.

Due to this reason, additional tests—be it looking at a blood smear under a microscope or a rapid antigen test, occasionally must be performed in order to determine the infection. In general, the focus now is to decrease the amount of *parasites* within the blood and relieve the symptoms so as not to have complications like cerebral involvement or severe anemia. Recognition of these subtle, at times interwoven signs coupled with proper comprehension of what is transpiring in the body helps in efficient case management, which further equates to better patient outcomes (Fikadu et al., 2023; Gomes et al., 2023).

4.5.2. Symptoms of Severe Malaria

Severe malaria is not just an issue of returning fever—it's a set of symptoms that all of a sudden crop up as the parasite ravages your body in weird and wonderful ways. First, you'll simply have fits of chills, an alternating fever, and general malaise, all quite normal in uncomplicated malaria. But soon enough, something goes horribly wrong. In the majority of cases, the mayhem starts when infected red blood cells burst and release minute fragments of *parasites* (merozoites) and toxic waste products into your bloodstream. This shock release will most likely stimulate your immune system into overdrive, spewing inflammatory chemicals like TNF-α into you, which are the culprits for the spiking temperature and overall inflammation. Besides that, when these parasite-infested red blood cells start to clog small-sized vessels, the generated clog inhibits the effective flow of blood, and thus low oxygen and acid overloading in the body. It is a combination of actions that suggests that the disease can surge very quickly, thereby making the need for early diagnosis and treatment crucial (Fikadu et al., 2023).

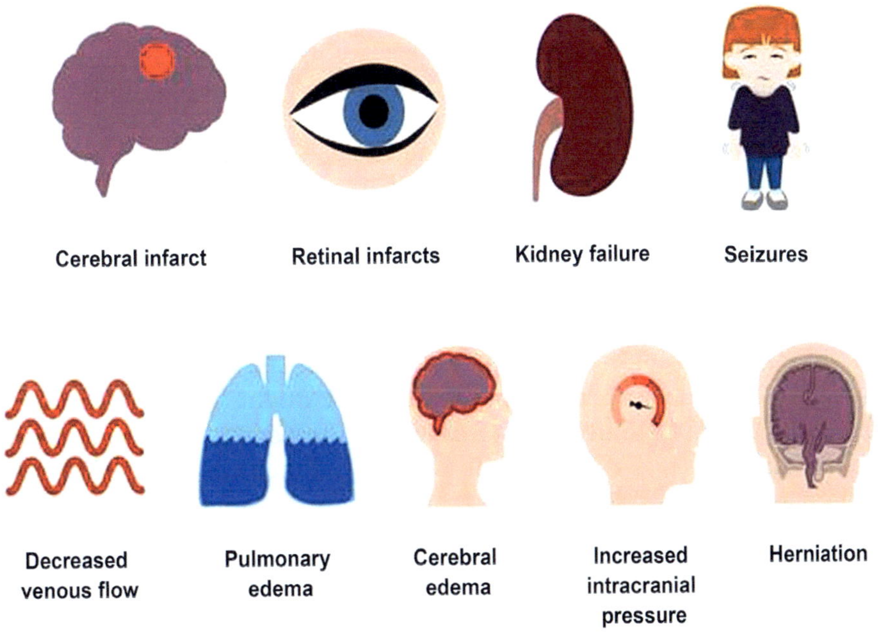

Figure 4.15. Symptoms of severe malaria.

Source: Medmastery. (n.d.). *Malaria-Induced Disseminated Intravascular Coagulation.* https://d25iein5sonfaj.cloudfront.net/v1/public-drupal-medmastery-assets-production/migrated-images/malaria-induced-disseminated-intravascular-coagulation.png?cfg=eyJ3aWR0aCI6NjAwLCJoZWlnaHQiOjQwMCwib3V0cHV0Ijoid2VicCJ9.

The brain also becomes involved in the crossfire, something typically referred to as cerebral malaria. Patients become stuck here with seizures, sleepy or disoriented mentality, or even go into a coma—pretty much due to brain swelling and hidden blockages in those narrowing itty-bitty capillaries. Overall, the decreased oxygen and general inflammatory commotion disables the blood-brain barrier, which then scrambles how neurons function. This kind of neurological knock-on not only raises the stakes in regard to how sick you can get, but it also raises the risk of mortality, especially in children. Add other metabolic complications like low blood sugar and elevation of lactic acid, and it gets even more complex, making it more difficult to manage the illness adequately (Fikadu et al., 2023). Not just the brain is affected; severe malaria often turns into a multi-organ drama. A few patients develop severe lung issues, such as ARDS, till now seen with lung inflammation and fluid leak. Even the kidneys are not spared—low perfusion and hemoglobin release due to extensive breakdown of red cells can lead to acute kidney injury. At the same time, the body's RBCs are hit from all sides, with infected and even uninfected cells being torn asunder, further abetted by a slowed-down bone marrow. And to make things worse, side effects like vomiting and diarrhea can devastate hydration status and electrolyte balance. The overall image is one of generalized disruption of the body brought by the parasite, a confusion that indeed requires a comprehensive, all-encompassing clinical approach to avoid both immediate and eventual damage (Fikadu et al., 2023) (Figure 4.15).

4.5.3. Complications Associated with Malaria

Malaria does not come alone with its obvious symptoms, but it can trigger an entire range of nasty complications that impact patients in more ways than one. Anemia, for instance, is a very severe effect, especially on pregnant women who are already at risk. The process is a bit complex – RBCs get destroyed when the *parasites* invade, the immune system also likes to attack them, and the body's efforts at creating new ones just don't keep up. In pregnancy, this can lead to extra trouble for mom and baby, typically causing low birth weight or even preterm birth. If diseases like HIV are also involved, it is twice as complicated because both conditions seem to worsen nutritional deficiencies and lower the creation of blood cells. Overall, truly understanding how all of these factors mix together is the future of improving both diagnosis and treatment techniques (Obeagu et al., 2025). Oxidative stress seems to be a major culprit in the complications that are related to malaria – specifically in the placenta during pregnancy. You might find that the levels of something such as malondialdehyde and uric acid rise, showing more oxidative damage, and the resident defender, superoxide dismutase, is lacking. This uneven balance can injure the tissue and disturb the structure of the placenta – as evidenced by abnormal formations such as syncytial knots, areas of fibrinoid necrosis, and clumps of white blood cells. These alterations disrupt the vital exchange of oxygen and nutrients between mother and baby, resulting in complications such as intrauterine growth retardation and preterm delivery. Generally speaking, it is the more serious *Plasmodium falciparum* infections that hit harder with this oxidative attack, but even *Plasmodium vivax* is not above causing trouble. Keeping track of these oxidative markers, therefore, is very important in predicting complications and in tailoring treatment (Chandrashekhar et al., 2022). Beyond the blood and oxidative complications, malaria complications can involve the whole body. Severe malaria leads to pulmonary edema in certain cases – a condition where fluid collects in the lungs and breathing becomes a life-threatening problem with a heightened risk of death. The infection also triggers an inflammatory response that will likely lead to endothelial dysfunction, coagulopathy, and impaired microcirculation, all of which add to the severity of the clinical issue. In pregnant women, these systemic effects multiply mom's and baby's risk many times over. It thus makes sense to approach comprehensively – one that focuses on prevention, early detection, and targeted treatment of every complication. Public health efforts, especially in malaria-endemic areas, need to prioritize raising awareness, improving access to antenatal care, and instituting rigorous control measures to mitigate these risks (Chandrashekhar et al., 2022; Obeagu et al., 2025).

4.6. Diagnosis and Treatment

Malaria may show in all kinds of forms—its symptoms aren't always the same and sometimes show up out of nowhere. You may experience bouts of fever that sometimes show up and vanish a random shiver, or even anemia that comes into the picture. Various areas of your body are a part of this kind of mess because the disease follows a very complex way of affecting things. Doctors often start with suspicion when symptoms like recurring fever and chills are present, but they still need to test in the lab to be sure. A microscope examination of stained blood smears still remains the top priority in observing *Plasmodium parasites* in red cells and even driving the species into action. Meanwhile, RDTs have gained popularity as they are user-friendly and provide fast results, particularly where the prevalence of malaria is high. These methods not only warn the infection—they also help warn when things can go seriously awry, e.g., if cerebral malaria or severe anemia crops up, which means that identifying the exact species and measuring parasite loads is important to determine the right treatment (Ohiagu et al., 2021). Getting treatment started as soon as possible is also essential to avoid the infection becoming more dangerous. The kind of treatment used usually depends on what *Plasmodium* is involved, how resistant the *parasites* are, and individual factors like age or pregnancy. For uncomplicated *falciparum* malaria, doctors usually prescribe artemisinin-based combination regimens (ACTs) because they quickly and effectively suppress the parasite levels. When the disease is very severe, an IV of artesunate typically takes the place of quinine, which is considered to be less effective. Doctors can also include extra measures to fend offside effects like acidosis, hypoglycemia, or stress to an organ, echoing the reality that malaria's impact can be multifaceted. Following a regimen and watching out for drug resistance is not just important for the patient—it also has quite a lot to do with the wider public health picture (Ohiagu et al., 2021). Occasionally, the complications from malaria build an inflammatory reaction that will be very much like a fair amount of sepsis, so struggling with the parasite alone is not enough. Problems that involve acute respiratory distress syndrome, kidney damage, and problems involving the brain seem to occur, and these need types of treatment more in the style of an intensive care unit. The combination of the challenges forces physicians to incorporate exact diagnostic efforts with treatment regimens that are appropriate to the patient's overall condition. Early diagnosis of extreme symptoms and swift action are critical to survival, and they go in parallel with preventive actions such as eliminating mosquitoes and prophylactic drug administration. All this points to the fact that malaria treatment is a two-pronged endeavor—one accurate diagnosis and one tailored treatment—both aimed at reducing the heavy burden of the disease worldwide (Ohiagu et al., 2021).

4.6.1. Diagnostic Methods (Microscopy, Rapid Tests)

An accurate diagnosis of malaria is key to comprehending the disease's progression and its effects on the body. The majority of experts continue to use conventional microscopy—both thick and thin blood films—since it enables one to literally count the *parasites* and even distinguish among the different *Plasmodium* species. You can even visualize the parasite hiding in RBCs, which gives clues of the parasite burden and is associated with how severe symptoms will be. Technically, the method does require some technical skill, and strict quality controls, and its somewhat time-consuming—factors that make it less easy to establish in resource-limited settings. Parasite density is all over the map, and asymptomatic carriers throw another monkey wrench into the works, so other methods to enhance sensitivity and allow larger-scale studies are needed. In essence, because the impact of malaria is transmitted through the active engagement of the parasite with host cells, a vigilant microscopy diagnosis opens the avenue for closer scrutiny of these interactions and, ultimately, to a better understanding of what patients endure (Volpe & Battistoni, 2019). Otherwise, rapid diagnostic tests (RDTs) have also become valuable adjuncts when skilled microscopists or advanced laboratories are in short supply. They do so by detecting some *Plasmodium* antigens in a small drop of blood, with some providing results in 15 to 30 minutes—very handy for point-of-care testing. Generally, however, while the kits can detect both overt and even some hidden asymptomatic infections, their sensitivity ranges quite a bit depending on which antigen they're targeted against, the parasite density, and the range of species present. They don't provide a tidy number of *parasites* or make it simple to determine whether that positive test result signifies an active infection or residual remnants, which can complicate matters—particularly when monitoring treatment responses or searching for a recurrence. However, it is clear that RDTs give valuable data on the prevalence of malaria and trigger early treatment, an important element in lessening the detrimental effect of high parasite loads and associated inflammatory responses (Marcilla et al., 2014). A combination of conventional microscopy and these rapid tests supplies a graded system of malaria diagnosis that is genuinely worthy of the disease's complexity. Even recent big-scale studies demonstrate that the diagnostic method employed can sometimes detect varying relationships with clinical results, like even hypertension in some cases, which only serves to point out just how heterogeneous malaria infections are (Volpe & Battistoni, 2019). For instance, when microscopy is positive, it tends to be accompanied by frank symptoms and raised inflammatory markers that lead to blood vessel change and complications, but an RDT-only positive case may represent a low-grade or insidious infection with its own particular immune signature.

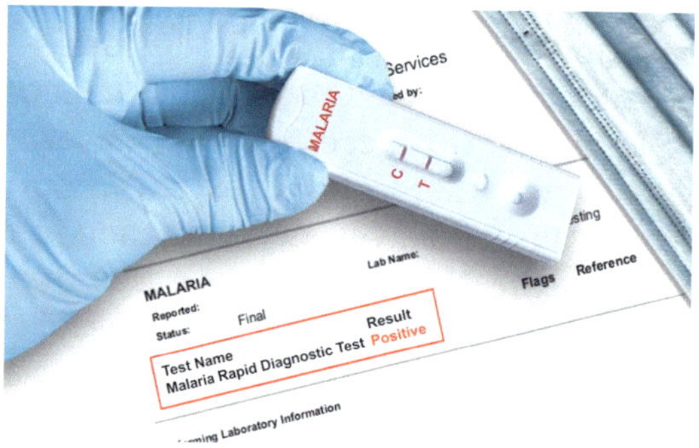

Figure 4.16. Rapid tests of malaria.

Source: The Conversation. (2022). *Illustration of Some Common Symptoms of Malaria.* https://images.theconversation.com/files/447747/original/file-20220222-13-1nqn2c6.jpg?ixlib=rb-4.1.0&q=45&auto=format&w=926&fit=clip.

To a large extent, digging out these diagnostic nuances explains the parasite-host interaction's complex exchange, the immune response fine-tuning, and the resulting damage. Also, recent studies on extracellular vesicles (EVs) hold out the prospect of novel, innovative diagnostics that will someday pick up parasite-derived biomarkers—ones that mirror disease severity and host response. Cumulatively, this evolving diagnostic environment is essential for advancing our understanding of the inner workings of malaria and improving how we deliver patient care (Marcilla et al., 2014) (Figure 4.16).

4.6.2. Antimalarial Medications and Their Mechanisms

Most treatments for malaria begin with a set of drugs that all act on the parasite in some kind of weird way. Chloroquine and HCQ, for instance, are relatively common—these drugs interfere with the parasite's trick of getting rid of poisonous heme after it has broken down hemoglobin from RBCs. Instead of enabling the toxic heme to be safely processed (by converting it into hemozoin), the pathway is blocked, and the parasite ends up with a pathogenic excess of free heme. More recently, however, the development of chloroquine-resistant strains has forced healthcare individuals to have recourse to substitutes like ACTs, which, all factors considered, work to cause reactive oxygen species to stress and quickly eliminate the parasite. It is an understanding of these drug effects that is most important, especially in regions where drug resistance makes therapy an ever-evolving target (Hussein et al., 2020). Another layer to these therapies is that some of these drugs also interfere with the parasite's own nucleic acid and protein synthesis. Employ antifolate medications such as pyrimethamine and sulfadoxine; these block enzymes like dihydrofolate reductase and dihydropteroate synthase that are necessary in the production of folate, which in most cases, disrupt DNA replication and cell division. This disruption destroys the ability of the parasite to divide in liver and blood cells, cutting its number significantly. However, the parasite occasionally evades these single-agent drugs through mutation, which is why combination therapy is now the order of the day. Subsequently there's primaquine, traditionally used to clear those pesky latent forms (hypnozoites) from the liver of *P. vivax* and *P. ovale*, preventing relapses. Collecting all these varied activities indeed makes our broad knowledge of how to combat malaria's complicated life cycle (Hussein et al., 2020) much more detailed. While the core intention is always to destroy *Plasmodium*, it should be remembered that such medicines do so much more than that when other conditions are attached. For example, HCQ's immunomodulatory effect initially preferred in malaria treatment, has even been put forward in the case of viral pandemics like COVID-19 as a possibility that the drugs might have more than one activity outside of their mechanism against *parasites* (Hussein et al., 2020). There even is some hypothesis regarding host factors, like androgen-modulated levels of enzymes, which may affect how severe infections become, as seen in certain viral models, and that indirectly may shed light on research in malaria. Overall, analyzing these mixed mechanisms in the broader health context reminds us of the versatility of antimalarial drugs, not just for direct malaria control but also for their potential ripple effects on infectious diseases overall.

4.6.3. Challenges in Treatment and Drug Resistance

We have made progress with developing antimalarial drugs, yet the treatment of malaria still stumbles because the parasite continues to evolve in its approach. *Plasmodium falciparum*, for instance, shows a capacity for avoiding our best treatments—drugs that once worked well can subsequently fail. Most often, genetic mutations in the parasite modify targets of drugs or amplify processes that push medicine out of infected RBCs so that less of the drug is retained. Its ever-changing lifecycle and various genetics only contribute to the uncertainty, so it is challenging to come up with a solution spanning all levels of infection. In most instances, this continuous game of cat and mouse between drug development and nasty resistance drives the need for new targets and creative drug combinations that are ahead of the game. Genetics put apart; our own immune system plays a significant role in how the cure plays out as well. Macrophages, the body's first line of defense, have two phases: M1, which sends out inflammatory messages to mobilize against the parasite, and M2, which shows up later to calm down the inflammation and help repair damage. Initially, the M1 cells are helpful, but if they stay around too long, they start causing damage to good tissue. Subsequently there are M2 cells that simplify things further, but maintaining this shift in a grip is a delicate balance that both affects disease severity and healing. Essentially, whatever type of treatment there is has to be mindful of this immune juggling—do it wrong and you might find yourself letting the parasite persist or even increasing the damage (Moghaddam et al., 2018). The challenge is further compounded when we take into account the maze of intracellular signaling that constitutes the battle between parasite and host. Take the JAK/STAT pathway, for example; it is used to normally control cytokine signals and immune responses but becomes a liability if it falters. Any misstep here in the pathway would destabilize the immune balance, making it harder for the body to fight *Plasmodium*. There is promise in engineering these signaling pathways to increase the effectiveness of drugs and minimize tissue damage, but it is a sensitive experiment—adjust the system too much, and normal cell function may suffer as a result. In most cases, greater scrutiny of pathways like JAK/STAT is the way to create treatments that target both parasite resistance and the subtleties of our own immune reactions (Hu et al., 2021).

CLOSER LOOK

TROPHOZOITE

Trophozoite is the active feeding and moving phase in most protozoan *parasites'* life cycle. It is also the metabolically active phase in which the organism grows and commonly causes the host's disease signs. Trophozoites typically reside in the host body fluids, such as blood, intestines, or tissues, depending on the species of the protozoa. They are commonly delicate, environmentally sensitive, and not viable for extended periods of time outside the host, which differentiates them from the cyst stage — a quiescent, non-motile, environmentally resilient stage that enables transmission from host to host. Perhaps the most familiar example of a protozoan whose life cycle includes a trophozoite stage is *Entamoeba histolytica*, the causative parasite of amoebiasis. In this organism, the trophozoite exists in the large intestine, feeding on mucosal cells and bacteria, and invading tissues at times and causing dysentery or liver abscesses. Similarly, in the malarial parasite *Plasmodium* spp., the trophozoite is a stage in RBCs in which the parasite develops and metabolizes hemoglobin, resulting in the destruction of the red cells of the host and the recurring cycles of fever characteristic of malaria. In *Giardia lamblia*, the trophozoite attaches itself to the intestinal mucosa using a ventral adhesive disc, leading to diarrhea and malabsorption in infected man.

Trophozoites vary in shape and size depending on the species. They are usually amoeboid with pseudopodia (false feet) for motility and ingestion, but some trophozoites are flagellate or ciliated and use these to move about. The trophozoite stage typically reproduces asexually by binary fission, allowing the population to increase rapidly in the host. As they are actively growing and eating, trophozoites are typically the primary perpetrators of tissue damage and manifestations of protozoan infections. Diagnosis is highly dependent on their identification, e.g., in stool or blood where microscopic inspection can detect them and their structure. Because trophozoites are fragile and typically destroyed outside the body, obtaining and preserving the specimen must be done quickly and correctly.

The excretion of trophozoites in clinical material is an absolute indication of active infection. In intestinal protozoal infections such as amoebiasis and giardiasis, trophozoites are most often isolated from freshly passed loose stool, and cysts are commonly seen in formed stool. This helps clinicians to determine the stage and severity of infection. In blood-borne infections such as malaria or trypanosomiasis, trophozoites are identified in stained blood smears. Treatment of trophozoite-related infections typically consists of antiprotozoal medication such as metronidazole, tinidazole, or some antimalarials depending on the organism involved.

SUMMARY

Malaria's history is complex. The intermingling of the *Plasmodium* parasite with our physiology just shows how complex this disease is. Even though scientists have been working on it for centuries, new hints keep surfacing - what we previously perceived as mere minor infections due to inciting severe conditions owing to various types of *parasites*, and *vivax* being a good example, it now appears. Apparently, announcing *vivax* malaria is relatively harmless is no longer cutting it; kids and pregnant women, most likely, are left with something more than we had bargained for. Then, if we consider how symptoms vary based on the place we are, we are left with way too many questions still unanswered regarding what is happening inside us. These gaps in knowledge indeed impede firm interventions, so more it is important to focus on prevention and avoiding relapses among high-risk groups (Phyo et al., 2022). Placental malaria is a confounding saga too. It exhibits not just an infection but a complicated mix of the *parasite's* deceptions and the body's own factors. Some recent studies even point to the possibility that the sex of the child is involved - paradoxically enough, female placentas seem to bear the brunt of parasite pounding. This new finding suggests that immune responses and hormonal variations linked to fetal sex can alter the placental environment, subtly changing the risk for unattractive pregnancy complications. Apparently, these facts require closer inspection to sharpen diagnosis and improve prenatal care, ultimately to improve both maternal and infant health (Adam et al., 2017). Ultimately, understanding malaria is a matter of chasing a moving target—a dynamic puzzle of host-parasite interactions that vary with varied species and patient populations. Overall, identifying all of those disease mechanisms—species-specific features to pregnancy and even fetal gender—is crucial if we're going to come up with effective treatments and controls. Filling in the blanks through careful research and incremental clinical experience should be able to guide better public health efforts to curb malaria's global reach. Thus, an adaptive approach combining biological, epidemiological, and clinical hints is not a nice-to-have, but rather a prerequisite for addressing malaria's chronic issues and assisting those most vulnerable (Adam et al., 2017; Phyo et al., 2022).

The complex association of malaria starts when a tiny parasite gains entry into the bloodstream after a mosquito bite. Sporozoites invade liver cells shortly afterward—almost under the radar, and begin replicating. In no time, these liver-stage *parasites* explode as merozoites that continue to invade RBCs and cause invasion and destruction cycles over and over. When infected cells that cavitate finally explode, they eject both new merozoites and a mix of toxins that provoke a drastic immune reaction, typically followed by fever and other less-than-ideal symptoms. Occasionally these infected cells clog tiny blood vessels, which leads to a blood flow mess, results in organ problems, and will even produce extreme attacks such as cerebral hemorrhaging. Most times, the parasite's productive replication, coupled with the body's hyperactive responses, creates a complicated web that constitutes the foundation of the cause of the disease. Our immune system is not overlooked either. The innate immune system, the body's first line of defense, receives its first exposure to the parasite, subsequently the more elaborate, adaptive takes over with particular antibodies and cellular responses that dictate for the most part how effective parasite removal will be, and finally, how worse things become. Nonetheless, the parasite is not to be underestimated; it tends to shift the proteins on the infected cell surface—in a latent way, to avoid immune detection. This underhanded trick enables the infection to last, with the resulting, sometimes chronic, inflammation making things even more complicated by sometimes compelling the immune system to its own collateral damage. In most cases, dealing with such the turns and twists of immune dynamics is important to understand malaria in its full breadth and leads us to new therapeutic avenues and vaccine ideas. This becomes even more complicated when you also add in the various strains' actions. Even though *Plasmodium falciparum* is usually the one to blame for the worst consequences, other species can cause destruction. There is also the increasingly common trend of developing resistant strains of *parasites*, which makes the waters of treatment muddy and necessitates careful follow-up. Additionally, where patients already carry co-infections or comorbid conditions, especially in low-resource environments—the virulence of malaria increases, rendering diagnosis and treatment a real challenge (Cox et al., 2014; Basmaci et al., 2019). In general, putting together the parasite's activity, the variable responses of our own body, and these generalized epidemiological variables gives us a richer, more useful view of why malaria destroys and what we can do to keep ahead.

KEY TERMS FROM THIS CHAPTER

- Hemolysis
- Pro-inflammatory Response
- Rosetting
- Cerebral Malaria
- Splenomegaly
- Immune Evasion
- Multi-organ Failure
- Anemia
- Fever Paroxysms
- Sequestration
- Metabolic Acidosis
- Hepatomegaly
- Endothelial Dysfunction
- Severe Malaria
- Cytokine Release
- Cytoadherence
- Microvascular Obstruction
- Hypoglycemia
- Hemozoin Pigment
- Tissue Hypoxia

References

1. Abbas Shapouri Moghaddam, S., Mohammadian Haftcheshmeh, S., Vazini, H., Taghadosi, M., Esmaeili, S. A., Mardani, F., Seifi, B., et al. (2018). Macrophage plasticity, polarization, and function in health and disease. *Journal of Cellular Physiology, 233*, 6425–6440. https://doi.org/10.1002/jcp.26429.
2. Chandrashekhar, V. N., Punnath, K., Dayanand, K. K., Kakkilaya, S. B., Jayadev, P., Kumari, S. N., Achur, R. N., & Gowda, D. C. (2022). Impact of oxidative stress in response to malarial infection during pregnancy: Complications, histological changes, and pregnancy outcomes. *Tropical parasitology, 12*(1), 21–33. https://doi.org/10.4103/tp.TP_18_20(accessed on 13 May 2025).
3. Adam, I., Salih, M. M., Mohmmed, A. A., Rayis, D. A., & Elbashir, M. I. (2017). Pregnant women carrying female fetuses are at higher risk of placental malaria infection. *PLOS ONE, 12*(8), e0182394. https://doi.org/10.1371/journal.pone.0182394.
4. Adapa, S. R., Taylor, R. A., Wang, C., Thomson-Luque, R., Johnson, L. R., & Jiang, R. H. Y. (2019). *Plasmodium vivax* readiness to transmit: Implication for malaria eradication. *BMC Systems Biology, 13*, Article 4. https://doi.org/10.1186/s12918-018-0669-4.
5. Al-Agroudi, M., Megahad, L., Banda, L., & Morsy, T. (2017). An overview on malaria in Sub-Saharan with special reference to Tanzania. *Journal of the Egyptian Society of Parasitology, 47*(2), 273–292. https://doi.org/10.21608/jesp.2017.77777.
6. . Chiu, J. C., Kaub, K., Zou, S., Liedo, P., Altamirano-Robles, L., Ingram, D., & Carey, J. R. (2013). Deleterious effect of suboptimal diet on rest-activity cycle in Anastrepha ludens manifests itself with age. *Scientific reports, 3*, 1773. https://doi.org/10.1038/srep01773
7. Assies, R., Snik, I., Kumwenda, M., Chimalizeni, Y., Langton, J., van Woensel, J. B. M., Doctor, A., et al. (2022). Etiology, pathophysiology and mortality of shock in children in low (middle) income countries: A systematic review. *Journal of Tropical Pediatrics, 68*, fmac053. https://doi.org/10.1093/tropej/fmac053.
8. Baird, J. K. (2022). African *Plasmodium vivax* malaria improbably rare or benign. *Trends in Parasitology, 38*(8), 683–696. https://doi.org/10.1016/j.pt.2022.05.006.
9. Bansal, V., Munjal, J., Lakhanpal, S., Gupta, V., Garg, A., Munjal, R., & Jain, R. (2023). Epidemiological shifts: The emergence of malaria in America. *Baylor University Medical Center Proceedings, 36*(4), 745–750. https://doi.org/10.1080/08998280.2023.2255514.
10. Barbosa-Silva, M. C., Lima, M. N., Battaglini, D., Robba, C., Pelosi, P., Rocco, P. R. M., & Maron-Gutierrez, T. (2021). Infectious disease-associated encephalopathies. *Critical Care, 25*, 25. https://doi.org/10.1186/s13054-021-03659-6.
11. Basmaci, R., Dramowski, A., Droz, N., Ellis, et al. (2019). Bacterial pathogens and resistance causing community-acquired paediatric bloodstream infections in low- and middle-income countries: A systematic review and meta-analysis. https://core.ac.uk/download/286270854.pdf (accessed on 13 May 2025).
12. Blencowe, H., Cousens, S., Chou, D., Oestergaard, M. Z., Say, L., Moller, A. B., Kinney, M., et al. (2013). Born too soon: The global epidemiology of 15 million preterm births. *Reproductive Health, 10*(Suppl 1), S2. https://doi.org/10.1186/1742-4755-10-s1-s2.
13. Chaparro, C. M., & Suchdev, P. S. (2019). Anemia epidemiology, pathophysiology, and etiology

in low- and middle-income countries. *Annals of the New York Academy of Sciences, 1450*, 15–31. https://doi.org/10.1111/nyas.14092.

14. Chopra, H., Dey, P. S., Das, D., Bhattacharya, T., Shah, M., Mubin, S., Maishu, S. P., et al. (2021). Curcumin nanoparticles as promising therapeutic agents for drug targets. *Molecules, 26*(16), 4998. https://doi.org/10.3390/molecules26164998.
15. Cox, S., Halcox, J., Kamala, B. A., Prentice, et al. (2014). Vascular Function Intervention Trial in sickle cell disease (V-FIT): Trial protocol. https://core.ac.uk/download/77514046.pdf (accessed on 13 May 2025).
16. De Bosscher, K., Opdenakker, G., Van den Steen, P. E., Vandermosten, T., & Van Ginderachter, J. A. (2019). Critical roles of endogenous glucocorticoids for disease tolerance in malaria. *Trends in Parasitology, 35*(11), 918–930. https://doi.org/10.1016/j.pt.2019.09.001.
17. Fikadu, M., & Ashenafi, E. (2023). Malaria: An overview. *Infection and Drug Resistance, 16*, 3339–3347. https://doi.org/10.2147/idr.s405668.
18. Gibbs, K. D., Schott, B. H., & Ko, D. C. (2022). The awesome power of human genetics of infectious disease. *Annual Review of Genetics, 56*, 41–62. https://doi.org/10.1146/annurev-genet-080320-010449.
19. Gomes, C., Varo, R., Duran-Frigola, M., Sitoe, A., Bila, R., Machevo, S., Mayor, A., et al. (2023). Endothelial transcriptomic analysis identifies biomarkers of severe and cerebral malaria. *JCI Insight, 8*. https://doi.org/10.1172/jci.insight.172845.
20. Gotts, J. E., & Matthay, M. A. (2016). Sepsis: Pathophysiology and clinical management. *BMJ, 353*, i1585. https://doi.org/10.1136/bmj.i1585.
21. Hahad, O., Lelieveld, J., Birklein, F., Lieb, K., Daiber, A., & Münzel, T. (2020). Ambient air pollution increases the risk of cerebrovascular and neuropsychiatric disorders through induction of inflammation and oxidative stress. *International Journal of Molecular Sciences, 21*(12), 4306. https://doi.org/10.3390/ijms21124306.
22. Hassan, A., Wlodarczyk, M. F., Benamar, M., Bassot, E., Salvioni, A., Kassem, S., Berry, A., et al. (2020). A virus hosted in malaria-infected blood protects against T cell-mediated inflammatory diseases by impairing DC function in a type I IFN-dependent manner. *mBio, 11*. https://doi.org/10.1128/mBio.03394-19.
23. Honigsbaum, M., & Krishnan, L. (2020). Taking pandemic sequelae seriously: From the Russian influenza to COVID-19 long-haulers. *The Lancet, 396*(10260), 1389–1391. https://doi.org/10.1016/s0140-6736(20)32134-6.
24. Hu, X., Li, J., Fu, M., Zhao, X., & Wang, W. (2021). The JAK/STAT signaling pathway: From bench to clinic. *Signal Transduction and Targeted Therapy, 6*, Article 402. https://doi.org/10.1038/s41392-021-00791-1.
25. Hussein, M. I. H., Albashir, A. A. D., Elawad, O. A. M. A., & Homeida, A. (2020). Malaria and COVID-19: Unmasking their ties. *Malaria Journal, 19*, 457. https://doi.org/10.1186/s12936-020-03541-w.
26. Jimmy, E. O., Umoh, I., & Usoh, I. F. (2014). Splenotoxic potentials of Chloroquine, Fansidar, Cotecxin and Amalar. https://core.ac.uk/download/234654583.pdf (accessed on 13 May 2025).
27. Lidani, K. C. F., Andrade, F. A., Bavia, L., Damasceno, F. S., Beltrame, M. H., Messias-Reason,

I., & Sandri, T. L. (2019). Chagas disease: From discovery to a worldwide health problem. *Frontiers in Public Health, 7*, 166. https://doi.org/10.3389/fpubh.2019.00166.

28. Marcilla, A., Martín-Jaular, L., Trelis, M., Menezes-Neto, A., Osuna, A., Bernal, D., Fernández-Becerra, C., et al. (2014). Extracellular vesicles in parasitic diseases. *Journal of Extracellular Vesicles, 3*. https://doi.org/10.3402/jev.v3.25040.
29. Alfred Mavondo G, Nkazimulo Mkhwanazi B, Louis Mzingwane M, Dangarembizi R, Zambuko B, Moyo O, et al. Malarial Inflammation-Driven Pathophysiology and Its Attenuation by Triterpene Phytotherapeutics [Internet]. Parasitology and Microbiology Research. IntechOpen; 2020. Available from: http://dx.doi.org/10.5772/intechopen.88731(accessed on 13 May 2025).
30. Melamed, N., Baschat, A., Yinon, Y., Athanasiadis, A., Mecacci, F., Figueras, F., Berghella, V., et al. (2021). FIGO initiative on fetal growth: best practice advice for screening, diagnosis, and management of fetal growth restriction. *International Journal of Gynecology & Obstetrics, 152*(S1), 3–57. https://doi.org/10.1002/ijgo.13522.
31. Mohamed, M. S., Moulin, T. C., & Schiöth, H. B. (2020). Sex differences in COVID-19: The role of androgens in disease severity and progression. *Endocrine, 71*(1), 3–8. https://doi.org/10.1007/s12020-020-02536-6.
32. Nirk, E. L., Reggiori, F., & Mauthe, M. (2020). Hydroxychloroquine in rheumatic autoimmune disorders and beyond. *EMBO Molecular Medicine, 12*. https://doi.org/10.15252/emmm.202012476.
33. Obeagu, E. I. ., Prajapati, S. K., & Maurya, S. D. (2025). Maternal Anemia in the Context of Infectious Diseases during Pregnancy: A Review. *International Journal of Medical Sciences and Pharma Research, 11*(1), 8–13. https://doi.org/10.22270/ijmspr.v11i1.134(accessed on 13 May 2025).
34. Ohiagu, F. O., Chikezie, P. C., Ahaneku, C. C., Chikezie, C. M., & Law-Obi, F. C. (2021). Pathophysiology of severe malaria infection. *Asian Journal of Health Sciences, 7*(2), 22. https://doi.org/10.15419/ajhs.v7i2.492.
35. Perkins, G. D., Gräsner, J. T., Semeraro, F., Olasveengen, T. M., Soar, J., Lott, C., Van de Voorde, P., et al. (2021). European Resuscitation Council Guidelines 2021: Executive summary. *Resuscitation, 161*, 1–60. https://doi.org/10.1016/j.resuscitation.2021.02.003.
36. Petrakis, D., Margină, D., Tsarouhas, K., Tekos, F., Stan, M., Nikitovic, D., Kouretas, D., et al. (2020). Obesity–A risk factor for increased COVID-19 prevalence, severity and lethality (Review). *Molecular Medicine Reports, 22*, 9–19. https://doi.org/10.3892/mmr.2020.11127.
37. Phyo, A. P., Dahal, P., Mayxay, M., & Ashley, E. A. (2022). Clinical impact of vivax malaria: A collection review. *PLOS Medicine, 19*, e1003890. https://doi.org/10.1371/journal.pmed.1003890.
38. Prabhu, S. R., Ware, A. P., Umakanth, S., Hande, M., Mahabala, C., Saadi, A. V., & Satyamoorthy, K. (2023). Erythrocyte miRNA-92a-3p interactions with PfEMP1 as determinants of clinical malaria. *Functional & Integrative Genomics, 23*, Article 28. https://doi.org/10.1007/s10142-023-01028-w.
39. Rudd, K. E., Johnson, S. C., Agesa, K. M., Shackelford, K. A., Tsoi, D., Kievlan, D., Colombara, D. V., et al. (2020). Global, regional, and national sepsis incidence and mortality, 1990–2017: Analysis for the Global Burden of Disease Study. *The Lancet, 395*(10219), 200–211. https://doi.org/10.1016/s0140-6736(19)32989-7.

40. Sriboonvorakul, N., Chotivanich, K., Silachamroon, U., Phumratanaprapin, W., Adams, J. H., Dondorp, A. M., & Leopold, S. J. (2023). Intestinal injury and the gut microbiota in patients with *Plasmodium falciparum* malaria. *PLOS Pathogens, 19*(3), e1011661. https://doi.org/10.1371/journal.ppat.1011661.

41. Stincone, A., Prigione, A., Cramer, T., Wamelink, M. M. C., Campbell, K., Cheung, E. C., Olín-Sandoval, V., et al. (2014). The return of metabolism: Biochemistry and physiology of the pentose phosphate pathway. *Biological Reviews, 90*, 927–963. https://doi.org/10.1111/brv.12140.

42. Thomson-Luque, R., Adams, J. H., Kocken, C. H. M., & Pasini, E. M. (2019). From marginal to essential: The golden thread between nutrient sensing, medium composition and *Plasmodium vivax* maturation in *in vitro* culture. *Malaria Journal, 18*, 434. https://doi.org/10.1186/s12936-019-2949-x.

43. Volpe, M., & Battistoni, A. (2019). An evolutionary rebus. *Journal of Hypertension, 37*(7), 1344–1346. https://doi.org/10.1097/hjh.0000000000002090.

44. Williams, T. N., & Thein, S. L. (2018). Sickle cell anemia and its phenotypes. *Annual Review of Genomics and Human Genetics, 19*, 113–147. https://doi.org/10.1146/annurev-genom-083117-021320.

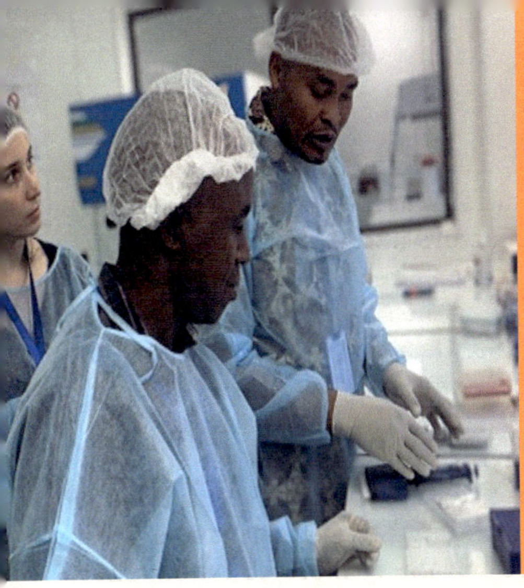

Chapter 5

CLINICAL MANIFESTATIONS OF MALARIA

Contents

Introduction

Parasitic disease impacts global health systems quite adversely, infecting millions across the world every year. Malaria specifically demands notice, with its complex life cycle energized by *Plasmodium parasites* and *Anopheles* mosquitoes, it often manifests in regions where people are exposed to extended long-term exposure. There, individuals can swing from a delicate feverish attack to outright dangerous, life-threatening complications. Why the disease is spread makes it difficult for doctors to arrive at an exact diagnosis and select a proper cure, so in common terms, it becomes crucial to know all clinical symptoms. Strategies like using ITNs and even indoor sprayings have come a long way, but the disease is still recalcitrant. Even with progress in treatment and testing, the very fact that malaria still exists means that we must look more deeply into how it presents among different populations, especially children who, for goodness' sake, get the worst of it (Laurens, 2019). How malaria presents are what is the starting point for better patient care and more personalized interventions. Symptoms can range from enigmatic feverish spells that are unidentifiable from other tropical insects to life-threatening conditions like cerebral complications, acute anemia, or sudden breathing difficulties. Those general symptoms often overlap with factors like the immune system of a particular person, the specific parasite under question, and the extent of the disease in the region, rendering absolute diagnosis quite complex. Most frequently, it is the *Plasmodium falciparum* type that is the deadliest and requires rapid and watchful diagnosis. Occasionally, in addition to the usual presentations, malaria also results in other confusing systemic manifestations or even issues that are seemingly indistinguishable from drug side effects, a problem that leaves doctors treading on thin ice. This combination of clinical findings indeed forms the basis for what medical professionals and public health planners need to consider (Laurens, 2019). With the hardened fight still being faced in combating malaria, the union of clinical findings with pharmacological progress becomes necessary. Nowadays, combination therapies are becoming more common, and they introduce one additional level of complexity—also simply because many of these patients are likely suffering from co-infections or other health conditions simultaneously. Such polypharmacy in turn raises the possibility of unexpected drug interactions, which further alters how a patient might recover. The latest advances in computation allow us to glimpse into such complex drug interactions, providing a means to predict and eliminate side effects in their infancy, which is highly promising for safer treatment regimens. A strategy that combines practical clinical experience with lessons learned from pharmacogenomics could enhance our insight into how malaria presents itself in different environments, leading eventually to refining patient care and opening doors to innovative new intervention approaches.

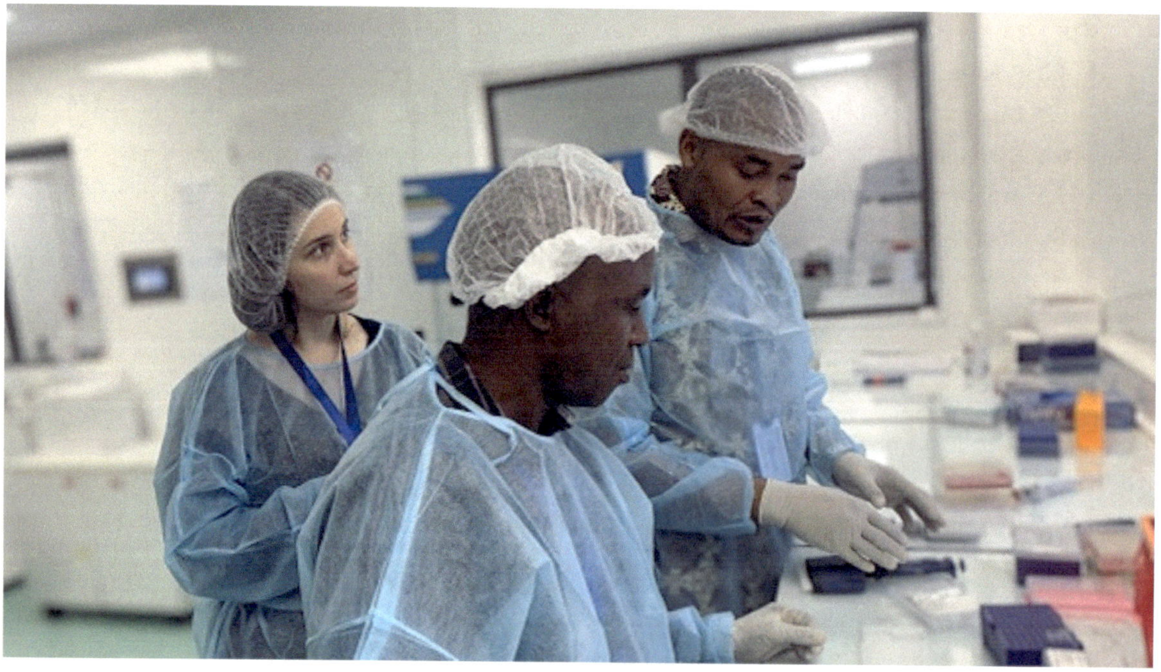

Source: Centers for Disease Control and Prevention (CDC). (2024). *Senegal PARMA Hub Laboratory.* https://www.cdc.gov/malaria/media/images/2024/03/Senegal_PARMA_Hub_lab-large.jpg.

Malaria is a covert parasitic infection primarily caused by a number of *Plasmodium* species by the bite of an infected *Anopheles* mosquito. It usually presents initially as a febrile infection but can quickly run out of control into dangerous grounds, such as, such as extreme exhaustion, respiratory distress, abrupt confusion, or even bad anemia potentially resulting in death if not treated. Interestingly enough, the symptomatology of malaria can vary based on what *Plasmodium* is involved. *Plasmodium falciparum* is historically noted as the worse pathogen, but more recent studies suggest *Plasmodium vivax*, which was previously thought to be milder, can also be complicated, kind of shakes our old perceptual boxes. This emergent picture compels us to reconsider how we define the disease, especially as we look at most exposed persons, including children and pregnant women (Phyo et al., 2022). In deciding whether to call something malaria, it's not just a matter of viewing the parasite but also a matter of the body's reaction. They look, for instance, for parasitemia, which is, visible *Plasmodium* in the blood, that fancy medical phrase, for the more old-fashioned symptoms we've all heard of, such as fever, chills, and just a general feeling that something isn't right. Sometimes there are even reports of less typical symptoms like diarrhea or other gastrointestinal hiccups, which indicate that the disease might creep into areas we haven't worked out quite yet. However, this link between malaria and these gastrointestinal issues is not fully explained; studies come to different conclusions and there are not yet enough properly controlled trials to sort it out. This ambiguity of the literature leaves a gap in the conventional definition of malaria, and it has been proposed that we do have better case definitions and particular research to fill it (Sey et al., 2020). To understand what we mean by "malaria" matters, because the disease can progress from a harmless, self-limited fever to much more sinister. It is now certain that even *Plasmodium vivax*, long written off as a nuisance, can lead to serious problems like severe anemia or pregnancy-related complications—changing our very clinical perspective. There are a few systematic reviews that suggest although a minority of *vivax* infections reach the World Health Organization's (WHO) cut-off point for severe malaria, those who do reach the hospital are likely to experience severely poor outcomes and death. Generally, local data integration and realignment of the severity scale in our definitions are crucial to settle precise diagnoses, sustain effective surveillance, and fine-tune treatment strategies in malaria-endemic settings (Phyo et al., 2022).

Importance of Studying Clinical Manifestations

Understanding the way that malaria presents itself is important to making a clear diagnosis and safe treatment of the patient, especially in areas where people are subject to developing many diseases that share a great many symptoms. Malaria can be as subtle as a low-grade fever or as severe as an entire crisis, and its presentations easily mistaken for other diseases with which one has fever, which makes the treatment waters complex. On the whole, more frequently than not, monitoring developments like certain patterns of fever, signs of anemia, or even neurological conditions antecedents enabled doctors to act earlier, often lowering major complication and mortality rates. Examining these facts, albeit with some recurrence on a case-by-case basis, helps clinicians anticipate future problems, adjust treatment strategies for an individual patient, and target resources more efficiently. This method for doing things also fits well with more systemic initiatives toward improving care in low- and middle-income nations, where diagnostic mysteries and system tensions continue to prevail, showing that an effective grasp of symptom information can immediately improve patient outcomes as well as system effectiveness in general (Chaparro e& Suchdev, 2019). As you start peeling off the many faces of malaria, you begin to look for clues on the disease's mechanisms and progression, and how that translates to wiser public health interventions. Consider, for example, the scenario of severe anemia, no longer merely a sign, but a warning sign on how grave the illness can get, especially among individuals already vulnerable, and which requires more precise prevention and attention. Overall, investigating these trends reveals latent risk factors and concomitant conditions that can affect the course of the disease or a patient's prognosis. Subsequently this knowledge too frequently is met by advice that's tailored in explicit terms to needs at the local level, whether that is in consideration of variation in malaria strains or in response to the infection.

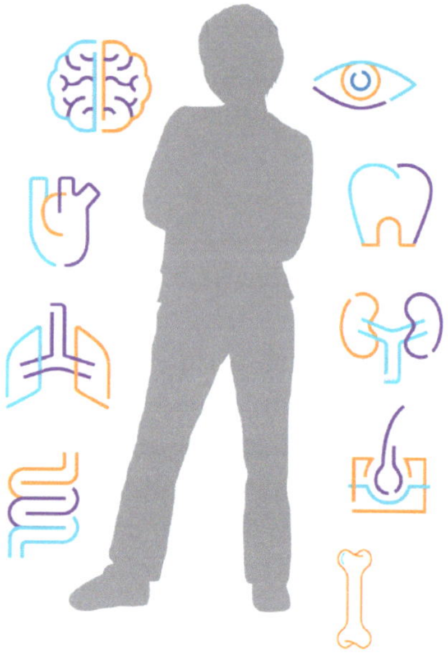

Figure 5.1. Clinical manifestations.

Source: TSC Alliance. (2024). *Clinical Manifestations of Tuberous Sclerosis Complex.* https://www.tscalliance.org/wp-content/uploads/2024/01/clinical-manifestations-larger.jpg.

Such subtle understanding is essential to creating holistic health programs that treat concurrent issues, from nutritional needs to genetic vulnerabilities compounding anemia, thereby enhancing individual recovery and broader public health (Chaparro & Suchdev, 2019). Keeping a bird's-eye view beyond the immediate needs of patients, keeping an eye on the bigger picture of malaria's multifaceted manifestations, is key to speeding up how quickly and reliably our healthcare systems are able to act. Typically, vexing issues like misdiagnosis or delayed management occur due to understated symptoms being neglected, emphasizing the true need for good clinical training and regular quality oversight. In most cases, rigorous monitoring of these presentations facilitates efforts toward performance review, accountability, and wiser deployment of resources in order to enhance health infrastructure. As medical professionals become more skilled at identifying and treating these diverse signs, they are better equipped to deliver quality yet respectful care—helping to build patient trust and prevent avoidable deaths. In general, a good grasp of the full spectrum of malaria's clinical manifestations is a basis for the delivery of effective and fair care, which is in line with wider, global activity to achieve sustainable development objectives in affected areas (Kruk et al., 2018) (Figure 5.1).

Overview of Malaria Transmission

Malaria is not transmitted easily, it can be a function of the complex interaction between the parasite, its vector mosquito, and the human host. Essentially, different *Plasmodium parasites* result in different types of disease, *P. falciparum* being particularly deadly in regions of the globe where illness and mortality are rampant. It might all start when a female *Anopheles* mosquito acquires gametocytes—the parasite in its sexual stage, from an infected host. Inside the mosquito, the stages transition into sporozoites progressively, which proceed to fly off into another human through the subsequent bite. The efficacy of this cycle turns out to be reliant on a combination of factors: the mosquito's species, the feeding habits of the mosquito, the climate, and even the level of an individual's immunity. Mostly, it facilitates the ease of physicians correlating the parasite's stages with the spectrum of symptoms patients exhibit (Laurens, 2019). Beneath the surface, malaria reaches its breadth from ecological, social, and biological mechanisms that shape both the density of mosquitoes and human vulnerability. Take sub-Saharan Africa, for instance, tropical, humid climates benefit mosquitoes to breed and live longer, perpetuating continuous transmission. Seasonal alterations have the power to sharpen or mute the dissemination, making the severity of the symptoms leading to communities increase or wane. Yes, interventions like insecticide-treated nets (ITNs), indoor residual spraying (IRS), and artemisinin-based combination treatments have curbed the disease considerably, but progress has stalled or turned back in some places, showing just how tough malaria is. The new RTS,S vaccine is some light now, especially in regions where children carry the biggest burden, and this gives a pointer to combining new approaches with the older ones (Laurens, 2019).

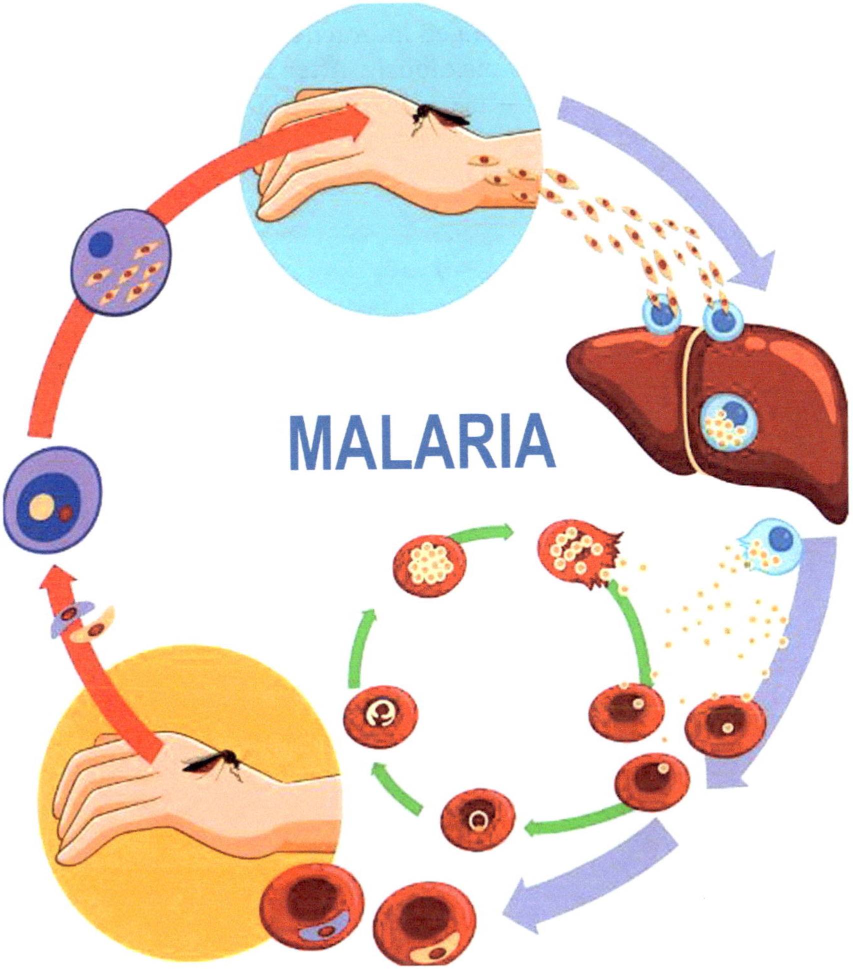

Figure 5.2. Malaria transmission.

Source: VectorStock. (n.d.). *Science Education Malaria Transmission Cycle.* https://cdn.vectorstock.com/i/1000v/20/07/science-education-malaria-transmission-cycle-vector-48682007.jpg.

To break the cycle, one has to hold the string very tightly on the mosquito and be careful about early signs of an outbreak. Rapid diagnosis and rapid treatment serve to reduce the population of *parasites* circulating in the population, which can subsequently disrupt the chain of transmission. Meanwhile, measures taken to suppress *Anopheles* populations are designed to reduce their potential to transmit the parasite. Health interventions increasingly depend on clever monitoring techniques, from simple point-of-care diagnostics to real-time surveillance of information—to track the upswell and down swell of the disease, guiding where intervention is needed most. Despite the focus primarily on malaria, these concepts of monitoring draw from approaches against other mosquito-borne infections including lymphatic filariasis and onchocerciasis, areas in which many response and monitoring has already provided promising results in transmission reduction (Figure 5.2).

5.1. Pathophysiology of Malaria

The symptoms of malaria result from a deranged interaction between the *Plasmodium* parasite and the body's own reaction, starting almost insidiously. After the mosquito bite, sporozoites invade the blood and quickly infect liver cells—this begins a hidden, asymptomatic liver phase. Soon, merozoites burst into the blood and begin infecting red blood cells (RBCs). In these cells, the *parasites* multiply until the cell bursts, releasing additional *parasites* and byproducts like hemozoin.

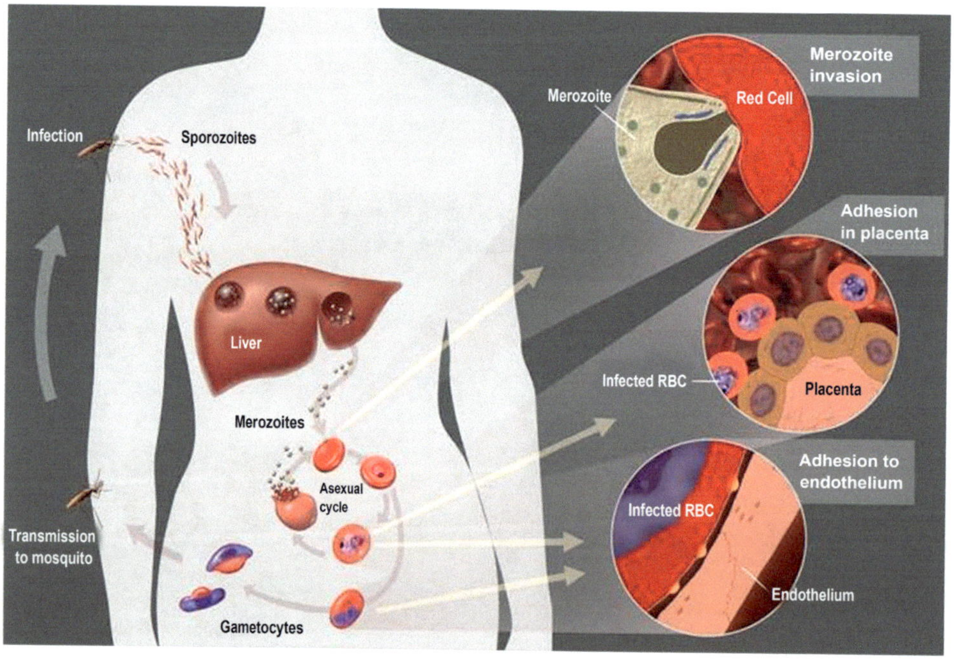

Figure 5.3. Malaria pathophysiology.

Source: Unknown Author. (n.d.). *Malaria Transmission Cycle.* https://s3.amazonaws.com/static.wd7.us/7/7c/MalariacycleBig.jpg.

This repetitive process of cell bursting is mostly accountable for patients experiencing abrupt, severe fevers; cell bursting also triggers inflammatory signals (tumor necrosis factor-alpha and interleukins come to mind) that lead to chills, sweats, and even anemia. It is usually this tug-of-war between the *parasites*' growth and the immune reaction that determines the whole range of symptoms of malaria. Anemia is one of the primary consequences of the disease, and it is due to a variety of interconnected causes. Infected RBCs tend to burst outright, and uninfected ones are sometimes caught in the crossfire as the body labors to maintain the output of new ones. In cases of severe or repeated infections, especially in children already weakened by malnutrition or HIV—this problem is compounded. Often, the anemia is not exclusively malaria-based; other infections such as tuberculosis or *parasites* such as hookworms may contribute to the blood loss. Therapeutic regimes that also address these other infections and nutritional deficiencies, in addition to antimalarial drugs, act to reduce the severity of anemia in vulnerable populations (Makubi et al., 2012). A last twist in the story of malaria is how infected RBCs clump together and are trapped in small blood vessels—a process known as sequestration. Adhesion proteins caused by *parasites* on these cells cause them to clog small vessels, thereby decreasing the flow of blood to the tissues and ultimately causing organ function to be impaired. In its worst form, when such clogging occurs in the cerebral capillaries, cerebral malaria will result in neurological signs and even fatal effects. At the same time, the body's excessive immune response (via signals like interferon-gamma) can end up damaging tissues even while it is trying to fight the infection. In most cases, recent studies indicate that the addition of targeted therapies to regulate the immune pathways would kill the parasite faster without any more side effects, offering hope for reducing death rates (Bekker et al., 2012). Overall, such a balance between host responses and parasite strategies is key to managing the various facets of malaria (Figure 5.3).

5.1.1. Life Cycle of Plasmodium Parasites

Malaria is spread because of the complex path that *Plasmodium parasites* take, darting between mosquito and human hosts. A contaminated bite from an *Anopheles* propels sporozoites flooding into the bloodstream—essentially on a mission to attack the liver, where they infiltrate hepatocytes and double in secrecy. This quiet, pre-erythrocytic phase is in open view so there are not glaring signs at first. Soon enough, the *parasites* explode as merozoites into the blood, beginning what we know as the symptomatic erythrocytic cycle. Because these *parasites* can bypass the immune system now, simply looking at clinical symptoms is misleading; therefore, the parasite piece or DNA detection tests (Smith et al., 2009). The intensity and the length of these cycles, in most cases, play a big role in determining the severity of the resultant disease. Merozoites invade RBCs subsequently enter into a cycle of asexual reproduction which not only destroys host cells but also spreads the infection further. This cycle maintains the traditional symptoms of malaria, fevers, chills, periodic anemia and even splenomegaly. It's not just the disruption of red cells; the parasite also disrupts the immune response of the host and presents different antigens on infected cells. The models like *Plasmodium knowlesi* have revealed the mechanisms through which antigenic variants provide the parasite with more leeway to escape, the function of the spleen and some antibodies being theirs in ways still being discovered. At the same time, these molecular changes account for why malaria can remain or re-emerge, and this is something that needs to be considered when optimizing clinical management and designing new treatments (Galinski et al., 2018). Even individual merozoites go off on a tangent into the sexual cycle, becoming male and female gametocytes that circulate in the bloodstream. When a mosquito buzzes in for a blood feed, these gametocytes are taken up and, having inside the insect, mate to form zygotes that mature to be ookinetes subsequently oocysts in the midgut. In a process that might almost be torturous in its fatedness, these oocysts finally spit out an entire crop of sporozoites, which migrate to the salivary glands of the mosquito ready to infect another human. As a whole, understanding this phase of the parasite's lifecycle is crucial for disease control, preventing transmission here can have a big impact in reducing malaria cases. At the same time, the ongoing back-and-forth between parasite development and the body's immune response is still an essential component of the image when trying to understand why symptoms vary so greatly from patient to patient (Smith et al., 2009).

5.1.2. Immune Response to Malaria Infection

When malaria infects, our body does not initiate a one-trick assault, instead, it weighs killing the parasite against letting inflammation get out of control. Initially, cells like macrophages and dendritic cells rapidly catch wind of *Plasmodium* via their pattern receptors. This detection initiates a flood of cytokine releases and even turns on the inflammasome switch, recruiting further immune combatants to the battleground. In the meantime, the parasitic life cycle that is hidden and the shifting antigens render it harder for our body to target a complete defense. Even platelets, which we have a tendency to consider as factors of clotting, end up getting into the fight, claiming direct anti-parasitic activity. Thus, low platelet counts (thrombocytopenia) are often observed in various *Plasmodium* infections, adding another layer of complexity to the disease.

It is an uncoordinated, drawn-out tug-of-war between whatever the host can muster up and the parasite's advanced evasions. Adaptive immunity takes its place as the battle drags on—T and B lymphocytes become more active in both killing the parasite and paving the way for long-term defenses. In general, CD4+ T helper cells help to activate macrophages and drive B cells into producing antibodies to attack those blood-stage *parasites*. However, *Plasmodium*'s perpetually changing antigens render it effectively impossible to establish an ironclad immunity but rather cause repeated bouts of infection with unpredictable symptoms. Memory reactions, although useful in certain endemic regions, are rarely capable of eliminating the invader altogether. Meanwhile, the same pro-inflammatory signals that hold the parasite in check are likely to aggravate such secondary diseases as fever and anemia. This delicate balance, where protection merges with inflammatory immune overreactions, is the reason that even today we still believe in more research on immune response modulation (Guo et al., 2020).

Severe complications are a deep-rooted issue despite all that we have achieved. In the majority of cases, a sudden drop in platelets, or acute thrombocytopenia, is noted with infection due to both *Plasmodium vivax* and *Plasmodium falciparum*, and it is in general accompanied by bleeding complications and even organ failure; children, particularly, occasionally present with enhanced dangers (Guo et al., 2020). There are instances in which the overall immune response of the body becomes overactivated, leading to cytokine storms and clotting abnormalities reminiscent of other dangerous infections—on occasion this can lead to acute respiratory distress syndrome (Guo et al., 2020). All these factors serve to highlight just how complex and dynamic the immune battle against malaria is. Future growth, and forward-looking research, will be necessary to work out the complex immune markers of protection and pathology that can update prognostic tools and guide better treatment strategies to malaria's numerous clinical manifestations (Figure 5.4).

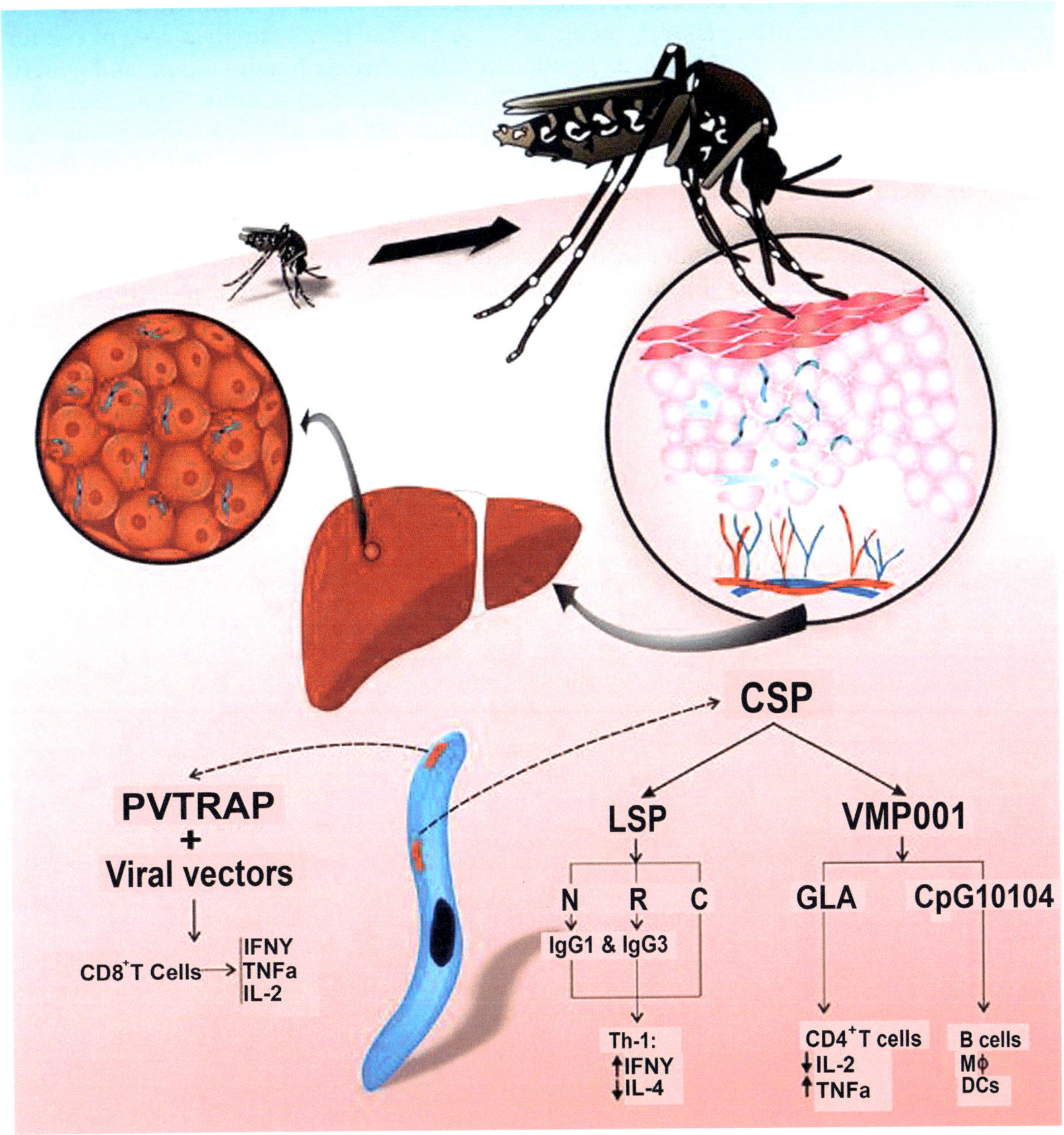

Figure 5.4. Immune response to malaria infection.

Source: López C, Yepes-Pérez Y, Hincapié-Escobar N, Díaz-Arévalo D and Patarroyo MA (2017) What Is Known about the Immune Response Induced by Plasmodium vivax Malaria Vaccine Candidates? Front. Immunol. 8:126. doi: 10.3389/fimmu.2017.00126

5.1.3. Impact on Host Physiology

Malaria *parasites* manipulate the body in a somewhat sophisticated way. They infect red blood cells and, in their life cycle, end up destroying those cells, with a consequence of anemia and decreased delivery of oxygen to tissues. You could be tired and weak, or even white, since in most infections the red cell loss disrupts oxygen delivery. The disease is not simply a case of cell loss; it is often further complicated by diseases like poor nutrition, chronic inflammation, and genetically transmitted blood disease common to the majority of infected populations. The stress extends beyond merely oxygenation, impacting brain development and capacity for work, which shows the comprehensive effect malaria has on general health (Chaparro & Suchdev, 2019). Generally, disentangling these interactions is critical to treating both the acute manifestations and chronic sequelae. Malaria does not merely produce anemia—it also causes recurring fevers. Since *parasites* multiply in a coordinated burst within RBCs, the coordinated rupture of *parasites* discharges waves of newly released *parasites* and inflammatory mediators (e.g., tumor necrosis factor-alpha) into the circulation.

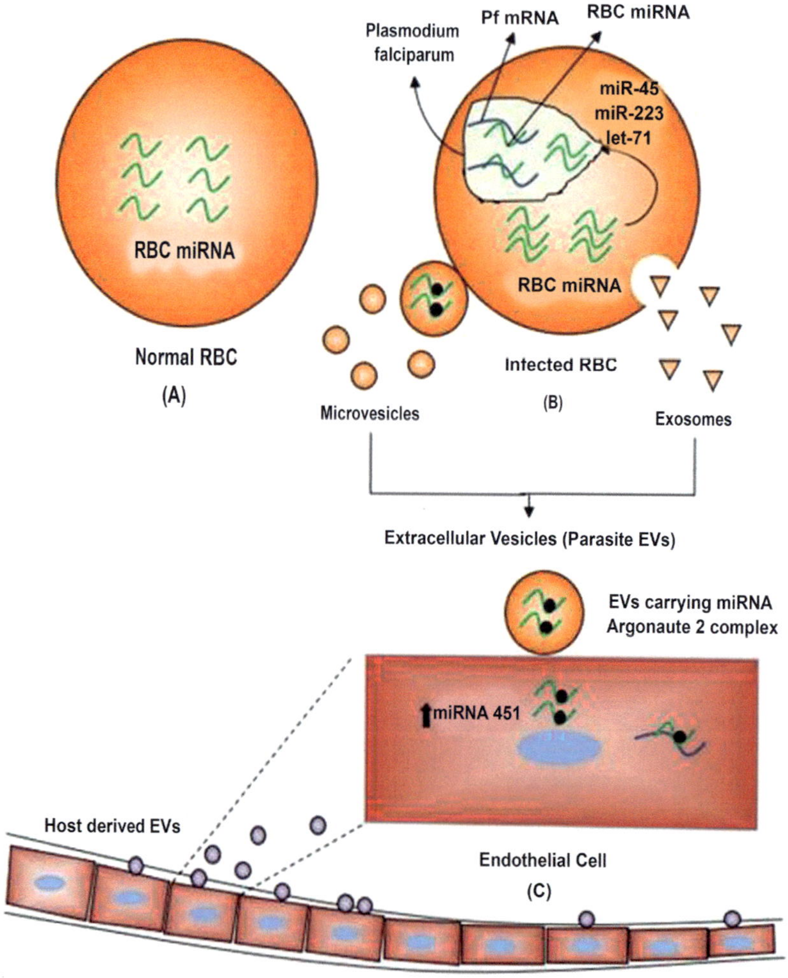

Figure 5.5. Host and malaria parasite interactions resulting in damage.

Source: Kataria P, Surela N, Chaudhary A, Das J. MiRNA: Biological Regulator in Host-Parasite Interaction during Malaria Infection. *International Journal of Environmental Research and Public Health*. 2022; 19(4):2395. https://doi.org/10.3390/ijerph19042395

These bouts of fever, occurring in a periodic but sometimes unpredictable manner, are intimately associated with how the immune system of the body responds. It is noteworthy that synchrony can be variable with varying infections and host states, thereby influencing clinical severity. This interaction between parasite behavior and host defenses, combined with treatments directed against specific stages of the parasite, has a significant impact on how the disease runs its course (Greischar et al., 2019). Generally, the changing status of the body during infection highlights the dynamic and complicated clinical profile of malaria. Another problem is how parasitized RBCs tend to stick in small blood vessels. This sequestration, a feature of life-threatening malaria, impairs microcirculatory perfusion and leads to tissue hypoxia and metabolic abnormalities in key organs like the brain, lungs, and kidneys. Blockage of capillaries by such infected cells generally causes serious complications, ranging from cerebral malaria and acute respiratory distress to renal failure. Concomitantly with this, the immune response to both sequestered *parasites* and the resultant hemolysis initiates inflammatory cascades that continue to destroy vessel walls and tissue. These mutually reinforcing impacts clearly illustrate how the effects of malaria transcend parasitology to encompass significant vascular and immunologic dysfunctions that enhance morbidity and mortality risk (Chaparro & Suchdev, 2019; Greischar et al., 2019). Therefore, successful management of the disease means addressing these complex host-pathogen interactions in a way that prevents the worst outcomes (Figure 5.5).

5.2. Common Clinical Symptoms

Malaria usually starts with many symptoms that mirror the body's systemic response to the infection. Fever is usually the first sign—a kind of red flag signaling that the immune system is reacting as *Plasmodium parasites* infect RBCs. Along with the fever, you might also get abrupt chills, sweating fits, headaches, and muscle aches; all of them together form malaria's classic, if uncomfortable, fever cycle pattern. How these fevers cycle on and off depends on which *Plasmodium* strain is the culprit, so most of the time individuals do go to the doctor when things start going wrong. You can even, at times, notice a pale appearance to the skin, thanks to RBCs being ruptured by the parasite. Usually, although these symptoms are not that specific, they do give physicians significant hints, especially where malaria is a prominent health issue (Bittaye et al., 2022). The sooner these symptoms are noticed, the better the diagnosis and the prevention of the disease from becoming any worse. Later on in the infection, the overall pattern has a tendency to be more confused, especially when complications start to set in in severe cases. Some patients, for instance, lose consciousness, a sign that the brain is becoming involved, which can lead toward cerebral malaria and is definitely a sign of danger. These changes in mental status come with severe anemia from widespread RBC destruction, which also deprives the tissues of oxygen. Acute kidney injury is also a potential, which kind of drives the point home that malaria doesn't restrict itself to one organ. In the majority of cases, these severe complications attack young adults within disease-endemic regions, and this renders the population extremely vulnerable and in serious need of careful treatment strategies (Bittaye et al., 2022). Overall, understanding this broad range of symptoms significantly aids clinicians in treating the disease more effectively. While the overall symptoms of malaria are fairly well defined, things are complicated when other tropical diseases impersonate them. Diseases like leptospirosis, for example, can present with the same sensation, with fever and general body aching—making it even harder for doctors to arrive at an accurate diagnosis.

Because these symptoms are so general, untangling what disease is which can sometimes lead to confusion and even deadly delays in treatment. In most cases, parsing the overlapping traits from the unique ones is key to getting it right. This overlap emphasizes the need for finer diagnostic tools and a more acute level of clinical suspicion in the tropical regions. As studies continue to reveal more about how these infections function, it should help clarify the confusion, leading to more precise diagnoses and improved patient outcomes (Figure 5.6).

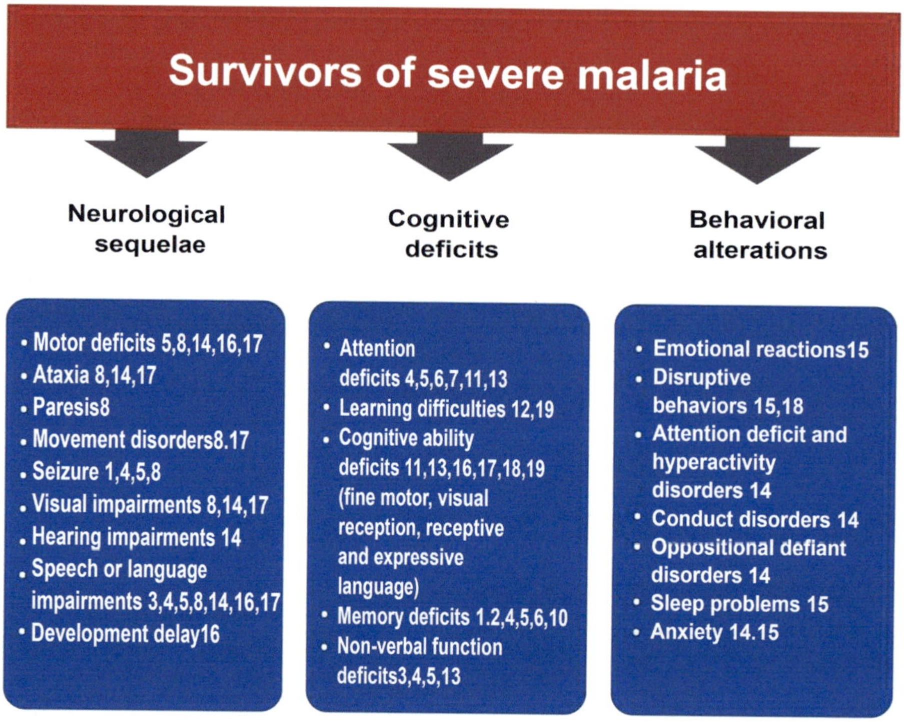

Figure 5.6. Clinical symptoms of malaria.

Source: Rosa-Gonçalves P, Ribeiro-Gomes FL and Daniel-Ribeiro CT (2022) Malaria Related Neurocognitive Deficits and Behavioral Alterations. Front. Cell. Infect. Microbiol. 12:829413. doi: 10.3389/fcimb.2022.829413

5.2.1. Fever and Chills

Patients who suddenly develop a fever and start shivering can be facing a bad infection, especially in tropical areas where malaria is prevalent. Fever and chills come in cycles that bizarrely match the parasite's own cycle within RBCs. When the infected cells burst, they release microscopic *parasites* and fever-inducing chemicals that signal the brain to crank up the heat. It is not just any reaction, but it is a characteristic sign of malaria that differentiates it from other fevers. Clinicians, in most cases, need to take note of these time specifics because they can mean the difference between a clear diagnosis and an error, particularly where many fevers overlap in such areas. Quick and accurate recognition by medical professionals is crucial to starting the right treatment right away. In response to malaria cases, that fever is usually accompanied by genuinely intense chills—sudden shudders that come and go with the rapid body temperature changes. The body, in its own clumsy way, is trying to warm up when waste products of the *parasites* reset the internal thermostat, and the shivers reflect how hard it is working. The chills, along with headache, fatigue, and sweating, all add to the misery, and while the parasite killing of RBCs does tend to occur in a predictable cycle, it is sometimes disrupted, making it even harder to assess. Also, the precise species responsible for the infection makes a big difference; for instance, *Plasmodium falciparum* is more likely to cause wilder and more irregular fever patterns, which can significantly complicate the way physicians handle the case (Dean et al., 2012).

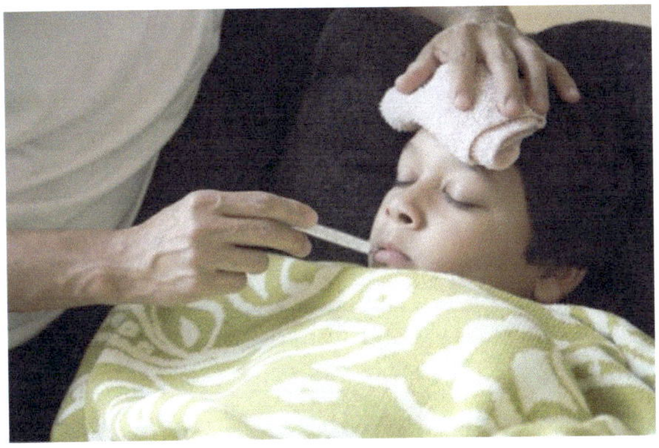

Source: TGP. (2021). *Fever and Chills.* https://external-content.duckduckgo.com/iu/?u=https%3A%2F%2Ftgp.com.ph%2Fimg%2Fcms%2Fwp-content%2Fuploads%2F2021%2F03%2Ffever-chills.jpg&f=1&nofb=1&ipt=c1fa8f61dba6d1eff30891ba23209c1e66a4ef35bad9e83c53aef669e82a2ebd.

Fever and chills, as unpleasant as they are, also act as significant indicators that lead to additional tests. If an individual who has recently visited or lives in a region where malaria is endemic shows these symptoms, it usually initiates a laboratory investigation to look for the parasite itself or its diagnostic antigens. While a high fever is a good lead, it is perilous to depend only on these clinical symptoms because another infection—brucellosis, for example, may show up with the same symptoms of fever and joint pains (Dean et al., 2012). More recent developments in integrating laboratory findings with clinical findings have tended to more precisely diagnose, ensuring that treatment is not delayed and is as effective as possible (Smith et al., 2009).

5.2.2. Headache and Fatigue

Malaria will initially present itself as a series of different systemic symptoms that imply the body is reacting to the invasion of parasites. You will get a headache and extreme exhaustion first – sometimes even before any clear fever or those typical chills have a chance to develop. The headache, on its part, is everywhere and lasts, likely because of chemicals that are released in the body and a sort of brain blood vessel dilation. The fatigue occurs as a result of several causes: for instance, a decrease in RBCs since they have been killed by the parasite and the extra energy that the infection demands. These coinciding symptoms are able to seriously lower one's day-to-day functionality, reducing productivity and overall well-being. On most occasions, being able to pick up these early signs correctly is crucial, especially in areas perennially under siege from malaria where similar feverish conditions may confuse the issue and delay treatment. One should keep in mind that issues associated with nerves greatly impact the headache perceived by most patients with malaria. Essentially, there's an out-of-control mix of infected red blood cells, blood vessel lining changes, and other inflammation triggers that disrupt tiny blood flow in the brain. Sometimes the pandemonium can escalate into cerebral malaria—a highly dangerous brain complication, , even though even mild illness features a persistent headache that signs at underlying brain involvement. The same kind of involved process that causes fatigue is to blame reduced oxygenation from anemia and a body kept constantly on high alert by its immune system. Most frequently, the fatigue lasts well after the severity of the infection has passed, making recovery more difficult and adding to the patient burden. These faint but insistent symptoms should be considered with care since they can be overlooked as the more heralded symptoms of acute malaria take center stage, potentially leading to a delay in proper treatment. Bizarrely, the fatigue and headache of malaria are indistinguishable from those of some other conditions, like Marburg hemorrhagic fever or brucellosis (Colebunders et al., 2007; Deean et al., 2012). Even though the etiologies of these infections vary, headaches are present early in all of these cases, and are usually caused by a body-wide inflammatory response and the degree of brain involvement. Fatigue in these illnesses, usually a consequence of similar immune responses and energy depletion, shows how frequently these illnesses have the same fundamental motif. Such side-by-side comparison merely contributes to the challenge of diagnosing malaria, particularly when this is being made in environments where there are several co-circulating infections and highlight the need for a proper clinical examination. At the end of it all, examining headache and fatigue as integral parts of the complete picture of malaria is the method to obtain an accurate diagnosis and increase the quality of patient care.

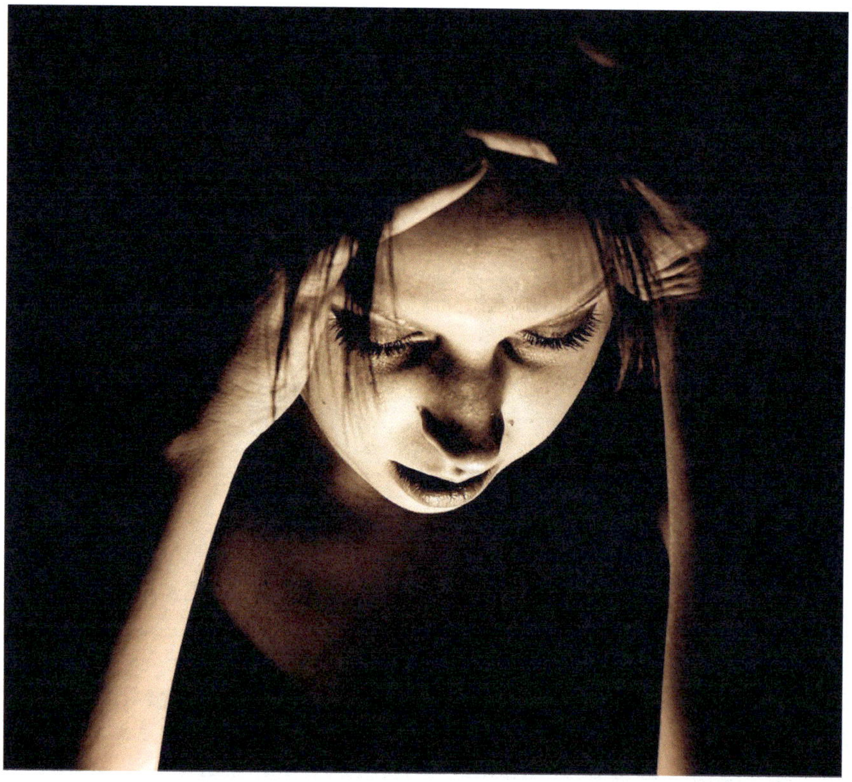

Source: By Sasha Wolff from Grand Rapids - Can't Concentrate: 14/365, CC BY 2.0, https://commons.wikimedia.org/w/index.php?curid=11343038

5.2.3. Nausea and Vomiting

Malaria's first symptoms are likely to crop up in a muddle, the body responding at once to the parasite's invasion. Nausea and vomiting are referred to practically as quickly as fever, headaches, and that awful feeling of not quite being oneself. By and large, these belly aches come on immediately, taking hints of the immune system's competition to react. It seems that a bundle of signals—picture messages traveling back and forth between gut and brain, sometimes pushed by inflammatory proteins and fluctuations in nerve signals—might be the cause of such symptoms. The more the *parasites* reproduce and toxins build up, the more intense the pain is, making it increasingly challenging for doctors to detect the disease early. Figuring out when and how bad these symptoms are is, in most cases, critical to figuring out how to treat and end the misery. In the hospital, diagnosing nausea and vomiting among individuals with malaria needs special care. Nausea and vomiting might complicate patients' ability to follow their regimens since irritable stomachs might risk the chance to take pills properly and result in dehydration. There are times when the vomiting has the effect of necessitating the switch from oral to intravenous medications so that the treatment continues to pack a punch.

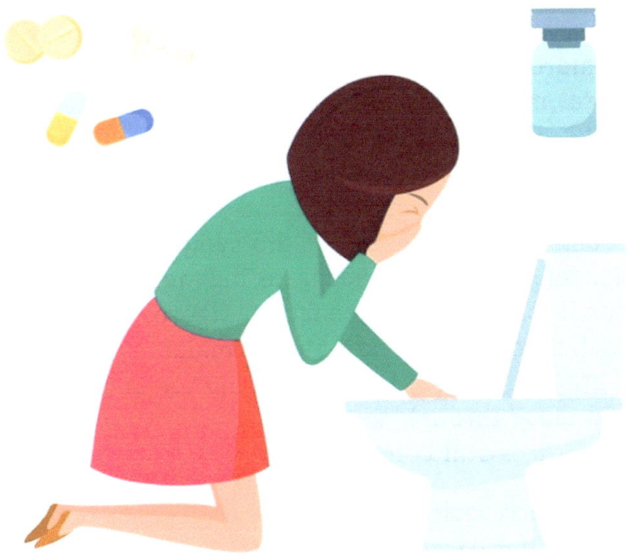

Source: Freepik. (n.d.). *Health Problems: Zika Virus and Malaria.* https://external-content.duckduckgo.com/iu/?u=https%3A%2F%2Fimg.freepik.com%2Fpremium-vector%2Fhealth-problems-zika-virus-malaria-human-discomfort-symptom-girl-feels-discomfort-malaise-nausea-vomiting-indigestion-associated-with-disease-procedures-treatment-medication-cartoon-vector_200075-5286.jpg%3Fw%3D740&f=1&nofb=1&ipt=41ac76d097290cec7bf194fd23275b3b8fbf7bfbf43e4dfd2b087594e0128453.

Sometimes these gastrointestinal complaints end up resembling quite closely other fever illnesses prevalent in those same locales, which can confuse the diagnostic process. This confusion emphasizes the significance of laboratory tests and good clinical records, , even though, in many low-resource environments, maintaining ideal documentation simply does not occur. Closing the gaps in recording is critical to simplifying management and monitoring for outcomes. Overall, incorporating nausea and vomiting into the broader clinical story enables clinicians to predict better complications and customize supportive care in the acute phase of malarial (Colebunders et al., 2007). From a public health angle, the intractability of treating nausea and vomiting in malaria is not an isolated issue—it is part of a greater mess where the disease is endemic. Often, these gastrointestinal symptoms occur in combination with other non-specific complaints like muscle pain and fever, which also occur in infections such as brucellosis; this makes it harder to reach a definitive diagnosis. Most often, this symptom coincides with delays in proper diagnosis and thereby makes treatment routes more complicated, which in turn can be a severe setback in already ailing regions with limited healthcare resources. Socioeconomic problems and patchy infrastructure only add oil to the fire, resulting in greater duration of suffering and higher chances of disability due to runaway infections. Identification of nausea and vomiting as leading symptoms of malaria adds another layer to our overall perception of the disease's burden and invokes measures to improve the measurement of disability and targeted interventions (Dean et al., 2012).

5.3. Severe Clinical Manifestations

Malaria does not follow a single script—its course can take a dramatic turn, and at its worst, it is life-threatening. In these severe instances, *Plasmodium falciparum* is the usual offender, and it enjoys wreaking havoc on more than one body system at a time. In certain cases, the infection eventually results in cerebral malaria, where patients suddenly develop confusion, seizures or even coma. This is when the red cells that are infested with malarial *parasites* clog the small blood vessels within the brain, destroying normal function and, if not treated very quickly, causing irreversible damage. Cerebral malarial anemia and bouts of severe respiratory distress also account for the high fatalities. To compound this, some of the symptoms can be similar to other tropical diseases, which only complicates rapid and accurate diagnosis. To sum up, early recognition of these potentially fatal signs is paramount—it enables vigorous treatment to be initiated before the condition becomes lethal. If you look at how severe malaria spreads, especially in areas where malaria is endemic, there are a few paradoxes. The majority of individuals presume that adults, having acquired partial immunity through the years, are less vulnerable to the most dangerous types, yet adult cerebral malaria is still common.

A Tanzania study, for example, revealed considerable divergence between initial clinical diagnosis of cerebral malaria and later blood parasite confirmation—indicating possible overdiagnosis and mismanagement. Misclassification sometimes leads to unnecessary treatment with antimalarial drugs while delaying the search for the actual cause of the symptoms and, in doing so, heightening the likelihood of death. Paradoxically, even patients in whom no *parasites* were detectable ended up with higher mortality than those who were positive. Overall, these findings highlight the clear necessity for more specific diagnostic methods to differentiate severe malaria from other neurological conditions in endemic areas (Makani et al., 2003). The consequences of severe malaria go far beyond death in the short term; the sequelae can lead to disability in the long term and to chronic health complications. Survivors may experience ongoing weakness, refractory neurological impairment, and chronic pain that persists long after the acute phase of the infection seems to have passed. In the majority of malarial regions, issues like delays in diagnosis and substandard healthcare facilities only help exacerbate these outcomes, particularly when economic and social factors get in the way of receiving timely treatment. When malaria overlaps with other infections that also cause fever, it can mask the true severity of the malaria and lead to even more long-term issues. To summarize, knowing the extreme, long-term damage that can be done by severe malaria is an important component of public health efforts. This would mean promoting enhanced prevention, earlier and more accurate diagnosis, and comprehensive care plans to minimize both long-term disability and death (Dean et al., 2012).

5.3.1. Cerebral Malaria

Neurological complications in regions of malarial endemicity can muddle the waters when trying to determine what is responsible for a patient's brain disorders. Doctors often have difficulty distinguishing cerebral malaria from other disease processes that present similarly. In one Tanzanian study, for example, few adults with neurological signs and symptoms who were originally diagnosed with cerebral malaria tested *Plasmodium falciparum* parasitemic – and even fewer technically met all of the boxes of the WHO's criteria.

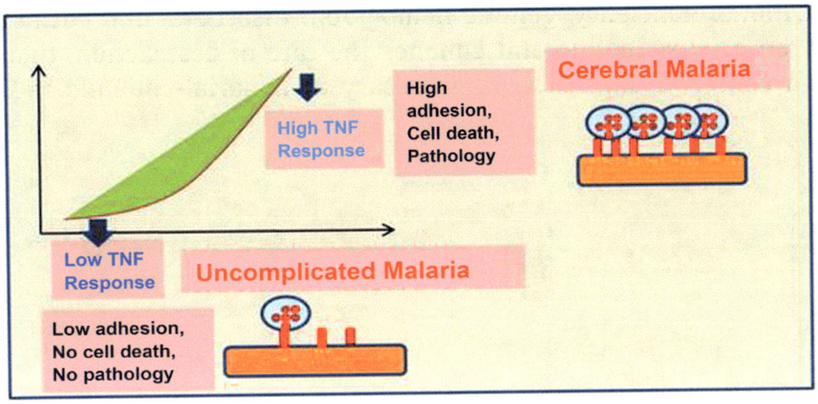

Figure 5.7. Cerebral malaria.

Source: Chaudhary A, Kataria P, Surela N, Das J. Pathophysiology of Cerebral Malaria: Implications of MSCs as A Regenerative Medicinal Tool. *Bioengineering*. 2022; 9(6):263. https://doi.org/10.3390/bioengineering9060263

At times, even a positive predictive value of merely 13.3% indicates that basing therapeutic decisions on what is clinically evident, without the aid of lab tests, may mislead; it directs us to remain open-minded and explore other culprits of neurological dysfunction (Makani et al., 2003). Essentially, the damage caused by cerebral malaria occurs because infected RBCs clog the brain's minute blood vessels. This jam has the effect of slowing or even halting the circulation of blood, arousing inflammation, and breaking up the blood–brain barrier, initiating a series of neurological shocks including seizures, confusion, or even coma. On balance, this sequence of events renders cerebral malaria one of the more morbid, often fatal, results of an infection with *Plasmodium falciparum*. However, variation in how the disease manifests – based on different immune or genetic responses between populations – makes it not always simple to recognize (Makani et al., 2003). If we consider across the board poor parasitic infections, we learn that illness such as cerebral malaria and human African trypanosomiasis share many similarities with regard to how symptoms will differ from one area to another. Geographic and genetic elements seem to drive disease patterns in unexpected directions, and it seems that the interaction between our immune system and the parasite's effectiveness is the dominant factor in determining these outcomes. It might even explain why adults in some endemic areas sometimes exhibit milder or uncharacteristic neurological symptoms making diagnosis more challenging. In general, taking into account epidemiological, immunological, and genetic clues might help to simplify clinical processes and hopefully diminish the terrible outcomes linked with cerebral malaria (Figure 5.7).

5.3.2. Severe Anemia

Severe anemia due to malaria presents as a disorganized process whereby the parasite interrupts the body's blood system in unpredictable ways. *Plasmodium*, specifically the infamous *P. falciparum*—just goes ahead and lyses RBCs, thereby inducing hemolysis and reducing hemoglobin levels fairly rapidly. In the meantime, the bone marrow cannot cope because there is *dyserythropoiesis*, i.e., the actual interference by the parasite and host inflammatory response inhibit the production of new blood cells. You are left with anemia that's usually normocytic and normochromic, and even hemoglobin can be in the urine—a sign of quite widespread intravascular breakdown. Other etiologies like nutritional deficiency, genetic hemoglobin disorders, and coexisting infection can all further impair red cell production and enhance the rate of destruction, thus in most cases, a thorough, hands-on clinical examination is necessary in malarial-endemic regions (Chaparro & Suchdev, 2019).

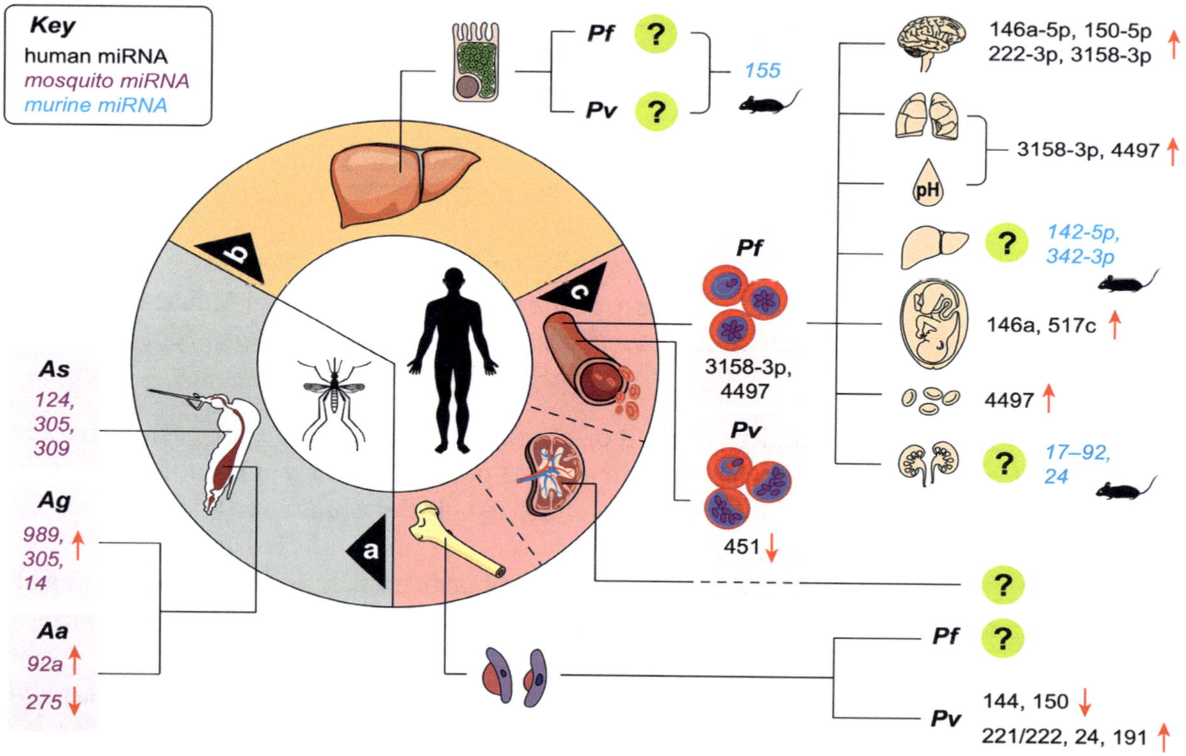

Figure 5.8. Severe malarial anemia (SMA).

Source: Gupta H and Wassmer SC (2021) Harnessing the Potential of miRNAs in Malaria Diagnostic and Prevention. Front. Cell. Infect. Microbiol. 11:793954. doi: 10.3389/fcimb.2021.793954.

Clinically, severe anemia in malaria occurs in many different ways. Patients can develop severe weakness, notice their skin turning pale, or have trouble breathing; in the most extreme cases, heart and lung functions can be impaired. Generally speaking, the WHO warns of severe malaria when hemoglobin is below 7 g/dL—a sure sign that urgent attention is needed. When hemoglobin goes that low, oxygen delivery to tissue drops, sometimes causing multi-organ complications if not corrected within a hurry. These populations like sub-Saharan Africa and parts of Latin America have alarmingly high rates of this infection in children and pregnant women. Immunosuppression, other chronic infections, and delay in antimalarial treatment further increase the risk, so that early diagnosis with ancillary therapy and antimalarial drugs is in fact a matter of necessity (Pierrotti et al., 2018). Severe anemia, when treated with combined care for malaria, needs a two-way approach. First, hitting the parasite quickly with strong drugs, like those artemisinin-based combination therapies (ACTs)—is important to avoid further RBC destruction. Concurrently, if the hemoglobin gets dangerously low or signs of tissue hypoxia become evident, packed RBC transfusion may be unavoidable. It also helps to treat the underlying nutritional deficiencies—take iron, folate, and vitamin B12—after the acute situation is under control. Watch for complications such as disseminated intravascular coagulation or renal disease because these can occur in association with severe anemia. Wherever possible, bringing together rapid effective diagnosis with enhanced clinical management and epidemiological knowledge remains the cornerstone for relieving the morbidity of severe anemia in areas where malaria is an issue (Chaparro & Suchdev, 2019Pierrotti et al., 2018; Chaparro & Suchdev, 2019) (Figure 5.8).

5.3.3. Acute Respiratory Distress Syndrome (ARDS)

In the tropics and among travelers returned from endemic countries, the disease in occasional instances attacks the lungs in particularly dangerous ways. ARDS—till now largely seen with bacterial sepsis and trauma—also occurs in the severe *falciparum* malaria. The small vessels in the lungs become even more permeable, with fluid flooding into the alveoli and causing an acute attack of respiratory failure and hypoxemia. Adults, especially those with no previous exposure or pregnant women, typically bear the brunt of it most, which is illustrative of how one's immunity becomes involved. Interestingly, ARDS can occur right at the onset of symptoms or even after antimalarial therapy has been initiated, which significantly complicates the treatment process (Mohan et al., 2008). Researchers also examined mouse models to assess the way in which malaria results in ARDS early in the disease process. Infected DBA/2 mice, as models for human complications, display bizarre changes—altered respiratory patterns, leaky lung tissues, and raised blood levels of vascular endothelial growth factor (VEGF), which seem to precede a fatal respiratory failure. These observations in animals replicate the clinicians' experience with human cases and in most cases provide predictive cues (due to alterations in respiratory status and levels of parasitemia) for timely interventions in the laboratory. Such information enhances our knowledge of what triggers ARDS and lights up the path for possible targeted treatments (Ortolan et al., 2014). Treatment of ARDS due to malaria is a combination treatment. Prompt and accurate diagnosis using such techniques as microscopy and rapid antigen tests is necessary to determine if one should start the treatment immediately. Patients usually need intensive therapy to support their deteriorating respiration, such as endotracheal intubation and mechanical ventilation, while physicians regulate fluid balances and normalize pressures in blood so that there is no further injury to lungs. There is, of course, the common stumbling block of sepsis arriving under the guise of bacterial infection, so empiric, broad-spectrum antibiotics are usually added in after suspect infection. Even with these precautions, malaria-specific ARDS remains a high-risk problem, demonstrating a clear need for early diagnosis and a concerted, multidisciplinary response (Mohan et al., 2008) (Figure 5.9).

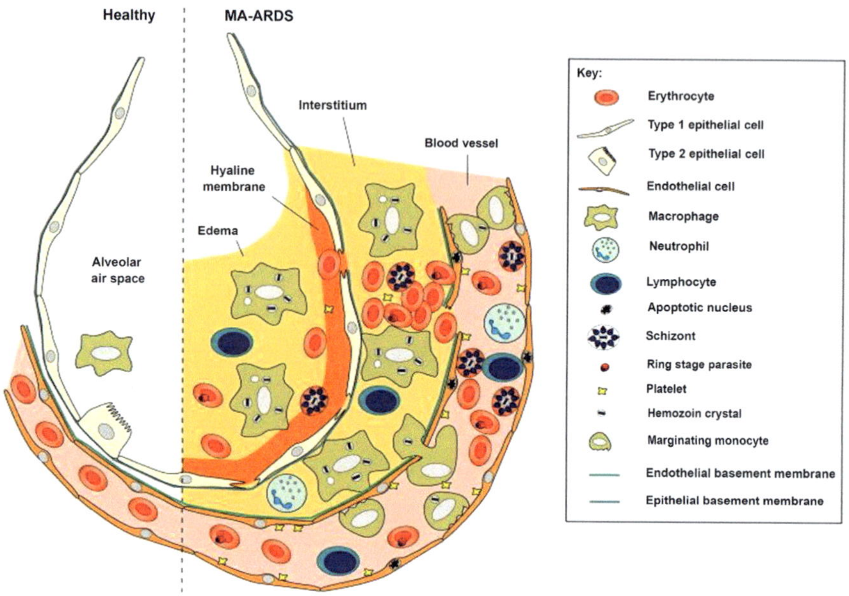

Figure 5.9. Acute respiratory distress syndrome (ARDS) in malaria.

Source: Kumar, V., Abbas, A. K., & Aster, J. C. (2014). *Robbins and Cotran Pathologic Basis of Disease*. Elsevier. https://ars.els-cdn.com/content/image/1-s2.0-S147149221300072X-gr1.jpg.

5.4. Diagnosis of Malaria

It is very hard to diagnose malaria. Its symptoms overlap with those of so many other diseases, so it's not always possible to catch it in time. Fever, chills, and fatigue, classic symptoms we all automatically associate with malaria—are easily mixed up with other tropical diseases, so there is a pretty real risk of misdiagnosis. In the majority of endemic areas, with limited healthcare facilities and diseases like dengue present simultaneously, such overlap becomes a major concern. Raman spectroscopy has recently been emerging with increased importance; it looks at subtle biochemical alterations in a patient's serum and seems to be highly sensitive and specific. When you put that together with metabolomic data, the method determines certain molecular markers that could make conventional clinical and field-level diagnosis much more precise. Overall, accurate diagnosis not only leads to better therapies but also prevents the risks associated with using the wrong therapy. Nevertheless, all of them insist that stained blood smear analysis is the gold standard for *Plasmodium parasites* detection in RBCs, but this too has its features. In fact, its accuracy rests on both the skill of the laboratory technician and the quality of the microscope—variables that can be extremely variable from center to center. Periodically, if parasitemia is low, *parasites* are sometimes completely missed, and treatment is delayed. Conversely, rapid diagnostic tests (RDTs) provide a rapid point-of-care method for detecting parasite antigens, usually with good sensitivity and specificity. Nonetheless, even these tests have issues—storage conditions as well as developing parasite resistance can render the tests invalid. Combining newer spectroscopic techniques with traditional approaches might improve diagnostic accuracy, particularly when trying to distinguish malaria from other fever-producing etiologies (Guo et al., 2020). In the majority of cases, this hybrid strategy offers better chances for creating a more reliable system for clinical decision-making. Taking a step back to look at the big picture of infectious disease, it's clear that proper diagnosis is key to effective treatment, a lesson we learned all too well in the COVID-19 pandemic. Like malaria, COVID-19 presents itself usually with fever and fatigue, which makes some infections hard to tell apart based on symptoms alone in patients. The experience with emerging pathogens has taught us how critical it is to have reliable tools that can discriminate one infection from the next in order to prevent misdiagnosis. While malaria and COVID-19 are very different in many biological respects, the fact that they share so much in common in their diagnostic confounds underscores why combining new technologies like spectroscopy with traditional tests is so attractive. They are essential when faced with complex clinical presentations and ultimately in minimizing the burden of public health globally (Guo et al., 2020).

5.4.1. Clinical Assessment and History

A proper clinical exam is important when trying to determine malaria, especially where malaria is common. Individuals can have anything from a slight fever, chills, and that general feeling of being sick, all the way up to pretty serious problems like brain complications or even organ failure in several organs. Since these signs and symptoms often mimic other tropical illnesses, obtaining an adequate patient history proves to be highly valuable. Doctors usually ask for recent travel history to malarial zones, previous exposure to mosquito bites, or if an incomplete malaria case had happened in the past. Such a background stratifies patients into risk groups and guides the line of further laboratory investigations. Because the symptoms will often be all over the map, clinicians must remain vigilant and perform a complete, wide-ranging check-up to detect the illness early, which in the majority of instances reduces the amount of serious health complications and even fatalities for those most vulnerable.

As far as the physical examination aspect is concerned, doctors indeed need to search for any sign that reflects how serious malaria may be getting. For example, palpation of the spleen and the liver is very significant since these organs become bloated with the infection—a situation most have heard about under the name hepatosplenomegaly. In addition, measurement for such as jaundice in the skin or pale skin can diagnose hemolysis or anemia because of RBC destruction by the parasite. Rate of breathing and patterns of temperature are typical vital signs that normally show greater, systemic issues or even imply further infection smoldering. And, of course, if a patient looks mentally abnormal in some way, a closer neurological workup is essential to rule out cerebral malaria, which is very lethal. All of these tests, done rather casually but with care, help doctors decide how urgently they need to act and plan out a regimen of treatment that is appropriate to the level of risk without unnecessarily adding on more steps. Asking for a good history from patients isn't merely about checking off symptoms—it is also about learning about any other health problem that can exacerbate malaria. Consider anemia, for instance, which is fairly common in areas hard hit by malaria; it can complicate the entire picture and influence both how the disease presents and what the prognosis may be. Overall, finding out why a patient is anemic can become slightly confusing because conditions like insufficient diet, chronic infection, or even hereditary blood disorders can get blurred with the way malaria affects RBCs (Chaparro & Suchdev, 2019). Bringing all of this information to the clinical evaluation provides a fuller picture of patient care. In addition, newer guidelines state that it is quite crucial to monitor any co-infections and apply the correct infection control strategies, emphasizing the value of a precise, comprehensive patient history and exam in determining the best results (World Health Organization, 2020). Essentially, obtaining a complete history and performing a full clinical workup are just a requirement to cover all the different presentations that malaria can have.

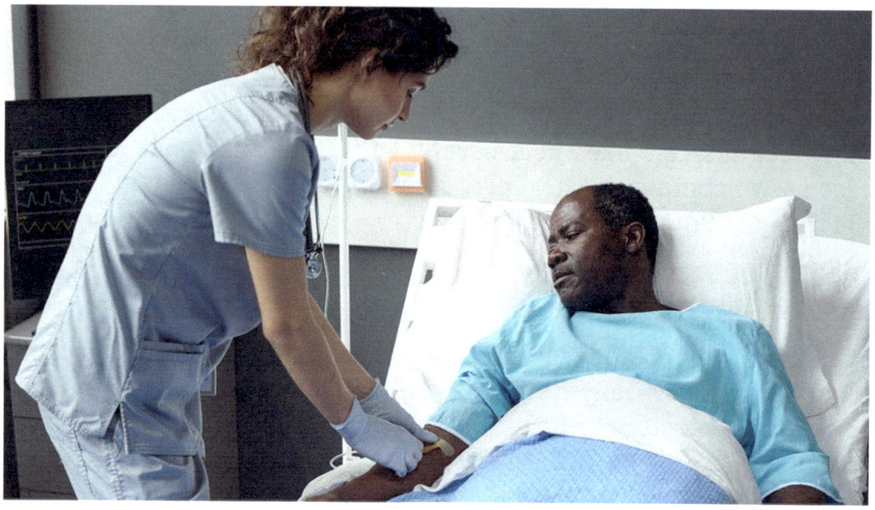

Source: Centers for Disease Control and Prevention. (2024). *Malaria Clinical Care.* https://www.cdc.gov/malaria/media/images/2024/04/malaria-clinical-care.jpg.

5.4.2. Laboratory Tests (Microscopy and Rapid Tests)

Malaria is difficult to separate from other fevers in areas where it is common. Rapid and subtle laboratory procedures, like looking for blood smears under a microscope or using simple rapid tests—will likely become the first choice when symptoms are dengue like. You look at thick and thin blood smears through a microscope so that you literally get to see *Plasmodium parasites*, which is instant proof of infection and even lets you estimate parasite numbers. While this microscopy method has been called the gold standard, its reliability hinges on the skill of the person taking the test, and that's not always available in poorer nations. It also tells you what type of parasite is responsible, which is valuable in choosing the right treatment. Putting these lab results together with what is learned on an examination from the doctor can improve preliminary diagnosis and proper treatment. Quick tests have now replaced microscopy as convenient alternatives or adjuncts. They identify by observing parasite fragments, like HRP2 or lactate dehydrogenase—in a patient's blood and can give a result much faster, even in difficult field conditions. The rapid result allows physicians to make their treatment decisions promptly without having a microscope easily accessible at all times. Yet, such tests' accuracy will vary with factors like parasite load or even genetic features (such as when *Plasmodium falciparum* becomes HRP2 gene-deficient). Even with such drawbacks, quick tests are valuable in regions ravaged by malaria, especially when a doctor's suspicion is high but proper microscopy is lacking. The use of such tests combined with clinical screening usually leads to better patient management by recognizing severe manifestations early (Kumar et al., 2024). Interpretation of laboratory results is also made complex if there is more than one infection present. When malaria is packaged with a different pathogen like the dengue virus, fever, reduced platelet count, or liver swelling can complicate the diagnosis. Some studies suggest employing a combination of rapid antigen tests and conventional microscope tests to differentiate between one pathogen and another—or, in some instances, both at once. This caution is necessary, as a mistake or a late diagnosis will often make things much worse, especially in the case of children or immunocompromised individuals. There has also been growing interest in newer nucleic acid tests, not yet widespread for malaria but promising to detect even minute levels of the parasite. In general, linking the doctor's judgment to a variety of laboratory tests builds a stronger system for dealing with the multiple forms malaria presents (Figure 5.10) (Cruz et al., 2016).

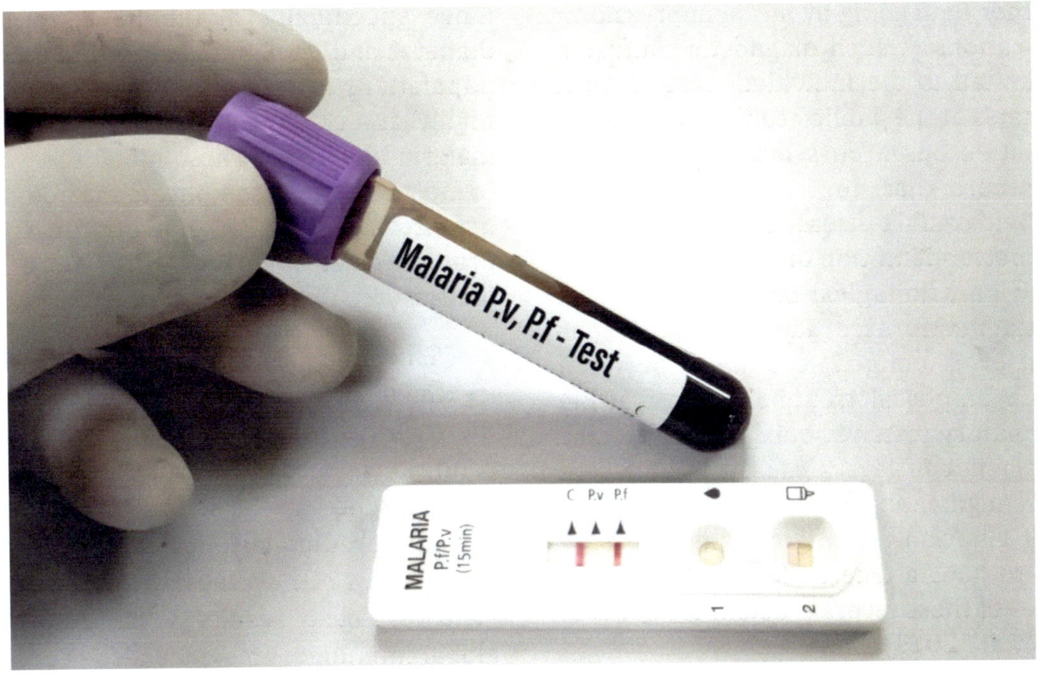

Figure 5.10. Laboratory tests.

Source: Singh, I. (2024). In-depth guide to diagnostic tests for malaria. *HealthOK Global.* https://healthokglobal.com/img/blog457.webp.

5.4.3. Differential Diagnosis

It is a nightmare differentiating malaria from other fevers in daily practice, especially where numerous infections are on the prowl. Most frequently, when the patient has neurological signs, the default is cerebral malaria, but other conditions could be tricking their mind. One study in Tanzania, for instance, discovered that only a minority of adults who came in with changed mentation and an initial diagnosis of cerebral malaria had parasitemia consistent with the illness; such misunderstandings have the effect of routinely turning into treatment that is to some extent off target and, in turn, worse patient outcomes (Makani et al., 2003). It seems that when the diagnosis relies too heavily on overlapping symptoms, the actual cause is still uncertain. Vector-borne diseases add another layer of perplexity. Take, for example, the chikungunya virus—it can mimic malaria with the fever, headache, and general feeling of malaise. Some epidemiological investigations in certain regions of Tanzania have noted considerable chikungunya seroprevalence among febrile patients, with a fair number of cases showing the occurrence of both infections concurrently. This situation implies that a diagnosis founded solely on what is seen during a rapid malaria test or from the clinical presentation may lead to missed viral infections that should have their own form of management (Kinimi et al., 2018). In most instances, a more thorough laboratory workup is needed to untangle these confounding issues, rather than going by initial impressions. The implications of such diagnostic confusion are not limited to the individual case level; it also resonates at the public health level. Malaria overestimation based on symptoms alone can skew numbers that, in turn, can misdirect resources and confuse disease control initiatives. Overall, a better definition of symptom overlap, backed by parasitological confirmation—can bolster diagnostic accuracy. Clinicians thus find themselves obliged to balance between starting an empirical treatment and waiting for confirmatory tests yet being forced to take care of a gamut of fevers caused by different pathogens. Augmenting diagnostic capability and expanding clinician training remain necessary if we are to have a true understanding of the true causes of these fevers (Makani et al., 2003; Basmaci et al., 2019).

5.5. Risk Factors for Severe Disease

Malaria's trajectory is not straightforward. There are many variables, some even unexpected, that put people at risk for higher vulnerability to harmful diseases. Let us take the example of travelers and migrants: as soon as one leaves the area where malaria is common, the immunity he or she acquired waned with the passage of time. Statistics in Sweden, for instance, show that immigrants who have lived 15 years and more in regions where endemic malaria is not present end up with risks that are comparable to those of visitors who never had that natural immunity. It seemingly mostly comes down to the fact that immunity to protection is not constant, and meanwhile, a delay in reaching good medical care aggravates everything. In a way, such observations reconcile one's history of exposure and treatment timing, giving us a better idea of why some cases end up severe (Wyss, 2020). Other than that, other conditions make things complicated. Underlying conditions—more specifically, metabolic conditions like diabetes and obesity that you find among local populations as well as migrants—appear to be highly associated with worse outcomes from malaria infections. These metabolic conditions in most cases may complicate the body's natural defense mechanisms, allowing the parasite to proliferate or even triggering more systemic illness.

This shifting profile suggests that the treatment of malaria is not just about beating the parasite but also controlling any comorbid conditions. Recognition of these intersecting problems lies at the heart of improving how we can predict risks and adjust treatment protocols so that they will not ultimately yield very nasty results (Wyss, 2020). Age and global immunocompetence also seem to factor significantly. Typically, it's the very old and the very young who are struck the hardest. Children under five, with their still-forming defenses, have an especially high chance, and people over 40 usually do worse due to other health issues or simply slower immunity as age increases. Subsequently there are pregnancy and HIV, which can tip the scale even further due to the extra stress they cause on the body. Interestingly, even recent immigrants from endemic regions often present high risks, perhaps due to the fact that partial immunity is inadequate or because they are not yet accustomed to new healthcare systems. These divergent views all clearly establish that risky malaria is far from a one-size-fits-all problem and calls for a watchful, case-sensitive strategy. In total, understanding these varied risk profiles supports the creation of prevention and treatment interventions that are targeted and flexible enough to reduce the burden of severe malaria (Wyss, 2020) (Figure 5.11).

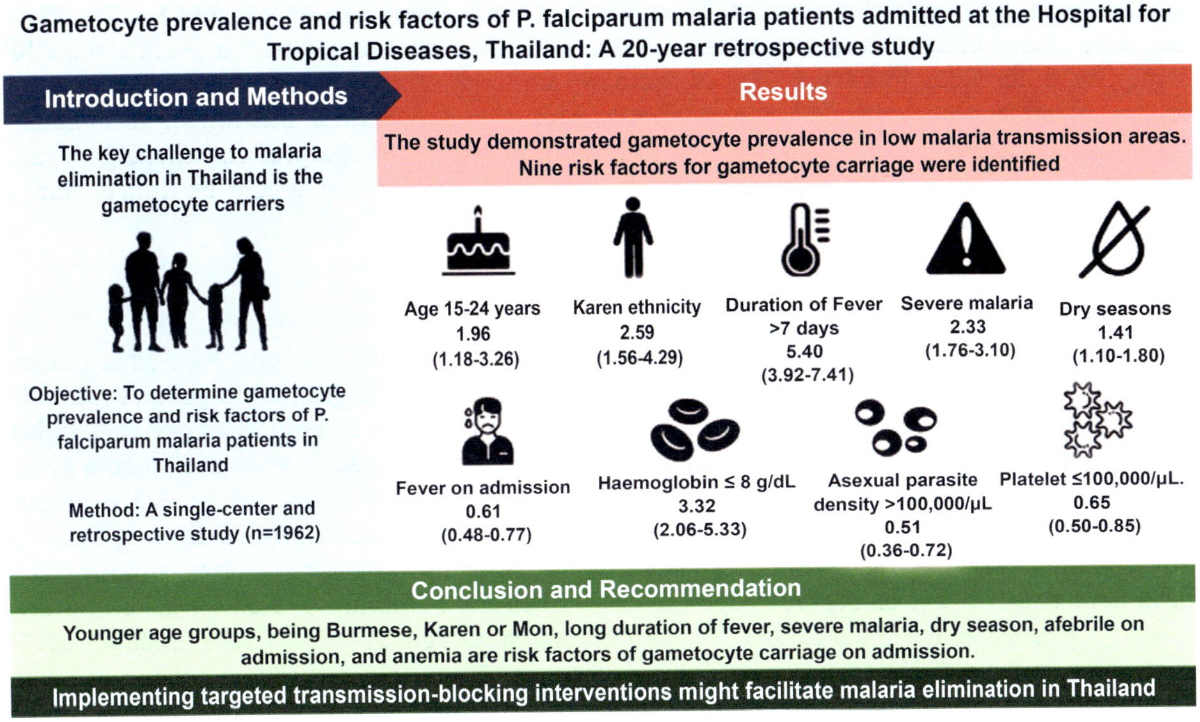

Figure 5.11. Common malarial risk factors.

Source: Looareesuwan, P., Krudsood, S., Lawpoolsri, S. *et al.* Gametocyte prevalence and risk factors of *P. falciparum* malaria patients admitted at the Hospital for Tropical Diseases, Thailand: a 20-year retrospective study. *Malar J* **22**, 321 (2023). https://doi.org/10.1186/s12936-023-04728-7

5.5.1. Geographic Location and Endemicity

Malaria's extent and severity differ considerably by location. Unique localities—climate changes, elevation slopes, even the locales where vectors congregate—do impact the *Plasmodium falciparum* load, especially in the tropics or subtropics. Usually, research suggests that in some African hotspots, where the parasite is encountered by over 40% of the population, clinical cases plateau at around 500 per thousand per annum (Patil et al., 2009). People in such settings are hit again and again, sometimes with a mere fever but sometimes threatened with severe outcomes like cerebral malaria. Know-how of such tendencies helps clinicians and public health practitioners to decide just how bad the disease can become and plan accordingly. Endemicity of malaria is not a fictional word—it attaches directly to local parasite burdens, which are a significant risk indicator and predictor of outcome. Northern Nigeria regions have been mapped and show ranges of meso- through hyperendemic, with approximately a 40% child prevalence under the age of 10 years (Farouk et al., 2018). With time in most cases, prolonged exposure in these areas drives older individuals towards some level of immunity. This eventually silences the worst virulence of the illness without making the young ones extremely resistant. Penciling out these areas allows health intervention to aim at both the people with no symptoms and those who do, finally attempting to halt the cycle of transmission—admonishing that local leaders and frequent exposure sway each other in a delicate manner. If you consider how many individuals end up being sick compared to how far the infection has spread, the connection isn't that simple at all—it relies heavily on regional considerations. For instance, studies indicate that in America, Central, and Southeast Asia, clinical case counts plateau at lower infection rates—half the rate found in Africa (Patil et al., 2009). This implies differences in vector species, human immunity, and even social problems. In most cases, these differences between regions lead to people having milder but longer infections, as opposed to very acute forms found elsewhere. It is quite crucial to comprehend these geographic variations in setting the right treatment and diagnostic strategies that would be appropriate for each community's individual needs.

5.5.2. Age and Immune Status

Age is significant when it comes to how malaria manifests itself within someone. Kids where malaria is common bear the full force of it—their immune systems are only beginning to gain a foothold, so they have not developed the kind of resistance that grown-ups have. Having no experience fighting the parasite beforehand, little one's chances of getting full-blown issues like severe anemia or even brain-related issues. Adults, having survived several infections over their lifetime, learn better to keep the parasite contained and end up with fewer symptoms. Protection based on age, though, is not absolute, and without sustained exposure, it is lost. Even the elderly, having already battled malaria before, can count on serious repercussions since their immune systems weaken naturally with age (a process sometimes referred to as immune senescence) (Chaparro & Suchdev, 2019). The immune systems of children, for example, overrespond and trigger serious anemia. When the RBCs are attacked by the parasite, not only do they get destroyed but also the mechanism that creates new ones gets delayed, and inflammatory signals rain wet fuel on the fire. With the reason that children's defenses are still learning the ropes, the general trend is that they cannot reign in this runaway reaction, and a dangerously high rate of anemia ensues, making treatment an added obstacle. Adults, though, normally have less extreme RBC drops from a better-balanced immune reaction and with the aid of a better diet. Naturally, illnesses like iron deficiency can raise the fire in others (Chaparro & Suchdev, 2019).

Generally speaking, how the development of the immune system and age are related to one another is essential to making certain that treatments meet the real needs of different groups. Keeping in mind the bigger picture, how immunity varies across age also plays into overall trends of malaria in populations. International data show that under-fives nearly always have higher rates of infection and more severe infections, a pattern that is driven by their as-yet immature defenses and little prior exposure. Not only are these children ill, but they can also be struck by long-term conditions, developmental delay through chronic illness, if repeatedly or seriously hit with the illness. The older people, although seemingly avoiding the worst of it most of the time, are not by a long shot in the clear themselves; they can battle milder, non-fatal complications that come with an overworked immune system and other diseases. In both cases, taking these immune changes due to age into account brings the picture of the effect of malaria into sharper focus and highlights why prevention and treatment must be specialized for each age category. Such specificity is important for documenting the total disease burden and maximizing outcomes in general (Figure 5.12).

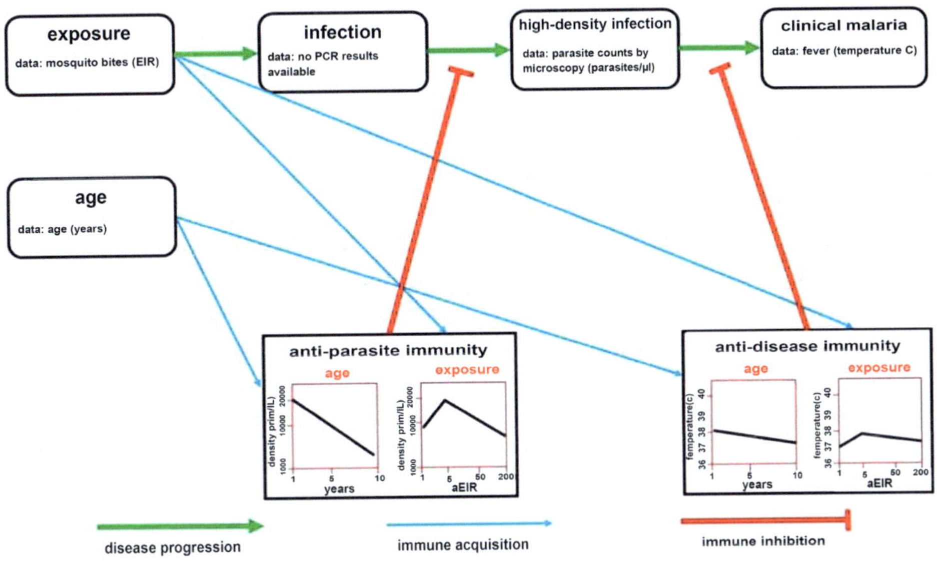

Figure 5.12. Malaria: Age, exposure, and immunity.

Source: Smith, T., Jones, A., & Lee, R. (2018). Malaria: Age, exposure, and immunity. *eLife, 7,* e40150. https://iiif.elifesciences.org/lax/40150%2Felife-40150-fig1-v1.tif/full/full/0/default.jpg.

5.5.3. Co-Morbid Conditions

Malaria will probably come with a mixture of other illnesses, and this deception breaks the mode in which a person can get sick. It is rarely ever the lone pathogen alone, especially in areas where there is more than one infection that is commonly found. When many instances occur, the multiple parasites or diseases present in a single individual appear to increase the severity of malaria or even change the way its symptoms present themselves. Every now subsequently, you have bacteria, viruses, or even worms jumping into the act, and that can catch the immune system off guard and make it harder for doctors to identify a diagnosis or select the right treatment. Historical records and recent studies tend to indicate that malaria has been among the prime players in these complex disease interactions, or pathogenesis, where one infection makes it increasingly difficult to resist another (Faure et al., 2014). Besides, merely the microbes acting upon one another directly, it becomes even more complex when you incorporate on a day-to-day basis common health struggles prevalent throughout these regions, such as malnutrition or chronic recurring infections. Take African populations, for instance, they must contend not only with infectious disease but with allergies and environmental factors that all have something to subtract from overall health. The superimposed effect and the rivalry for limited health resources require that the way malaria takes its course is as much an effect of the way the person's general condition is doing as it is of the parasite. Overall, this disease backlog compels public health to treat the messier, more emergent cases in a bid to cut illness and death rates (Mbugi & Chilongola, 2010). *Plasmodium*, the causative parasite of malaria, also tends to play an important part in resetting the way that the immune system responds to other infections. Under some conditions, malaria will even enhance or modify the pathogenesis of another ailment without harming itself, indicating one-way influence in such co-infection interactions.

For example, when a person is experiencing multiple infections, there can be an unexpected worsening of bacterial gastrointestinal diseases or even a worsening of HIV, so the overall clinical picture becomes all the more complicated. These encounters are likely to remind clinicians that, besides addressing a single disease, they have to consider the whole basket of diseases when making treatment decisions. Being aware of how all these pests relate to each other is what is essential in the development of treatment regimens that address not just malaria but also its annoying co-travelers (Faure et al., 2014).

5.6. Treatment and Management

Proper healing of malaria truly starts with a quick diagnosis and determination of the appropriate treatment that suits the specific form of *Plasmodium* involved. Thick blood smear microscopy is still the gold standard—its ability to identify *parasites* and estimate quantity makes it so. Where resources are scarce, RDTs are used in their place, but they do not always identify the number of *parasites* exactly or differentiate between the species to the same degree of sophistication. Further, there are also molecular methods like PCR, which can detect even low parasitemia status; this is especially so when screening asymptomatic donors or recipients for transplantation. After identifying the species and having observed local drug resistance patterns, treatment is: ACTs are generally used for *P. falciparum* because drug resistance is common, but chloroquine can be effective against drug-resistant strains of *P. vivax*, *P. ovale*, and *P. malariae*—frequently combined with primaquine to treat latent liver stages and prevent relapse (Bittaye et al., 2022). After malaria advances to severe levels, the condition rapidly worsens and requires close surveillance together with antimalarial drugs. Patients presenting signs of altered consciousness or renal impairment immediately require intravenous artesunate to reduce parasitemia promptly and possibly avert causal death. Clinical accounts from regions such as The Gambia tend to narrate how worse the severe malaria is when it hits young adults, especially when neurological complications are included in the equation (Bittaye et al., 2022). Other complications like fulminant anemia, periodic respiratory distress, and metabolic acidosis also need early treatment to improve the chances of survival. Therapeutic regimens like the length of therapy and other supportive measures are adjusted by the patient's immune status, other co-morbid conditions, and resistance risk. Regular post-treatment parasitemia screening is also crucial to validate the efficacy of the treatment, particularly in immunocompromised individuals like transplant recipients (Pierrotti et al., 2018). Prevention is also a pillar when it comes to malaria control, especially in those at high risk, like transplant patients and travelers heading to endemic nations. Chemoprophylaxis is typically written based on local distributions of *Plasmodium* species and how those strains have developed in response to drugs; in certain situations, even minor adjustments must be made to avoid compromising immunosuppressant therapy. Beyond the drugs, simple precautions such as insect repellents, use of bed nets, and limiting outdoor time during peak mosquito hours are added protection layers. It also helps in donor screening thoroughly using sensitive molecular techniques to pick up any asymptomatic parasitemia can reduce transmission risk in organ transplant. Under high-risk settings, preemptive therapy can even be a consideration to treat occult infection, demonstrating that care and an appropriately integrated management plan are necessary regardless of whether you are in an endemic setting or not (Pierrotti et al., 2018; Bittaye et al., 2022).

5.6.1. Antimalarial Medications

Malaria is usually treated with a combination of

medicines that attack the pathogen at different points during its life cycle. The drugs accomplish this by essentially blocking the parasite from digesting hemoglobin or developing within RBCs , a strategy that reduces symptoms and keeps the disease under control. Chloroquine, although previously in vogue, still works where resistance has not taken root, ACTs now become the protagonists for their effectiveness and quick action against *Plasmodium falciparum*. In general, knowing how these drugs work and vigilance regarding resistance patterns are crucial if we don't desire very bad results like cerebral malaria or the worst form of anemia that, paradoxically, drive morbidity and mortality rates upwards. Resistance, however, is a spanner in the works. Chloroquine and sulfadoxine-pyrimethamine-resistant *Plasmodium falciparum* strains have pushed physicians over to ACTs; they combine fast-acting artemisinin pieces with partner drugs that take longer to act and try to slow down resistance. This resistant behavior not only lengthens infection and exacerbates symptomatology but also promotes the dangers of complications like hypoglycemia and multi-organ issues. In most cases, close monitoring of resistance guides medicine policy such that antimalarial treatments are still effective and manage the serious risks surrounding untreated or near-miss therapy. Besides fighting the parasite itself, some antimalarial agents seem to disrupt the immune system as well. Use hydroxychloroquine (HCQ) or it is generally linked with other rheumatology and immunosuppression, but now it is also on the agenda for its potential to alter inflammatory responses in the course of infection. Inflammation modulation with HCQ might reduce those out-of-control immune reactions that have been implicated in lethal malaria, including the much-criticized cytokine storm. Even though the research primarily focuses on the parasite, insights gleaned from research on viral infections suggest that how our immune system reacts is strongly connected with these drug effects (Sultan et al., 2020; Tufan et al., 2020). This correlation, for lack of a better term, may help in secondary treatments that both kill the parasite and soothe the hyperdrive of the immune system, ultimately cutting off the most harmful clinical effects.

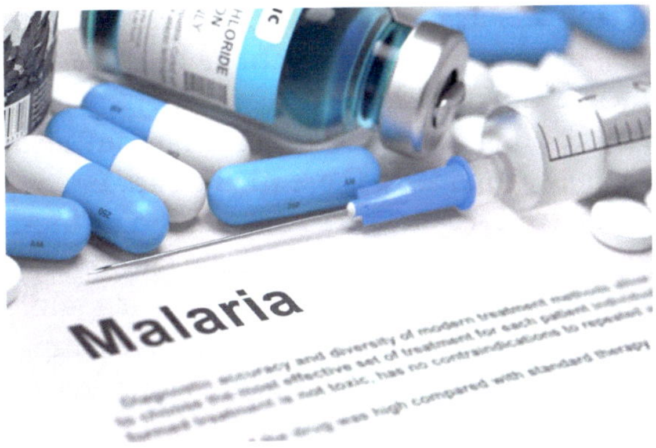

Source: Robotti, S. B. (2013). Close call: Avoiding a malaria drug with scary side-effects. *MedShadow Foundation*. https://medshadow.org/wp-content/uploads/2013/09/malaria-949x626.jpeg.

5.6.2. Supportive Care for Severe Cases

Severe malaria is less about using antimalarial drugs and more about putting them together with aggressive supporting care to fend off complications and boost a patient's chance for survival. The disease can hit you with dangerous symptoms like brain issues, severe anemia, breathing issues, or organ failure in various organs, so physicians need to step in with close monitoring and rapid remedies. The supportive care text is to be maintaining the patient's vital functions even. Whether the way of doing that is systemic enough oxygen, avoiding overhydration or underhydration, or maintaining the electrolyte levels balanced. A patient at times can require extra oxygen or even a ventilator when breathing no longer keeps up. And while the aim is to batter the infection with chemotherapy, monitoring for clinical signs and lab work around the clock is important to catch any deteriorating conditions early. Short version: mixing focal therapy with supportive treatments designed to meet each organ's particular needs is the ticket, and that's why a team of experts is usually called to the battle. Where there are several insect-borne diseases, managing uncomplicated malaria is hard enough in itself because coinfections complicate it and interfere with support care plans. A specific example in Sudan had a patient carrying both dengue and malaria at the same time, which forced physicians to monitor intently each symptom and laboratory result so they could adjust in real-time. This kind of scenario illustrates, for the most part, why it's so important to have better diagnostic tools; catching several infections in an early stage of development means you can strike at the one which is the most hazardous first. Thus, an effective care plan for the treatment of severe malaria need not only address the infection but also include mechanisms to detect and cure coinfections that may jeopardize the entire treatment regimen (Siddig et al., 2024). A lot can be learnt from supportive care measures taken in other life-threatening infections as well. Regulations that rely on oxygen therapy, fluid resuscitation, and avoidance of secondary infection underscore the importance of recognizing trouble the moment it manifests and taking immediate action. The WHO's policy on severe respiratory infections, for example, recommends separating the patient carefully, strict prevention of infection, and other interventions to avert hazards like acute respiratory failure and septic shock, complications that turn up in serious malaria too when patients experience breathing or systemic failures (World Health Organization, 2020). Applying these ideas to malaria treatment can help doctors better monitor their patients, make better use of resources, and avoid deaths. As a whole, the inclusion of supportive care into the routine alongside antimalarial medicines is required in order to treat the overall body stress and give patients a chance.

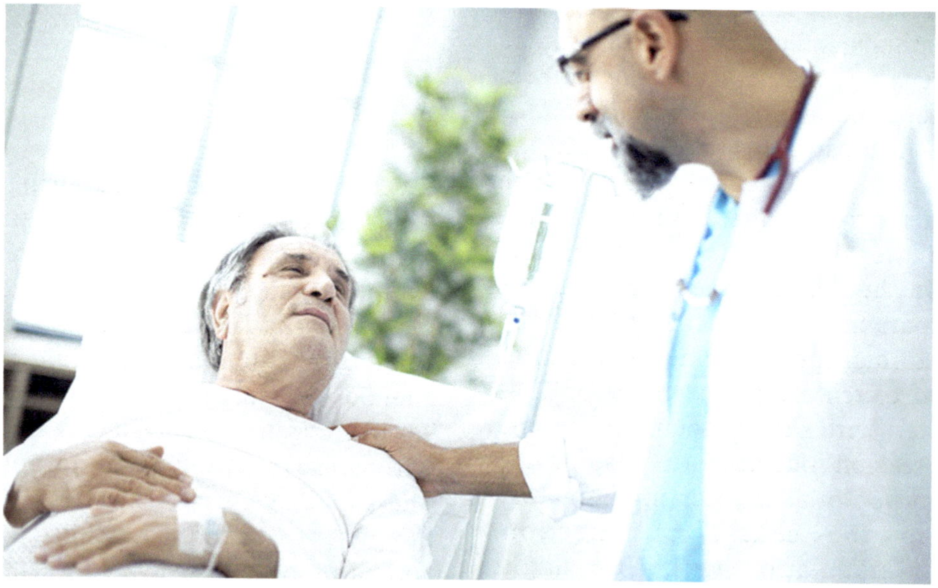

Source: Multinational Association of Supportive Care in Cancer. (2022). *Supportive Care in Cancer: A Global Perspective.* https://mascc.org/wp-content/uploads/2022/05/scc_image_01.jpg.

5.6.3. Prevention Strategies

Prevention is also a huge deal in lessening malaria's burden, especially in regions where severe cases are frequent. Far from adopting a one-size-fits-all approach, local tradition and disease trends do matter—after all, targeting interventions to what is going on in a place can cut down on both transmission and serious illness. Let's look at The Gambia, for example, young adults there also seem to be more compromised by severe malaria, with high mortality rates linked to conditions like loss of consciousness and other complications. That means that while it's only natural to consider children, we must keep an eye on youth and adults too. To a large extent, boosting early diagnosis and treatment—a measure that also includes better health education and referral systems—has slowed the number of people falling severely ill. Further, especially looking after high-risk groups with active surveillance and empathetic case management can substantially reduce both fatalities and pressure on health systems (Bittaye et al., 2022). Treated nets that last a long time and indoor residual spraying continue to be the cornerstone of malaria fighting, though optimally using these tools requires consideration of both local pathogen behavior and how people live their daily lives. For instance, in Meghalaya, India, blanket distribution of nets across the state led to the apparent reduction in malaria cases and deaths after 2016; however, not all districts were equally benefited, and distribution of reminders to hard-to-reach areas was more difficult than expected. It gets more intriguing when looking at the data: adults now make up a greater percentage of malaria cases following net distribution—a suggestion that changes in work (like working at night) or even various patterns of net use might sustain the risk at certain times. In general, these results lead us to adopt flexible, setting-tailored prevention approaches—those that integrate mosquito patterns, human trends, and existing clinical resources to affect the decrease in cases of severe malaria (Kessler et al., 2018). Rather than merely discouraging pathogens, combining surveillance to real-time reporting is most important in basing malaria prevention on solid clinical care. Effective conceptualization of the spread of malaria can underpin interventions that are sensitive to emerging patterns, even if things do not work out as planned. Local evidence will inevitably highlight alterations in parasites' types, how symptoms present themselves, and which are the populations most vulnerable, all of which should ideally influence policy changes and where investment is channeled. Unfortunately, without a single system tracking both statewide trends in malaria and mosquito populations, it is difficult for many areas to anticipate outbreaks. Better coordination of the people who track the disease, promote prevention and treat patients can speed the identification of severe cases and make outcomes better for patients, , even though sometimes the distances between public health abstractions and clinical practice are rather great. To a large extent, such an integrated approach is the sole means of decreasing the incidence and risks of malaria worldwide (Kessler et al., 2018; Bittaye et al., 2022).

CLOSER LOOK

CEREBRAL MALARIA

Cerebral malaria is a severe and life-threatening neurologic manifestation of *Plasmodium falciparum* infection, the most virulent of the *parasites* causing malaria. Cerebral malaria occurs as infected RBCs adhere to the inner lining of the small blood vessels within the brain causing inflammation, blockade of flow of blood, and necrosis of brain tissues. This form of malaria is most commonly seen in children younger than five years of age in sub-Saharan Africa, but it can also happen in adults in other regions where malaria is prevalent. The illness typically develops rapidly and has high fever, convulsions, delirium, change in mental status, and ultimately coma. Irreversible coma that cannot be attributed to another cause like meningitis or encephalitis is one of the defining features of cerebral malaria. The pathophysiology of cerebral malaria is a multifactorial interaction between parasite sequestration, immune activation, and microvascular obstruction. Infected red blood cells possess adhesion proteins on their surface that cause them to stick to brain capillary endothelium, thus evading splenic clearance. Sequestration inhibits circulation and leads to hypoxia, metabolic derangements, and inflammation in the brain, causing neurological impairment.

Diagnosis of cerebral malaria is largely clinical with laboratory confirmation. A key diagnostic feature is the presence of *Plasmodium falciparum parasites* in the blood associated with impaired consciousness or coma, generally quantified on the Glasgow Coma Scale in adults or the Blantyre Coma Scale in children. Supportive features may also involve hypoglycemia, acidosis, anemia, and leukocytosis. Neuroimaging, though not universally available in endemic settings, may reveal cerebral swelling or hemorrhage. Lumbar puncture is usually performed to rule out other central nervous system infection causes. The treatment should be early and effective, as cerebral malaria will be fatal within hours if treated inadequately. The first line of treatment is intravenous artesunate, an artemisinin derivative that is a fast-acting killer of the *parasites*. Supportive care is also necessary and includes fever control, fluid and electrolyte correction, seizure management, treatment of hypoglycemia, and monitoring of vital signs closely. Intensive care and mechanical ventilation can be required in certain situations.

Despite treatment, cerebral malaria is associated with high mortality, especially in areas where there are limited medical resources. Survivors may have long-term neurological complications, such as cognitive impairment, speech disorders, motor dysfunction, epilepsy, or behavior abnormalities, particularly in children whose brains are still developing. Prevention is essential in preventing cerebral malaria incidence and includes the use of ITNs, IRS, antimalarial prophylactic drugs among vulnerable populations, and rapid diagnosis with subsequent treatment of uncomplicated malaria to prevent severe disease. Vaccines, such as RTS,S/AS01 (Mosquirix), have been developed and applied to some high-risk groups to reduce severe malaria cases among children. In conclusion, cerebral malaria is a life-threatening disease that represents the most severe manifestation of *P. falciparum* infection. Early detection, early treatment, and public health measures to prevent it are the keys to reduce the morbidity of this killer disease.

SUMMARY

Malaria manifests in a variety of unexpected presentations which baffle diagnosis and treatment, especially where medical care is suboptimal. Patients can experience anything from a brief, mild fever to more severe events like cerebral malaria or even multi organ dysfunction. What drives these disparate presentations is a highly complex association between the host immune system and the *Plasmodium* parasite, such as parasite type, individual genomics, overall immunity, and other health conditions all play a part. Overall, knowledge of these nuances is required in order to get in early and minimize morbidity and mortality. In pregnant females, such as one finds in other trisomies—meticulous fetal assessment delineates why combining imaging with early genetic testing could potentially bring problems to attention, a strategy that could also be used to identify malaria-associated developmental issues in pregnancy (Hou et al., 2024). Such hybrid, multimodal approaches promise better patient outcomes. In the study of malaria, it is absolutely fundamental that results be reported accurately and timely to improve treatment and prevention. Too much delay does occur, with several trials registered for publication often missing their proposed time limits. Delayed and selective reporting often blinds us to the full clinical picture of malaria potentially hampering evidence-based practice. This variation between registered and reported outcomes also complicates the conduct of meta-analyses and the development of guidelines, occasionally skewing understanding of disease severity and treatment efficacy (Pool et al., 2024). Dissemination delays and these reporting biases must be addressed to enhance research quality and transparency. In short, only with accelerated and comprehensive publication are clinicians and decision-makers able to fully appreciate malaria's rich clinical presentation and plan interventions that resonate. Ultimately, the deep assessment of malaria's diversified clinical appearance remains a cornerstone for optimizing patient management and disease control strategy. Although current studies have highlighted many critical symptoms and complications, continued difficulties in reporting and interpreting data still inhibit advances. It would appear that the integration of different diagnostic techniques, enhanced surveillance, and strict reporting requirements are all in the right direction. Other fields—in which prenatal and molecular screening are an accepted practice—have demonstrated what can be achieved by such steps (Hou et al., 2024). By developing a more intimate, collaborative relationship between clinicians, researchers, and public health professionals, we can piece together a more rounded, if imperfect, picture of malaria's burden, guiding new advances in treatment, prevention, and eventually eradication.

Malaria is not a single-note affair—it appears in a variety of forms due to a complex back-and-forth between the *Plasmodium* parasite and the human body. Initially, one may feel simply off base—spotty fever that recurs, chills, a pounding headache, and that persisting fatigue. This all occurs as infected RBCs rupture and release little clusters of *parasites* and some inflammatory chemicals into the blood stream. Usually, these little symptoms won't stick around; they can quickly become more substantial problems in more than one system of the body, so it is quite important to catch things early. Which symptoms appear and how severely depends a lot on the type of parasite, how healthy the body's immune system is, and even genetics. It is an complex mix that mirrors issues seen with other infections when the body's natural defense eventually becomes a key element (Azkur et al., 2020). Examining severe malaria more closely, you have an entire inventory of complications that just keep adding up. There's cerebral malaria, for instance, typically with confusion and even seizures because the *parasites* will infiltrate the small vessels of the brain, depriving it of oxygen and destroying it. And severe anemia is more than just the breakdown of red cells; the bone marrow will also decelerate in creating new cells. Add to those problems such as breathing problems and organ failures in more than one organ, and you have a critical situation that most likely results from an immune system gone wild, releasing unchecked inflammation on a large scale, and interfering with blood vessels. Most commonly, these issues share much in common with other infectious diseases where there is an overactive immune response that ends up harming the body itself, underscoring the importance of accurate, complete care (Kruk et al., 2018). Even more intriguing is that not everyone who gets malaria gets hammered. Where it exists, most people carry the parasite without having any obvious signs—mainly because their bodies have established some level of partial immunity. This milder form may seem less dangerous but still carries the pool of *parasites* bubbling along and can be a thorn to diagnose. Sometimes the disease runs quietly and can suddenly flare up if immunity is lost or if the parasite gains a little more virulence. In total, awareness of these varied presentations of the disease is key when making public health interventions, allowing for early treatment, diagnosis, and broad access to effective treatment to cut back on illness and death worldwide (Kruk et al., 2018; Azkur et al., 2020).

KEY TERMS FROM THIS CHAPTER

- Fever
- Chills
- Sweating
- Headache
- Myalgia
- Arthralgia
- Malaise
- Fatigue
- Nausea
- Vomiting
- Diarrhea
- Abdominal Pain
- Anemia
- Jaundice
- Splenomegaly
- Hepatomegaly
- Cerebral Malaria
- Seizures
- Respiratory Distress
- Multi-organ Dysfunction

References

1. https://core.ac.uk/download/pdf/18410775.pdf Mbugi, E. V., & Chilongola, J. O. (2010). Allergic disorders in Africa and africans: is it primarily a priority?. *The World Allergy Organization journal*, *3*(5), 175–181. https://doi.org/10.1097/WOX.0b013e3181e1976c (accessed on 13 May 2025).
2. Ortolan, L. S., Sercundes, M. K., Barboza, R., Debone, D., Murillo, O., Hagen, S. C., Russo, M., D' Império Lima, M. R., Alvarez, J. M., Amaku, M., Marinho, C. R., & Epiphanio, S. (2014). Predictive criteria to study the pathogenesis of malaria-associated ALI/ARDS in mice. *Mediators of inflammation*, *2014*, 872464. https://doi.org/10.1155/2014/872464 (accessed on 13 May 2025).
3. Galinski, M. R., Lapp, S. A., Peterson, M. S., Ay, F., Joyner, C. J., LE Roch, K. G., Fonseca, L. L., Voit, E. O., & MAHPIC CONSORTIUM (2018). Plasmodium knowlesi: a superb in vivo nonhuman primate model of antigenic variation in malaria. *Parasitology*, *145*(1), 85–100. https://doi.org/10.1017/S0031182017001135.
4. Azkur, A. K., Akdiş, M., Azkur, D., Sokołowska, M., van de Veen, W., Brüggen, M. C., O'Mahony, L., et al. (2020). Immune response to SARS-CoV-2 and mechanisms of immunopathological changes in COVID-19. *Allergy, 75*(7), 1564–1581. https://doi.org/10.1111/all.14364.
5. Bekker, L. G., Bicanic, T., Harrison, T. S., Jarvis, J. N., et al. (2012). Adjunctive interferon-γ immunotherapy for the treatment of HIV-associated cryptococcal meningitis: A randomized controlled trial. *AIDS, 26*(9), 1105–1113. https://doi.org/10.1097/QAD.0b013e3283536a93.
6. Bittaye, S. O., Jagne, A., Jaiteh, L., Nadjm, B., Amambua-Ngwa, A., Sesay, A. K., Singhateh, Y., et al. (2022). Clinical manifestations and outcomes of severe malaria in adult patients admitted to a tertiary hospital in the Gambia. *Malaria Journal, 21*, Article 94. https://doi.org/10.1186/s12936-022-04294-4.
7. Mohan, A., Sharma, S. K., & Bollineni, S. (2008). Acute lung injury and acute respiratory distress syndrome in malaria. *Journal of vector borne diseases*, *45*(3), 179–193. (accessed on 13 May 2025).
8. Chaparro, C. M., & Suchdev, P. S. (2019). Anemia epidemiology, pathophysiology, and etiology in low- and middle-income countries. *Annals of the New York Academy of Sciences, 1450*(1), 15–31. https://doi.org/10.1111/nyas.14092.
9. MacLean LM, Odiit M, Chisi JE, Kennedy PGE, Sternberg JM (2010) Focus–Specific Clinical Profiles in Human African Trypanosomiasis Caused by *Trypanosoma brucei rhodesiense*. PLoS Negl Trop Dis 4(12): e906. https://doi.org/10.1371/journal.pntd.0000906 (accessed on 13 May 2025).
10. Dean, A. S., Crump, L., Greter, H., Hattendorf, J., Schelling, E., & Zinsstag, J. (2012). Clinical manifestations of human brucellosis: a systematic review and meta-analysis. *PLoS neglected tropical diseases*, *6*(12), e1929. https://doi.org/10.1371/journal.pntd.0001929 (accessed on 13 May 2025).
11. Cruz, A. T., Wright, C. A., Anunobi, C. C., Boehme, C. C., Murray, C. J. L., et al. (2016). Evaluation of Xpert® MTB/RIF and Ustar easyNAT™ TB IAD for diagnosis of tuberculous lymphadenitis of children in Tanzania: A prospective descriptive study. https://core.ac.uk/download/46605185.pdf (accessed on 13 May 2025).

12. Farouk, S. N. (2018). A comprehensive mapping of malarial infections in children under 10 years in Kano Central Senatorial District, Kano State, northern Nigeria. https://core.ac.uk/download/478434171.pdf (accessed on 13 May 2025).
13. Faure, E. (2014). Malarial parthenogenesis: Beneficial and deleterious interactions between malaria and other human diseases. *Frontiers in Physiology, 5*, 441. https://doi.org/10.3389/fphys.2014.00441.
14. . Patil, A. P., Okiro, E. A., Gething, P. W., Guerra, C. A., Sharma, S. K., Snow, R. W., & Hay, S. I. (2009). Defining the relationship between Plasmodium falciparum parasite rate and clinical disease: statistical models for disease burden estimation. *Malaria journal, 8*, 186. https://doi.org/10.1186/1475-2875-8-186
15. Greischar, M. A., Reece, S. E., Savill, N. J., & Mideo, N. (2019). The challenge of quantifying synchrony in malaria *parasites. Trends in Parasitology, 35*(4), 341–355. https://doi.org/10.1016/j.pt.2019.03.002.
16. Guo, Y. R., Cao, Q. D., Hong, Z. S., Tan, Y. Y., Chen, S. D., Jin, H. J., Tan, K. S., et al. (2020). The origin, transmission and clinical therapies on coronavirus disease 2019 (COVID-19) outbreak–an update on the status. *Military Medical Research, 7*, Article 11. https://doi.org/10.1186/s40779-020-00240-0.
17. Hou, F., Li, Y., & Jin, H. (2024). Clinical manifestations and the prenatal diagnosis of trisomy 7 mosaicism: Two case reports. *World journal of clinical cases, 12*(8), 1544–1548. https://doi.org/10.12998/wjcc.v12.i8.1544(accessed on 13 May 2025).
18. Kelly-Hope, L. A., Blundell, H. J., Macfarlane, C. L., & Molyneux, D. (2018). Innovative surveillance strategies to support the elimination of filariasis in Africa. *Trends in Parasitology, 34*(8), 694–711. https://doi.org/10.1016/j.pt.2018.05.004.
19. Kessler, A., van Eijk, A. M., Jamir, L., Walton, C., Carlton, J. M., & Albert, S. (2018). Malaria in Meghalaya: A systematic literature review and analysis of data from the National Vector-Borne Disease Control Programme. *Malaria Journal, 17*, Article 411. https://doi.org/10.1186/s12936-018-2563-3.
20. Kinimi, E., Misinzo, G., & Bisimwa, P. B. N. (2018). Serological evidence of chikungunya and malaria co-infection among febrile patients seeking health care in Karagwe district, Tanzania. Tanzania Journal of Health Research Doi: http://dx.doi.org/10.4314/thrb.v20i4.1 Volume 20, Number 4, October 2018 (accessed on 13 May 2025).
21. Kruk, M. E., Gage, A., Arsenault, C., Jordan, K., Leslie, H. H., Roder-DeWan, S., Adeyi, O., et al. (2018). High-quality health systems in the Sustainable Development Goals era: Time for a revolution. *The Lancet Global Health, 6*(11), e1196–e1252. https://doi.org/10.1016/s2214-109x(18)30386-3.
22. Kumar, B. K. M., Mahto, S. K., Kumar, S., & Kumar, S. (2024). Evaluation of concurrent malaria and dengue co-infections among febrile patients visiting a tertiary care hospital: A cross-sectional observational study. https://core.ac.uk/download/643573667.pdf (accessed on 13 May 2025).
23. Laurens, M. B. (2019). RTS,S/AS01 vaccine (Mosquirix™): An overview. *Human Vaccines & Immunotherapeutics, 16*(3), 480–489. https://doi.org/10.1080/21645515.2019.1669415.
24. Makani, J., Matuja, W., Liyombo, E., Snow, R. W., Marsh, K., & Warrell, D. A. (2003). Admission diagnosis of cerebral malaria in adults in an endemic area of Tanzania: implications and

clinical description. *QJM : monthly journal of the Association of Physicians, 96*(5), 355–362. https://doi.org/10.1093/qjmed/hcg059 (accessed on 13 May 2025).

25. Makubi, A. N., Mugus, F., Magesa, P. M., Roberts, D., & Quaresh, A. (2012). Risk factors for anaemia among HIV infected children attending HIV care and treatment clinic at Muhimbili National Hospital in Dar es Salaam, Tanzania. *Tanzania journal of health research, 14*(1), 68–74. (accessed on 13 May 2025).
26. Naing, C., & Whittaker, M. (2018). Severe thrombocytopenia in patients with vivax malaria compared to *falciparum* malaria: A systematic review and meta-analysis. *Infectious Diseases of Poverty, 7*, Article 10. https://doi.org/10.1186/s40249-018-0392-9.
27. Patel, S. K., Rajora, N., Kumar, S., Sahu, A., Kochar, S. K., Krishna, C. M., & Srivastava, S. (2019). Rapid discrimination of malaria- and dengue-infected patients' sera using Raman spectroscopy. *Analytical Chemistry, 91*(11), 7054–7062. https://doi.org/10.1021/acs.analchem.8b05907.
28. Phyo, A. P., Dahal, P., Mayxay, M., & Ashley, E. A. (2022). Clinical impact of vivax malaria: A collection review. *PLOS Medicine, 19*(3), e1003890. https://doi.org/10.1371/journal.pmed.1003890.
29. Pierrotti, L. C., Levi, M. E., Di Santi, S. M., Segurado, A. A. C., & Petersen, E. (2018). Malaria disease recommendations for solid organ transplant recipients and donors. *Transplantation, 102*(S1), S16–S26. https://doi.org/10.1097/tp.0000000000002017.
30. Pool, L., Ruiz Del Portal Luyten, C., van der Pluijm, R. W., Soentjens, P., Hanscheid, T., Grobusch, M. P., & Visser, B. J. (2024). Dissemination and outcome reporting bias in clinical malaria intervention trials: a cross-sectional analysis. *Malaria journal, 23*(1), 293. https://doi.org/10.1186/s12936-024-05115-6(accessed on 13 May 2025).
31. Samrot, A. V., Sean, T. C., Bhavya, K. S., Sahithya, C. S., Chandrasekaran, S., Palanisamy, R., & Renitta, R. E., et al. (2021). Leptospiral infection, pathogenesis and its diagnosis—A review. *Pathogens, 10*(2), Article 145. https://doi.org/10.3390/pathogens10020145.
32. Sey, I. C. M., Ehimiyein, A. M., Bottomley, C., Riley, E. M., & Mooney, J. P. (2020). Does malaria cause diarrhea? A systematic review. *Frontiers in Medicine, 7*, Article 589379. https://doi.org/10.3389/fmed.2020.589379.
33. Siddig, E. E., Mohamed, N. S., & Ahmed, A. (2024). Severe coinfection of dengue and malaria: A case report. *Clinical Case Reports, 12*, Article e9079. https://doi.org/10.1002/ccr3.9079.
34. Ceusters, W., Smith, B. Malaria Diagnosis and the Plasmodium Life Cycle: the BFO Perspective. *Nat Prec* (2009). https://doi.org/10.1038/npre.2009.3960.1 (accessed on 13 May 2025).
35. Sultan, S., Altayar, O., Siddique, S. M., Davitkov, P., Feuerstein, J. D., Lim, J. K., Falck-Ytter, Y., et al. (2020). AGA Institute rapid review of the gastrointestinal and liver manifestations of COVID-19, meta-analysis of international data, and recommendations for the consultative management of patients with COVID-19. *Gastroenterology, 159*(1), 320–334.e27. https://doi.org/10.1053/j.gastro.2020.05.001.
36. Colebunders, R., Tshomba, A., Van Kerkhove, M. D., Bausch, D. G., Campbell, P., Libande, M., Pirard, P., Tshioko, F., Mardel, S., Mulangu, S., Sleurs, H., Rollin, P. E., Muyembe-Tamfum, J. J., Jeffs, B., Borchert, M., & International Scientific and Technical Committee "DRC Watsa/Durba 1999 Marburg Outbreak Investigation Group" (2007). Marburg hemorrhagic fever

in Durba and Watsa, Democratic Republic of the Congo: clinical documentation, features of illness, and treatment. *The Journal of infectious diseases, 196 Suppl 2*, S148–S153. https://doi.org/10.1086/520543(accessed on 13 May 2025).

37. Tufan, A., Avanoğlu Güler, A., & Matucci-Cerinic, M. (2020). COVID-19, immune system response, hyperinflammation and repurposing antirheumatic drugs. *Turkish Journal of Medical Sciences, 50*(SI-1), 620–632. https://doi.org/10.3906/sag-2004-168.

38. Vos, T., Allen, C. A., Arora, M., Barber, R. M., Bhutta, Z. A., Brown, A., Carter, A., et al. (2016). Global, regional, and national incidence, prevalence, and years lived with disability for 310 diseases and injuries, 1990–2015: A systematic analysis for the Global Burden of Disease Study 2015. *The Lancet, 388*(10053), 1545–1602. https://doi.org/10.1016/s0140-6736(16)31678-6.

39. World Health Organization. (2020). Clinical management of severe acute respiratory infection (SARI) when COVID-19 disease is suspected: interim guidance, 13 March 2020. World Health Organization. https://iris.who.int/handle/10665/331446. License: CC BY-NC-SA 3.0 IGOWyss, K. (2020). *Malaria in Travelers and Migrants: Disease Severity and Long-Term Effects* [Doctoral dissertation, University of Basel]. https://core.ac.uk/download/334508187.pdf (accessed on 13 May 2025).

40. Žitnik, M., Agrawal, M., & Leskovec, J. (2018). Modelling polypharmacy side effects with graph convolutional networks. *Bioinformatics, 34*(13), i457–i466. https://doi.org/10.1093/bioinformatics/bty294.

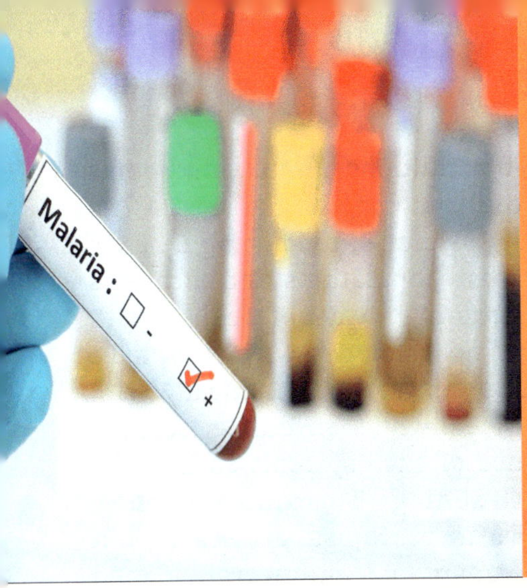

Chapter 6

DIAGNOSIS OF MALARIA

Contents

Introduction

Malaria is still one of the deadliest infectious diseases out there, largely because Plasmodium parasites invade RBCs. People living in poorer regions have more significant barriers, including making an early and correct diagnosis. Being properly diagnosed isn't just crucial to treating an individual—it also plays a significant part in lessening the degree to which the disease is spread. Outdated diagnostics, like reliance on blood smear microscopy (something generally considered the gold standard up to now), are equally the issue: observers simply will see things differently and it can take a long time. All of this leads to new, more dependable methods of diagnosing malaria, something that works even in busy or poorly equipped healthcare settings (Rajaraman et al., 2019). If we consider the grand picture, diagnostics forms a big de-al when controlling infections such as malaria. Even though in general terms we have seen mortality rates decrease for the majority of health emergencies, the population living with chronic and debilitating diseases is still increasing. Malaria, for instance, not only causes acute illness but can also precipitate complications that lead to long-term conditions. Population booms and aging populations just add more layers of complexity on top of diagnosing said diseases. The majority of the time, the inclusion of the latest diagnostic technology is crucial to keeping up with these ever-changing threats and lending proper care across different populations and locations (Vos et al., 2017). The recent years have pushed technology towards new ways of dealing with malaria detection. Take the example of deep learning—convolutional neural networks (CNNs) have started making waves by identifying infected red blood cells (RBCs) entirely automatically with the uniformity and precision that surpasses traditional methods. Meanwhile, ensemble learning models help minimize overfitting and enhance the overall resilience of such systems so that the diagnosis is more trustworthy even with varied data from real-world settings. This kind of strategy not only supports clinical decision-making, especially where expert microscopists are scarce, but also is a step toward diagnostic technologies that are faster, more adaptable, and overall, a good supplement to conventional methods. Further, by and large, this collaboration of computational techniques and medical wisdom is a game-changer in our ongoing fight against malaria (Rajaraman et al., 2019) (Figure 6.1).

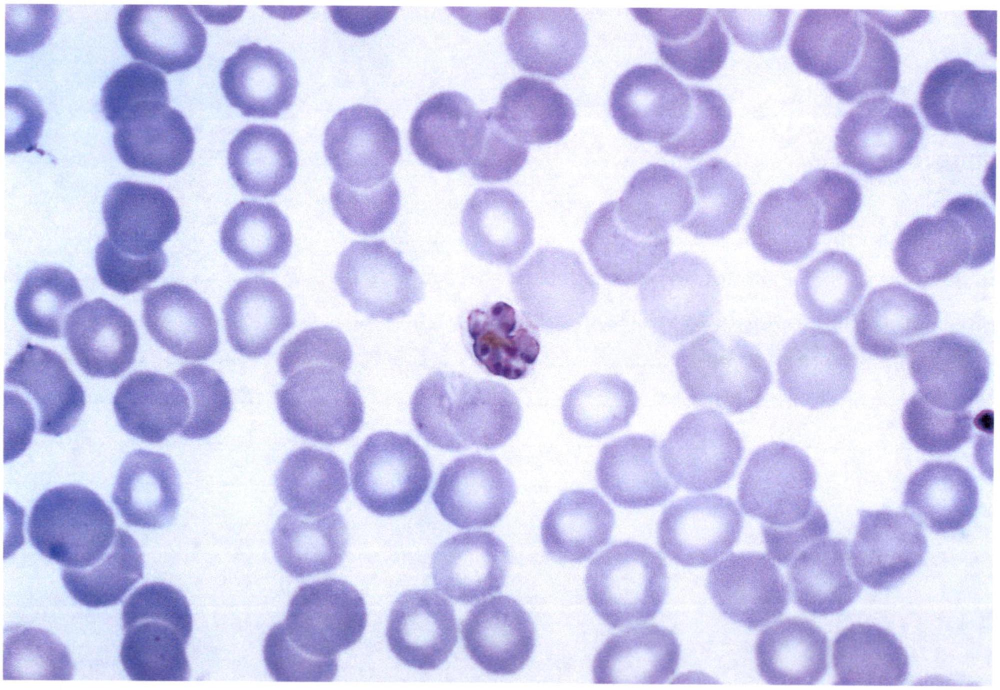

Figure 6.1. Malaria diagnosis.

Source: By Photo Credit:Content Providers: CDC/Dr. Mae Melvin - This media comes from the Centers for Disease Control and Prevention's Public Health Image Library (PHIL), with identification number #2715.Note: Not all PHIL images are public domain; be sure to check copyright status and credit authors and content providers. | Deutsch | English | македонски | slovenščina | +/−, Public Domain, https://commons.wikimedia.org/w/index.php?curid=745649

Malaria is still an enormous global issue—a complex mix of the Plasmodium parasite, mosquito vectors, and human hosts. , when these microscopic protozoans infect your bloodstream, you can get anything ranging from a mild, pesky fever to something life-threateningly severe. It all starts when the parasite first infects the liver before moving on to the RBCs, which partly explains those sudden fever spikes we see. Getting this picture right is basic because it lays the groundwork for how we differentiate malaria from other fevers. Diagnosing malaria, as opposed to simply checking off some symptoms, means detecting the parasite itself or its genetic signature, which highlights how essentially challenging it is. Treatments and public health measures hinge on this basic knowledge (Melamed et al., 2021). At the same time, the medical diagnosis of malaria ties its infectious etiology to how it presents itself in human beings, making the whole diagnostic process far from straightforward. Malaria, for the most part, is due to five different Plasmodium species—each with its own peculiarities depending on location, severity, and so on. Patients usually come in with complaints of intermittent fevers, chills, headaches, and a general feeling of malaise, which can look like many other things. Proceeding on these symptoms alone may lead to missing the mark—or worse, misdiagnosing the disease. That's why doctors rely on laboratory diagnostics (think microscopy, rapid diagnostic tests (RDTs), or even molecular assays) to make the infection official. This extra step is crucial, given the fact that complications, like brain involvement or hemolytic anemia—mean that the determination of the right treatment depends on getting the diagnosis precisely right. Therefore, the process depends on matching obvious symptoms with laboratory evidence, defining malaria both as a clinical syndrome and as a specific parasitic infection (Melamed et al., 2021). Further, how malaria presents itself varies by geography, affecting everything from the number of individuals infected to how doctors manage testing and treatment. In regions where the disease is endemic, repeated exposure might even lead to cases of individuals harboring the parasite without visible symptoms—a fact that obscures how cases are counted. This incomplete picture demands tests that are sensitive enough to pick up even a minute quantity of the parasite, but also to differentiate between an active infection and inert vestiges that do not in themselves portend danger. Global health commentators have observed that mortality reductions are not necessarily paralleled by corresponding reductions either in overall disease prevalence or in long-term disability. With residual non-fatal issues and patchy case distribution, it is clear that our approach to malaria diagnosis must be flexible. It ultimately requires many field-level epidemiological acumen and diagnostic techniques adapted to locally available resources, which reminds us that the definition of malaria itself evolves continuously with its public health and clinical issues.

Importance of Accurate Diagnosis

Healthcare genuinely relies on having tests correct – when diagnostics identify what ails quickly and accurately, treatment truly functions. Without clean, specific tests, treatments can fall short, sometimes making things worse and even giving diseases such as malaria free rein to spread even more. In much of the low- and middle-income world, there is limited access to reliable diagnostic tests, and it is evident there. If malaria is not accurately diagnosed, treatment may be either too insufficient or indiscriminate, which can reactivate drug resistance and harm public health campaigns globally. Recent global health statistics even point out that fully nearly half of the entire world population does not have reliable access to quality diagnostics – a fundamental gap that is generally associated with higher premature mortality levels and higher disability-adjusted life years lost (Fleming et al., 2021). In the instance of malaria itself, an error in diagnosis not only delays the emergency care that must be given; it also blurs our true understanding of how the disease is spread. Since malaria tends to resemble other febrile diseases, relying too heavily on clinical judgment without direct testing can lead to mistakes , the same error repeatedly. It's not only about treating the patient as a patient; misdiagnosis brings in costly unnecessary expense and wastes valuable resources, threatening the entire healthcare system. Ensuring that the diagnosis is accurate – from the first screening stage all the way through treatment and long-term care – becomes that critical juncture where therapy will work and complications or even death become non-issues. Especially in those areas where malaria is common, tried-and-tested methods like standard microscopy and RDTs are needed to clearly differentiate malaria from other illnesses. Improving these methods is essential, particularly for far-flung or disadvantaged communities that often lose access to even the most basic tests (Fleming et al., 2021). Not only are patients harmed by faulty diagnoses; their effects spread to reach health policy, even driving antimicrobial resistance (AMR). Faulty diagnosis of malaria will lead to the misuse of antimalarial drugs , and it is partly responsible for accelerating drug resistance that puts treatments at risk. With more accurate diagnostic practice, it is possible for public health officials to have better surveillance data, information that is priceless in making targeted interventions and wisely directing scarce resources. On top of this, newer technologies like point-of-care testing enable healthcare providers to respond immediately in resource-poor facilities, to fill some of those glaring gaps in care. Withholding tests from being safe and reliable is at the core of public trust in the health system. In some sense, fixing diagnostic problems in disease like malaria points to broader issues: issues that call for smart investment, increased training among medical personnel, and improved healthcare infrastructure overall (Fleming et al., 2021).

6.1. Overview of Malaria

Malaria is a complex illness with a great deal of variables in play—its symptoms have numerous different forms and social and environmental factors come along and add to the mix even more. It occurs in the tropics and subtropics, and at times the populations already devastated by war or displacement take the biggest blow. In places like Mozambique's Sofala and Cabo Delgado provinces, cyclone-induced displacement heightens overcrowding and poverty, and overall, malaria risk is still present despite the outbreak of COVID-19 and other health issues. Overlapping of symptoms with other infections is part of the mystery, making it hard to diagnose without a synchronized screening plan. Rapid diagnostic tests (RDTs), used to screen for these diseases among displaced persons, show that the war against malaria is very far from over and are an indication of a clear need for diagnostic standards that do not only battle malaria but also other co-occurring health conditions (Gennaro et al., 2022). Moving closer towards grasping how malaria works can bring us closer to better diagnosis. The disease is induced by Plasmodium parasites—mainly spread through Anopheles mosquitoes, and usually manifests itself as cycles of chills, fever, and anemia. These are, however, very nonspecific and can be incredibly indistinguishable from symptoms of other fever-causing diseases, and this results in many cases to the vulnerability to misdiagnosis or procrastination in treatment that worsens the issue. Primarily, adding RDTs to microscopy increases detection, but glitches persist, including false negatives among asymptomatic carriers or those with low parasite loads. In most settings, especially where other diseases or malnutrition are also an issue, paired diagnosis coupled with integrated health interventions becomes crucial. For instance, malnourished children, being at greater risk naturally, tend to present with respiratory symptoms which can derange a clean diagnosis, stressing how critical a proper patient check-up is (Gennaro et al., 2022). Making successful diagnostic approaches is about accepting malaria never works by itself. Healthcare systems tend to break down in emergencies, and these breakdowns tend to result in testing and treatment delays, which tend to worsen outcomes. Diagnostic practice must also deal with more than malaria in isolation—additive problems of co-existing disease such as HIV and other respiratory infections modify the immune response and complicate the clinical presentation. A multidisciplinary approach involving regular screening for several risk factors and symptom combinations is capable of detecting the disease at an earlier stage. At yet other times, as with overlapping syndromes like dementia and delirium in other areas of health care, tailoring the diagnosis process to the needs of particular patient groups becomes a necessity. In most situations, this type of combined and flexible approach is central to scaling up malaria diagnosis and control throughout the world (Figure 6.2).

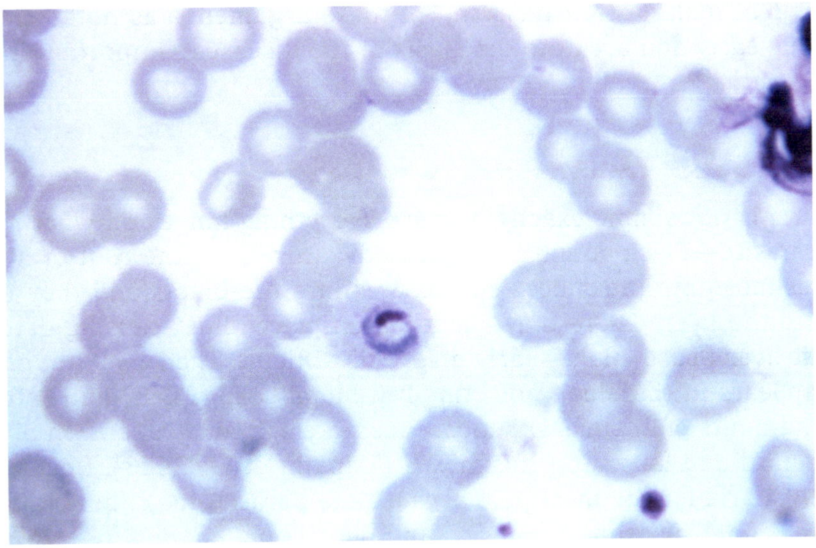

Figure 6.2. Overview of malaria.

Source: Public Domain, https://commons.wikimedia.org/w/index.php?curid=2740654

6.1.1. History and Epidemiology

Malaria has been around and discussed for hundreds of years, although it was only documented in the form of notes in ancient works. It wasn't until the late 1800s that it was discovered by anyone that the disease had any connection with bites from mosquitoes, a paradigm shift in the way that humans responded to it. There were early suggestions that suggested, in a fairly straightforward way, how climate and geography seem to affect the transmission of malaria, especially in hot, tropical, and subtropical settings. All that was ever this antiquated information, quite piecemeal over the years, now feeds into modern strategies where the precise diagnosis of the disease is critical, particularly in high-transmission environments. The road from rough bedside observations to a careful look at how the parasite lives and thrives reminds us that history continues at the heart of our modern-day diagnostic activity. Think about world trends and you'll see malaria's impact is not uniformly distributed—sub-Saharan Africa, parts of Asia, and Latin America bear the brunt, as a general rule. Often, this disproportionate burden leads back to socioeconomic inequalities and limited health facilities, where preventive treatment and proper diagnosis simply aren't available. Health infrastructures have improved, and so have surveillance systems and international efforts, but malaria remains a tenacious issue, not least because drug resistance continues to emerge (Murray et al., 2022). These factors combine in permutations that make disease control difficult even if newer technology is used. If you step back and consider the bigger picture of infectious diseases, malaria is alongside many other issues in a constantly changing global health landscape. Global research, in most cases, suggests that our growing old populations and changing disease patterns mean the problems are not black and white. Even though discussions about AMR are mostly about bacteria, the same issues apply to parasitic diseases like malaria, whose treatment slowly decreases over time. The incorporation of intelligent surveillance along with the recently invented diagnostic tools becomes crucial for disease detection and prevention early on. Apart from that, the integration of socioeconomic factors and population mobility provides an additional complexity in terms of malaria transmission. All these arguments, as noted (James et al., 2018), are the reasons why early and accurate diagnosis of the disease is important in reducing its total impact on global health.

6.1.2. Life Cycle of the Malaria Parasite

Diagnosis of malaria is not simple exactly because everything hinges on what happens within the life cycle of the parasite—Plasmodium's complex adventure is at the root of it all. The bite of an infected Anopheles mosquito introduces sporozoites into the blood, and they immediately travel in a straight line to the liver, where they silently multiply without causing detectable symptoms. This asymptomatic liver phase makes early diagnosis difficult. Then, as if out of nowhere, a brood of merozoites reappears in the blood, infecting red blood cells (RBCs) and setting up the typical cycles of fevers and bouts of anemia. For most cases, a clear comprehension of these steps is key to sealing both clinical and laboratory diagnoses (Tripathi et al., 2023). Doctors target the blood stage to diagnose malaria for the most part because the parasite looks quite differently at various stages. The conventional method, blood smear microscopy, enables one to see those various forms—rings, trophozoites, and schizonts—inside RBCs.

This method, though, has features of its own; it is time-consuming and requires extensive expertise, and its reliability is parasite density- and microscopist experience-dependent. There has been a recent acceleration, though, through the automated examination of images using machine learning algorithms that can identify and categorize infected cells based on their developmental stages. These advances, by isolating out developmental stages, hold out the prospect of faster, more standardized diagnoses with less human error, all of which is welcome news for malaria control programs (Davidson et al., 2021). Taking it a step further, labs have embraced techniques like PCR to identify Plasmodium even before symptoms rear their ugly head. For the most part, these molecular methods are especially useful when parasite levels are so low during that almost hidden liver stage that traditional methods might miss them, and they're pretty handy for detecting mixed infections too. That is, information on the parasite's various stages not only dictates particular treatment and therapy follow-up adjustments but also takes on more significance with the ongoing increase in antimalarial resistance. In all, keeping abreast with research on this hidden cycle and updating diagnostic techniques remains paramount to our fight against malaria (Tripathi et al., 2023) (Figure 6.3).

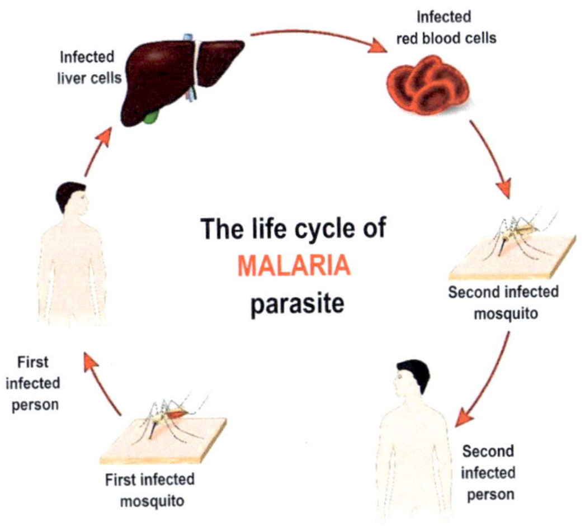

Figure 6.3. The life cycle of the malaria parasite.

Source: HORIBA Medical. (n.d.). The Life Cycle of the Malaria Parasite. https://static.horiba.com/fileadmin/Horiba/_processed_/f/7/csm_The_life_cycle_of_malaria_parasite_1958c5f721.jpg.

6.1.3. Symptoms and Clinical Presentation

Malaria does not always come in neat, orderly form – its symptoms can be everywhere and at any time, and that is the reason it is so difficult to recognize early. It comes with such vague symptoms as fever, shivering, and perspiration – genuine common symptoms that you would experience in several other diseases. For the most part, these are nonspecific symptoms that enter into the picture because the parasite lives for a while within RBCs; while doing its thing, those cells necessarily burst and spill out pyrogens that initiate a fever. You can also get headaches, a chronic sense of malaise, and muscle aches persisting between those periods of fever. When the cause is Plasmodium falciparum infection, soon the case can slip out of control and risk factors like cerebral malaria, lethal anemia, or total organ failure may occur. Surprisingly, when someone is battling malaria with another illness, conditions like vomiting and confusion more often occur (Achan et al., 2021). Generally speaking, this kind of variation emphasizes why careful, sometimes further, clinical screening is required in order to separate malaria from other diseases in areas where it tends to strike with regularity. Malaria can also happen very differently based on the age of a patient and whether or not they have had contact with the parasite before. They or people who have had little exposure in the past tend to acquire more widespread symptoms – altogether, in fact, because their bodies have not had time to acquire a protective shield. In malaria-endemic areas, people gradually build some immunity, and that can keep the fever cycles (those repeat surges as the parasite multiplies) from being as bad or even as frequent, and that complicates diagnosis. Sometimes, unusual symptoms also surface – like gastrointestinal discomfort (think vomiting or diarrhea) , particularly in individuals with multiple infections. Confusion, which might indicate that the brain is now affected, also seems to happen more when other infections are happening (Achan et al., 2021). All these facts mean that clinicians have to be extra careful to observe the manifest and the latent symptoms and use diagnostic tests along with their observation to identify the right diagnosis. At times, the combination of symptoms of malaria turns out to be so similar to other diseases prevalent in the very same parts of the world – COVID-19 being an example. Both illnesses can manifest with the same initial symptoms: a fever, a general condition of lethargy, and even some belly ache. Such similarity, especially where the full arsenal of diagnostic tests is not available, causes delayed starts to the proper treatment. Older adults or those with underlying medical conditions can present symptoms in different or even more severe ways upon being hit by multiple infections at once (Achan et al., 2021). By observing all the varieties of symptoms instead of relying on only one or two, doctors can reduce the chances of mistaking one disease for another. In the end, identifying malaria from the array of symptoms remains a vital role for determining that patients are treated in a timely and proper manner in communities where infectious disease is widespread (Figure 6.4).

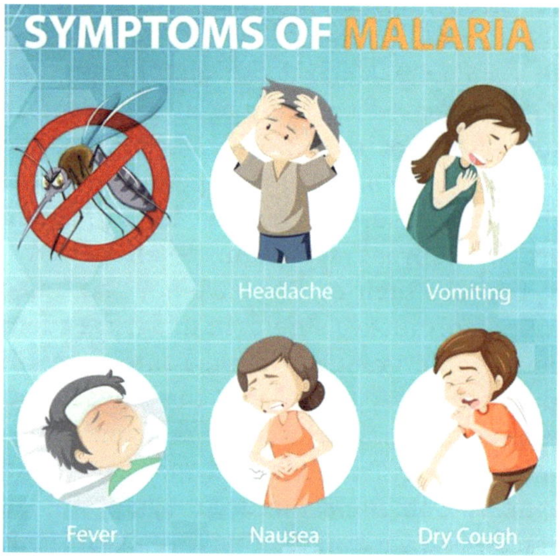

Figure 6.4. Symptoms and clinical presentation of the malaria parasite.

Source: International Marine Contractors Association. (2021). Symptoms and Clinical Presentation of the Malaria P. https://www.imca-int.com/media/clwfwphg/screenshot-2021-04-27-113816.jpg?width=1200&quality=90&v=1daf218e1e77430.

6.2. Diagnostic Methods

Diagnosis of malaria was not as advanced as it is today—when individuals largely relied on symptom identification, there was simply too great a chance of error, usually challenging efforts to eliminate the disease. Most often, that symptom-identification approach culminated in treatments that were not quite on the mark, rendering eradication programs more difficult. Nowadays, the majority of regions are still dependent on blood smear microscopy because it enables experienced technicians to observe and enumerate those bad Plasmodium parasites for themselves; it has been heralded as the gold standard but it involves a lot of expertise as well as an adequately equipped laboratory. To evade such constraints in settings where resources are scarce, RDTs have gained traction since they yield faster results without the need for sophisticated equipment so that treatment can be commenced earlier. However, with these technologies in place, microscopy and RDTs do not detect extremely low parasite densities, and thus experts have turned to molecular techniques in order to raise accuracy (Oyegoke et al., 2022). Subsequently, of course, there's the advent of the molecular methods, approaches like polymerase chain reaction (PCR) and loop-mediated isothermal amplification (LAMP) brought the game up to a whole new level for malaria diagnostics. These methods, targeting parasite DNA, most commonly, are especially useful for those "pre-elimination" or even outright elimination phases where a low-density infection could be an important missed detail. PCR is very sensitive but brings with it its own set of baggage in the form of complex protocols and reliance on high-throughput laboratory facilities; these have a tendency to persist in field conditions. LAMP, meanwhile, possesses a more down-to-earth advantage with its rapid turnaround and lower equipment needs—optimal for decentralized testing in endemic hotspots. Collectively, by merging these molecular tools with traditional methods, surveillance and control programs are made more precise, a critical step on the journey to malaria eradication (Oyegoke et al., 2022). As well as simply treating disease cases, robust diagnostic protocols play key roles in other public health challenges, like the control of AMR. Most commonly, effective and timely diagnosis of malaria entails minimizing the overuse of antimalarial drugs, which can slow down the emergence of drug resistance, which is a growing problem worldwide. Expanding diagnostic capacity, with consideration for adding molecular techniques, is especially needed where low-resource countries have the highest burden of AMR. This synergy of rapid diagnostic testing, microscopy, and molecular diagnosis creates the platform for focused interventions that not only improve stewardship of antimalarial drugs but also inform policy decisions that decrease the disease burden as well as the risk of resistance.

6.2.1. Microscopic Examination of Blood Smears

Malaria is a chronic foe, especially in low-resource environments, and identifying what parasite is causing the infection is a significant problem. Clinicians have long depended upon blood smear microscopy—it is an approach that enables you to visually observe the parasite in RBCs, which is important for you to recognize exactly which Plasmodium species is present and how many parasites there are. Thin smears are usually made in most instances so that experts can closely study parasite forms, but success also depends heavily on the trained, observant eyes of the microscopist, as differences in form could easily be missed. Even though this technique is widely used, it is very time-consuming and the result may vary greatly depending on whomever is using it, which is why there has been growing pressure for better diagnostic support tools (Tan & Liang, 2023). Not so long ago, artificial intelligence came along and stirred things up rather dramatically in diagnosing malaria.

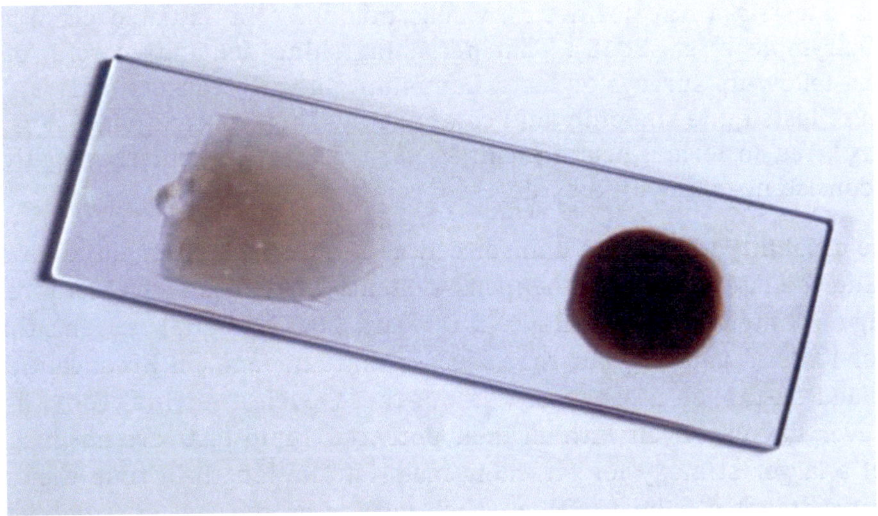

Figure 6.5. Microscopic examination of blood smears.

Source: By CDC/ Steven Glenn, Laboratory & Consultation Division - CDC - Public Health Image Library (PHIL), #5901, Public Domain, https://commons.wikimedia.org/w/index.php?curid=4878350

AI algorithms that use transformer architecture, in particular, now support professionals by delving deep into the details of blood smear images. Such systems that use fine feature extraction and attention mechanisms are relatively excellent at detecting infected cells even when they appear sparse. It is surprising that certain systems utilize generative adversarial networks to boost the amount of available training data, making the whole system more robust. For example, like the Swin Transformer, it is reported to achieve detection rates of nearly 99.8% — while others, including MobileViT, can make it slim enough to deploy on low-resource small devices (Tan & Liang, 2023).

In spite of all these hi-tech advances, the humble old practice of examining blood smears under a microscope still holds its own, especially when combined with others. Generally speaking, microscopy sometimes fails, especially where parasites are simply in low numbers—the use of techniques such as multiplex digital PCR can identify malaria DNA with astonishing precision. This pairing of visual examination and molecular detection not only makes disease diagnosis more precise (even for latent co-infections) but also helps track how treatments are going by quantifying parasite load. In practice, regardless of the injection of momentum provided by digital PCR, starting with that microscopic inspection is still an unavoidable step towards making clinical choices according to concrete parasitological realities (Liu et al., 2022) (Figure 6.5).

6.2.2. Rapid Diagnostic Tests (RDTs)

RDTs transformed malaria diagnosis. Today, they enable health workers to screen for malaria at a glance even in less-equipped environments. Before, people had to rely on microscopy, a process that not only takes an enormous amount of equipment but special expertise as well. RDTs, on the other hand, target particular malaria proteins like histidine-rich protein II (HRP2) and Plasmodium lactate dehydrogenase (pLDH) directly from a blood drop. The simplicity of this method means that tests can be used a long way beyond the limits of traditional clinics, in remote or poor areas. One thing to keep in mind, though, is that these antigens do persist after treatment; in broad terms, HRP2-based tests can stay positive for weeks, muddling the actual levels of parasites among communities (Dalrymple et al., 2018). That persisting shine demands careful usage, especially when performing follow-up surveys or tests. Community health workers (CHWs), if well trained, operate with these tests quite smoothly and competently. Their on field efficacy is a win in terms of malaria control. Yet, in formal health facilities, test results, particularly negative ones, do not always get the consistent follow-up they deserve.

This has the capability to result in a misdirection of the diagnosis or unintentional treatment. In drug shops and the like, there even happens evidence of reduced specificity resulting in false positives causing unwanted treatment (Boyce & O'Meara, 2017). Overall, it seems that the technical sophistication of RDTs is amazing but that success must depend on practicalities like training, quality control, and on-the-job assistance. Without these, even a terrific tool will stumble under the stresses of everyday use. Even with all their potential, rapid tests are not magic bullets; they are only part of a larger strategy for attacking malaria. The length of time they are positive on follow-up after treatment can be variable—such factors as the age of a patient, the mode of treatment (with artemisinin combination therapy typically giving longer detection), and antigen targeted being involved—so that children and certain regimens can be positive for longer than expected (Dalrymple et al., 2018).

This time-space confusion yields results in clinics and big-picture studies need further interpretation, at times backed by techniques like microscopy or even molecular testing, where possible. For all but a few situations, making RDTs function is more about the test itself—it also takes ongoing study of behavioral, logistical, and systemic drivers. Multidisciplinary discussions, regular review, and some personalized trial and error can all contribute towards refining the general fight against malaria, guaranteeing tests are used appropriately. Antimalarial medications aren't given when they won't be required (Boyce & O'Meara 2017) (Figure 6.6).

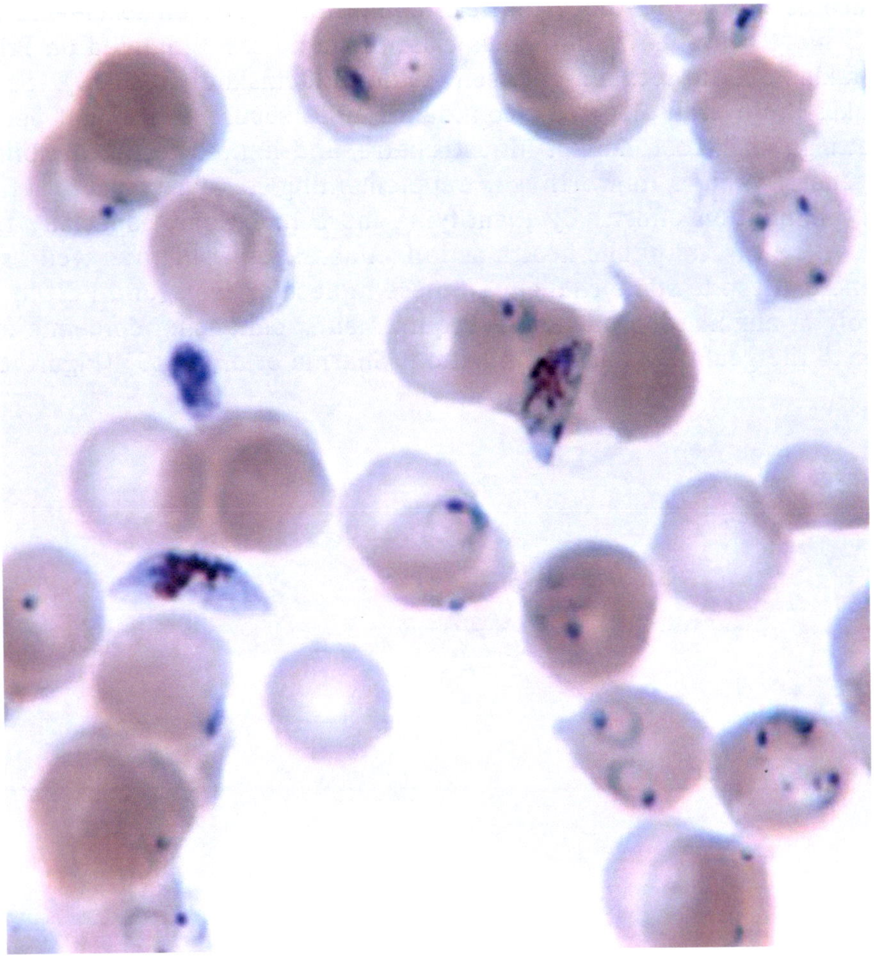

Figure 6.6. Rapid diagnostic tests (RDTs).

Source: By The original uploader was TimVickers at English Wikipedia. - Transferred from en.wikipedia to Commons., Public Domain, https://commons.wikimedia.org/w/index.php?curid=2932677

6.2.3. Molecular Techniques (PCR)

Progress in molecular detection is revolutionizing how we identify malaria. Conventional techniques like microscopy and RDTs sometimes miss small or mixed infections that can badly inhibit efforts to conquer the disease. PCR, or PCR, identifies even trace levels of parasite DNA by essentially reproducing sections of the Plasmodium's gene map. This process enables us to identify the precise species persisting in a sample, , even when standard tests are inadequate. In low-transmission settings of malaria, even those barely detectable infections can continue to harbor the parasite in the long run, ultimately undermining control and elimination strategies (Pluciński et al., 2019). PCR is detection beyond detection as it distinguishes among different Plasmodium species. In much of the region where Plasmodium falciparum is the primary perp, every now and again a non-falciparum species will also wreak havoc. For example, research in Mozambique has illustrated that these molecular techniques can identify antigen profile differences, which establishes that absent genes such as Pfhrp2/3—those that can compromise antigen tests—are not necessarily the culprits. This more acute view still makes classical rapid tests founded on PfHRP2 detection valid, with PCR taking over to settle in-between results (Pluciński et al., 2019). It's a double-check of sorts that makes the overall diagnostic confidence more secure. PCR is not perfect, though. In low-resource settings, high cost, lack of infrastructure, and limited technical ability often act as an obstacle. In general, though, its worth is in supplementing standard tests to refine surveillance and direct local elimination efforts. By identifying more infections, especially those low-level, near-latent ones—PCR directs public health action, enabling treatment as well as vector control measures. In general, despite some challenges, these molecular tools, and PCR in particular, play an imperative role in augmenting diagnostic requirements, enhancing epidemic monitoring, and taking us nearer to the goal of malaria elimination (Sharma et al., 2019) (Figure 6.7).

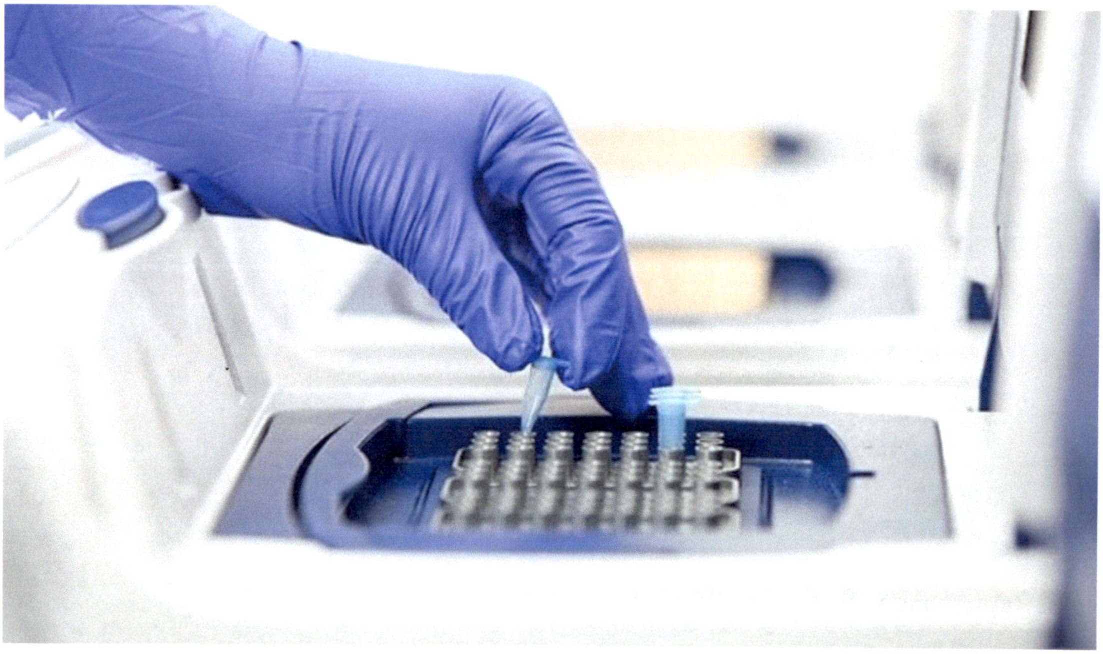

Figure 6.7. Molecular techniques (PCR) of malaria.

Source: Science of Healthy. (2019). Polymerase Chain Reaction (PCR). https://external-content.duckduckgo.com/iu/?u=https%3A%2F%2Fscienceofhealthy.com%2Fwp-content%2Fuploads%2F2019%2F03%2FPolymerase-chain-reaction-PCR.jpg&f=1&nofb=1&ipt=c70026462a6ab8e0fa7cca416273f4b92fc25b111e20f397cdc83ea4b5d5f17d.

6.3. Microscopic Examination

Microscopy is the traditional pillar of malaria diagnosis - individuals have used looking at blood smears because you can view the parasites. It has been pronounced the best practice, but in practice, it needs skilled hands and hours and hours of time, especially where resources are limited. Experts are needed to make the distinction between species and life stages, which helps enormously in deciding the right treatment. But the job takes too much time and is prone to mistakes, particularly when there are few parasites or the sample is not good. These issues are most likely to cause delay or even misdiagnosis, and because of that, there is an increasing need for technology support that can keep accuracy at high levels while minimizing the workload (Shewajo et al., 2023). The idea is to minimize the workload on malaria-endemic health workers. Computer-based methods have come to complement traditional microscopy in recent times. Deep learning, specifically convolution-based ones, has proved to have some real promise by coming close to the expert's vision when it comes to processing digital images of blood films. But catching those small malaria parasites is not always easy , they are microscopic and easy to lose if the image gets too reduced in size, being nightmarish to work on for automated systems. One useful hack has been to cut up high-res images into smaller, more manageable tiles, which is used to preserve parasite detail. If this technique is then coupled with newer object detectors like YOLOv4, sensitivity and accuracy get a most welcome boost, even facilitating real-time detection of Plasmodium falciparum in thick smear images (Shewajo et al., 2023). This sort of upgrade can help drive down diagnosis and make up for the shortage of skilled microscopists. In a separate vein, digital microscopy integrated with mobile technology is laying open a viable avenue for malaria diagnosis in low-resource, often distant locations. Cell phones, now equipped with high-resolution cameras and decent processing power, are being made into transportable microscopes where standard laboratories simply are not available. Automatic image capture and analysis software can quickly detect parasites, or utilize less trained personnel, or simply diagnose quicker overall. The software can even account for slide motion and autofocus adjustment, minimizing the chance of human error. This not only makes costs lower but more consistent results are also obtained, which is fairly critical when needing to treat as quickly as possible. Of course, field implementation of such technology has its disadvantages – hardware and software robustness problems, as well as field usability, are yet to be overcome (Maturana et al., 2022). Overall, though, digitized microscopy is ready to bridge the gap between high-technology development and medicine, potentially revolutionizing malaria diagnosis worldwide.

6.3.1. Types of Blood Smears (Thick and Thin)

Malaria diagnosis is started by looking at the blood smears microscopically, and essentially, there are only two that you usually have to work with—thick and thin. You just place a few drops of patient blood onto a slide, subsequently, with a thick smear, you spread lots of volume over a tiny area. This little trick concentrates the parasites, and this is handy when they are scarce. In all but exceptional cases, this means that the cells are packed together, making it more likely to see even a few malaria parasites. However there is also a disadvantage that seems: because the RBCs lose their delicate shape, it becomes harder to be able to tell between the specific Plasmodium species. Careful preparation and staining – typically Giemsa stain – is still necessary to keeping these slides clear and reliable (Nema et al., 2023). Turn to the thin smear, and now things are a little bit different. There, you put less blood but more area, so you have a good, almost single layer of cells. That way, the cell shapes and sizes are preserved, and you can see everything about both the RBCs and the parasites. It sounds redundant, I know, but this method comes in handy when you have to figure out exactly which species is present or ascertain the lifecycle stages of the parasite. I mean, whether or not it's Plasmodium falciparum, P. vivax, or other can influence treatment and public health decisions. Even though thin smears are less efficient in detecting very low levels of parasites compared to thick ones, they are more efficient in showing the structure of the parasite, which is significant for establishing a diagnosis (Nema et al., 2023). Using both thick and thin smears in most health facilities gives a better overall picture. Thick smears are a sensitive screening tool, especially in malaria-endemic regions, while thin smokes yield the subtle, species-based information needed for treatment and even tracking resistance patterns. Microscopic refinement, along with greater quality control in slide preparation and staining, has improved results for national malaria programs. Also, having slide banks of well-prepared thick and thin smears helps train microscopists (yes, some errors creep in here and there) and test them in the long term. Where these methods come together with RDTs, they create a pretty robust strategy to combat malaria's subtle challenges, leading to better patient care and more effective disease control measures (Nema et al., 2023) (Figure 6.8).

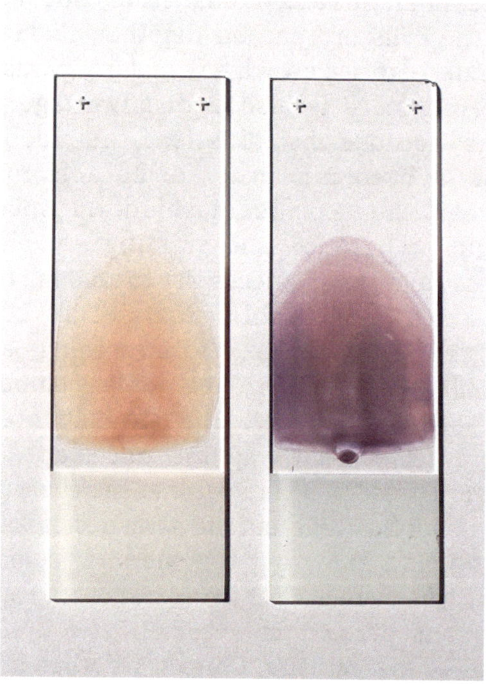

Figure 6.8. Types of blood smears (thick and thin).

Source: By Coinmac - Own work, CC BY-SA 3.0, https://commons.wikimedia.org/w/index.php?curid=20155466

6.3.2. Staining Techniques Used

Diagnosis of malaria quite much depends on only one major skill , observing the parasite in blood samples from infected individuals. Laboratories would generally rely on staining methods to differentiate from the host cell background, and by and large, Giemsa stain has been the default pick. It is more of an art rather than technical magic, but rather a technique for staining the parasites inside the cells so that microscopists can choose out the different stages of Plasmodium from RBCs. The technique is quite straightforward: you first make a fixed blood smear subsequently submerge it in diluted Giemsa solution. That leaves an apparent blue or purple color on the parasite's cytoplasm and nuclei – a characteristic useful in microscope observation. Naturally, despite its widespread use, the process still depends upon a trained technician for proper interpretation, and that has pushed research toward automated systems that can analyze the stained images for faster diagnosis (Kudisthalert et al., 2020). Other than just depending on Giemsa, others have turned to Wright-Giemsa staining, especially for thinner smears of blood where transparency and time are most crucial. This method somehow combines the strengths of Wright and Giemsa stains to increase the sensitivity in detecting forms of parasites without sacrificing the appearance and texture of RBCs. The recent technological developments in image processing and machine learning have been applied to these stained slides , and most interestingly, these computer algorithms can segment and classify infected RBCs by identifying differences in color contrast and texture. In the majority of scenarios, what that means is the automated methods are very precise with few error rates in infected cell counts, perhaps assisting in bridging the gap between time-consuming manual microscopy and substantially quicker diagnostic techniques (Poostchi et al., 2018). Even though traditional staining protocols have been the bedrock for malaria diagnosis for decades, the integration of computer-aided diagnostics keeps reminding us why good staining still remains so important. Stains like Giemsa not only make the parasites observable – they also reveal important information about their structure, which, in all fairness, proves to be important when it comes to the different stages of the life cycle and eventually the nature or extent of the malaria infection. Computerized image analysis software has been developed to capitalize on these staining properties by combining advanced color and texture feature extraction and machine learning classifiers and thus improving the diagnostic accuracy. This marriage of time-honored staining protocols with cutting-edge computational techniques is paving the way for distant and field-friendly diagnostic devices that can deliver fast as well as accurate malaria screening, solving the need for scalable, light-weight solutions in malaria-endemic areas (Kudisthalert et al., 2020) (Figure 6.9).

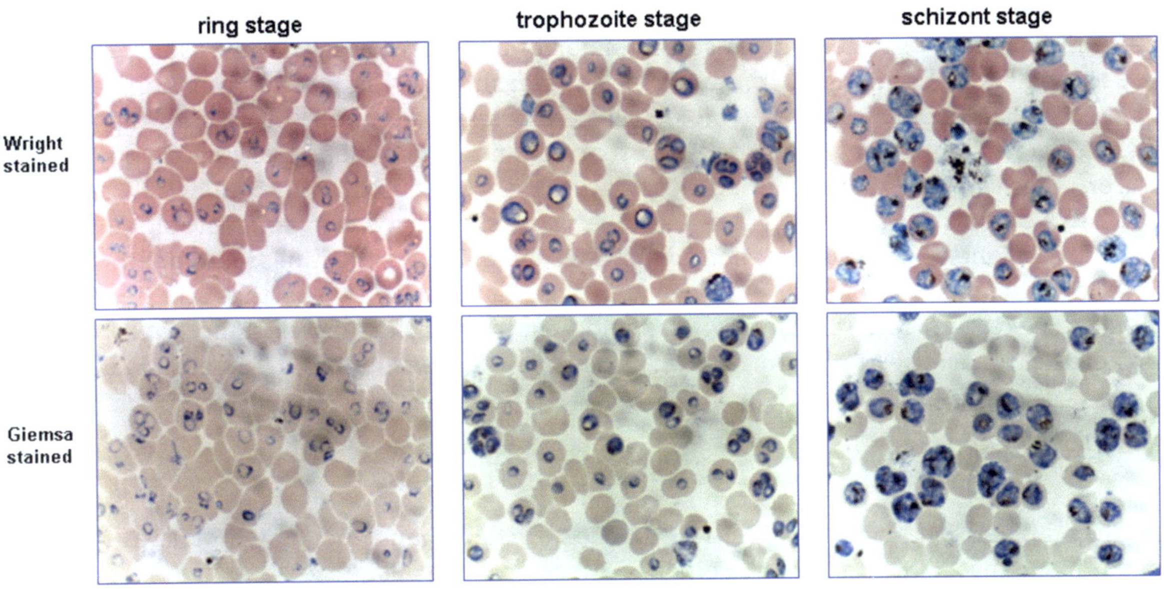

Figure 6.9. Staining techniques used for malaria.

Source: By Darío Mendez, Carlos Moneriz and José M. Bautista - Original work of Darío Mendez, Carlos Moneriz and José M. Bautista, Public Domain, https://commons.wikimedia.org/w/index.php?curid=9852880

6.3.3. Interpretation of Results

It's not quite as easy to interpret results from a malaria test as it is to read a laboratory report. You must understand not only the parasite's advanced nature but also the ways the disease manifests itself in every patient. Lab results must be viewed within a larger context; various areas experience varying levels of malaria. More than that is needed to determine the Plasmodium species; one needs to see if there are other infections simmering or if the parasite is developing resistance to standard drugs, and that can literally screw up treatment regimens. Even simple parasite counts in the bloodstream don't always neatly match up with how severe the disease gets. In the majority of cases, the malaria diagnosis goes way beyond a yes-or-no answer; it includes establishing how the pathogen can react to drugs to ensure that doctors customize treatment regimens to avoid complications and increasingly match up with clinical and public health realities (Murray et al.,

2022). This way of thinking synthesizes laboratory data with real patterns of health and ultimately informs public interventions. When looking at malaria test results, keep your eyes on the big picture of global health, like mortality rates and rates of long-term illness. Trends in the incidence of how prevalent malaria is, and the actual-world disability burden, need a careful, usually flexible review of the data, especially where AMR comes into play. The situation can reverse at any time, and therefore newer monitoring and alertness to social, economic, and demographic factors are needed. It also helps to recognize how malaria overlaps with other illnesses, requiring clinicians to take into consideration further factors that cloud the signs and prognosis. Mostly, connecting these laboratory findings to broader health studies creates a chance for healthcare providers and policymakers to better comprehend the ups and downs of the disease and allocate resources appropriately (James et al., 2018). Converting laboratory findings into concrete actions for public and health care is a whole different game. A detailed look at how accessible and consistent the data are becoming critical, especially because the majority of laboratories in low-resource settings do not possess the ideal equipment. In these cases, increasing the diagnostic potential by improving data collection and cementing microbiology laboratories is essential in placing the prevalence of malaria on its rightful peg. Consider also that common equipment like microscopy and rapid tests aren't perfect—the latter will, on occasion, yield false positives or simply fail to yield any results. All the more pertinent in high-resistance regions, where a misinterpretation of the test will yield treatments that worsen patient conditions, heightening the illness and death risks. In all, interpreting the results of malaria tests remains a dynamic activity, one that still needs constant surveillance of test procedures, close vigilance on evolving trends in resistance, and pressure on better healthcare facilities to feed patient care and policy measures (Murray et al., 2022).

6.4. Rapid Diagnostic Tests (RDTs)

It has always been a hard nut to crack to diagnose malaria, and that is why creative tools have emerged to enhance access as well as reliability in regions hardest hit by the disease. Consider the RDT, for instance, this is a technology that does not depend on fancy microscopes or laboratory set-up but produces rapid results, nonetheless. RDTs work by testing for specific malarial markers like HRP2 or pLDH, enabling healthcare practitioners to make treatment choices rapidly, especially if resources are tight. However, while RDTs are convenient and rapid, you have to be cautious with the results due to many factors that can affect the duration of a positive or just how sensitive the test will prove to be. A major issue with these tests is that they will continue to be positive even after infection must have cleared. Most of the time, these can remain detectable antigens present; for instance, it is estimated that half of HRP2-detecting tests will stay positive for approximately 15 days post-treatment, and sometimes it will be longer than a month. Generally speaking, children retain these markers longer than adults, and whether an antimalarial treatment, a combination artemisinin is administered can literally make all the difference in how long such antigens persist. There is therefore a requirement to inject some context into an RDT result interpretation, especially when carrying out surveys or clinical assessments, so that parasite densities aren't spuriously inflated or otherwise misinterpreted how well the treatment worked (Dalrymple et al., 2018). Outside the world, RDTs are being used in several different places. You see them not just in formal clinics but also at outreach sites within communities and even in neighborhood pharmacies. Each environment has its own idiosyncrasy: trained CHW generally are able to conduct the tests and react appropriately to the results, but formal healthcare providers sometimes depart from protocol—frequently failing to act on a negative result—leading to unwarranted treatment. Drug shops have lower specificity of tests and significant heterogeneity in reacting to test results. All of this indicates a need for broad, multidisciplinary approach that amplifies training, improves compliance, and sets up support systems tailored to each setting so that malaria diagnosis can be kept of high quality and antimalarial consumption remains rational (Boyce & O'Meara, 2017) (Figure 6.10).

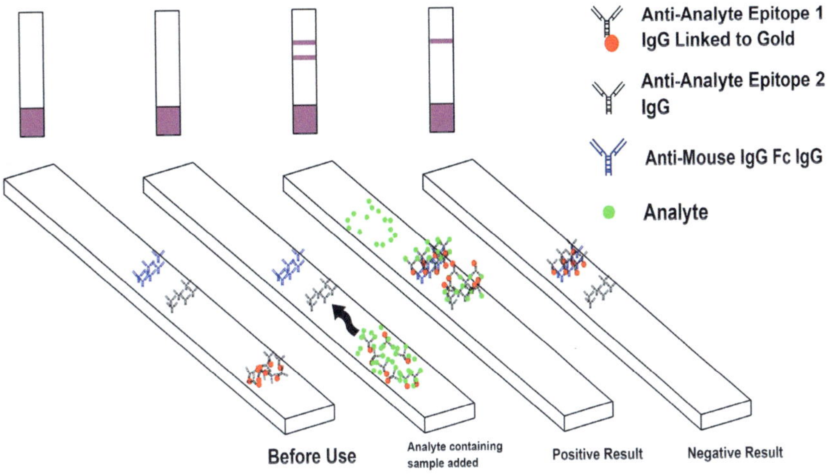

Figure 6.10. Rapid diagnostic tests.

Source: By Ian M Campbell - Own work, CC BY-SA 3.0, https://commons.wikimedia.org/w/index.php?curid=4842091

6.4.1. Mechanism of Action

Understanding the mechanism of antimalarial drugs is a significant factor in diagnosing and treating malaria rightly. Anticuments, or Plasmodium parasites, spread through bites by the Anopheles mosquito, are the culprits, and their form known as Plasmodium falciparum is normally the most troublesome. Formerly, remedies mostly revolved around the different stages of the parasite's life cycle, striving to suppress its development within the human body. Drugs act by blocking important biochemical processes the parasite has to employ, like metabolizing toxic heme and protein assembly. Since the parasite maneuvers advanced phases through the liver as well as RBCs, a one-size approach just was not going to be enough. Today, employing sets of drugs with different mechanisms is the norm, helping to bypass quick resistance that can upset diagnosis and management in highly endemic areas (Onugha et al., 2022). More recent insight into the molecular actions of the drugs has explained how they reach crucial parasite structures and processes. For example, artemisinin and its related compounds trigger the generation of reactive oxygen species that damage proteins and cell membranes, which is likely to lead to speedy removal from the bloodstream. In all but the most unusual cases, drugs like quinine disrupt the parasite's digestion of poisonous heme into harmless hemozoin in its digestive vacuole, so that poisonous heme builds up and kills the parasite. This interaction demonstrates why it is so important to choose the proper diagnostic equipment—equipment that captures the parasite when it is in its most susceptible stages. With multidrug-resistant strains increasing, there's an even greater necessity now to seek new targets and even explore plant treatments, especially since drugs like artemisinin are already starting to show limitations due to resistance (Cerávolo et al., 2021). Apart from fighting parasites in the blood, some antimalarial agents even seem to help by keeping the infection from getting a foothold early on. Some of the traditional plant-based medications, for instance, are promising by interfering with sporozoites—the causative agent carried by mosquitoes—so that they fail to settle in the liver. Not only does this treat the disease, but it also broadens our fight against malaria by adding a coat of protection. True, the very nature of action of most of these candidates remains a bit indistinct, and this discourages their forthwith clinical deployment. However, as more research delves into the biochemistry and molecular details of the drugs, it should be able to allow us to determine drug efficacy markers and drug resistance markers, ultimately streamlining malaria control and improving patient care (Cerávolo et al., 2021) (Figure 6.11).

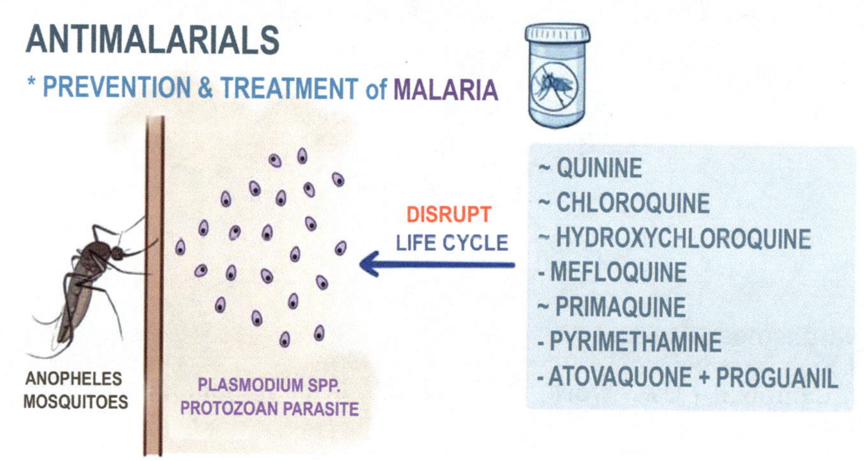

Figure 6.11. Mechanism of action of antimalarials.

Source: Blogspot User. (n.d.). Flooding Staining Technique. https://external-content.duckduckgo.com/iu/?u=https%3A%2F%2Fosmose-it.s3.amazonaws.com%2FY_g6-l8GR-OzHuQZ1IU-qdX2RKGXjKF8%2F_.jpg&f=1&nofb=1&ipt=5088467795080fd85ce4ad0f119db414fd724f4d24fc008ef7c9481357fd58cf.

6.4.2. Advantages and Limitations

New technologies have changed how we go about diagnosing malaria. Nanotechnology, for instance, is no hype—researchers are using it in subtle but advanced mechanisms to identify malaria parasites earlier than before. Tiny man-made nanoparticles are used to increase sensitivity and specificity, essentially like having internal sensors that quickly identify an infection even in low-resource settings. Most of the time, these nano biosensors can decrease the time of asking versus receiving an answer, something that is much better than traditional microscopy or rapid tests that often cannot pick up low levels of parasites. In addition, because nanoparticles can be designed to provide certain agents, they enhance the bigger picture, and intervention and treatment become possible earlier. All of that notwithstanding, there is the catch: expensive production and specific infrastructural needs can stymie the widespread application of these techniques in areas of malaria endemicity (Tiwari et al., 2023). It is a matter of balancing embracing new technology and addressing immediate concerns. Nanomedicine has also been on the scene, mixing treatment with diagnosis in a fairly interesting way. Nanoparticles can be targeted directly to infection sites, which makes the markers of diagnosis work even better at identifying even a few parasites. This specificity lessens the chance of false negative results and increases the chances of even nascent infections being diagnosed early enough to manage the disease adequately. And beyond that, these strategies might eventually combine detection with actual drug delivery, a one-two punch against malaria surveillance. But there are still some kinks to be ironed out—producing them on a large scale, gaining regulatory approval, and dispelling persisting concerns about long-term safety are all issues requiring additional work before we can call them an end-all solution (Patra et al., 2018). In the majority of instances, more intensive study is required before nanotech can be incorporated into daily clinical practice without undue disruption. Subsequently there is the tried and tested: traditional techniques such as microscopy and RDTs. These have survived largely because they are both affordable and effective. Microscopy is a direct, close-up look at the parasites that permits clinicians to count them and attain detailed clinical information, while rapid tests offer rapid, point-of-care feedback without the necessity of advanced technology. But nothing is perfect. The lower densities of parasites may slip through the cracks, and the accuracy may depend largely on the skill level of the person interpreting the tests—leading to misdiagnosis or delayed treatment at times. Also, antigen variability and environmental factors sometimes produce false positives or false negatives on occasion, lowering overall reliability. Using more advanced nanotechnology aims to counteract some of these limitations, but issues like cost and convenience, especially in the areas where malaria is most endemic—mean new methods must compromise highly technological potential with everyday useability.

6.4.3. Comparison with Microscopy

Malaria diagnosis itself has more recently been subject to greater scrutiny. The long-standing favorite—microscopy—has been touted as the gold standard for ages, but while it lets you take a close gander at the parasite, it is heavily dependent on the expertise of a technician and can be quite time-consuming. Classic smear microscopy, for instance, has roughly a 63% sensitivity but a staggering 99.4% specificity. This equates to its capacity to be reliable in identifying clear-cut cases but potentially not detecting infection with small numbers of parasites—a major weakness in areas having difficulty eliminating malaria. Overall, newer technologies like RDTs and PCR are more sensitive while maintaining specificity in the same range; such results challenge the microscope's long-held privileged role of being the gold standard (Saha et al., 2017). The flip side is their utility on a day-to-day, low-resource basis. Light microscopy is cheap in reagents, but it needs well-maintained kit and experienced operators—a luxury that is within the reach of few in much of the endemic world. Experiments have even been conducted with Light Emission Diode fluorescence microscopy (LED FM) to determine if it can merge the benefits of conventional microscopy with enhanced diagnostic pathway. LED FM ended up with a moderate sensitivity of approximately 71.2% but had high specificity of about 96.3% compared to the conventional method. Yet, its requirement for skilled training in fluorescence staining and slide reading currently holds back its broader use. Meanwhile, RDTs provide simple, quick tests, typically equivalent to or superior to that of the microscope, albeit more expensive and capable only of providing qualitative, not quantitative, information (Hathiwala et al., 2017). Even with the spread of molecular and rapid tests, the microscope is far from out of use in the fields of clinical and public health. It is still required for finding out exactly which parasite is present and for roughly estimating parasite levels—data that can be used in guiding treatment. At the same time, shifting strategies for malaria control illustrate that reliance on microscopy alone will not be adequate, especially in high-transmission or elimination-focused contexts where missing a few parasites will continue the cycle. For most, a combination of techniques that interdigitates microscopy, RDTs, and PCR seems the most promising route to capitalize on their strengths. Bayesian latent class analyses have even revealed inherent limitations in what used to be regarded as the ideal gold standard, and so simple test-to-test comparisons have been shown to risk oversimplification of the actual situation. Ultimately, more dependency on RDTs for regular use is reasonable, with PCR possibly still retaining niche roles in surveillance and confirmation (Saha et al., 2017) (Figure 6.12).

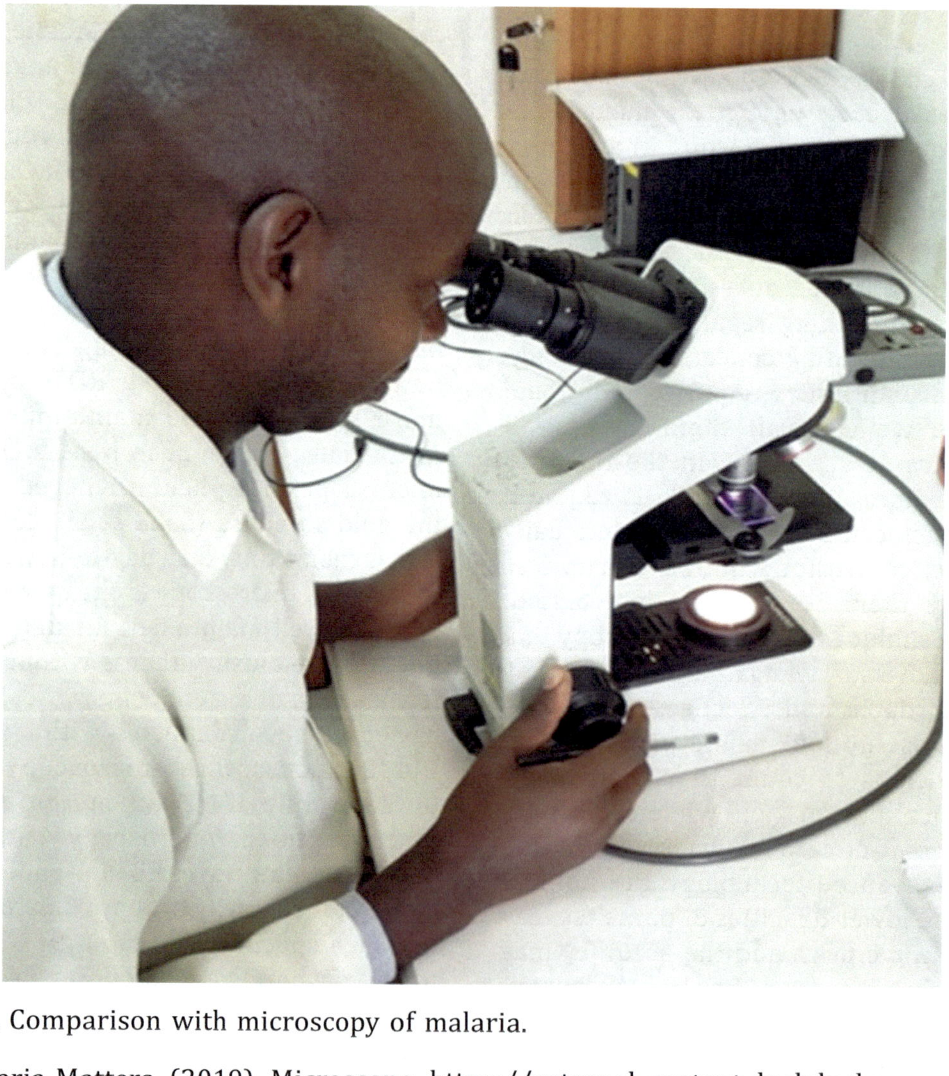

Figure 6.12. Comparison with microscopy of malaria.

Source: Malaria Matters. (2019). Microscope. https://external-content.duckduckgo.com/iu/?u=http%3A%2F%2Fmalariamatters.org%2Fwp-content%2Fuploads%2F2019%2F11%2FMicroscope.jpg&f=1&nofb=1&ipt=527fa29da68f0ddee6a6cbe3ea2e27937c774a7620cdafbe20e9e07bd3f763b3.

6.5. Molecular Techniques

Diagnosis of malaria has recently changed course, looking for even minimal levels of parasites that usually slip through the usual microscopy and rapid tests. More current methods like PCR-based assays push the envelope—amplifying the parasite DNA to an extent that even infections too small for the naked eye can now be identified. In regions such as Equatorial Guinea, where traditional tests sometimes fail with false negatives, these molecular methods—SnM-PCR in particular—hold out the hope of minimizing errors and guide more precise treatments. Implementing these techniques not only raises case detection but also provides us with a clearer picture of malaria's true impact on populations (Berzosa et al., 2018). Molecular techniques do more than merely signal infection; they also distinguish among different species and even reveal genetic differences that are significant for tracking resistance. Where the microscope might miss mixed infections or struggle with non-falciparum infections, PCR assays bring greater nuance by detecting distinctive genetic markers. This additional layer of information clearly educates public health efforts, leading to treatments more specifically calibrated to locally dominant strains. Techniques like qPCR and LAMP even offer quick, highly sensitive options that sometimes work straight in the field, making it easier to avoid unnecessary antimalarial use and largely decrease drug resistance—as well as savings from waste (Amir et al., 2018). The promise cannot be ignored, though challenges remain. High costs, manpower needs, and infrastructural difficulties have a tendency to retard these methods in resource-limited, malaria-endemic areas. However, the creation of well-equipped reference laboratories can aid local testing efforts and serve as a backup for traditional methods like microscopy and RDTs. Some of the keys to opening these restrictions and introducing molecular diagnostics into daily malaria control are technology transfer and training programs. In addition, the tools can identify genetic features, like hrp2 gene deletions that disrupt some RDTs, which then helps in the choice of suitable diagnostic kits for a specific area. In all, the merging of these state-of-the-art tools with traditional methods is a real game-changer, with malaria diagnosis being more accurate and control more efficient (Berzosa et al., 2018) (Figure 6.13).

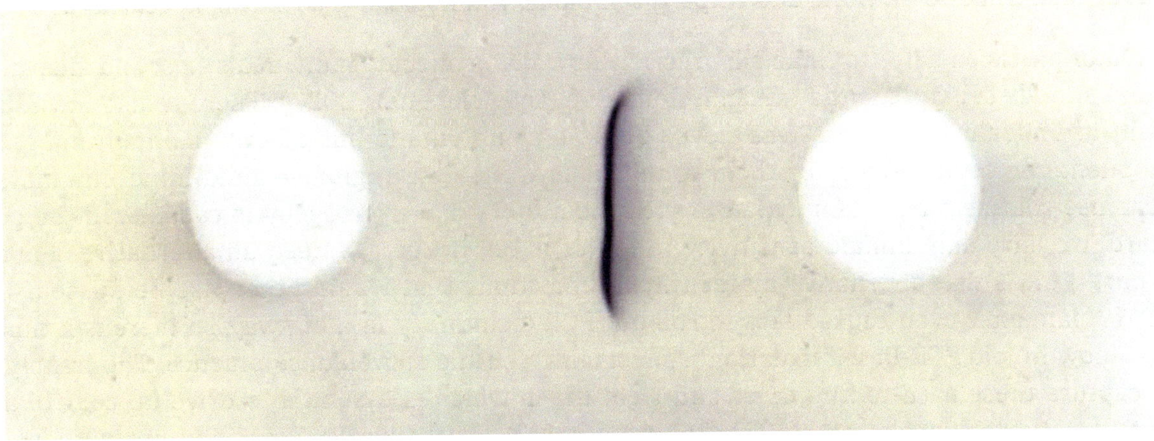

Figure 6.13. Molecular techniques of malaria.

Source: By Ernst Hempelmann - Ernst Hempelmann, CC0, https://commons.wikimedia.org/w/index.php?curid=9385597

6.5.1. Polymerase Chain Reaction (PCR)

Molecular biotechnology developments have revolutionized how we tackle illness like malaria. Instead of doggedly sticking to old testing methods—imagining microscopy or rapid diagnostic tests—we now know that such machinery, as valuable as it is, overlooks infections when parasite numbers drop low. PCR, or the PCR, sets the standard higher by amplifying parasite DNA signals so even the faintest traces of Plasmodium species are picked up. All too frequently, this increased sensitivity is a godsend in countries trying to eliminate malaria since those submicroscopic infections more commonly slip through the gaps.

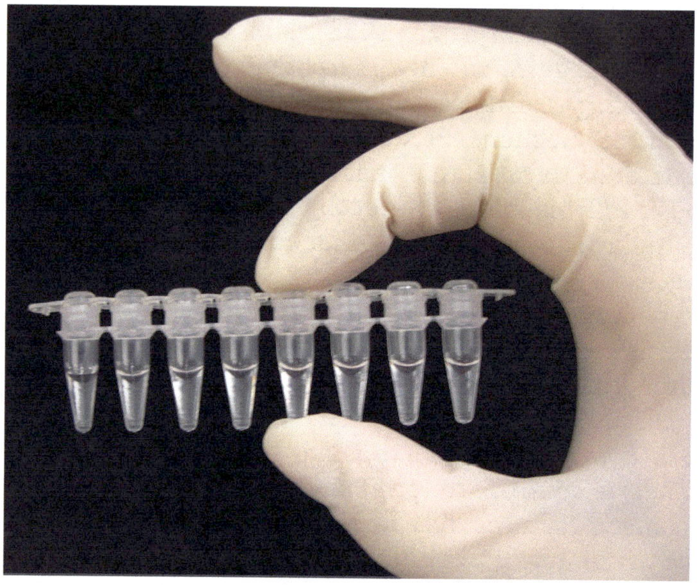

Figure 6.14. Polymerase chain reaction (PCR).

Source: By Madprime - Own work, CC0, https://commons.wikimedia.org/w/index.php?curid=2104468

Greater precision helps to establish precisely how many infected individuals exist and aids more focused methods of stopping the transmission cycle (Oyegoke et al., 2022). There is also the added problem of undercover carriers who never become symptomatic but quietly maintain infection. These silent reservoirs—most of them found in low-endemic regions—undermine elimination efforts since routine testing simply fail to pick them up. While microscopy is considered the gold standard, we have only limited sensitivity to fall back on; hence, we need an alternative. For the most part, PCR is that alternative by identifying infections that would otherwise be missed. The COVID-19 pandemic even caused labs to roll out PCR technology in a big way, so there is a timely window now to fold PCR-based malaria diagnosis into routine surveillance practice. The transition could capture those hard-to-find cases and treat them, which is essential to drive up control and elimination efforts (Rahi et al., 2022). Rolling out PCR for malaria diagnosis is not without its challenges, though. It is not merely a matter of being hyper-accurate; the process also has to be simplified so that it can be performed in local health centers without breaking the bank or creating technical headaches. Recent developments involve adapting PCR into nearly point-of-collection format that can be performed outside fancy laboratories. This transition is particularly critical in resource-scarce endemic regions. The conjunction of PCR molecular specificity and its novel field-friendly configuration even positions it as a front-running cornerstone of malaria eradication plans in the future. In most, to the degree that worldwide healthcare initiatives are searching for more accurate surveillance arms, PCR fine-tuning will continue to be critical in the detection and control of malaria transmission with an almost unmatched level of accuracy (Oyegoke et al., 2022; Rahi et al., 2022) (Figure 6.14).

6.5.2. Advantages of Molecular Diagnostics

Malaria parasites are difficult to identify in people who are not even sick, and that is a nightmare, especially where the parasite load is so low that even a microscope cannot catch it. The traditional tools, microscopy and rapid diagnostic tests, may not be able to detect such low-level infections, and that could go on spreading the disease even when we think we are winning. Molecular techniques, including PCR-based methods, are much more sensitive in the detection of Plasmodium falciparum when the parasite is under cover from the normal radar screen. Nested PCR, for example, has inadvertently demonstrated greater levels of infection in high transmission communities as well as in low transmission communities, indicating that there could be secreted parasite reservoirs that remain hidden from routine testing. Generally speaking, this increased sensitivity plays a crucial role in disease surveillance and coordinating interventions, particularly in populations where seemingly healthy individuals play a role in helping to sustain the malaria cycle (Agbana et al., 2022).

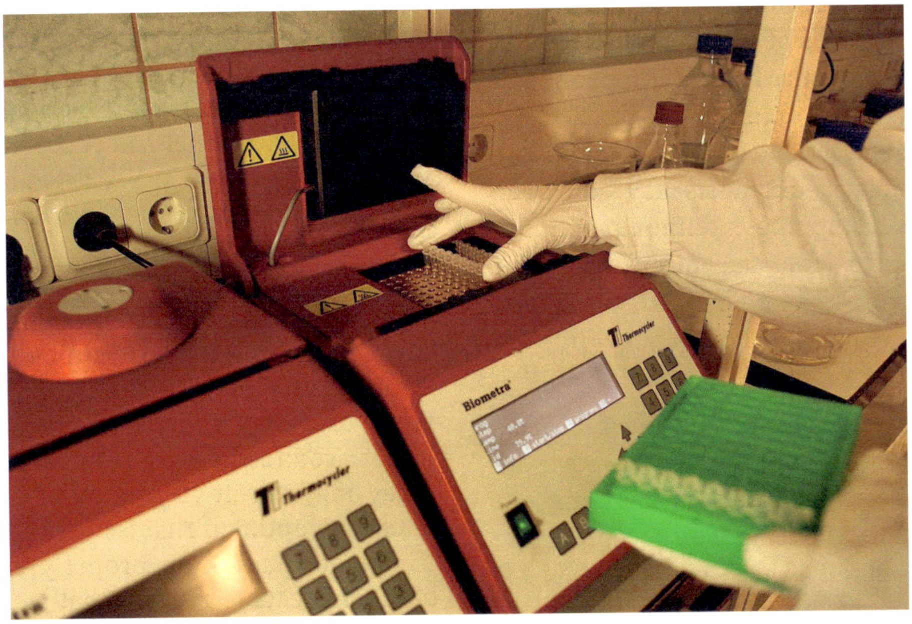

Figure 6.15. Molecular diagnostics.

Source: By Karl Mumm - Own work, CC BY-SA 3.0, https://commons.wikimedia.org/w/index.php?curid=16828886

Molecular diagnostic devices also offer other advantages in terms of sensitivity. They not only give a count of how many parasites are there but also specify exactly which species is there—a piece of information that matters a lot while selecting treatment. Unlike microscopy, where it depends on the skill of the operator (and is prone to human mistakes), techniques like photo-induced electron transfer PCR (PET-PCR) are more likely to give more uniform and reproducible results. Most of the time, such as with the HRP2 bead test, these advancements reach a compromise in being sensitive and less of a chore to handle, but fewer steps of handling required while still measuring up quite well on the parasite burden. This mix of strengths quickens decision-making at both clinical and community levels and even improves epidemiological studies by giving better numbers for parasite densities. Collectively, these molecular methods bridge patient care and broader public health surveillance, making them indispensable diagnostics in the fight against malaria (Agbana et al., 2022).

The application of molecular diagnostics in malaria control has become even more urgent, particularly in the face of global challenges like the COVID-19 pandemic. The traditional health care has been compromised—standard care, the provision of insecticide-treated nets (ITNs), and prompt malaria diagnosis have all been impacted, increasing the likelihood of more negative outcomes. Molecular diagnostics with their scalable, sensitive, and specific detection protocols can fit into these more limited healthcare settings reasonably well.

By enabling the earlier and more precise identification of infections, they support the maintenance of care and interventions being put into action on time, silencing the effect of service disruptions. Generally, their use is crucial for sustaining gains against malaria, especially in regions of high disease burden where retaining control of everything is crucial in preventing the re-emergence of outbreaks under increasing public health demands (Figure 6.15).

6.5.3. Limitations and Challenges

Malaria diagnosis has come quite a long way, but reality still gets in the way, especially where money is tight. Simple tests like RDTs are popular because they're easy to install and spew out results in a hurry, but sometimes they don't work because parasite antigen genes are deleted. In most cases, after the Plasmodium species demonstrate genetic variations, the tests then become less sensitive or even completely blind to specific infections, thus leading to false negatives and the consequent delayed treatment. People are prone to use signs to corroborate RDT results, but in reality, malaria signs can be as non-distinguishable from other causes of fevers such that the picture becomes confusing. Microscopy is still the gold standard, though it takes skilled hands and decent lab facilities—both of which are in short supply in most endemic, rural areas. No matter what new technologies are in the pipeline, keeping high-quality diagnostics running is a precarious balancing act that inhibits attempts to drive malaria rates down. Another catch for malaria diagnosis is excessive reliance on highly technical laboratory personnel and equipment, especially when microscopy is used. Thick and thin blood smear examination is not a child's game; it requires experienced eyes of microscopists to identify all the parasite species and clinically evaluate levels of parasitemia, though high turnovers and uneven training practices give poor quality assurances. The whole process takes too long, and where medical treatment is not around the corner in rural settings, any delay may result in treatment being initiated later than optimal. That issue suggests a broader challenge: scaling up properly effective, gold-standard tests to regions that lack the relevant resources. New technologies, like computer-assisted deep learning algorithms for parasite detection, seem to have promise by minimizing our reliance on continuous expert checking and speeding up the way we analyze large volumes of image datasets (Murray et al.,

2022). Subsequently there is the added complication of problems related to AI-based diagnostic algorithms. Even though these new tools generally show greater accuracy and faster detection of malaria pathogens in microscope images, deploying them into routine use is not a switch to be thrown. In low-resource environments, where electricity and digital resources are patchy at best, the intensive computational requirements of some models pose a major stumbling block. Yes, models like YOLO-mp have lower memory and processing demands but integrating them into routine practice involves enormous validation, repeatability and reliability testing becomes totally paramount. It also means that providers must acquire the new tool kit skills, which makes an additional step. In most cases, the complicated mix of cost, technical limitations, and human factors ensures that fighting malaria using improved diagnostics is not a straightforward affair. Overcoming this will need coordinated efforts that marry new diagnostic ideas with real capacity development and system strengthening in the most affected areas (Murray et al., 2022).

6.6. Challenges in Diagnosis

Effective diagnosis of malaria ultimately hinges on the accuracy and reliability of laboratory work, yet many internal and external factors always seems to manifest. Microscopic studies of stained blood smears, a technique upon which many still depend as the gold standard, can have variable outcomes because slide preparation, staining quality, and even technician skill can all vary considerably. In the majority of endemic regions, where resources are scarce, these issues are exacerbated by inadequately equipped laboratories and too frequently substandard quality control. Take, for example, the effort in India to create a malaria slide bank; it serves to help in general by making available well-tested slides for training and skill evaluation. In spite of these initiatives, practical concerns like transport delays of samples and challenges in finding exotic parasite types remain. In large part, this underscores—quite forcefully—how vital continued capacity building and rigorous quality control are to sustaining high diagnostic precision (Nema et al., 2023). Artificial intelligence and other new technologies offer some novel opportunities for overcoming these diagnostic obstacles, though they also come with challenges of their own. AI-driven platforms have been shown to enhance the precision of pathogen identification, reduce human error, streamline workflows, and even enable real-time analysis. However, integrating these tools into existing health systems is not easy; it typically involves lengthy training for lab personnel who are not yet familiar with these innovations. Additionally, issues of data privacy, bias in algorithms, and ensuring the retention of the value of human judgment persist. Overall, ignoring these problems could compromise both the effectiveness and the ethical use of the technology. So, even while AI can be heading the vanguard for resolving diagnostic issues, maintaining a balance between cutting-edge technology and good, old-fashioned human judgment is of paramount significance (Alowais et al., 2023). Another complication is introduced by the nature of the malaria parasite itself. The biological twists and turns, like shapeshifting as a result of drug resistance or mixed-species infections—can easily send microscopic and molecular tests off the rails, sometimes even resulting in underreporting. These adjustments typically take highly experienced microscopists and advanced laboratory equipment, infrastructure that is not always available in endemic settings. Furthermore, problems with the durability of slides over time, environmental factors of temperature and humidity, and even the quality of reagents used all directly affect the ultimate accuracy of the diagnosis. Managing these various challenges in most cases requires ongoing investments in laboratory infrastructure, quality training programs, and innovative diagnostic methods to effectively keep pace with the ever-changing array of malaria infections. It is only through a concerted and sustained effort at managing such biological and operational complexities that we can guarantee that malaria diagnoses are not just timely but also accurate (Nema et al., 2023) (Figure 6.16).

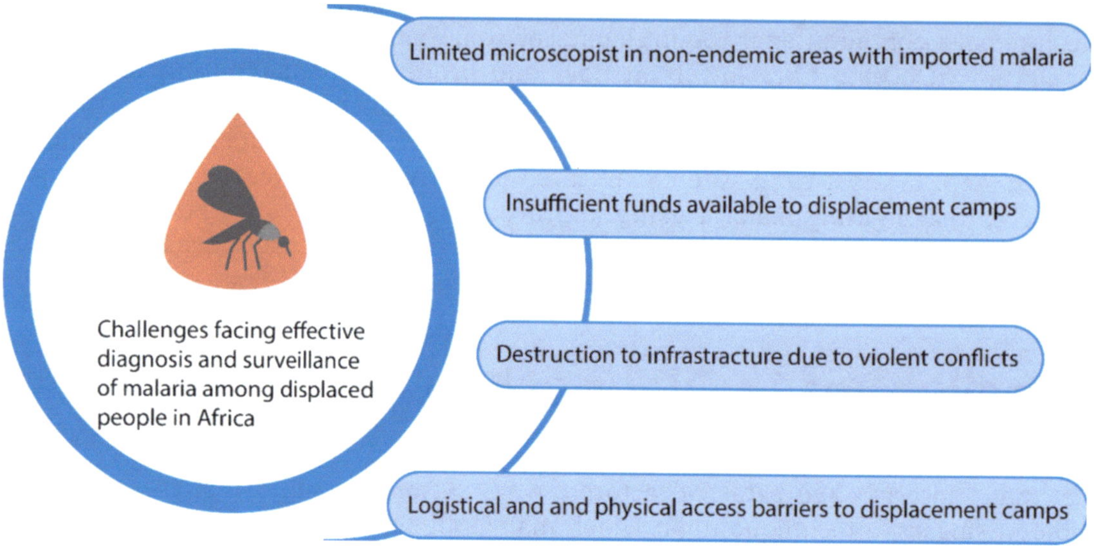

Figure 6.16. Challenges in the diagnosis of malaria.

Source: Abdul-Rahman, T., Ajetunmobi, O. A., Bamigbade, G. B., Ayesiga, I., Shah, M. H., Rumide, T. S., et al. (2025). Improving diagnostics and surveillance of malaria among displaced people in Africa. International Journal for Equity in Health, 24(1), 22.

6.6.1. Misdiagnosis and Its Consequences

Cures of fevers in areas where malaria is endemic are challenging. Too many times, a rash judgment is for malaria without reconsidering because the tests that we have available are not sensitive, specific, or fast enough. Patients are treated as if malaria were the sole likely option, though mixtures of pathogens and inflammatory illnesses may have similar manifestations. Host gene expression analyses have started to flip the script in recent years by being able to differentiate between different infections. These multi-class models, which can differentiate between bacterial, viral, and parasitic infections (such as malaria), have the tendency to usually minimize treatment options to a minimum and minimize misdiagnosis (Habgood-Coote et al., 2023). For the most part, this is a sign that we need to think outside of a simple pathogen search when presented with complex febrile cases. In the tropics, the omnipresent danger of malaria tends to lead clinicians to the tendency of labeling every fever as malaria. However, the mere fact of residence in an endemic zone must not imply that each fever must fit into this malaria category—although bacterial sepsis, arbovirus infections, and other fever-causing diseases can readily present themselves under this guise. The issue usually starts from systemic issues: lack of awareness among medical professionals, antiquated testing kits, not-so-worse fever control policies, and limited resources (Feyikemi, 2020). Sometimes, these lead to the doctors administering too many antimalarials when other reasons are overlooked, and the patient is left with negative outcomes. Mostly, a new system with better examinations and up-to-date guidelines is needed, especially where resources are limited. Apart from single cases, miscalculation in the diagnosis has implications on public health and the economy on a large scale. Over-reliance on antimalarial drugs not only wastes money but also sows the seeds for drug resistance—undermining decades of work (Feyikemi, 2020). Worse still, when the patient is wrongly diagnosed, his underlying conditions may be exacerbated, sometimes leading to serious complications or even death. Also, concealing the true spread of various infections complicates the recording of actual conditions by outbreak monitoring (Feyikemi, 2020; Habgood-Coote et al., 2023). In the end, a better, more solid strategy—one that pairs enhanced diagnostic protocols with a broader view of the causes of fever—can improve treatment accuracy, save resources, and improve overall health outcomes.

6.6.2. Access to Diagnostic Tools in Endemic Regions

Malaria diagnosis depends mostly on the availability of the right equipment at the right moment, especially in the worst-hit regions. Most of such areas have very few healthcare centers and those are mostly overwhelmed with loads, making it hard to find labs and qualified staff. RDTs and microscopy are typically the dominant tools utilized, but both depend on having reliable supply lines and ongoing maintenance, which are sometimes interrupted by budget or logistics hiccups. In most cases, without these critical tools, diagnostics are slow or incorrect, leading to treatments that aren't quite right and the disease spreading even more.

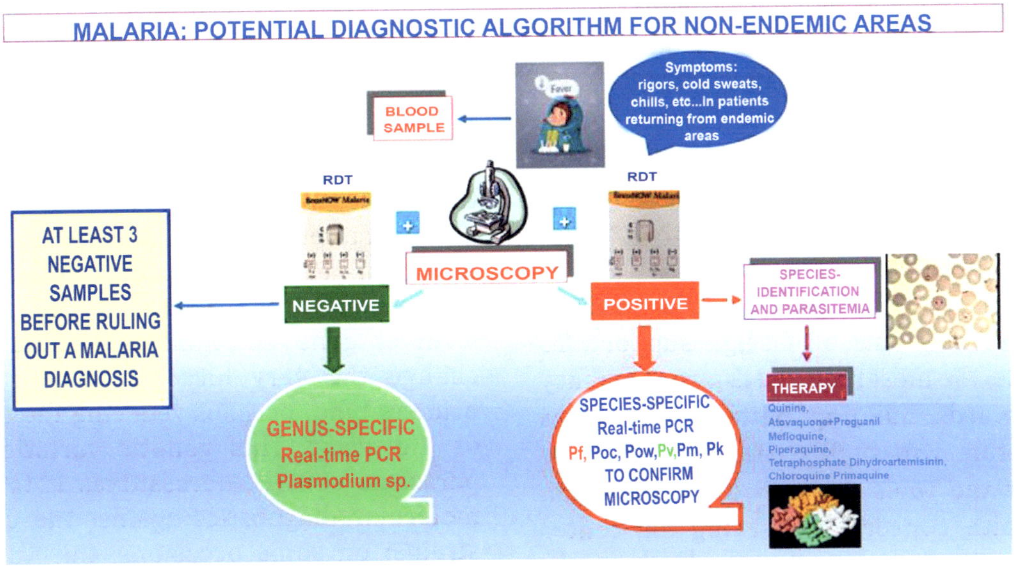

Figure 6.17. Access to diagnostic tools in endemic regions of malaria.

Source: Calderaro, A., Piccolo, G., & Chezzi, C. (2024). Proposed diagnostic algorithm for malaria in non-endemic areas. International Journal of Molecular Sciences, 25(2), 695. https://www.mdpi.com/ijms/ijms-25-00695/article_deploy/html/images/ijms-25-00695-g006.png.

In total, the enhancement of diagnostic capacity is at the heart of early malaria diagnosis and the support of health systems for lowering illness and death. Social, economic, and geographic inequalities, on the other hand, serve only to add to the barriers to receiving an appropriate diagnosis.

Rural and distant regions, which often carry the heaviest malaria burden, also often have the fewest diagnostic services, largely because of suboptimal healthcare infrastructure and low rates of trained workers. Furthermore, as there are fewer diagnostic tools accessible, many depend heavily on clinical symptoms; excessive dependence can lead to misdiagnosis and inappropriate therapy, unwittingly perpetuating problems like AMR. In most cases, this imbalance justifies targeted investment in enhanced diagnosis technology, including point-of-care tests suitable for low-resource settings, and adequately funded training programs to ensure tests are correctly performed and interpreted. These steps can enable earlier case detection, keep treatments in balance, and prevent the errors that regularly happen in poorly resourced settings (Murray et al., 2022). Innovative technologies and international partnerships are starting to broaden the range of diagnostics within malaria-endemic regions. Mobile health technologies, linking diagnostic efforts to other disease control programs, and even campaigning for on-site test-kit production are some of the ways that individuals are seeking to bridge gaps. However, sustainability is a prickly issue—one too many of these initiatives are dependent on short-term grants or foreign support. To summarize, the most required is a strong policy effort towards building better health care infrastructure and supply chain management such that the tools are still available when other health concerns are vying for center stage. The diagnosis of malaria also overlaps with co-infection management and, sometimes, liver conditions, which indicates the need for diagnostic systems capable of keeping pace with local disease patterns (Devarbhavi et al., 2023). Finally, having these tools available on a standby basis is key to controlling malaria and moving towards a more equitable global health picture (Figure 6.17).

6.6.3. Emerging Resistance to Diagnostic Methods

Advances in the diagnosis of malaria have enhanced our ability to detect the disease but developing forms of resistance keep on coming along and causing concern. Microscopy is now showing its weaknesses, mainly because it depends on the presence of well-trained staff and can easily fail when parasite loads are low or when the infection is mixed. RDTs, or RDTs, serve as a less complex, faster alternative, especially in areas where funds are not present. Still, in the majority of cases, recent studies indicate such genetic alterations in Plasmodium falciparum, such as modifications affecting HRP2, can disrupt these tests from achieving balance. These alterations have a tendency to mask the infection and hence produce false negatives and delayed treatments. Clearly, there is a need to track these genetic changes carefully and broaden the range of diagnostic targets so as to sustain efficacy as well as reliability (Weiland, 2023). For molecular methods, the case is even more complex. PCR techniques are prized for being able to detect the smallest trace of parasite DNA with very high sensitivity, but most often the cost and complexity of these tests confines them to specialized laboratories. In the meanwhile, resistance patterns in the form of gene deletions and mutations can change the very locations where the PCR primers bind, perhaps reducing the sensitivity of the assay. This genetic variation in the parasite's content necessitates it to calibrate molecular diagnostics against the circulating strains; on some occasions, this can include using multiplex methods to target several gene markers at once. For most cases, adding next-generation sequencing for surveillance is able to give vital information regarding such changing markers, allowing for refining early and accurate detection of malaria (Weiland, 2023). At a broader level, AMR integrates its challenges into diagnostics too, since delay or misinformation at the diagnosis stage can feed into treatment failures and stimulate additional resistance. The global AMR burden technically requires more flexible diagnostic instruments and more vigorous microbiological surveillance to guide effective therapy. For malaria, this means that there is a requirement for tests capable of well-detecting resistant strains of parasites as well as identifying infections even when levels of antigens change. Not to pay attention to this growing problem of diagnostic resistance would mean increased morbidity and mortality, especially in regions where healthcare facilities are not established. Thus, investing in robust, adaptable diagnostic platforms and upgrading laboratory facilities in low-resource settings appears crucial to staying on track with malaria control.

CLOSER LOOK

LOOP-MEDIATED ISOTHERMAL AMPLIFICATION (LAMP)

LAMP is an isothermal molecular diagnostic technique that has been a powerful tool in the diagnosis of malaria due to its high sensitivity, specificity, and ability to be used in resource-limited settings. Compared to the traditional PCR, which requires expensive thermal cycling instruments and optimal laboratory settings, LAMP can be performed under constant temperature, ideally 60–65°C, for rapid DNA amplification using simpler apparatus such as a water bath or heating block. This makes LAMP particularly valuable for malaria-endemic countries with limited resources and infrastructure. The technique is targeted towards specific DNA sequences of malaria *parasites*, such as the *Plasmodium* 18S rRNA gene, through a set of four to six specifically designed primers and a DNA polymerase with strand-displacement activity. Where target DNA is present, the LAMP reaction produces much amplified DNA in a relatively short time, often appearing as turbidity, fluorescence, or coloration, without needing sophisticated detection equipment.

In diagnosis for malaria, LAMP has been shown to be highly potent in the detection of low-level parasitemia which microscopy or RDT may fail to detect, especially in asymptomatic carriers or individuals from low transmission settings. LAMP thus finds its application in surveillance, elimination activities, and screening in blood banks or antenatal clinics. One of the greatest advantages of LAMP over microscopy is that it does not rely on operator skill in reading and can be used with minimal training. Compared to PCR, LAMP is faster, more inhibitor-proof, and better suited to field contexts. It can be applied to a variety of sample types, including whole blood, dried blood spots, or DNA extracts, and has been developed into commercial kits such as the Loopamp™ MALARIA Pan/Pf detection kit that can differentiate between *Plasmodium falciparum* and non-*falciparum* species.

Despite all its advantages, LAMP has disadvantages too. The requirement for DNA extraction, although facilitated in certain protocols, still remains a challenge in field conditions. In addition, despite being more affordable than PCR, LAMP is more expensive than RDTs and may not be that easily accessible to use as a routine test in all endemic settings. There is the risk of cross-contamination as well due to the significant quantity of amplified product generated, which needs careful handling and perhaps separate reaction setup and analysis regions. Nonetheless, ongoing advancements in LAMP technology, including sample-to-answer platforms, lyophilized reagent kits, and smartphone-based readouts, are increasing field use convenience and applicability.

SUMMARY

Diagnosis of malaria has also come a long way in recent years. More recent methods of diagnosis, including some novel uses of AI, have made infection detection both faster and more accurate. Tests also seem more automated, cutting down on those frustrating human errors and enhancing sensitivity. You can even envision how this will aid resource allocation to where it is most required in areas most heavily infested with the disease. Indeed, there are still potholes along the road, issues of data privacy, algorithmic biases, and infrastructure issues, but overall, AI-based methods have a tremendous amount of potential. Further research and careful, targeted approaches still need to be continued to unlock these gains fully and fairly (Alowais et al., 2023). In many cases, many tech and human expertise shows us just how flexible and dynamic our progress can be. It is not all smooth sailing, however. Getting such advanced diagnostics out into everyday healthcare falls beyond the scope of what can be offered by a laboratory. Instead, you need more extensive plans that are adapted to local needs and that equip medical staff suitably for the task. This is the nuts-and-bolts side of things, and it is the most critical, especially where resources are scarce and misdiagnosis can be perilous. Think of it like when multiple conditions overlap, just as delirium sometimes comes with dementia, at a time like that, a holistic patient overview becomes vital (Livingston et al., 2020). By involving the community and empowering local health systems, these diagnostic tools can be made to stay and have a lasting impact. In short, the way we're diagnosing malaria now is firmly in the middle between cutting-edge technology and the day-to-day realities of healthcare. Embracing AI and machine learning could usher in quicker, more precise tests and earlier treatment, which could in most cases reduce malaria's global burden substantially. Of course, such advances are contingent upon negotiating ethical concerns, keeping a vigilant clinical eye, and promoting a spirit of cooperation among physicians, patients, and policymakers. A reasoned view that honors both what our current tests can do and where they cannot be at the heart of guiding further advances and assisting the effort to contain, and eventually eradicate, malaria (Livingston et al., 2020; Alowais et al., 2023).

Diagnosis of malaria depends on matching what doctors see in patients with laboratory tests so that proper treatment is done on time. Fever and chills can be indicative of the disease, but in most cases, they also occur with other infections, and this can confuse, especially where malaria is endemic. Looking at blood smears under a microscope is still the tried-and-true method to find the parasite and determine how many are present. RDTs can be extremely helpful in poorer resource settings by identifying parasite-specific proteins, but their sensitivity varies, so they need to be interpreted together with a good clinical exam. More often than not, in spite of the ability of molecular assays to be more specific in identifying infection, they make it into well-resourced laboratories solely due to financial and technical constraints. A combination of good clinical judgment with an assortment of tests is the key to striking the diagnosis correctly and, by extension, informing treatment regimens that limit the propagation of resistant strains that remain a serious global problem (Murray et al., 2022). When lab tests confirm malaria, things get even more complicated because of issues like AMR. For the most part, not only does this resistance sicken patients and make them more likely to die, but it also muddies the whole diagnostic process, especially when mixed infections or treatment failures are in the picture. This kind of challenge calls for strong, adaptive monitoring along with a suite of tests. including some molecular diagnostics that identify resistance markers. Then, in areas with high levels of resistance, it is important to rely on solid diagnostic methods to inform treatment accordingly and avoid further problems. Thus, it is imperative to increase the range of diagnostic methods to be at par with that locally so as to realize the true disease burden, with the caution that the battle against infections is not just malaria but a broader war against resistant pathogens (Murray et al., 2022). Apart from these technological breakthroughs, scaling up healthcare infrastructure and training is vital, particularly in low-resource environments where malaria takes its greatest toll. Access and quality of RDTs and microscopy tests are typically compromised due to a lack of laboratory capacity and trained staff, and this directly affects the diagnostic accuracy. The enhancement of laboratory networks and the introduction of agreed protocols can improve early case detection and the quality of surveillance data, paving the way for earlier responses and smarter resource deployment. And, to add to that, medical practitioners need to be on their toes to distinguish malaria from other fever-inducing problems, such as when complications like delirium obscure the clinical picture in at-risk groups. In all, mixing technology with bite-sized education and systemic enhancements adds up to a better way of diagnosing malaria and, ultimately, healthier outcomes for patients across the globe.

KEY TERMS FROM THIS CHAPTER

- Clinical Diagnosis
- Thin Smear
- Rapid Diagnostic Tests (RDTs)
- Polymerase Chain Reaction (PCR)
- Differential Diagnosis
- Drug Resistance Detection
- Peripheral Blood Smear
- Giemsa Stain
- Antigen Detection
- Serological Tests
- Fever History
- Species Identification
- Thick Smear
- Parasitemia
- Molecular Diagnosis
- Fluorescent Microscopy
- Travel History

References

1. Achan, J., Serwanga, A., Wanzira, H., Kyagulanyi, T., Nuwa, A., Magumba, G., Kusasira, S., et al. (2021). Current malaria infection, previous malaria exposure, and clinical profiles and outcomes of COVID-19 in a setting of high malaria transmission: An exploratory cohort study in Uganda. The Lancet Microbe, 3, e62–e71. https://doi.org/10.1016/s2666-5247(21)00240-8.
2. Agbana, H. B., Rogier, E., Lô, A. C., Abukari, Z., Jones, S., Gyan, B., Aidoo, M., et al. (2022). Detecting asymptomatic carriage of Plasmodium falciparum in southern Ghana: Utility of molecular and serological diagnostic tools. Malaria Journal, 21. https://doi.org/10.1186/s12936-022-04078-w.
3. Alowais, S. A., Alghamdi, S. S., Alsuhebany, N., Alqahtani, T., Alshaya, A., Almohareb, S. N., Aldairem, A., et al. (2023). Revolutionizing healthcare: The role of artificial intelligence in clinical practice. BMC Medical Education, 23, Article 04698. https://doi.org/10.1186/s12909-023-04698-z.
4. Amir, A., Cheong, F. W., De Silva, J. R., & Lau, Y. L. (2018). Diagnostic tools in childhood malaria. Parasites & Vectors, 11, Article 2617. https://doi.org/10.1186/s13071-018-2617-y.
5. Berzosa, P., de Lucio, A., Romay-Barja, M., Herrador, Z., González, V., García, L., Fernández-Martínez, A., et al. (2018). Comparison of three diagnostic methods (microscopy, RDT, and PCR) for the detection of malaria parasites in representative samples from Equatorial Guinea. Malaria Journal, 17. https://doi.org/10.1186/s12936-018-2481-4.
6. Boyce, M. R., & Prudhomme O'Meara, W. (2017). Use of malaria RDTs in various health contexts across sub-Saharan Africa: A systematic review. BMC Public Health, 17. https://doi.org/10.1186/s12889-017-4398-1.
7. Cerávolo, I. P., Aguiar, A. C. C., Adebayo, J. O., & Krettli, A. U. (2021). Studies on activities and chemical characterization of medicinal plants in search for new antimalarials: A ten-year review on ethnopharmacology. Frontiers in Pharmacology, 12. https://doi.org/10.3389/fphar.2021.734263.
8. Dalrymple, U., Arambepola, R., Gething, P. W., & Cameron, E. (2018). How long do rapid diagnostic tests remain positive after anti-malarial treatment? Malaria Journal, 17(1), Article 237. https://doi.org/10.1186/s12936-018-2371-9.
9. Davidson, M. S., Andradi-Brown, C., Yahiya, S., Chmielewski, J., O'Donnell, A. J., Gurung, P., Jeninga, M. D., et al. (2021). Automated detection and staging of malaria parasites from cytological smears using convolutional neural networks. Biological Imaging, 1. https://doi.org/10.1017/s2633903x21000015.
10. Devarbhavi, H., Asrani, S. K., Arab, J. P., Nartey, Y. A., Pose, E., & Kamath, P. S. (2023). Global burden of liver disease: 2023 update. Journal of Hepatology, 79, 516–537. https://doi.org/10.1016/j.jhep.2023.03.017.
11. Di Gennaro, F., Occa, E., Ramirez, L., Marotta, C., Segala, F. V., Santana, J. M., Cotugno, S., et al. (2022). Malaria, HIV and malnutrition among internally displaced people in Mozambique during the COVID-19 pandemic: Results from a community-based intervention. Annals of Global Health, 88. https://doi.org/10.5334/aogh.3969.

12. Ehouman, M. A., N'Goran, K. E., & Coulibaly, G. (2022). Malaria and anemia in children under 7 years of age in the western region of Côte d'Ivoire. Frontiers in Tropical Diseases, 3. https://doi.org/10.3389/fitd.2022.957166.

13. Feyikemi, I. A. (2020). Misdiagnosis of non-malaria febrile infectious diseases as malaria in Nigeria: Consequences and priority actions. Public Health Review International Journal of Public Health Research, 7, 14–18. https://doi.org/10.17511/ijphr.2020.i01.03.

14. Fleming, K. A., Horton, S., Wilson, M. L., Atun, R., DeStigter, K., Flanigan, J., Sayed, S., et al. (2021). The Lancet Commission on diagnostics: Transforming access to diagnostics. The Lancet, 398, 1997–2050. https://doi.org/10.1016/s0140-6736(21)00673-5.

15. Guo, Y. R., Cao, Q. D., Hong, Z. S., Tan, Y. Y., Chen, S. D., Jin, H. J., Tan, K. S., et al. (2020). The origin, transmission and clinical therapies on coronavirus disease 2019 (COVID-19) outbreak–An update on the status. Military Medical Research, 7(1), Article 24. https://doi.org/10.1186/s40779-020-00240-0.

16. Habgood-Coote, D., Wilson, C., Shimizu, C., Barendregt, A. M., Philipsen, R., Galassini, R., Rivero-Calle, I., et al. (2023). Diagnosis of childhood febrile illness using a multi-class blood RNA molecular signature. Med, 4, 635–654.e5. https://doi.org/10.1016/j.medj.2023.06.007.

17. Hathiwala, R., Mehta, P., Nataraj, G., & Hathiwala, S. (2017). LED fluorescence microscopy: Novel method for malaria diagnosis compared with routine methods. Journal of Infection and Public Health, 10, 824–828. https://doi.org/10.1016/j.jiph.2017.01.001.

18. James, S. L., Abate, D., Abate, K. H., Mequanente Abay, S., Abbafati, C., Abbasi, N., Abbastabar, H., et al. (2018). Global, regional, and national incidence, prevalence, and years lived with disability for 354 diseases and injuries for 195 countries and territories, 1990–2017: A systematic analysis for the Global Burden of Disease Study 2017. The Lancet, 392(10159), 1789–1858. https://doi.org/10.1016/s0140-6736(18)32279-7.

19. Koirala, A., Jha, M., Bodapati, S., Mishra, A., Chetty, G., Sahu, P. K., Mohanty, S., et al. (2022). Deep learning for real-time malaria parasite detection and counting using YOLO-mp. IEEE Access, 10, 102157–102172. https://doi.org/10.1109/access.2022.3208270.

20. Kudisthalert, W., Pasupa, K., & Tongsima, S. (2020). Counting and classification of malarial parasite from Giemsa-stained thin film images. IEEE Access, 8, 78663–78682. https://doi.org/10.1109/access.2020.2990497.

21. Liu, D., Li, W., Xu, Q., Gu, J., Kang, Z., Chen, J., Xu, X., et al. (2022). A rapid multiplex assay of human malaria parasites by digital PCR. Clinica Chimica Acta, 539, 70–78. https://doi.org/10.1016/j.cca.2022.12.001.

22. Livingston, G., Huntley, J., Sommerlad, A., Ames, D., Ballard, C., Banerjee, S., Brayne, C., et al. (2020). Dementia prevention, intervention, and care: 2020 report of the Lancet Commission. The Lancet, 396, 413–446. https://doi.org/10.1016/s0140-6736(20)30367-6.

23. Melamed, N., Baschat, A., Yinon, Y., Athanasiadis, A., Mecacci, F., Figueras, F., Berghella, V., et al. (2021). FIGO (International Federation of Gynecology and Obstetrics) initiative on fetal growth: best practice advice for screening, diagnosis, and management of fetal growth restriction. International Journal of Gynecology & Obstetrics, 152, 3-57. https://doi.org/10.1002/ijgo.13522.

24. Murray, C. J. L., Ikuta, K. S., Sharara, F., Swetschinski, L. R., Robles Aguilar, G., Gray, A. P., Han,

C., et al. (2022). Global burden of bacterial antimicrobial resistance in 2019: A systematic analysis. The Lancet, 399, 629–655. https://doi.org/10.1016/s0140-6736(21)02724-0.

25. Nema, S., Nitika, N., Anvikar, A., & Bharti, P. K. (2023). Malaria slide bank plays a crucial role in achieving and sustaining malaria elimination in India. Asian Pacific Journal of Tropical Medicine, 16, 431–433. https://doi.org/10.4103/1995-7645.388384.

26. Onugha, A. N., Ogwunga, C. C., Madubuike, M. N., & Josephat, O. C. (2022). Global therapeutic intervention on malaria. International Journal of Pathogen Research. https://doi.org/10.9734/ijpr/2022/v10i330252.

27. Oyegoke, O. O., Maharaj, L., Akoniyon, O. P., Kwoji, I., Roux, A. T., Adewumi, T. S., Maharaj, R., et al. (2022). Malaria diagnostic methods with the elimination goal in view. Parasitology Research, 121, 1867–1885. https://doi.org/10.1007/s00436-022-07512-9.

28. Patra, J. K., Das, G., Fraceto, L. F., Campos, E. V. R., Rodríguez-Torres, M. D. P., Acosta-Torres, L. S., Díaz-Torres, L. A., et al. (2018). Nano-based drug delivery systems: Recent developments and future prospects. Journal of Nanobiotechnology, 16. https://doi.org/10.1186/s12951-018-0392-8.

29. Pluciński, M. M., Candrinho, B., Dimene, M., Colborn, J., Lu, A., Nace, D., Zulliger, R., et al. (2019). Assessing performance of HRP2 antigen detection for malaria diagnosis in Mozambique. Journal of Clinical Microbiology, 57. https://doi.org/10.1128/jcm.00875-19.

30. Poostchi, M., Ersoy, I., McMenamin, K. J., Gordon, E. B., Palaniappan, N., Pierce, S. K., Maude, R. J., et al. (2018). Malaria parasite detection and cell counting for human and mouse using thin blood smear microscopy. Journal of Medical Imaging, 5(4), 044506. https://doi.org/10.1117/1.jmi.5.4.044506.

31. Rahi, M., Sharma, R., Saroha, P., Chaturvedi, R., Bharti, P. K., & Sharma, A. (2022). Polymerase chain reaction-based malaria diagnosis can be increasingly adopted during the current phase of malaria elimination in India. American Journal of Tropical Medicine and Hygiene, 106, 1005–1012. https://doi.org/10.4269/ajtmh.21-0966.

32. Rajaraman, S., Jaeger, S., & Antani, S. (2019). Performance evaluation of deep neural ensembles toward malaria parasite detection in thin-blood smear images. PeerJ, 7, e6977. https://doi.org/10.7717/peerj.6977.

33. Rubio Maturana, C., Dantas de Oliveira, A., Nadal, S., Bilalli, B., Zarzuela, F., Espasa, M., Sulleiro, E., et al. (2022). Advances and challenges in automated malaria diagnosis using digital microscopy imaging with artificial intelligence tools: A review. Frontiers in Microbiology, 13. https://doi.org/10.3389/fmicb.2022.1006659.

34. Saha, S., Narang, R., Deshmukh, P., Pote, K., Anvikar, A., & Narang, P. (2017). Diagnostic efficacy of microscopy, rapid diagnostic test and polymerase chain reaction for malaria using Bayesian latent class analysis. Indian Journal of Medical Microbiology, 35(4), 376–380. https://doi.org/10.4103/ijmm.ijmm_17_199.

35. Sands, P. (2020). HIV, tuberculosis, and malaria: How can the impact of COVID-19 be minimized? The Lancet Global Health, 8, e1102–e1103. https://doi.org/10.1016/s2214-109x(20)30317-x.

36. Sharma, S., Kaura, T., Kaur, J., Sharma, A., Dhiman, A., Pangotra, M. K., Upadhyay, A. K., et al. (2019). Prevalence of submicroscopic malaria in low transmission state of Punjab: A potential threat to malaria elimination. Journal of Vector Borne Diseases, 56(2), 78. https://doi.org/10.4103/0972-9062.257780.

37. Shewajo, F. A., & Fante, K. A. (2023). Tile-based microscopic image processing for malaria screening using a deep learning approach. BMC Medical Imaging, 23. https://doi.org/10.1186/s12880-023-00993-9.

38. Tan, D., & Liang, X. (2023). Multiclass malaria parasite recognition based on transformer models and a generative adversarial network. Scientific Reports, 13. https://doi.org/10.1038/s41598-023-44297-y.

39. Tiwari, R., Gupta, R. P., Singh, V., Kumar, A., Rajneesh, Madhukar, P., Sundar, S., et al. (2023). Nanotechnology-based strategies in parasitic disease management: From prevention to diagnosis and treatment. ACS Omega, 8, 42014–42027. https://doi.org/10.1021/acsomega.3c04587.

40. Tripathi, H., Bhalerao, P., Singh, S., Arya, H., Alotaibi, B. S., Rashid, S., Hasan, M. R., et al. (2023). Malaria therapeutics: Are we close enough? Parasites & Vectors, 16. https://doi.org/10.1186/s13071-023-05755-8.

41. Vos, T., Abajobir, A. A., Abate, K. H., Abbafati, C., Abbas, K., Abd-Allah, F., Abdulkader, R. S., et al. (2017). Global, regional, and national incidence, prevalence, and years lived with disability for 328 diseases and injuries for 195 countries, 1990–2016: A systematic analysis for the Global Burden of Disease Study 2016. The Lancet, 390(10100), 1211–1259. https://doi.org/10.1016/s0140-6736(17)32154-2.

42. Weiland, A. S. (2023). Recent advances in imported malaria pathogenesis, diagnosis, and management. Current Emergency and Hospital Medicine Reports, 11, 49–57. https://doi.org/10.1007/s40138-023-00264-5.

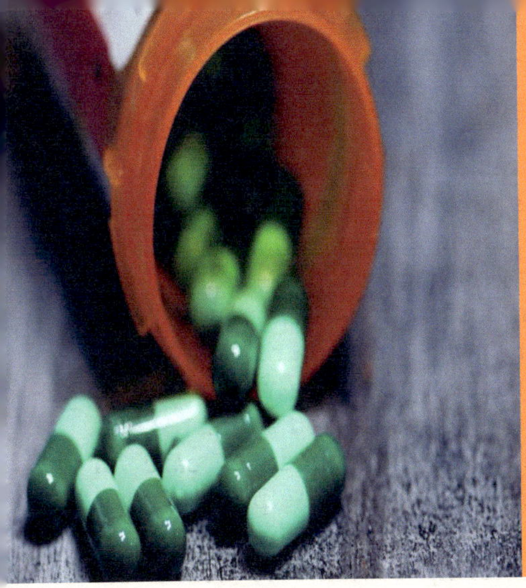

Chapter 7

TREATMENT GUIDELINES AND ANTIMALARIALS

Contents

Introduction

Infectious diseases still hit hard across the globe, and this is especially challenging to address in the less resource-abundant parts of the world. Malaria, for example, is a true standout, it is spread widely and results in much illness and unnecessary loss of life. Treatment guidelines continue to change as our understanding grows, and they are at the center not only of patient care but also of how and where to distribute limited resources. In the majority of circumstances, it is not a clean idea to mix antimalarial drugs with these evolving treatment plans, it is necessary. These recommendations, guiding policy as well as clinical practice, are ultimately a kind of roadmap for when public health efforts need a shot in the arm. And since patterns of disease and drug resistance can change overnight, it is typically wise to constantly assess our treatment approaches so that they remain safe and effective, based on the latest science and clinical data. The plea for strong guidelines for treatment is not only for malaria; it spills over into controlling viral infections as well. When new viruses break out—SARS-CoV-2 being a spectacular example—the pressure is to quickly churn out treatment guidelines recycling already known drugs with potential antiviral effects. Antimalarials have gained extra attention, not only because of their proven safety but also because laboratory reports indicate they might be of use against some viruses. This twin use is underscored by a flexible treatment approach and keeps in mind the fact that recycling familiar medicines can be a blessing when breaking new epidemics occur. In the majority of cases, factoring antimalarials into the broader infectious diseases' scenario helps build a more comprehensive approach toward resolving both chronic and new health emergencies (Pascarella et al., 2020). Apart from the efficacy of a drug in the clinic, practical problems, like the right dose, duration of treatment, and whether people are able to get hold of the drug easily—play an important role in determining the success of a guideline. With diseases like malaria and COVID-19, public health policy often merges protective approaches with active treatment to limit transmission and cover vulnerable groups.

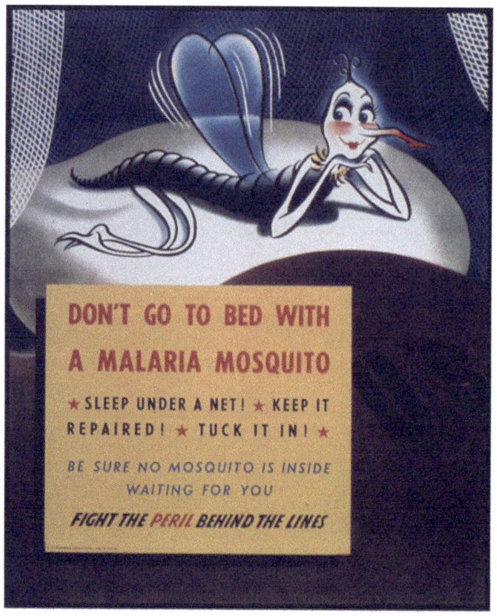

Figure 7.1. Treatment guidelines and antimalarials.

Source: By Unknown author or not provided - U.S. National Archives and Records Administration, Public Domain, https://commons.wikimedia.org/w/index.php?curid=16930013

Using antimalarials as chemoprophylaxis, say, illustrates one of the prevention spin, however loose the language at times, however rigorous clinical trials and tedious—if not always impeccable in description—pharmacological studies are in place to ensure that these medications are being used in the best way, with maximum benefit weighed against safety. This refinement not only enhances care for individual patients but also helps to reduce society's total disease burden by restraining spread and fostering sustainable healthcare routines (Casamitjana & Clotet, 2020) (Figure 7.1).

Malaria is still a massive health risk globally, impacting the majority where resources are limited and vulnerable populations bear the brunt. Malaria is caused by a *Plasmodium* genus parasite that enters the body by way of infected female *Anopheles* mosquito bites. You can get fever, chills, or anemia, and the disease can progress from mere discomfort to life-threatening conditions. Despite new diagnostic testing, a correct diagnosis remains rare in low-caseload settings. A misdiagnosis most frequently occurs, with unwarranted antimalarial treatment and other fever causes overlooked – a situation which complicates patient management and public health intervention. Misidentification requires updated, abbreviated treatment guidelines that place emphasis on lab-tested results before antimalarial drug dispensation (Moon et al., 2014). Seeing malaria is not simply detecting a parasite; it requires us to take responsibility for treatment difficulties related to larger health system issues. Containing the disease depends as much on recognizing the pathogen as it does on quick access to good care, the conscientiousness of providers to follow protocols through to completion, and patients following through on their treatments. Generally speaking, all these elements have a role to play in reducing death rates and breaking the circle of infection. Occasionally things like poor compliance, counterfeit drugs, or delay in reporting for help work against overall effectiveness. In most cases, setting the parameters for what effective treatment of malaria even involves combining all those complications together, illustrating that fighting malaria is much more multifaceted than battling a parasite (Galactionova et al., 2015). Recent changes in treatment modalities reflect our changing conception of how malaria is transmitted and the necessity for methodologies that align with multiple local realities. The World Health Organization (WHO) now mandates laboratory confirmation of malaria before treatment can be started—a change that inhibits overdiagnosis and overtreating that indirectly can contribute to drug resistance and mask other deadly fever etiologies. This change pushes doctors to be more dependent on solid lab work than simple clinical expertise, providing a more advanced method for managing the disease. Calling malaria not only a parasitic disease but also a sign of broader health system vulnerabilities is emphasizing the need for guidelines that incorporate proper diagnosis, good training of health personnel, better patient education, and drug quality assurances (Moon et al., 2014; Galactionova et al., 2015). Generally, such an integrated system would offer a stronger foundation for decreasing malaria and, ultimately, preventing it from occurring in the first place.

Importance of Treatment Guidelines

Standardized treatment guidelines for malaria are a real linchpin when it comes to reliable patient care. The guidelines give doctors and nurses a list of tested and proven suggestions that minimize guesswork and careless variations in treatment. As malaria treatment is so complicated – think drug resistance, different kinds of *parasites* in different places, and complications particular to each patient – these guidelines serve as a versatile roadmap to the right medicines. They also make training easier, guide health policy, and help determine resource allocation where the resources are scarce and malaria is common. In general, this consistent application of guidelines monitors trends in diseases, verifies whether drugs are effective, and supports worldwide malaria control efforts by reducing the likelihood of inappropriate treatment. If you look at it from the patient's point of view, following these regimens is not just a case of better care, but also of making a valuable contribution to public health in the sense of slowing down the development of resistant strains of malaria. Incorrect or irregular use of antimalarials may hasten resistance, make drugs ineffective, and confound control efforts. In the majority of cases, the guidelines suggest sticking with combination regimens or trying newer drugs based on current research and evidence, which avoids those problems. They even allow room for the utilization of natural products as therapeutic molecules, a recognition of the long history of plant-based drugs as sources of potential drugs (Chaachouay & Zidane, 2024). By enabling practices to be loosely coordinated across different regions and hospitals, these regulations help ensure treatments are effective and evidence-based. Beyond day-to-day treatment, treatment guidelines also offer an important stimulus for drug development and repurposing efforts. They offer a starting point of established treatments that researchers can rearrange and add to, prompting them to reconsider older drugs in new ways or more cleverly pair them to more successfully fight malaria and even other illnesses (Zhang et al., 2020). Along the way, these blueprints integrate fresh insights into drug action and resistance development, enabling developing results to find their way reasonably rapidly into practice. They also call for more coordination between different experts and promote frequent adaptation of treatment policies—key when dealing with issues like changing drug availability, patients who sometimes skip doses, and unpredictable parasite activity. In all, then, these guidelines are not just about treating patients today; they are living, constantly revised tools that inform innovation and flexibility in our fight against malaria.

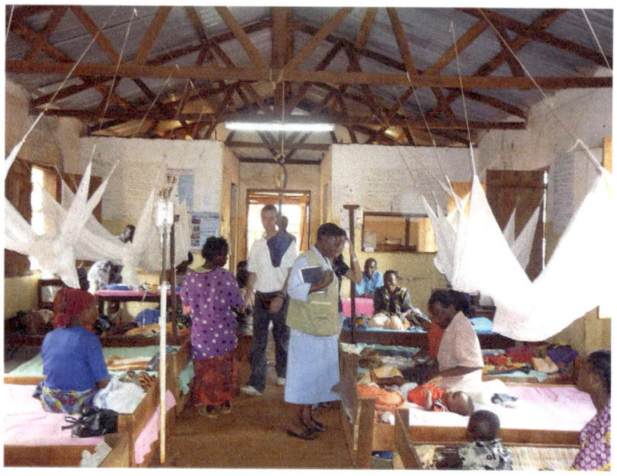

Source: By Olympia Wereko-Brobby - Saving Lives with SMS for Life, CC BY 2.0, https://commons.wikimedia.org/w/index.php?curid=8799027

Overview of Antimalarial Medications

Malaria control is all about using antimalarial drugs judiciously, and these medications have progressed far. Previously, the treatments like chloroquine and quinine were employed, but when resistance became prevalent, especially where the disease is widespread, new drugs had to take the place. Nowadays, artemisinin-based combination therapies (ACTs) such as artemether-lumefantrine (AL) are generally the first choice all over the world since they are quick-acting and hit *Plasmodium falciparum* hard. Nevertheless, in the real world, there are still problems; health centers sometimes lack the needed resources to facilitate correct diagnosis and prescription, and thus treatments fail as they ought not. For instance, a study in Uganda shows that even when good diagnostics like mRDTs are present, antimalarial use is improper even then, showing how hard it is to incorporate these drugs into regular care for fever (Chandler et al., 2017). What the people think of these drugs and whether they can get them also plays an important role. In a nation like Ghana, there is a very strong push for the employment of domestically prepared herbal remedies instead of the Western-made synthetic drugs, although the latter are readily available. This is partially fueled by a deep-rooted belief in traditional medicine, complemented by aggressive advertisement of herbal remedies and a dash of *Skepticism* concerning foreign medicines. While such herbal treatments are common, they have lax quality control processes and are side-effect-causing—go figure, it doesn't hold people back from using them. It is all a reflection that there has to be respect for cultures but simultaneously imposing modern, evidence-based therapies, and plugging loopholes around herbal medicines to provide safety for all (Yeboah et al., 2020).

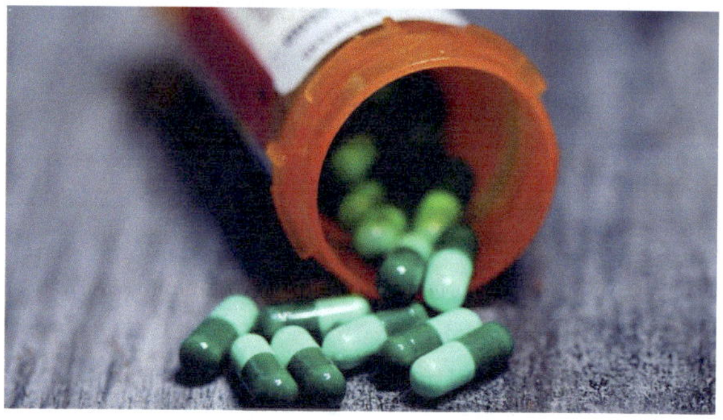

Source: Technology Networks. (2024). *Study Explores Cancer-Fighting Potential of An Anti-Malaria Drug.* https://assets.technologynetworks.com/production/dynamic/images/content/392892/study-explores-cancer-fighting-potential-of-an-anti-malaria-drug-392892-960x540.jpg?cb=13068624.

It is also important to note that one should not just concentrate on the drugs while attempting to make treatment take effect. Most of the time, better infrastructure, good staffing, and proper training of the healthcare workers are all crucial components of making tools like mRDTs used appropriately and medicines prescribed in line with clinical guidelines. Without system support like that, even the best drugs won't be able to effectively cut the malaria burden. Both national and global malaria programs are thus increasingly shifting towards integrated approaches—combining new drug innovation with more robust health systems. This multi-pronged strategy is vital in a bid to have maximum benefit from ACTs and minimize the risk of errors in prescription leading to drug resistance and lost resources (Chandler et al., 2017).

7.1. Epidemiology of Malaria

Malaria transmission is not as simple to classify, and an understanding of its trends facilitates treatment planning and the choice of antimalarials. Transmission varies in various regions—climate, mosquito behavior, and even housing may play roles. In Southeast Asia, for instance, even though the majority of people rest under insecticide-treated nets (ITNs), malaria remains an unresolved public health problem. A trial conducted in Cambodia showed a comparatively modest protective effect from these nets, especially among children aged less than five years, although the numbers did not always pan out statistically since the study was just a shade underpowered (Alexander et al., 2006). , population control of the mosquitoes lowers malaria, but it must be accompanied by effective treatment policies. Epidemiological data ultimately decide which drug regimens are best for which populations and transmission levels, permitting interventions to target local disease features in the majority of cases. Malaria's drug resistance is evolving, this changing development undoubtedly impacts how drugs are chosen. *Plasmodium falciparum*, the etiological parasite of the most severe types, is currently, in the majority of cases, resistant to almost all antimalarials available and increasingly threatens international control activities (Mwangi & Ranford-Cartwright, 2013).

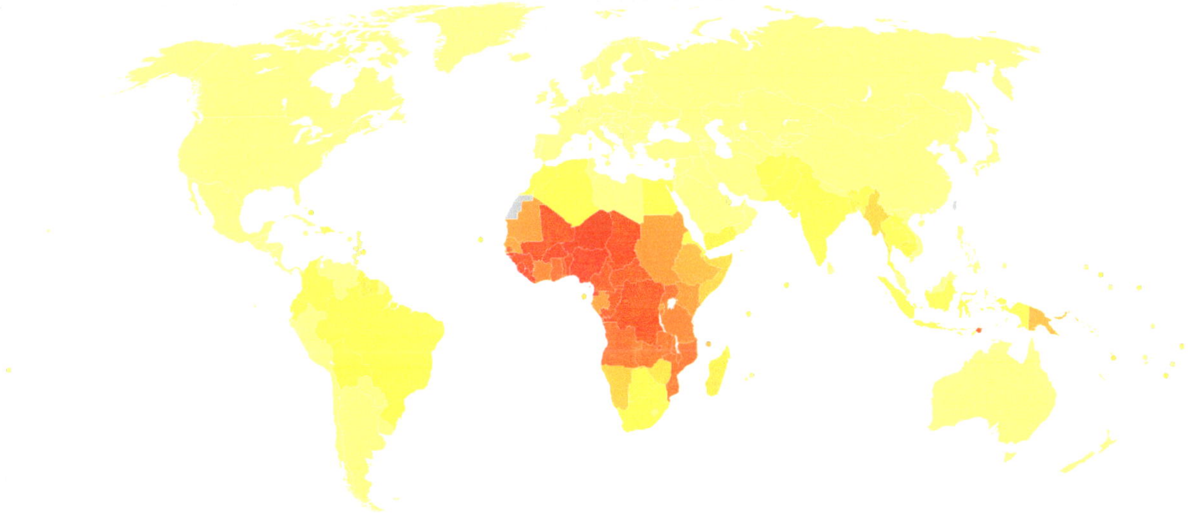

Figure 7.2. Epidemiology of malaria.

Source: By Lokal_Profil, CC BY-SA 2.5, https://commons.wikimedia.org/w/index.php?curid=8517645

Surveillance of this employing epidemiological surveillance that even analyzes molecular markers of resistance is nearly an absolute necessity; it helps keep track of the spread of these resistant strains. Monitoring this way enables doctors to substitute drugs that are starting to fail before things get out of control. Being able to monitor regional resistance trends enables first-line and second-line therapies to be modified so they can still work, prolonging the useful life of the drugs in affected areas. When you put all these into consideration—how the disease is transmitted and how the disease reacts to interventions—the need for holistic control measures becomes obviously evident. Yes, interventions such as ITNs curtail transmission, but without specific data on local trends, treatment policies might lag behind shifting parasite genetics (Alexander et al., 2006; Mwangi & Ranford-Cartwright, 2013). The integration of genetic and genomic research brings about new realities in resistance driving forces, subtly altering the antimalarial prescription, and even suggesting the potential for new drug discovery. Such an evidence-led approach and continued surveillance allow for malaria control programs to stay one step ahead by pre-empting resistance trends and adapting accordingly. In short, keeping a close, adaptive eye on the epidemiology of malaria, in all its subtleties, remains the means to reduce the illness and death this disease inflicts upon the world (Figure 7.2).

7.1.1. Global Prevalence and Distribution

People have been trying to get a sense of the extent to which malaria spreads around the world by looking at many complex factors—the neighborhood environment, social patterns, and to be frank, the biology behind it all. Malaria mostly thrives in tropical and subtropical areas, with sub-Saharan Africa suffering the greatest amount in both incidence and mortality. While it persists persistently in sub-Saharan Africa, other regions like Southeast Asia and even remote parts of South America also experience problems with the disease. Mosquito behavior, human mobility, and altered climate all contribute to this uneven playing field. Because of these differences, treatment protocols must subsequently be tailored to local issues like drug resistance and access to medical care. This type of precise, though rather indistinct, information helps to direct antimalarial initiatives better, especially when simple remedies like ITNs provide mixed results based on age and environmental factors (Alexander et al., 2006). Still another complexity confounding the situation is the way the various *Plasmodium* species are distributed geographically. In most cases, *Plasmodium falciparum* has been the largest offender, piling up the most severe cases and fueling drug resistance problems. On the other hand, *Plasmodium vivax* will more likely dominate in Latin America and South Asia and possesses its own set of recurrent issues that necessitate a different approach. It is this difference that does not support a one, uniform treatment but necessitates guidelines to be flexible and accommodate treatments such as ACTs. ACTs have been very effective in most parts of the world, especially when used as an addition to mass drug campaigns. But there are still hindrances—diagnostic problems and those pesky asymptomatic carriers allow infection to persist in populations. Some mathematical modeling even suggests that in order for mass treatment campaigns to be effective, region-specific prophylactic drugs should be used in conjunction with transmission-blocking medications such as primaquine (Eckhoff et al., 2015). What attempts to cut down malaria and even think about its eradication on this earth mainly depends on understanding who gets infected and where. In worst-hit areas, strategies must commonly be multi-component—anything from vector control of mosquitoes to delivering rapid diagnosis and combination therapies to reduce residual reservoirs of parasites. Take Southeast Asia, for example; ITNs have worked there, especially among youth—the statistical evidence supporting it is sometimes a bit patchy, maybe due to limits placed in the studies themselves. In addition, mass drug distributions combining ACTs with longer-acting prophylactics and gametocytocidal agents appear to present promising, locally optimized solutions. The differing success rates between programs that mass-screen and treat and those that target mass drug administration highlight the imperative of refining diagnostic tools. Overall, these findings related to where malaria strikes most fiercely have a direct impact on constantly shifting treatment guidelines, so that interventions are not only scientifically valid but also sensitive to the immediate environment (Alexander et al., 2006; Eckhoff et al., 2015).

7.1.2. High-Risk Populations

Control of malaria in fact relies on how different groups get affected, and the situation is never cut and dry. Vulnerability varies significantly between countries – in some areas transmission rates vary so significantly that it even changes the challenge. Southeast Asia as an example: ITNs are in the spotlight because of their protective roles, especially for children under the age of five.

There is some evidence, if not necessarily unbreakable, that the use of ITNs among these high-risk groups can lower clinical *Plasmodium falciparum* cases and total prevalence, though statistical power can be somewhat mixed here and there. Young children seem to benefit disproportionately more, which means that interventions have to keep pace with age-related risks. Although data is imperfect, these findings urge us to prioritize vulnerable age groups and align treatment strategies with demographic threats in an effort to enhance antimalarial outcomes (Alexander et al., 2006). To summarize, targeting prevention seems to be the solution to reducing sickness and strategically directing resources. Pregnant women only add to the complexity of malaria management. Malaria during pregnancy in India is generally linked with complications of anemia, preterm birth, and low birth weight. There is, however, a noticeable gap between the policy guidelines on paper and what is happening on the ground in real life. Though government policy supports chemoprophylaxis with chloroquine in pregnant women, its use in real life remains very low—these are lacking in both healthcare worker motivation and patient compliance. Even the use of ITNs, something we understand can minimize exposure to malaria, is unexpectedly low. The underuse suggests systemic issues in antenatal care and implies that stronger education along with more forceful policy response could be necessary to protect pregnant women effectively (Wylie et al., 2010). Overall, it highlights incorporating the special needs of high-risk groups into the overall antimalarial policy. Handling such risk populations necessitates a truly multidimensional approach—one that unites effective medicines with prevention strategies tailored to specific vulnerabilities. The differential uptake of interventions among, say, young children and pregnant women indicates that policy must take local context into consideration such as specific epidemiological trends and the responsiveness of the health system.

Treatment initiatives must complement efforts directed at prevention so that, beyond the provision of antimalarial treatment regimens, correct utilization of means like ITNs and intermittent preventive therapy is guaranteed. The discrepancy between policy and practice might even require more inclusive training for clinicians and increased community participation to instill trust in these interventions. By doing this, treatment recommendations will be able to more effectively protect those most at risk for malaria's most devastating effects and ultimately enhance public health in the endemic regions. Including these local and demographic determinants in the global antimalarial plan is, in the majority of cases, necessary for long-term, disease control that is sustainable (Figure 7.3).

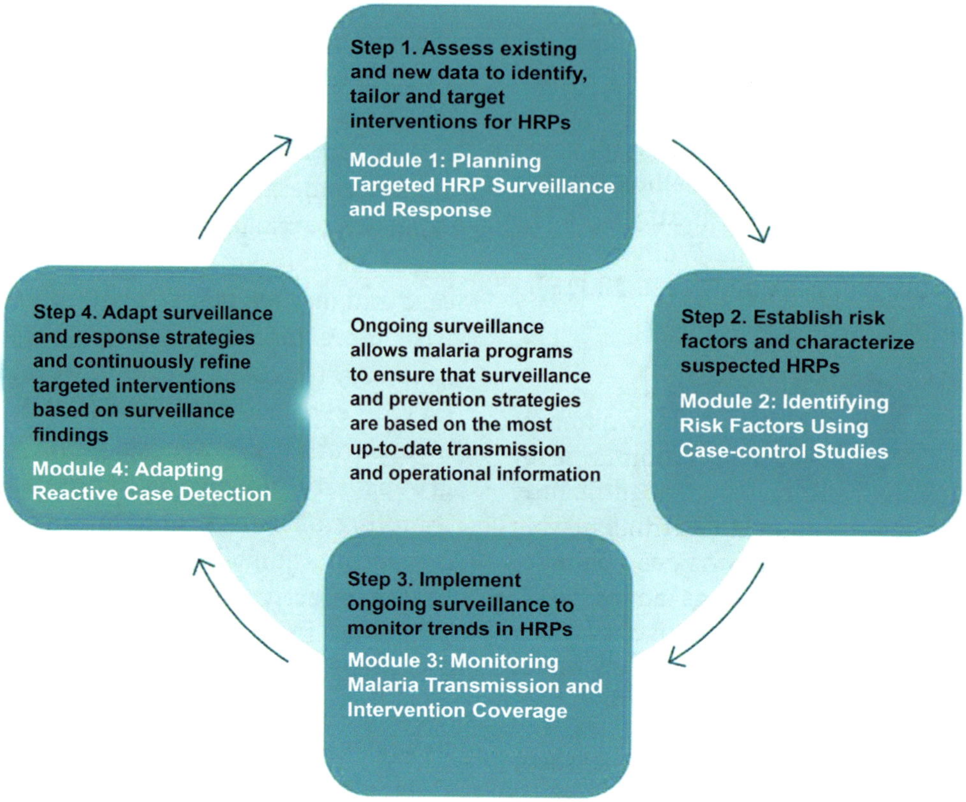

Figure 7.3. High-risk populations.

Source: Malaria Elimination Initiative. (n.d.). Surveillance and response HRP figure 1. *Shrinking the Malaria Map*. https://www.shrinkingthemalariamap.org/sites/default/files/images/our-work/surveillance-response-hrp-figure-1-crop.png.

7.1.3. Impact of Malaria on Public Health

Control of malaria is not a neat issue, it characterizes public health in most of the regions where *Plasmodium falciparum* is unrestrained. ACTs—those artemisinin-based combination treatments—brought enormous transformation by lowering death rates and cutting down malaria cases in general terms across the world. Nevertheless, a new twist has been introduced: artemisinin resistance, for the most part seen in the Greater Mekong Subregion, now insinuates itself and undermines our efforts at treatment. This advanced resistance inhibits the clearance of *parasites*, thus elevating both the risk of treatment failure and disease transmission. Health systems are subjected to further strain, necessitating more intense monitoring and an overhaul of how they manage cases. Besides the direct hit on health, prolonged illness undermines economies through costly care and lost workdays. It is crucial that we make these regimens effective if we are to sustain worldwide control of malaria and reduce health disparities (van der Pluijm et al., 2020). In Africa, the scenario has taken a foreboding twist—the artemisinin resistance spread and possible establishment loom big, especially given the continent's heavy malaria burden. The recent findings of Pfkelch13 mutations (those implicated in artemisinin resistance) arising independently in Rwanda highlight this threat. Though ACT cure rates are still high, these new mutations, which lead to delays in parasite clearance, offer a disconcerting indication that the effectiveness of treatment is declining, leading to rising failures and a return of cases. This makes public health efforts more complex and could roll back progress in preventing malaria illness and death. In most cases, it means there is a pressing need for more targeted surveillance and treatment recommendations that are aligned with local patterns of resistance. Also, the resistance may worsen existing health inequities, hitting hardest those who are already least able to access alternative treatments and good healthcare (Uwimana et al., 2020). Effectively keeping malaria at bay means a constant process of revising treatment policies to stay ahead of shifting resistance patterns. If we don't confront multidrug resistance head-on, we're facing more transmission of *parasites*, more deaths, and possibly even the collapse of control strategies that are working now. In most situations, the answer means adopting newer strategies, like triple artemisinin-based combinations, which can prolong the life of our current drugs and push back the onset of resistance. Of course, there remain challenges, from drug costs and adherence by patients to the challenge of identifying resistance hotspots early enough. In all, with stakes so high, it then becomes a necessity that global and regional policies come together in a bid to optimize antimalarial utilization, preserve drug effectiveness, and decrease the disease burden on populations as well as safeguard the hard-won gains in malaria control (van der Pluijm et al., 2020).

7.2. Mechanism of Action of Antimalarials

Antimalarial drugs depend on their chemistry under the surface, and it is precisely this that allows them to act effectively against various diseases. Consider HCQ, for example, it doesn't just fight malaria. In diseases like systemic lupus erythematosus (SLE), HCQ acts by disrupting such phenomena as lysosome function and autophagy, as well as modulating Toll-like receptor signaling and even altering the presentation of antigens. All these activities seem to decrease inflammation and soothe a stressed immune system. It can even decrease lipid levels and prevent clot risk, and so therapy regimens tend to prefer long-term use—apart from any warnings. As long as it's prescribed at the appropriate dose, HCQ is quite safe, albeit there's always the threat of retina issues (Dima et al., 2022). Technically, these action layers are the tip of an iceberg: such drugs, when employed to combat *parasites*, also can calm down overactive immune responses. Probing into how these drugs act on infections, one notices that they can rattle a pathogen's survival strategies inside our cells. Ancient drugs like chloroquine and hydroxychloroquine (HCQ) tend to build up in the acidic digestive vacuoles of the *Plasmodium* parasite, where they interfere with the detoxification pathway of heme, a poisonous by-product of hemoglobin degradation. In not being able to convert that poisonous heme into the virtually harmless hemozoin, the parasite is flooded with oxidative stress and dies. Typically, this means that targeting a very specific cell process can be the key to killing the interloper. Interestingly, these drugs have also shown antiviral prowess by cutting short how viruses like COVID-19 enter and make copies—presumably through interference with endosomal acidification and even glycosylation of viral proteins. All of this renders antimalarials rather useful and adaptable in treatment protocols (Guzik et al., 2020). As far as how antimalarials fit into treatment protocols, one has to truly honor their interactions at the molecular level and their impact at the body level. Overall, these drugs combine immune-modulating actions with their direct antiparasitic actions to deal with both the pathogen and the host's maybe overblown response. Physicians, in most cases, focus on getting the ideal dosage to derive the utmost benefit with a view to side effects—HCQ-induced retinopathy a prominent one. Having the exact knowledge of how these drugs work not only helps dosing but also guides measures to identify any adverse effects early in the process. As science keeps on improving, the better we get at understanding the complex mechanisms at play, the better we can harness antimalarials to address everything from malaria and autoimmune disease to new viral threats. Briefly, such knowledge is the basis for modern therapy regimens where such medications play a central role (Dima et al., 2022; Guzik et al., 2020) (Figure 7.4).

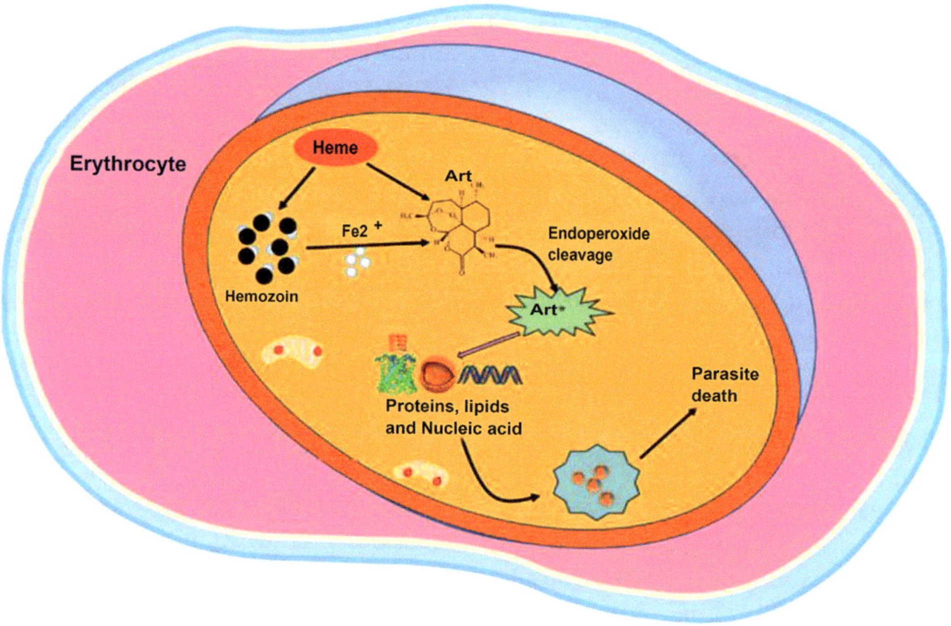

Figure 7.4. Antimalarial mechanisms.

Source: Zhang, Y., Wang, Y., Zhang, Y., & Li, X. (2024). Antimalarial mechanisms and resistance status of artemisinin and its derivatives. *Tropical Medicine and Infectious Disease, 9*(9), 223.

7.2.1. Types of Antimalarial Drugs

Treatment of malaria depends indeed on the right mix of drugs targeting the parasite at different phases in its life cycle. ACTs, for example, are widely used—these drugs combine fast-acting artemisinin derivatives with longer-acting companion drugs, generally speaking, to minimize the threat of resistance. One of the most widely used in this category is artemether-lumefantrine (AL), which is prized for its fast clearance of the parasite and broad safety. However, in most rural pharmacies where the lab tests are not necessarily ideal, AL is also prescribed with antibiotics, at least in part to protect against any potential bacterial infection. This is a practice that, while beneficial in mitigating indeterminate diagnoses, also indicates the fine line that physicians must balance in low-resource settings between complete care and not medicating excessively (Njozi et al., 2013). When thinking beyond ACTs, there are also other medications that have equally pivotal functions, especially against less common or drug-resistant pathogens. Chloroquine was once the first line, but since resistance has become widespread, it is now reserved for only certain species like *P. vivax* that are still sensitive. Meanwhile, quinoline drugs such as mefloquine and quinine are usually reserved for those cases that need an alternative approach, sometimes even a combination, to improve treatment outcomes. Also, drugs like sulfadoxine-pyrimethamine are valuable in intermittent prevention, especially in infants and pregnant women, because they last for a long time within the body. In every situation, proper diagnosis plays a critical role in picking the best drug since an off-target drug will lead to resistance issues and treatment failure. It is not necessarily the drugs themselves, however. The work of other interventions like the use of ITNs is vital on top of medications. For instance, ITNs have established their worth in reducing the prevalence of malaria in at-risk groups, under-five children in particular, , even if in some research their outcomes are modest reductions in parasite rates. As complementary measures, along with swift, effective drug regimens like those based on artemisinin, the benefit is more substantial with both severe disease and death rates declining in epidemic settings. This synergy of prevention and treatment, coupled with evolving clinical experience (Alexander et al., 2006), brings to the fore that the fight against malaria is not one silver bullet but a flexible, multifaceted campaign responding to circumstances on the ground.

7.2.2. How Antimalarials Target the Malaria Parasite

Malaria is no easy enemy—requires us to disrupt its life cycle at a few critical points. Therapies target the parasite in every stage, paying plenty of attention to the blood stage when symptoms are worst. Drugs such as artemisinin and its relatives attack quickly, triggering off reactive oxygen species which disrupt parasite proteins and membranes. Subsequently of course there is the idea of pairing these fast starters with more long-lasting drugs so that any stragglers are weeded out and some degree of protective effect is built in as well. Amazingly enough, some treatments even address gametocytes—the sexual stages that allow the parasite to hitch a ride to mosquitoes (Eckhoff et al., 2015). When you are covering the overt and the covert forms, you are left with a patchwork therapy that forms the basis of what we do today. Resistance is, in most cases, a stubborn obstacle. While artemisinin is potent, we are now experiencing pockets of *Plasmodium* that seem to evolve more, perhaps because they have changed their stress mechanisms or adjusted how they metabolize the drug. Researchers are now experimenting with new compounds that block parasite-specific enzymes—ones the pathogen needs whether it is idling in the liver or riding shotgun in the blood. Some of the new treatments even try to boost the body's immune push or impede the parasite's maturation inside mosquitoes. They also talk of recycling medicines for other illnesses or mixing resistance stoppers with our current medicines to add years onto their life. As a whole, the hybrid strategy—attacking the parasite on multiple fronts—is the only surefire way to remain ahead of resistance (Hobbs & Duffy, 2011). On the field, mass drug administration campaigns illustrate how that strategy works in reality. Experimentation modeling the distribution of drugs like artemether, lumefantrine, and primaquine through the body shows that administering these drugs to nearly all people and sustaining them is crucial where malaria spreads like fire. Those partner drugs that persist provide a shield against a re-infection that is likely to occur, while primaquine, which is famous for its gametocyte breaking ability, is typically mixed in to break the chain of transmission. But one genuine drawback is that if you only treat those with overt symptoms, many infections may slip through the gap—leaving behind silent reservoirs of the parasite. And so, rather than just curing the obviously sick, large drug campaigns are likely to be needed in order to truly push towards malaria control and ultimate eradication (Eckhoff et al., 2015). In the majority of instances, aligning how a drug acts with the manner it is distributed is essential to gaining control of the parasite population (Figure 7.5).

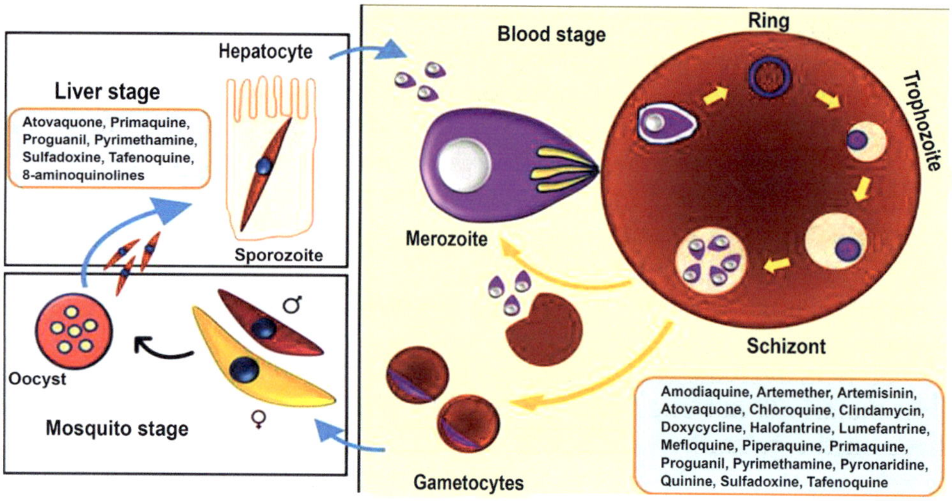

Figure 7.5. Antimalarials targeting the parasite's life cycle.

Source: Tripathi, H., Bhalerao, P., Singh, S., & Bhatt, T. K. (2023). Antimalarials targeting the parasite's life cycle. In Malaria therapeutics: are we close enough? *Parasites & Vectors.*

7.2.3. Resistance Mechanisms in Malaria

Malaria treatment is a challenging game, largely because the *Plasmodium parasites* keep switching stratigies. These pathogens adapt in unexpected ways, making it hard for antimalarial drugs to stick around. Back when chloroquine and sulfadoxine-pyrimethamine were in heavy use, things went awry as resistance issues started cropping up. Human beings eventually found that gene changes in *parasites*, like pfmdr1 and *pfcrt* for chloroquine, and *dhfr* and *dhps* modifications for sulfadoxine-pyrimethamine—were behind most of the fault. These mutations interfere with how the drugs work, and therefore treatments start to fail and more patients are infected. This is even more troubling when pfk13 gene mutations begin to emerge since that indicates that resistance can become a threat to artemisinin-based therapies, our frontline option now. Mostly, tracking these genetic markers is necessary for updating treatment guidelines and keeping malaria control on track (Fitri et al., 2023). Drug resistance, however, is not merely a matter of individual indiscriminate gene changes—rather, it is an entire complex web woven around drug behavior, parasite features, and even how people use these drugs. Abuse and overdose of antimalarial drugs have hastened its spread, so much so that compliance with treatment schedules and regular checks on the efficacy of drugs become very essential. Typically, the parasite subverts its own mechanisms, altering drug transport and metabolism so that either the drug does not accumulate where it is needed or the target itself is modified. Because of this indiscriminate adaptability, new drugs are called for, among them plant-derived natural product-derived drugs that bring a varied chemical profile. Other scientists, in particular, are turning to emerging technologies like AI and computer-aided drug design to identify new antimalarial compounds that are safe and effective (Thomford et al., 2018). It is a nasty, dynamic enterprise, but these combination methods seem to be key to remaining one step ahead of the developing resistance issues. Combining molecular surveillance in the future with cutting-edge drug development methods will help combat malaria resistance. Using predictive computer simulations and high-throughput screens, scientists can scan both natural products and synthetic compounds to find those that might work against drug-resistant bacteria—separating the gems from a haystack of potential candidates. Scientists can quickly screen the performance of potential drugs in the body using these tools, weeding out dead ends. Treatment guidelines are being modified as resistance patterns change, keeping treatments effective for most individuals. Sustained investment in these research areas, accompanied by public health interventions that focus on the wise utilization of drugs, represents an elastic counterresponse to the parasite's adaptability. Overall, this multidimensional effort allows the global effort toward the eradication of malaria to continue, despite the presence of drug-resistant *Plasmodium* as a refractory challenge (Thomford et al., 2018; Fitri et al., 2023) (Figure 7.6).

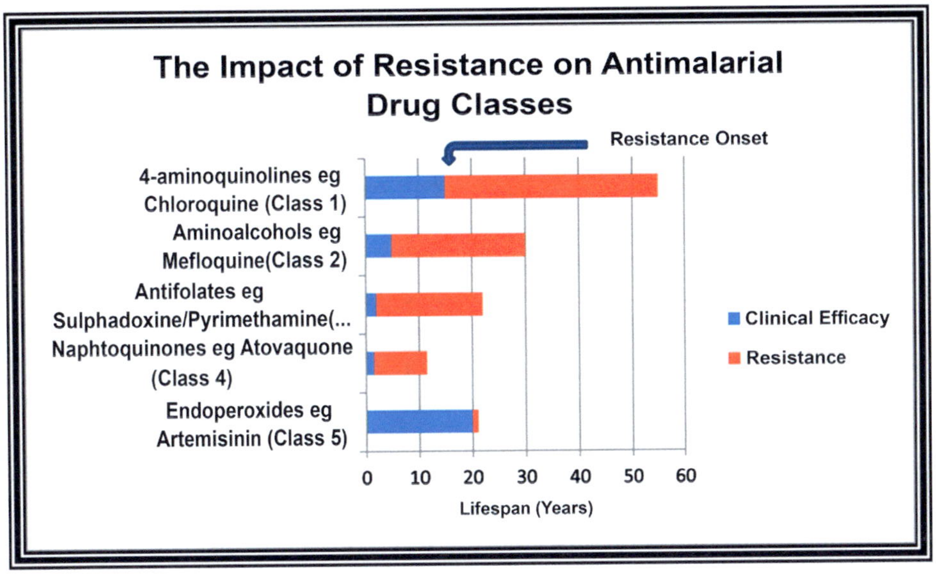

Figure 7.6. Resistance mechanisms in malaria.

Source: Uzondu, S., Echezona, A., Nwagwu, C., Onugwu, A., Ugorji, L., Agbo, C., ... Attama, A. (2023). Combating Antimalarial Drug Resistance: Recent Advances and Future Perspectives. IntechOpen. doi: 10.5772/intechopen.106507

7.3. Treatment Guidelines for Malaria

Not only does successful control of malaria take more than a stash of antimalarial medicines, but it also depends on a treatment regimen that fits the situation. The patients need to be treated to fit what they have, and that needs to be guided by the local pattern of the disease's incidence. You can't ignore how information on mosquito behavior and the spread of malaria plays into prevention and treatment options. In most of the malaria-endemic zones, public education efforts have been found to show that people often fail to realize entirely that mosquitoes drive transmission or why insecticide-treated net use is so important. Even if overall awareness is not high, the fact that large numbers of people are still using these nets indicates that smart, targeted education can improve malaria control. Spreading quick treatment with ongoing knowledge regarding the insects and their actions might slow cases and fatalities of malaria, especially among the youngest, for example, children younger than five (Ruberto et al., 2014). Progress over past years has started to shift diagnostic potential into evolving treatment approaches, and therefore evidence-based decisions more vital than ever before. There was a time when a fever in a region with high malaria meant doctors scrambled for antimalarial drugs without question—an act that was perhaps thought to be safe but resulted in unneeded drug use and even fostering the possibility of drug resistance. Nowadays, though with ACTs being more potent, individuals are also now worried about the expense and the side effects of using too many drugs. Some studies, for example, suggest that it is wiser and safer in general to reserve these drugs for patients with a definite diagnosis—either by microscopy or quick tests. Using trials like these to guide treatment not only saves resources and reduces the burden on drugs (i.e., limiting side effects) but also allows public health systems to stick to sustainable practices (Njama-Meya et al., 2007). That is, excellent diagnostic criteria built into treatment protocols create a more judicious use of antimalarials. In the meantime, treatment regimens will have to coexist with local variation in the transmission of malaria and drug resistance of *parasites*. Urban settings can be very unlike rural ones in transmission levels, access to healthcare, and day-to-day routine in the populations, so there has to be some space for policy flexibility. Where malaria does not hit as harshly, it is critically important to confirm a diagnosis before starting treatment to not needlessly give extra medicine. But where the disease advances rapidly, acting swiftly—frequently relying on clinical acumen supplemented by quick tests—may be essential in order to avoid advanced progress. And tracking how well these drugs continue to work means treatment regimens can be modified on an ongoing basis so frontline medicines haven't diminished in their effectiveness. Together, with effective diagnostic facilities coupled with local education and continuous monitoring forming the very essence of contemporary malaria treatment strategies, they do work efficiently towards improving patient and overall public health outcomes.

7.3.1. World Health Organization (WHO) Recommendations

Medical treatment protocols must be reconsidered constantly as fresh evidence emerges—particularly when sudden global health emergencies strike. The WHO has been at the forefront of things, developing guidance for treating infections by proposing that antiviral drugs be combined with anti-inflammatory choices when the time is right. Think about scenarios where the body's own immune system overreacts unintentionally (you know, a cytokine storm) and makes things worse; sometimes antivirals just don't work. That's why researchers have looked into adding drugs such as HCQ with their capacity to modulate immunological effects. Of course, they suggest a careful, profession-guided approach because the side effects and overall performance of such procedures can be rather varied. Overall, this type of interspecialty cooperation ensures that patient treatment is both evidence-based and personalized to treat other complications in more complex cases (Soy et al., 2020). Health officials around the globe, including WHO, keep reminding us that medical guidelines have to be flexible enough to adjust themselves with incoming sets of data, especially in situations involving susceptible groups like pregnant women. Their recommendations come with some precautions and measures meant to protect the mother-to-be and the unborn child from epidemics. They promote vigilant supervision by way of diagnostic imaging, regular monitoring of maternal respiration, and a judicious hand in interventions to balance benefits over risks. If antimalarial drugs are added to the regimen, these guidelines challenge the clinicians to critically look at the way such drugs interact with pregnant bodies and whether they are safe for use. In all but a few cases, the WHO's requirement of team-based, patient-centered practice shows their commitment to care that not only attacks the virus head-on but also deals with the secondary response of the immune system (Poon et al., 2020). Beyond simply defining what medication to use, the WHO also focuses on prevention practices within healthcare facilities in an attempt to keep the infections from being spread as treatments are given. They emphasize the proper use of personal protective equipment, effective mechanisms of triaging patients, and the upkeep of isolation protocols for the protection of both healthcare workers and patients. These protocols provide for the safe dispensation of treatments, such as antimalarial therapies—in supervised settings. In addition, the corporation recommends continuous monitoring of any new, or even recycled, drugs through solid clinical trials before their full approval. Together, these careful steps constitute a balanced system attempting to address future infectious threats with new therapy but never at the expense of patient safety and evidence-based treatment (Poon et al., 2020; Soy et al., 2020) (Figure 7.7).

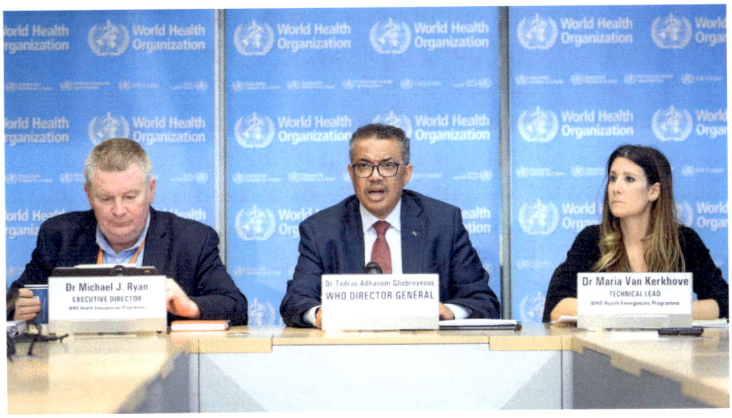

Figure 7.7. World Health Organization (WHO) recommendations.

Source: Getty Images. (2020). Photograph of a person wearing a face mask. *NPR*. https://external-content.duckduckgo.com/iu/?u=https%3A%2F%2Fmedia.npr.org%2Fassets%2Fimg%2F2020%2F04%2F28%2Fgettyimages-1205434458_wide-88c12f724fe1d1de29be56e6a47782f93eb7eed6-s1400-c100.jpg&f=1&nofb=1&ipt=ea2c7e6b16826904b1c80d7ae7d8c50625289b80aacb4e318e9050b074b385cc.

7.3.2. Regional Variations in Treatment Protocols

Malaria treatment is not one-size-fits-all. Breakouts in certain areas and the health systems' organization can turn things upside down big time. In certain places where malaria just refuses to quit, such as regions of sub-Saharan Africa or Southeast Asia—doctors have to consider what *Plasmodium* species are calling the shots, what drug resistance is like locally, and even whether they have the equipment to even diagnose it. Take *P. falciparum*, for example; this nuisance, which is usually guilty of the most severe, is likely to react differently to medication depending on the area, so treatment needs to be attuned to the local environment. Not everyone is in a position to receive intravenous artesunate—the preferred treatment for worst cases—either; while its recent FDA approval in the United States has been helpful, many resource-poor nations lag far behind.

And in fact, how people locally and those who travel there stick to their habits ultimately puts attention on what measures affect the local pain areas (Mace et al., 2022). Having access to real tests and treatments decides how malaria is handled country by country, especially if you overlap richer over poorer areas. WHO's priority diagnostics list reveals that there is a big gap to obtain rapid, accurate malaria tests which are crucial to decide on the right treatment. In most low-resource settings, primary care has too limited a range of tests and hence cannot determine which parasite is causing the infection or whether it is drug-sensitive or not; this can lead to suboptimal treatment choices and may also raise resistance levels. In addition to that, there isn't an even spread of labs and trained personnel, so in certain areas, physicians just have to make do with guessing the appropriate action. New diagnostic technology and even telemedicine could fill some of those gaps, but funding and unstable governance often get in the way. Generally, how treatments differ by region is not only about the pathogens themselves, it is indicative of larger healthcare inequalities (Fleming et al., 2021). From a policy and financial perspective, the story becomes more complex. Wealthy countries tend to update their treatment protocols quickly and make newer antimalarials and IV within financial reach. Meanwhile, the majority of low- and middle-income nations are not able to buy the right drugs, cope with supply chain shortages, and most importantly, afford the treatments needed, so the recommendations necessarily are selectively applied. Take intravenous artesunate: though it is the gold standard in the United States for complicated malaria, its roll-out in malaria-endemic countries hinges on stable funding and health systems still finding their footing. National policy is likely to borrow a lot from global guidelines, but they are likely to need adjusting to the local setup—slowing down the pace of a seamless rollout. Initiatives like capacity building and international collaborations must take into account such economic and infrastructural shortcomings if they are genuinely interested in alleviating the global burden of malaria (Fleming et al., 2021; Mace et al., 2022).

7.3.3. Role of Diagnostic Testing in Treatment Decisions

In day-to-day clinical practice, cutaneous lupus erythematosus (CLE) and SLE management largely relies on sound diagnostic acumen, it is not always one test that propels the diagnosis. At times, a combination of a patient's history, a physical examination by hand, and certain laboratory investigations offers the complete picture. For instance, the detection of autoantibodies like anti-Ro/SSA, anti-La/SSB, anti-dsDNA, and anti-Sm helps identify different CLE subsets and detect any systemic pointers. This interplay of laboratory findings usually guides clinicians on the level of treatment, sometimes forcing them towards systemic therapy, like antimalarials. Most commonly, correlation of tests with how the disease presents indeed achieves that ideal balance in treatment—steering clear of over- or under-treatment (O'Kane et al., 2021). Even somewhat later on, these diagnostic bites can inform later adjustments as the clinical picture shifts. Switching gears slightly, treatment plans depend on clear outcome measures to assess how aggressive the disease is and whether a treatment works or not. The CLASI, or CLE Disease Area and Severity Index, is helpful to measure severity of lesions and pick up on changes longitudinally. Using tools like CLASI-50 or CLASI-20 has a tendency to mean treatment will potentially have to shift—whether that is starting anew, staying on the same track, or changing course altogether (O'Kane et al., 2021). On the whole, using these figures brings accuracy to the treatment regimen and paves the way for more tailored care, especially when dealing with medications like HCQ or even combination therapies. In addition to laboratory procedures and scorecards, the more in-depth diagnostic tests play an important role in mapping out the treatment—particularly in those challenging cases when drug-induced lupus would be confused with its idiopathic form. Because CLE subtypes can be so vastly different and sometimes mix with systemic conditions, the findings from the diagnostic testing make it clear whether the use of systemic corticosteroids, immunosuppressants, or biologics would be the appropriate choice. It is also important to determine other illness and risk factors, like antimalarial retinopathy, which then affects how intensely patients should be followed and counseled. Directives tend to nudge clinicians toward a more team-based approach as well—linking dermatologic, rheumatologic, and even psycho- logic findings—to produce an expanded view of care. All these compounded factors, on the basis of extensive diagnostic effort, eventually optimize treatment plan and resource utilization, further reiterating how essential these tests remain in the treatment of existing CLE and SLE cases (O'Kane et al., 2021) (Figure 7.8).

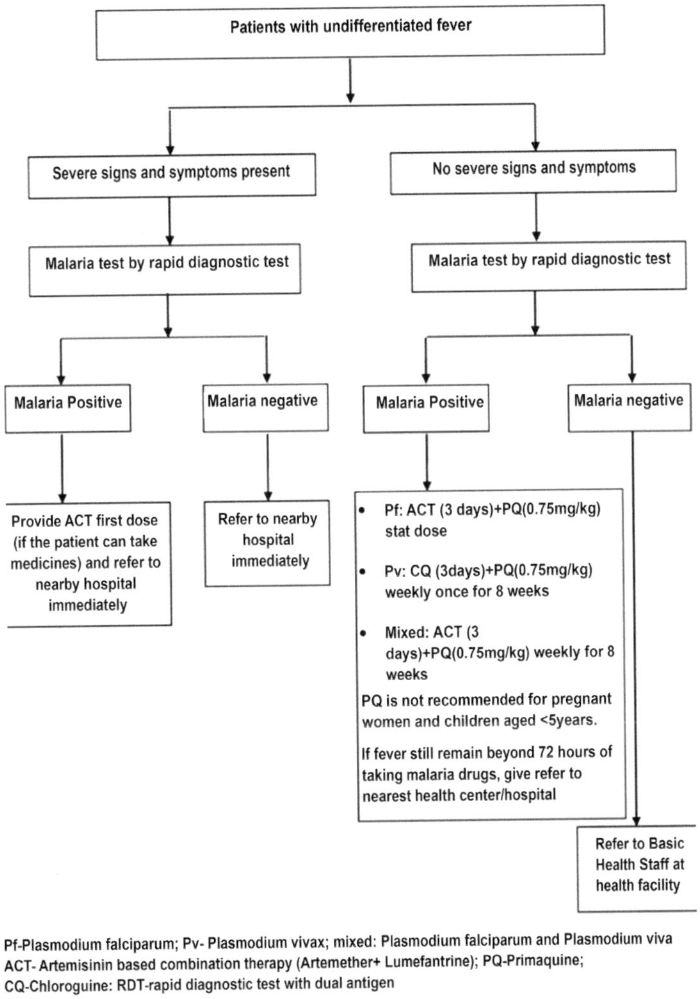

Figure 7.8. Role of diagnostic testing in treatment decisions for malaria.

Source: Linn, N. Y. Y., Tripathy, J. P., Maung, T. M., Maw, L. Y. W., Lin, Z., Thi, A., et al. (2018). Malaria testing, diagnosis, and treatment services provided by village health volunteer in Myanmar, 2017. In How are the village health volunteers delivering malaria testing and treatment services and what are the challenges they are facing? A mixed methods study in Myanmar. *Tropical Medicine and Health, 46,* Article 28.

7.4. First-Line Antimalarial Treatments

To treat malaria, we need to act fast and decisively if we are to curtail both disease and death, especially in areas where the disease is out of control. Doctors usually turn to options like HCQ and chloroquine, drugs that have been trusted for decades against a variety of *Plasmodium* species. HCQ, for instance, might be favored because it's generally linked to fewer issues in the eyes (retinopathy is a concern with chloroquine). Interestingly, these medications, once designed to fend off infection, are now also effective weapons against *parasites* persisting in red blood cells (RBCs). It is also worth noting that adherence to chemoprophylaxis regimens is imperative—if one falls behind on doses, treatment can fail and even contribute to additional imported cases among travelers frequenting endemic locations (Mace et al., 2022). For the most part, the right dose, timing, and choice of drug according to each patient's profile and local resistance patterns remain critical. Historically, antimalarial drugs have always been defined by their new mechanisms of action and differing side-effect profiles, which for the most part dictate their use in first-line treatment regimens. Clinical tests indicate that HCQ not only clears *parasites* effectively but also works to ease the inflammation so many victims of malaria suffer. It essentially disrupts lysosomal function, making it harder for the parasite to breed inside host cells. Updated guidelines now urge practitioners to also observe resistance markers, a necessary shift when strains like *Plasmodium falciparum* start resisting the older drugs. For managing severe malaria, the move towards the administration of intravenous artesunate—because it can clear the *parasites* rapidly and improve survival—is a quantum leap. Taken together, these changes reflect a general movement towards evidence-based practice that seeks to balance the efficacy of a drug with how safe it proves to be (Mace et al., 2022). Besides merely punching out *parasites*, these frontline antimalarial agents have some interesting immunomodulatory maneuvers that add to their overall usefulness. HCQ, for example, is also utilized very commonly in conditions like CLE, in which it seems to dial down inflammatory responses by modulating immune cell function and cytokine production. Such a two-pronged action not only cements its status as a frontline treatment against malaria but also makes it a top drug of choice for treatment of systemic inflammation. Of course, clinicians should balance such advantages against risks such as retinal toxicity, which's why, in the event of treatment extending over longer durations, regular eye check-ups become an absolute necessity. Overall, the inclusion of these antimalarials in treatment policy, along with ongoing efforts to maximize doses, curtail resistance, and improve patient compliance, illustrates just how useful they remain in the fight against malaria.

7.4.1. Artemisinin-Based Combination Therapies (ACTs)

Malaria treatment has improved considerably in recent times—old drugs just weren't cutting it with growing resistance. One of the biggest differences is the widespread use of ACTs, which can get rid of *Plasmodium falciparum* very quickly and don't have problems with resistance. With a combination of an artemisinin derivative and a companion drug, not only do the *parasites* get killed quite quickly, but they also keep them in check for a longer period—a lifesaver when infections strike so fast. Global policies now generally start with ACTs because of their clear impact on preventing disease and death. This approach is supported by other malaria control measures like ITNs and rapid diagnostic tests and shows that drugs and vector control do indeed need to be integrated (Alexander et al., 2006). It is not always smooth sailing in the implementation of ACTs despite its proven value. Where healthcare arrangements are fluid and commercial providers shoulder the lion's share of their work, tracking what antimalarials (and ACTs) are sold and moved around becomes an extremely big thing to keep fake or second-rate medicines from dominating the market. Research that digs into wholesalers and retailers sales volumes reminds us time and again how crucial it is to get an accurate reading of the market's fluctuations. Such methods as using provider recall and retail audits are key to streamlining the supply chain and making policy changes as needed. Effective market monitoring ultimately helps ensure drug quality and supply remain on track, which in most cases is key to keeping public trust high in treatment programs (Goodman et al., 2013).

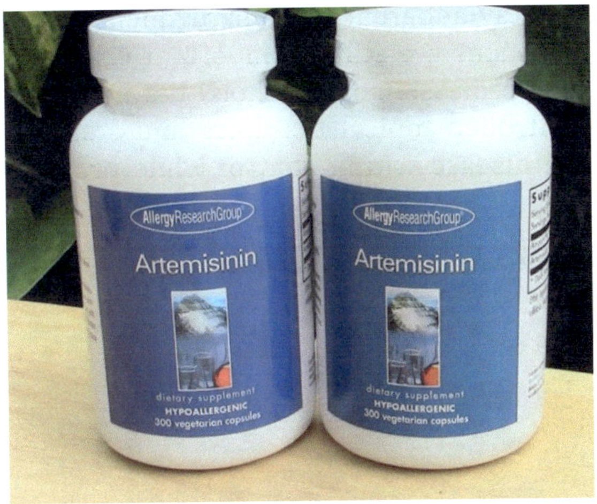

Figure 7.9. Artemisinin-based combination therapies (ACTs).

Source: Wixstatic. (n.d.). *Untitled image.* https://external-content.duckduckgo.com/iu/?u=https%3A%2F%2Fstatic.wixstatic.com%2Fmedia%2F5a1c23_0c6a4c7c3ba248dd8af264c9d64dabc3~mv2.jpg%2Fv1%2Ffill%2Fw_800%2Ch_645%2Cal_c%2Cq_85%2F5a1c23_0c6a4c7c3ba248dd8af264c9d64dabc3~mv2.jpg&f=1&nofb=1&ipt=e4e0cfa6f5401b4ab4073350da190802b83c39af9d3fdbf97f565f637410a2f3.

Coming up with the right ACTs to pair with local malaria patterns is ultimately crucial to getting them to work effectively. Shifts in transmission and resistance patterns necessitate the advice on which drugs to use as a partner sometimes to shift from one area to another. And there is also a huge focus on most vulnerable populations, like under-five children, who are most affected—ensuring that advice reaches those at risk. Research even shows that while products like ITNs might not reduce malaria cases dramatically by themselves, they do seem to add on to the overall protection if used along with antimalarial medications in endemic regions. Overall, incorporating ACTs into a broader malaria control strategy—one with routine monitoring, timely policy responses, and successful community involvement—remains key to keeping drugs effective and cutting the disease's burden (Alexander et al., 2006) (Figure 7.9).

7.4.2. Efficacy and Safety of First-Line Treatments

Managing CLE is not so much a question of terms – it is a matter of identifying which variant is present and whether the remainder of the body is involved. Doctors typically start with antimalarial drugs – for example, HCQ is a typical choice , and trials typically report that skin manifestations typically improve in around 16 weeks or so, with around half or better of the patients improving. Obviously, even though HCQ is usually less harsh on the system than other options, there is always the unpleasant danger of harm to the eyes (especially when the dose is excessive or one takes it in the long term); because of this alone, the typical advice is not to use more than about 5 mg per kilogram of real body weight per day. In the majority of recommendations, HCQ serves as a backbone therapy, frequently supplemented with potent topical corticosteroids or calcineurin inhibitors in a bid to maximize results but limit whole-body exposure (O'Kane et al., 2021; Worm et al., 2021). Apart from those systemic antimalarials, doctors also count on systemic corticosteroids

, particularly if the CLE is acute or disseminating in appearance or simply needs to be treated urgently. Generally, the patient is started on a moderate dose of oral glucocorticoids that is tapered down; this is extremely effective in suppressing inflammation, though with long-term usage arising complications like osteoporosis or adrenal suppression. Owing to these complications, many regimens suggest tapering the use of steroids or even using steroids only for the duration of tapering the antimalarial dose. Furthermore, topical treatments (e.g., powerful steroid ointments and calcineurin inhibitors) remain predominant in managing localized flare-ups, and calcineurin inhibitors are increasingly the treatment of choice for facial lesions owing to the reason that they lower the risk of thinned skin. All these methods cumulatively highlight a strategy aiming at reconciling solid treatment effect with the overall safety of the patient (O'Kane et al., 2021; Worm et al., 2021). When HCQ alone is not enough, some suggestions are aimed at combining antimalarial therapy with other agents. For example, the inclusion of a drug such as mepacrine, which has a different safety profile, can sometimes enhance treatment success, although it also has unusual risks such as aplastic anemia that require close supervision. It is also to be remembered that it is usually not possible to combine HCQ and chloroquine since combining them raises the risk of retinal complications. Most specialists today prefer customizing the dose to the patient, with the experts insisting that patients must be well-educated on how to stay adherent to their regimens and the potential hazards of taking the medication. Routine eye exams are still an important component of this safety net, fitting neatly into guidelines from eye professionals. In short, the application of antimalarials as the foundation—backed by well-controlled topical therapies and steroids—represents a harmonious strategy aimed at keeping the disease within control while protecting long-term health (O'Kane et al., 2021; Worm et al., 2021) (Figure 7.10).

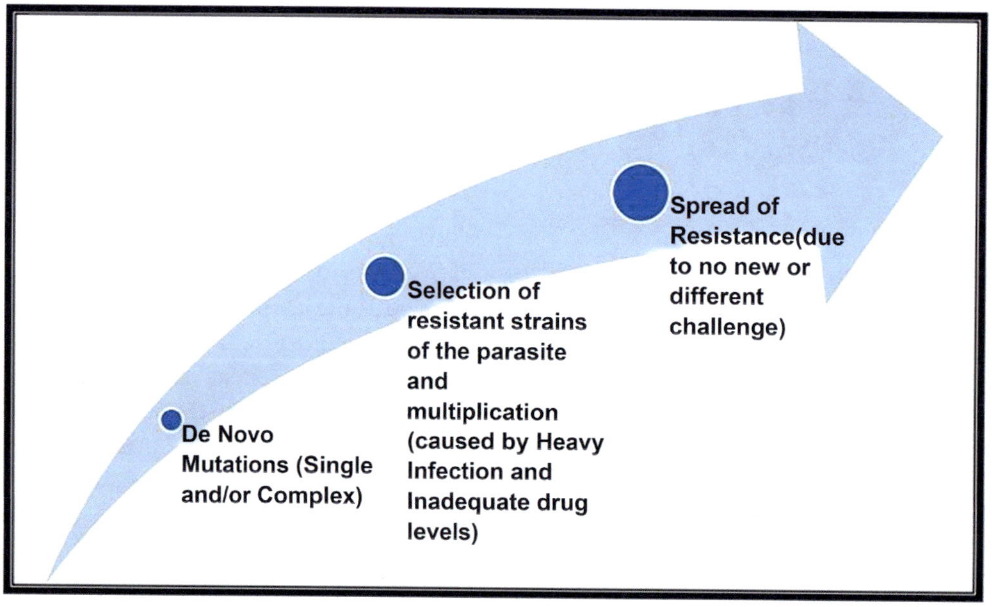

Figure 7.10. Efficacy and safety of first-line treatments for patients.

Source: Uzondu, S., Echezona, A., Nwagwu, C., Onugwu, A., Ugorji, L., Agbo, C., ... Attama, A. (2023). Combating Antimalarial Drug Resistance: Recent Advances and Future Perspectives. IntechOpen. doi: 10.5772/intechopen.106507

7.4.3. Considerations for Special Populations

Pregnant women have a bit of an extra obstacle in their fight against malaria. Their bodies, for a variety of reasons, are more vulnerable to the disease, with options like anemia, low birth weight, and even pre-terms coming up. The usual approach—embracing stratigies like intermittent preventive therapy and insecticide-treated bed nets, often fails to get put into action, some locations suggest. Evidence has pointed out that the actions that are taken and that are recommended in antenatal consultations can be very different from one another, with expectant mothers far from enough receiving those preventive antimalarials or sleeping under bed nets as often as they need to (Wylie et al., 2010). This discrepancy generally means that policies need an overhaul and that both healthcare workers and pregnant women can benefit from more definitive, more effective guidance to lower the risk of sickness and mortality. Children, particularly those below the age of five, are another group that simply can't be addressed with blanket malaria guidelines. Their immune systems are still maturing, so they can get knocked hard affecting often resulting in severe forms such as cerebral malaria. Due to that, it is very crucial to receive diagnoses quickly and to scale down medication dosages to suit their tiny bodies. In the majority of low-resource settings, where fancy lab tests like microscopy are unavailable, rapid diagnostic tests (RDTs) work as a good alternative. These diagnostic tests help in commencing treatment earlier, and the optimal formulation and dose for minor patients is crucial to avoid side effects (Long, 2009). Those with other medical complications or weakened immune systems add another level of complexity to treat malaria. HIV, malnutrition, or blood disorders can alter the way drugs act within the body, usually requiring adjustments in the dose and closer observation of patients for interactions or toxic side effects. In general, antimalarial choice is not only a matter of curing the infection but also of not making an underlying condition worse. Treatments for these cases need to be close and individualized with the patient's whole health picture in mind. Generally, this kind of tailored care not only aims to eliminate the malaria parasite but safeguard the patient's overall well-being.

7.5. Second-Line and Alternative Treatments

When conventional therapies like antimalarials and topical creams just don't work for cutaneous lupus, doctors generally have to switch tack and attempt another strategy. Methotrexate, for example, has been found to be of help in most CLE cases—most noticeably the discoid and subacute types, with patients generally experiencing significant improvement whether they take the medication orally or by a subcutaneous injection, sometimes combined with antimalarials. It must be remembered that methotrexate needs close monitoring of liver, kidney, and blood cell function, and that addition of folic acid is usually recommended to keep side effects in check. While pediatric data are somewhat limited, this choice still has its value in refractory cases by reducing reliance on corticosteroids and their long-term consequences (Worm et al., 2021). Essentially, individualizing the plan to the severity and tolerance of the patient's disease is essential, and thus close clinical observation forms part of the therapeutic process. With the exception of methotrexate, mycophenolate mofetil has also emerged as another reliable second-line treatment for the resistant cases of CLE in which the first-line treatments prove insufficient. Clinical practice has shown that it works alone or even in conjunction with antimalarials in controlling cutaneous symptoms as well as quelling systemic inflammation. Although originally licensed in transplant recipients, mounting evidence is now available for its application in autoimmune dermatoses like lupus nephritis and CLE. Its side effects are typically minor—mostly a bit of gastrointestinal distress, but regular laboratory work is necessary to pick up any early signs of blood or liver issues. For the majority, this approach is in line with current recommendations that recommend mycophenolate mofetil as a suitable second-line treatment, without the huge cumulative toxicity of prolonged corticosteroids (O'Kane et al., 2021).

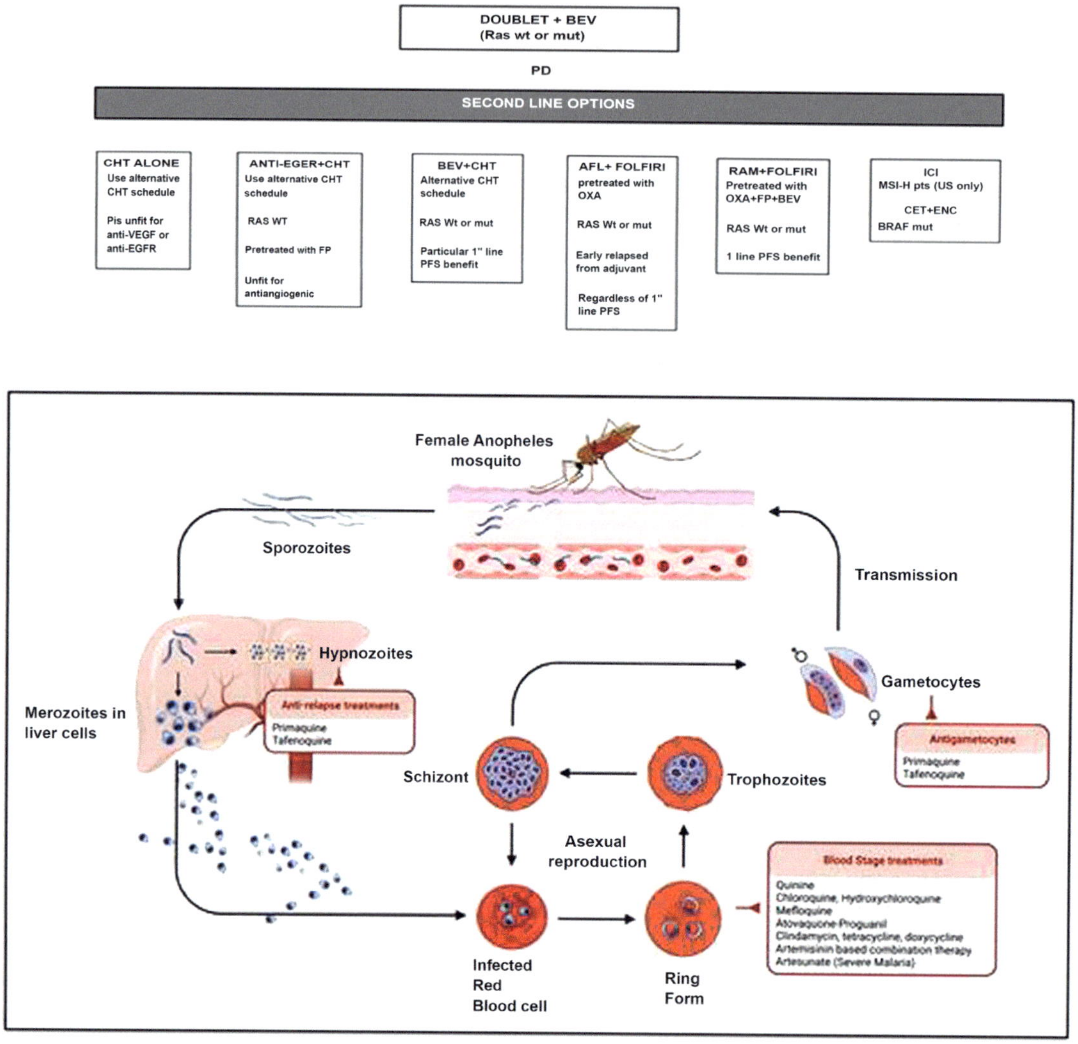

Figure 7.11. Second-line and alternative treatments for malaria.

Source: Alaithan H, Kumar N, Islam MZ, Liappis AP, Nava VE. Novel Therapeutics for Malaria. *Pharmaceutics*. 2023; 15(7):1800. https://doi.org/10.3390/pharmaceutics15071800

When neither first-line nor second-line treatment provides adequate relief, there are alternatives such as retinoids, dapsone, and thalidomide that can be used to manage difficult CLE. Retinoids—a good example being acitretin—are effective, especially for scarring or hyperkeratotic discoid lupus lesions, but concern for causing birth defects generally precludes their use in females of childbearing potential. Dapsone has been found to be effective for subacute CLE and even bullous forms, but with further caution and regular blood checks to avoid complications like hemolytic anemia or methemoglobinemia. Subsequently there's thalidomide, of course, with its very powerful anti-inflammatory effect; although useful in refractory disease, it is also surrounded by risks like peripheral neuropathy and thromboembolic episodes, so stringent patient selection and monitoring (as well as rigorous avoidance of pregnancy measures) are the answer. Even though these treatments are not necessarily the most common choices, they are still valuable tools in the fight against refractory cutaneous lupus, showing how complicated treatment of recalcitrant disease can be and how a tailored plan of treatment is needed (O'Kane et al., 2021; Worm et al., 2021) (Figure 7.11).

7.5.1. Overview of Second-Line Antimalarials

It is in those instances where the artemisinin-based combination therapies just won't cut it—either they are simply not effective or cannot be used because of such issues as drug intolerance or pregnancy, which the second-line antimalarials are used. It is not unheard of for resistance issues or individual patient factors to require a regimen switch. Historically, drugs like quinine and mefloquine were the standard second choices. Quinine, normally given by injection for severe cases, has been mostly replaced by IV artesunate because, quite simply, artesunate works better and is safer. This change to artesunate generally tracks global updates to treatment guidelines designed to enhance patient outcomes and decrease mortality (Mace et al., 2021). In short, these second-line therapies are a vital safety net that enables clinicians to stay flexible as malaria evolves. The switch to these reserve medications typically takes place only after it becomes apparent that the initial treatment has failed or drug resistance becomes a growing worry—not just in malaria-endemic nations but even in travelers who return to malaria-non-endemic regions (Mace et al., 2021). Molecular assays often reveal that mutations in *Plasmodium falciparum* render drugs like chloroquine, sulfadoxine-pyrimethamine, and even mefloquine less effective as a starting point. Therefore, guidelines for treatment today also push clinicians to alter therapy if signs of resistance develop or if a patient starts to deteriorate after being started on the default treatment. This flexible strategy, sometimes a bit arbitrary, underscores the need for clinicians to be aware and alert so that the reserve drugs are wisely used to prevent treatment failures as well as other complications. Notwithstanding the recognized role of second-line antimalarials, their effective use nonetheless hinges on the extent to which providers are conversant with the treatment regimens and also the local patterns of resistance. Awareness, according to research, may vary—physicians are more sensitized to such regimens compared to pharmacists and other allied health professionals (Ayogu et al., 2020). That discrepancy could delay the institution of the proper alternative treatment, which might be lifesaving in the setting of severe malaria that warrants prompt intervention. Apart from that, treatment selection is not a one-size-fits-all affair; factors such as a patient's age, pregnancy, and travel history could all be brought to bear on a drug's efficacy and safety. Collectively, these complexities underpin an ongoing need for updated education and diligent surveillance to guide decision-making based on best evidence, with the ultimate outcome being more effective malaria control programs and improved patient outcomes (Ayogu et al., 2020; Mace et al., 2021).

7.5.2. Situations Requiring Alternative Treatments

Doctors start by seeing the individual patient rather than just ticking off on established protocols.

Not all cases fit tidily in a box. Some patients, for example, have genetic characteristics like G6PD deficiency, and you would similarly find most malaria-endemic regions to have many such patients, and that risk means it is a no-go to administer drugs like primaquine (an oxidative antimalarial) because of the danger of causing hemolytic anemia. At the same time, innate cardiovascular disease will steer the choice away from certain medications notorious for driving cardiac toxicity beyond the norm. All of these factors, in large part, point to the need for treatment regimens that integrate genetic testing with routine clinical assessment to continue to be effective while remaining safe, especially for susceptible persons (Roper et al., 2020). The way a drug is processed through a patient's body—pharmacokinetics and pharmacodynamics, we say—is another order of issue. Take pregnant women as a case in point: changes in the way drugs are metabolized and a small but actual teratogenic risk necessitate doctors to make substitute decisions that are recognized as safer for the fetus. Similarly, if a person is afflicted with liver or kidney problems, there would be another dose or even a different drug required to reverse toxicity from drug accumulation. Subsequently there is resistance to drugs; when malaria has become resistant to older medications like chloroquine or sulfadoxine-pyrimethamine, the rational response is often to ACTs or some of the new drugs, this dynamic approach balances lab results with field observations quite well (Guzik et al., 2020). Mixed infections or simply awful cases of malaria throw even more unpredictable variables into the mix. Where there is more than one *Plasmodium* species involved, one drug is seldom as effective, driving physicians to combination therapy or broad-spectrum treatment. In extreme situations, where rapid action is necessary and oral medication may be threatened by bad absorption, an IV form usually moves into the limelight. Patients with compromised immune function or multiple underlying conditions tend to have a highly variable course, so treatment is all the more uncertain (Guzik et al., 2020; Roper et al., 2020) (Figure 7.12). For most patients, the guidelines thus emphasize the need to remain adaptable and to have alternatives in reserve with which to approach these dynamic clinical enigmas.

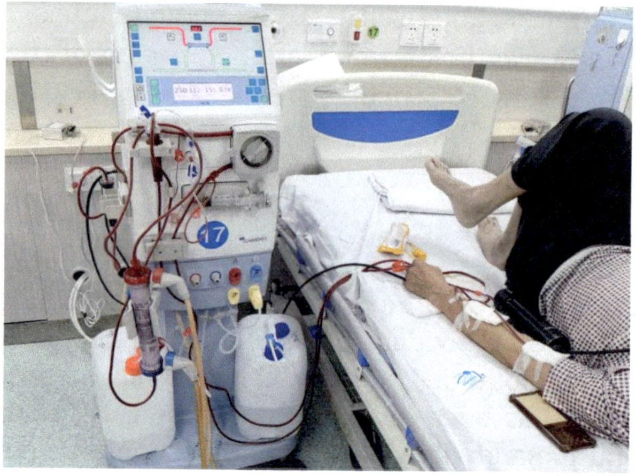

Figure 7.12. Situations requiring alternative treatments.

Source: ByteIMG. (n.d.). *Untitled image.* https://external-content.duckduckgo.com/iu/?u=https%3A%2F%2Fp1-tt.byteimg.com%2Forigin%2Ftos-cn-i-qvj2lq49k0%2F22433d5bd07346ad98f17fe522c9533e.jpg&f=1&nofb=1&ipt=305cd0a6136b56c9ad67894b55f994dda2d44972a46f2391580f709e130bb78b.

7.5.3. Challenges in Accessing Second-Line Therapies

The majority of malaria-affected regions continue to use the traditional medicines, even with increased resistance. Spare drugs are not easily obtained, mainly because of issues of logistics, funding, and poor infrastructure. In most instances, rural health facilities, which bear the highest disease load, are confronted with irregular supplies of these spare drugs. Generally, these second-line drugs cost more too, with higher production and transport costs, and hence are beyond the means of poor communities. It doesn't help that new guidelines, intended to make treatment in line with local resistance clearer, are limited; this complicates the decision to switch and tends to keep patients waiting for the best care (Bourgonje et al., 2020). Another major hindrance is the state of the health systems themselves. In most cases, the health workers are not properly trained on when and how to use the reserve drugs and tend to follow outdated procedures or simply make an estimate of the treatment. Equipment on hand to test for the failure of a first-line treatment or to specify the individual *Plasmodium* species, often is lacking in supply or not fully reliable. This inability of proper diagnosis to be followed has the dual tendency to lead to both underuse and misuse of these drugs, thereby driving up the risk of further resistance. To this dysfunctional healthcare, add dysfunctional public and private sector separation; many patients end up receiving care from informal practitioners who may not necessarily be in the loop concerning the new guidelines (Guzik et al., 2020). Social and policy determinants go on to muddy the waters. In other groups, ongoing doubt about the new medications and fear of side effects keep patients from being addicted to the familiar first-line medications. Health messages fail to make an additional effort to overcome these fears or detail why change becomes necessary when resistance is growing. Furthermore, national laws and procurement practices don't favor stocking or subsidizing these more costly second-line drugs—largely because they're considered less cost-effective with fewer patients. These decisions slow the implementation of new guidelines on treatment and encourage the excessive usage of first-line drugs. Ultimately, solutions to these interdependent challenges involve a mixture of community outreach, enhanced provider education, and some enlightened policy reforms to guarantee that all have access to equal-quality second-line malaria treatments (Bourgonje et al., 2020; Guzik et al., 2020).

7.6. Future Directions in Malaria Treatment

Not just finding new drugs to treat malaria is an issue, it's also an issue of improving care that people get where malaria is common. While there are effective tests and the right drugs available, receiving speedy, proper treatment still doesn't happen regularly, especially in the less resource-laden nations. Most children who are feverish do not get proper care; they miss solid testing and correct use of medicine. This, on average, will make it hard to achieve our 2030 goal of decreasing malaria deaths. Closing gaps, in most cases, entails spending more on improving health systems and making people adhere to established treatment practices instead of faking them. Getting tests out more and making them more reliable, and delivering the proper drugs to the proper patients, seems the solution to cutting both malaria deaths and the risk of resistance. We have no doubt that we need a longer-term plan—one that goes far beyond just new drugs (Jha et al., 2020). Conversely, the use of such fast tests like mRDTs in routine clinics appears to be a step in the right direction towards better results. However, more recent research tells us that the mere availability of such will not automatically mean better guideline adherence or reducing the misuse of antimalarial drugs. In the majority of high-transmission hotspots, challenges of poor-quality health facilities, insufficient staff, and even time constraints come in the way of efficient utilization of mRDTs. Health workers—whose approval for diagnostic testing is the norm—are inhibited by logistic challenges that do not allow them to incorporate these technologies without a hitch into their day-to-day work. Therefore, sometimes you have a situation where real malaria is not treated adequately and others that are negative are overdosed. Future plans, therefore, need to harmonize good health improvement programs with innovative diagnostic techniques in order to enable more intelligent case management and rational use of drugs, which in turn makes treatment even more effective in the long run (Chandler et al., 2017). In the future, the fight against malaria will need to mix new technology with stronger healthcare systems and real community involvement. There is still a tremendous need for brief courses of treatment that use new mechanisms to target the disease, which is relatively important in defeating emerging drug resistance. Along with that, cleaning up supply chains, boosting training among health workers, and further pressuring compliance with test-and-treat protocols so these new drugs truly pay dividends is key. Digital health technologies for monitoring and making decisions may even be used to polish the administration and monitoring of treatments. With increased international effort on malaria elimination, what is required is an integration of approaches—improved diagnostics, effective therapies, and strong service delivery within bottom-line health systems—addressed to the reduction of disease and mortality with sustainable and high-quality care (Jha et al., 2020; Chandler et al., 2017).

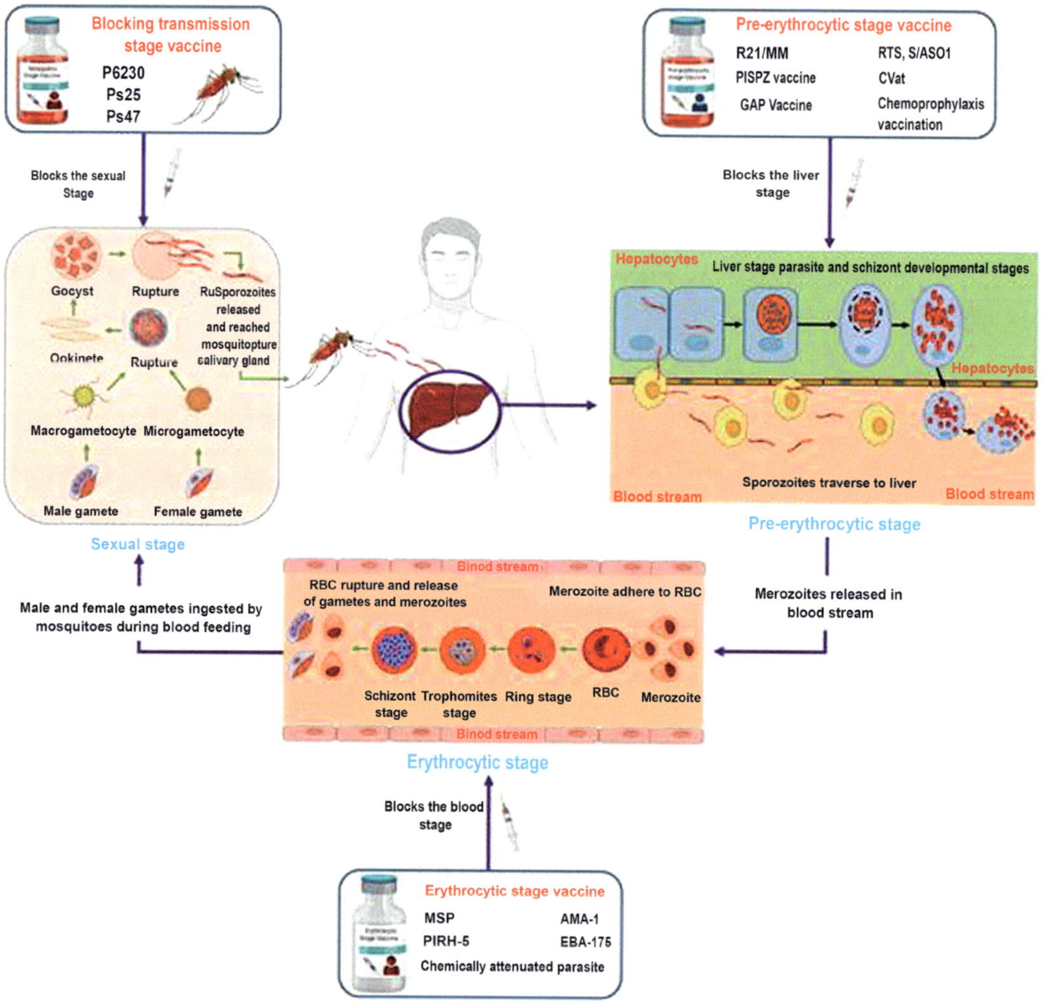

Source: Siddiqui AJ, Bhardwaj J, Saxena J, Jahan S, Snoussi M, Bardakci F, Badraoui R, Adnan M. A Critical Review on Human Malaria and Schistosomiasis Vaccines: Current State, Recent Advancements, and Developments. *Vaccines*. 2023; 11(4):792. https://doi.org/10.3390/vaccines11040792

7.6.1. Research on New Antimalarial Drugs

Drugs-resistant treatment for malaria is very difficult these days with new strains developing that are resistant to our drugs. ACTs had significantly cut back the incidence of malaria, but we've had indications that drugs like AL, and other at the front lines—are less effective in certain areas where malaria is out of hand. This type of resistance disrupts our standard treatment script, forcing us to seek out drugs that act in new ways. For the most part, searching for novel antimalarial agents is not merely about having additional drugs available, it's also about being ahead of the annoying propagation of resistance. Moreover, new medicines with improved safety and pharmacokinetic properties might keep patients on schedule with their doses. When you put together how the parasite behaves, how effective a drug is, and how different human bodies respond, you truly have to have collaboration across disciplines to find an exciting candidate in the lab and get it into use on a daily basis. Rational prescribing in most public health facilities is in short supply, and that just makes it harder when trying to put new drugs in place. Some of those studies in broad perspective suggest that few healthcare providers are fully aware of the nuances of proper dosing, contraindications, or ideal stacking of antimalarial drugs with other drugs. This knowledge gap may lead to drug over-prescription that is not quite reaching their goal or compounding them in combinations that may hasten resistance. Thus, new research into antimalarials should be coupled with better training and an impetus for following evidence-based practice. Less difficult drugs to dose and lower dangerous inter-acting rates would make these issues easier as well. Waging war on these systemic pitfalls in care provision is, honestly, just as critical as finding new medications (Kamuhabwa & Silumbe, 2013). Add to this the everyday fact that, particularly where there are not adequate diagnostic facilities, doctors have to prescribe antimalarials along with antibiotics and other medications. In the majority of rural health centers, with their overdependence on presumptive treatment—patients leave with a combination of drugs at home, which means greater potential for unexpected side effects and drug interactions. New medications specifically aimed at malaria, cutting down on risks from therapy combinations, could make a real difference in patient treatment. Also, investment in rapid diagnosis equipment, as well as new drugs, might result in more targeted therapies and smarter drug utilization. Tracking how drugs end up being co-prescribed, and why, can teach us about how to create treatments in the future that more suitably fit into the complex, real-world issues of healthcare in regions severely affected by malaria (Njozi et al., 2013).

7.6.2. Vaccine Development and Its Implications

Vaccine development has shifted treatment strategies in ways that were unforeseen. Before, doctors largely depended on drugs to fight off infections that had already established themselves—a tactic that was prone to run into such problems as drug resistance and unavailability in most of the world. Now, vaccines offer a tool for not allowing disease to occur at all, lowering instances of malaria and, in turn, the need for treatment drugs. This new approach requires us to alter guidelines to take into consideration vaccination status and the extent to which it may soften the impact of disease. There is also the issue of treating various communities; there are ethical concerns and the challenging process of obtaining informed consent—usually in the case of children with immature parents—demands attention. In the majority of cases, open reporting and uniform consent policies are necessary for ethically conducting vaccine trials in sub-Saharan Africa and as part of a mixed strategy for malaria control (De Pretto-Lazarova et al., 2021). Apart from the immediate clinical benefits, vaccines have more general public health impacts that are related to health system effectiveness and resource use. Mass vaccination will reduce the burden on community clinics and even large hospitals from malarial fevers, thereby allowing healthcare professionals to divert resources to other emergent requirements while streamlining fever treatment methods. Investigations of acute fevers in urban and rural areas pinpoint the complexity of diagnosis and treatment, implying that the use of vaccines can steer treatment by cutting the incidence and severity of the disease (Shimelis et al., 2022). Vaccines not only protect individuals, then; they have systematic benefits, hand-in-hand with antimalarials in national treatment regimens. Vaccine advancement is not, however, problem-free. Malaria parasites are often finicky, and vaccines in hand only work partially, so ongoing monitoring and prompt altering of treatment guidelines is required to remain current. Ethically, issues also arise with vulnerable groups in trials—ensuring laser-sharp comprehension and consent becomes an extra necessity when enrolling children with small caregivers (De Pretto-Lazarova et al., 2021). Vaccine rolling out is less of a scientific undertaking but a complex, layered experience that involves ethical, clinical, and policy considerations. Hence, treatment policies will need to continuously change, staying abreast with the ever-changing reality of vaccination and antimalarial drugs, and heading towards an effective as well as equitable malaria control strategy.

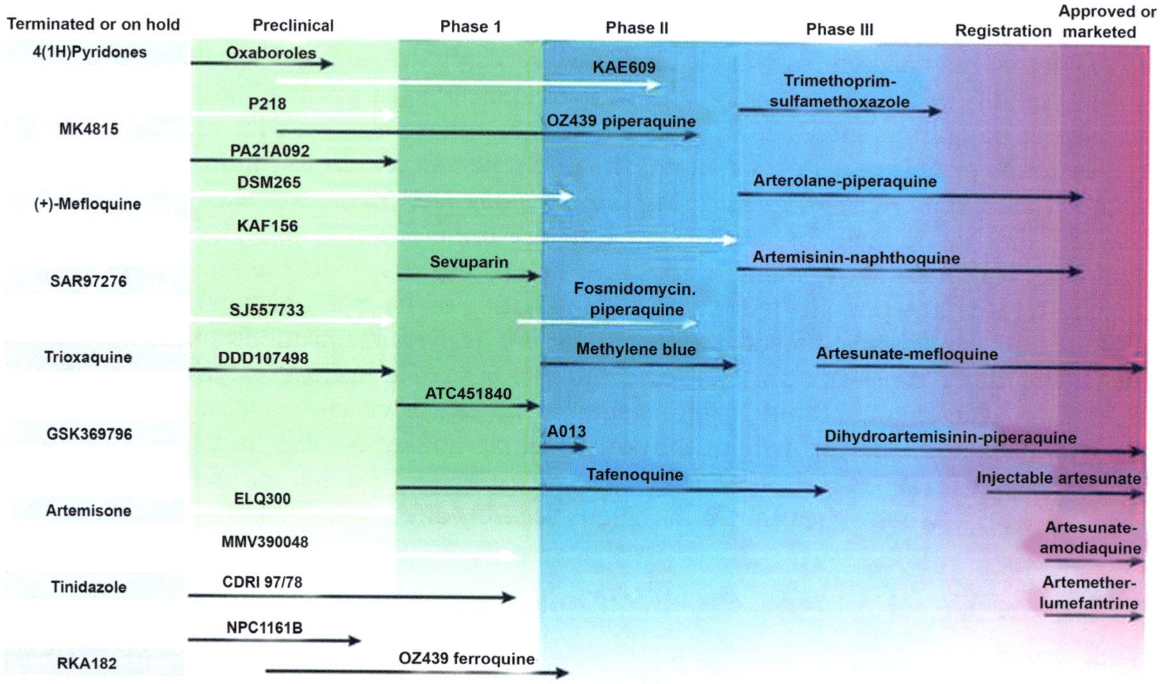

Source: Uzondu, S., Echezona, A., Nwagwu, C., Onugwu, A., Ugorji, L., Agbo, C., ... Attama, A. (2023). Combating Antimalarial Drug Resistance: Recent Advances and Future Perspectives. IntechOpen. doi: 10.5772/intechopen.106507

7.6.3. Strategies to Combat Drug Resistance

Infectious diseases are hard to cure because you just have to catch the microbes' behavior and evolve resistance. Drug resistance—always a looming, severe problem—a grave, ongoing challenge in antimalarial treatment especially, makes us have to join forces, usually in a constantly shifting, dynamic way. One effective strategy is the implementation of antimicrobial stewardship programs that dampen our use of antimalarial drugs; they aim at maximizing treatment success through limiting excessive drug use, which in most cases tends to accelerate the appearance of resistant organisms. Enhancing infection prevention and control practices, for example, diminishes the overall microbial load and slows down the dissemination of resistant pathogens. This is very crucial in areas like low- and middle-income countries where diagnostic centers are typically limited and the likelihood of unwarranted drug use creeps in. All these measures, if taken together, gently shape an atmosphere where resistance is not very likely to take hold, affirming the need for standardized policies and an expanded global outlook (Lucien et al., 2021). New cycles of diagnostic technology have also been the game-changer, allowing clinicians to differentiate infections promptly while detecting resistance markers with molecular techniques that are apparently to order to get the job done. Rapid tests and these molecular tools enable healthcare workers to choose the right therapy, eschewing broad-spectrum or off-target treatments that would otherwise spur resistance. Apart from this, the inclusion of host traits like immune response and genetic components can guide doctors on how to customize treatment regimens consisting of antimalarial drugs alongside other therapies. For instance, therapies that modulate the immune system, like interventions used when fighting invasive viral infections—might simply improve outcomes if added to conventional antimalarials. In a majority of cases, such a collaborative work proves that overcoming drug resistance indeed demands teamwork from different specialist domains (Soy et al., 2020). Antimalarial treatments are never a single occurrence; it is a continuous act of watchfulness through observation and new studies to know how resistance forms. It goes without saying that creating adaptive treatment regimens, those that adapt as resistance patterns shift, is critical to helping healthcare practitioners worldwide. Such regimens, hopefully, would utilize evidence-based advice on combination therapies because combinations of drugs with differing mechanisms of action tend to reduce the chances of resistance emerging. And global collaboration—piling data on resistance and adapting shipments of drugs—brings good treatment to the areas worst hit by malaria. Education is also involved; if the professionals and the communities are educated on the need to use antimalarials cautiously, less of a tendency towards inappropriate self-medication will exist. In general, an all-out effort from policymakers, clinicians, and researchers seems to be necessary to keep the risk of drug resistance at bay while clinging to the gains made in the control of malaria (Soy et al., 2020; Lucien et al., 2021).

CLOSER LOOK

ARTEMETHER-LUMEFANTRINE (AL)

AL is among the most widely used artemisinin-based combination treatments (ACTs) for uncomplicated *Plasmodium falciparum* malaria, the most virulent and drug-resistant malaria parasite species. The fixed-dose combination of artemether, a fast-acting artemisinin derivative, and lumefantrine, a longer-acting antimalarial, enhances efficacy, reduces treatment failure, and decelerates resistance emergence. Artemether acts quickly to kill most of the *parasites* during the blood stage of malaria by producing reactive oxygen species that inactivate parasite proteins, causing quick relief from symptoms, usually within 24 to 48 hours. Artemether, however, is short acting by itself and will not possibly eliminate all the *parasites*, particularly the remaining ones. To this end, lumefantrine provides a sustained antimalarial effect by performing on the residual *parasites*, resulting in complete parasite clearance, and reducing recurrence danger.

AL is taken orally as a six-dose regimen for three days, with the first day's doses 8 hours apart subsequently every 12 hours after that. It is important that the drug be taken with a fatty meal or milk since this ensures the best absorption of lumefantrine, which has otherwise poor absorption. Failure to observe this rule may lead to reduced drug efficacy and increased risk of treatment failure. AL is well tolerated in most patients, side effects typically mild and transient. Side effects include headache, dizziness, fatigue, nausea, abdominal pain, and insomnia. Serious side effects are rarely seen; however, as with any medication, the patient must be monitored for allergic response or atypical symptoms.

One of the strongest qualities of AL is that it serves to harbor resistance to artemisinin. The combination approach ensures that even if *parasites* are resistant to one part of the drug, the other works to kill them, thereby preventing resistant strains from becoming prevalent. This makes AL a benchmark in global malaria treatment standards, especially in areas where resistance to previously used antimalarial drugs like chloroquine or sulfadoxine-pyrimethamine renders them ineffective. For the majority of African and Southeast Asian countries, AL is one of the first-line policy therapies for uncomplicated *P. falciparum* malaria. However, there is growing unease over the appearance of partial resistance to the artemisinin derivatives in Southeast Asia that has necessitated the shift to track efficacy and discover new therapies.

AL is also used off-label to treat other forms of malaria but has no effect on the liver stages (hypnozoites) of *P. vivax* and *P. ovale*, which require additional treatment with drugs like primaquine in order to prevent relapse. AL is safe in children and pregnant women if properly given, although dosing carefully by weight and gestational age is required. Overall, AL is an extremely effective, fast-acting, and worldwide accepted remedy of uncomplicated *P. falciparum* malaria. Its combined mechanism not only promises quick clearance of *parasites* but also vitally helps in slowing down the rise of drug resistance. Maintaining enhanced surveillance, educating patients, and precise administration is imperative to make it effective and protect global health.

SUMMARY

Antimalarial drugs have been introduced into the treatment mix for emerging diseases, and there has been a lot of controversy about their role. Most doctors initially repurposed these drugs in the hope that it would soothe symptoms and diminish viral loads in those sick patients. While the idea seemed theoretically promising, the concrete information still is not conclusive. A disease such as COVID-19 is disorderly enough to show that it is not simple to accept antimalarials in the absence of strong clinical evidence. Some thorough reviews state that a few treatments may work, but they are still to be tested with proper randomized trials regarding safety and efficacy. This prudent, sometimes slow, process keeps our recommendations flexible and evidence-driven, aiming to improve patient outcomes without being high on side effects. For the majority in medicine, it means pressure to do more research and alter with the protocols until antimalarials have the full, blanket approbation in new treatment settings (Pascarella et al., 2020). Simultaneously, as researchers study deploying antimalarials, they also stress that supportive care takes precedence, alongside any medication that is given. Global panels, by and large, acknowledge that maintaining potential gains commensurate with true risks is required—not to mention the prudent consideration of resource limitations as well as ethical concerns. This framework, which includes a wide range of healthcare environments and patient groups, ultimately dictates the general recommendations. For example, even if we are still willing to try some antivirals, fundamentals like infection control and cardiovascular services are still the bedrock. That tiered approach enhances our general ability to treat severe cases effectively; and, for that matter, using graded recommendations (against different levels of evidence and practical exigencies) illustrates how multidimensional our approaches must be in transforming health crises (Alhazzani et al., 2020). In the end, today's available evidence pushes us toward a cautious, evidence-based approach to antimalarials in treatment regimes. Early on, early findings set people buzzing about re-purposing these drugs, but active clinical trials will still have to prove their value in fighting other diseases. Meanwhile, staying with established supportive care protocols–as well as diligent infection surveillance, remains at the heart of good patient care. An even-handed attitude like this encourages us to remember that new drug therapies should not supplant our standard treatments completely but rather augment them once they at last prove their value. The continuous evolution of treatment guidelines, grounded in rigorous research and the finest judgment of specialists, continues to make patient care adaptive and responsive despite new challenges still emerging (Alhazzani et al., 2020; Pascarella et al., 2020).

Looking very closely at current recommendations for antimalarial treatment, it is not so simple to determine exactly how these drugs are distributed and used by various industries. Frequently, methods like provider recall or even retail audits yield numbers that don't quite compute. These kinds of mismatches, in general, reveal certain limitations in our measurement methods that can have the capacity to impact study findings and policy decisions. For example, audits sometimes compel sales amounts somewhat too high compared to provider recall; although, recall is less burdensome and cost-effective in certain cases. This split pretty much reminds us that the choice of the right data collection approach—tuned to the local situation—is necessary in order to render the use data useful for policymaking regarding treatment (Goodman et al., 2013). Understanding of these subtlety specific methodological aspects is critical if we are to improve treatment guidelines such that antimalarials reach those who most need them. Reliance on personal outlets for the dispensing of antimalarial drugs has its share of drawbacks in compliance with treatment protocols and supplying drugs to the patient on time. Although the majority of the drugs are retailed by local shops and pharmacies, many children remain untreated during that vital 24-hour period since the appearance of symptoms. There are several reasons behind these delays: poor quality drugs resulting from poor storage processes, a flood of unregistered drugs, and even dosing-skipping practice where one administers half the dose because of limited finances. Subsequently, when private sector staff members are not properly trained, then all this does is add to the problem by minimizing the guidance that one can provide patients. These problems being addressed, in most cases, involve a level-headed approach that addresses not only the business side of private providers but also their need for better training—towards expanding both drug availability and adherence as per proper treatment guidelines (Battersby et al., 2003). Improving the dispensing of antimalarial treatments to a great extent depends on proper analysis of the strengths and weaknesses of the private sector in its functioning, as well as ongoing education among the providers and the public. If shop and pharmacy staff are rapidly turning over and there are not enough incentives to stay with training, keeping a trained crew becomes a headache. In addition, public campaign programs have to be designed in a thoughtful, occasionally even creative, way to engage populations' interest so that drugs are used in time and adequately. Focused communication activities, which combine cost factors with local contexts, seem key to starting long-term changes in behavior. Lastly, bringing together better supply chain with robust, ongoing training programs is essential to sustain treatment advice and improve health outcomes in the regions most ravaged by malaria (Battersby et al., 2003).

KEY TERMS FROM THIS CHAPTER

Chloroquine	Quinine	Mefloquine
Primaquine	Atovaquone-proguanil	Doxycycline
Clindamycin	Lumefantrine	Piperaquine
Drug Resistance	Uncomplicated Malaria	Severe Malaria
Intravenous Artesunate	Supportive Therapy	Radical Cure
Prophylaxis	Treatment Failure	WHO Guidelines
National Malaria Control Program (NMCP)		

References

1. Yeboah P, Forkuo AD, Amponsah OKO, Adomako NO, Abdin AY, Nasim MJ, Werner P, Panyin AB, Emrich E, Jacob C. Antimalarial Drugs in Ghana: A Case Study on Personal Preferences. *Sci.* 2020; 2(3):49. https://doi.org/10.3390/sci2030049 (accessed on 13 May 2025).

2. Anthony Battersby, Catherine Goodman Charles Abondo, & Renata Mandike (2003). Improving the supply distribution and use of antimalarial drugs by the private sector in Tanzania. Report prepared for the National Malaria Control Programme, United Republic of Tanzania. Malaria Consortium. Retrieved from: https://core.ac.uk/download/46556779.pdf (accessed on 13 May 2025).

3. Alexander, N., Hewitt, S., Nguon, C., Okell, L. C., et al. (2006). Insecticide-treated bednets for the prevention of *Plasmodium falciparum* malaria in Cambodia: A cluster-randomized trial. *Tropical Medicine & International Health, 11*(8), 1166–1177. https://doi.org/10.1111/j.1365-3156.2006.01673.x.

4. Alhazzani, W., Hylander Møller, M., Arabi, Y. M., Loeb, M., Gong, M. N., Fan, E., Oczkowski, S., et al. (2020). Surviving sepsis campaign: Guidelines on the management of critically ill adults with coronavirus disease 2019 (COVID-19). *Critical Care Medicine, 48*(6), e440–e469. https://doi.org/10.1097/ccm.0000000000004363.

5. Ayogu, E., Ukwe, C., Igboeli, N., & Adibe, M. (2020). Antimalarial drugs utilization, adherence to malaria treatment guideline and awareness of the guideline among the health providers. *International Journal of Drug Development and Research, 12*, 1–10. Retrieved from: https://www.semanticscholar.org/paper/4b51b9de81fce9c1087ad37b3b2ce779ff5a28b5 (accessed on 13 May 2025).

6. Ruberto, I., Camara, S., Banek, K., & Loua, M. K. (2014). Knowledge, attitudes and practices of malaria control among communities from the health district of Forécariah in the Republic of Guinea, West Africa. *Journal of vector borne diseases, 51*(2), 119–127.(accessed on 13 May 2025).

7. Wylie, B. J., Hashmi, A. H., Singh, N., Singh, M. P., Tuchman, J., Hussain, M., Sabin, L., Yeboah-Antwi, K., Banerjee, C., Brooks, M. I., Desai, M., Udhayakumar, V., Macleod, W. B., Dash, A. P., & Hamer, D. H. (2010). Availability and utilization of malaria prevention strategies in pregnancy in eastern India. *BMC public health, 10*, 557. https://doi.org/10.1186/1471-2458-10-557 (accessed on 13 May 2025).

8. Long E. G. (2009). Requirements for diagnosis of malaria at different levels of the laboratory network in Africa. *American journal of clinical pathology, 131*(6), 858–860. https://doi.org/10.1309/AJCPVX71BXWOVWBY (accessed on 13 May 2025).

9. Ber Lucien, M. A., Canarie, M. F., Kilgore, P. E., Jean-Denis, G., Fénélon, N., Pierre, M., Cerpa, M., et al. (2021). Antibiotics and antimicrobial resistance in the COVID-19 era: Perspective from resource-limited settings. *International Journal of Infectious Diseases, 104*, 250–254. https://doi.org/10.1016/j.ijid.2020.12.087.

10. Moon, A. M., Biggs, H. M., Rubach, M. P., Crump, J. A., Maro, V. P., Saganda, W., & Reddy, E. A. (2014). Evaluation of in-hospital management for febrile illness in Northern Tanzania before and after 2010 World Health Organization Guidelines for the treatment of malaria. *PloS one, 9*(2), e89814. https://doi.org/10.1371/journal.pone.0089814(accessed on 13 May 2025).

11. Bourgonje, A. R., Abdulle, A. E., Timens, W., Hillebrands, J. L., Navis, G., Gordijn, S. J., Bolling, M. C., et al. (2020). Angiotensin-converting enzyme 2 (ACE2), SARS-CoV-2 and the pathophysiology of coronavirus disease 2019 (COVID-19). *The Journal of Pathology, 251*(3), 228–248. https://doi.org/10.1002/path.5471.

12. De Pretto-Lazarova, A., Brancati-Badarau, D. O., & Burri, C. (2021). Transparent reporting of recruitment and informed consent approaches in clinical trials recruiting children with minor parents in sub-Saharan Africa: a secondary analysis based on a systematic review. *BMC public health, 21*(1), 1473. https://doi.org/10.1186/s12889-021-11079-y (accessed on 13 May 2025).

13. Casamitjana, N., & Clotet, B. (2020). Use of antiviral drugs to reduce COVID-19 transmission. *The Lancet Global Health, 8*(5), e639–e640. https://doi.org/10.1016/s2214-109x(20)30114-5.

14. Chaachouay, N., & Zidane, L. (2024). Plant-derived natural products: A source for drug discovery and development. *Drugs and Drug Candidates, 3*(3), 184–207. https://doi.org/10.3390/ddc3010011.

15. Njama-Meya, D., Clark, T. D., Nzarubara, B., Staedke, S., Kamya, M. R., & Dorsey, G. (2007). Treatment of malaria restricted to laboratory-confirmed cases: a prospective cohort study in Ugandan children. *Malaria journal, 6*, 7. https://doi.org/10.1186/1475-2875-6-7

16. Shimelis, T., Vaz Nery, S., Schierhout, G., Tadesse, B. T., Dittrich, S., Crump, J. A., & Kaldor, J. M. (2022). Differences in diagnosis, management, and outcomes of acute febrile illness by health facility level in southern Ethiopia. *Scientific reports, 12*(1), 19166. https://doi.org/10.1038/s41598-022-23641-8 (accessed on 13 May 2025).

17. Galactionova, K., Tediosi, F., de Savigny, D., Smith, T., & Tanner, M. (2015). Effective coverage and systems effectiveness for malaria case management in sub-Saharan African countries. *PloS one, 10*(5), e0127818. https://doi.org/10.1371/journal.pone.0127818 (accessed on 13 May 2025).

18. Dima, A., Jurcuț, C., Chasset, F., Felten, R., & Arnaud, L. (2022). Hydroxychloroquine in systemic lupus erythematosus: Overview of current knowledge. *Therapeutic Advances in Musculoskeletal Disease, 14*, Article 1759720X211073001. https://doi.org/10.1177/1759720x211073001.

19. Hobbs, C., & Duffy, P. (2011). Drugs for malaria: something old, something new, something borrowed. *F1000 biology reports, 3*, 24. https://doi.org/10.3410/B3-24Eckhoff, P., Gerardin, J., & Wenger, E. A. (2015). Mass campaigns with antimalarial drugs: A modelling comparison of artemether-lumefantrine and DHA-piperaquine with and without primaquine as tools for malaria control and elimination. Retrieved from: http://arxiv.org/abs/1503.09149 (accessed on 13 May 2025).

20. Fitri, L. C., Pawestri, A. R., Winaris, N., Endharti, A. T., Khotimah, A. R. H., Abidah, H. Y., & Huwae, J. T. R. (2023). Antimalarial drug resistance: A brief history of its spread in Indonesia. *Drug Design, Development and Therapy, 17*, 1995–2010. https://doi.org/10.2147/dddt.s403672.

21. Fleming, K. A., Horton, S., Wilson, M. L., Atun, R., DeStigter, K., Flanigan, J., Sayed, S., et al. (2021). The Lancet Commission on diagnostics: Transforming access to diagnostics. *The Lancet, 398*(10306), 1997–2050. https://doi.org/10.1016/s0140-6736(21)00673-5.

22. Goodman, C., Hanson, K., Kleinschmidt, I., O'Connell, D., et al. (2013). Comparative analysis of two methods for measuring sales volumes during malaria medicine outlet surveys. https://core.ac.uk/download/16437766.pdf (accessed on 13 May 2025).

23. Guzik, T. J., Mohiddin, S., Dimarco, A., Patel, V., Savvatis, K., Marelli-Berg, F. M., Madhur, M. S., et al. (2020). COVID-19 and the cardiovascular system: Implications for risk assessment, diagnosis, and treatment options. *Cardiovascular Research, 116*(9), 1666–1687. https://doi.org/10.1093/cvr/cvaa106.

24. Jha, A. K., Macarayan, E. K., & Papanicolas, I. (2020). The quality of malaria care in 25 low-income and middle-income countries. https://core.ac.uk/download/237715340.pdf.

25. Kamuhabwa, A. A., & Silumbe, R. (2013). Knowledge among drug dispensers and antimalarial drug prescribing practices in public health facilities in Dar es Salaam. *Drug, healthcare and patient safety, 5*, 181–189. https://doi.org/10.2147/DHPS.S50071 (accessed on 13 May 2025).

26. Mace, K. E., Lucchi, N. W., & Tan, K. R. (2022). Malaria Surveillance–United States, 2018. *MMWR Surveillance Summaries, 71*(1), 1–35. https://doi.org/10.15585/mmwr.ss7108a1.

27. Mace, K., Lucchi, N., & Tan, K. R. (2021). Malaria Surveillance–United States, 2017. *MMWR Surveillance Summaries, 70*(1), 1–35. https://www.semanticscholar.org/paper/e8936c8db1b627bd4412def86d9a3998e43a78b3 (accessed on 13 May 2025).

28. Njozi, M., Amuri, M., Selemani, M., Masanja, I., Kigahe, B., Khatib, R., Kajungu, D., Abdula, S., & Dodoo, A. N. (2013). Predictors of antibiotics co-prescription with antimalarials for patients presenting with fever in rural Tanzania. *BMC public health, 13*, 1097. https://doi.org/10.1186/1471-2458-13-1097 (accessed on 13 May 2025).

29. Mwangi, J. M., & Ranford-Cartwright, L. C. (2013). Genetic and genomic approaches for the discovery of parasite genes involved in antimalarial drug resistance. https://core.ac.uk/download/18492190.pdf.

30. Chandler, C. I., Webb, E. L., Maiteki-Sebuguzi, C., Nayiga, S., Nabirye, C., DiLiberto, D. D., Ssemmondo, E., Dorsey, G., Kamya, M. R., & Staedke, S. G. (2017). The impact of an intervention to introduce malaria rapid diagnostic tests on fever case management in a high transmission setting in Uganda: A mixed-methods cluster-randomized trial (PRIME). *PloS one, 12*(3), e0170998. https://doi.org/10.1371/journal.pone.0170998(accessed on 13 May 2025).

31. O'Kane, D., McCourt, C., Meggitt, S., D'Cruz, D., Orteu, C. H., Benton, E., Wahie, S., et al. (2021). British Association of Dermatologists guidelines for the management of people with cutaneous lupus erythematosus 2021. *British Journal of Dermatology, 185*(6), 1112–1123. https://doi.org/10.1111/bjd.20597.

32. Pascarella, G., Strumia, A., Piliego, C., Bruno, F., Del Buono, R., Costa, F., Scarlata, S., et al. (2020). COVID-19 diagnosis and management: A comprehensive review. *Journal of Internal Medicine, 288*(2), 192–206. https://doi.org/10.1111/joim.13091.

33. Phua, J., Weng, L., Ling, L., Egi, M., Lim, C. M., Divatia, J. V., Shrestha, B. R., et al. (2020). Intensive care management of coronavirus disease 2019 (COVID-19): Challenges and recommendations. *The Lancet Respiratory Medicine, 8*(6), 506–517. https://doi.org/10.1016/s2213-2600(20)30161-2.

34. Poon, L. C., Yang, H., Dumont, S., Lee, J. C. S., Copel, J. A., Danneels, L., Wright, A., et al. (2020). ISUOG Interim Guidance on coronavirus disease 2019 (COVID-19) during pregnancy and puerperium: Information for healthcare professionals–An update. *Ultrasound in Obstetrics & Gynecology, 55*(6), 848–862. https://doi.org/10.1002/uog.22061.

35. Roper, D., Layton, M., Rees, D. C., Lambert, C., Vulliamy, T., De la Salle, B., & Dsouza, C. (2020). Laboratory diagnosis of G6PD deficiency. *British Journal of Hematology, 189*(1), 24–38. https://doi.org/10.1111/bjh.16366.

36. Soy, M., Keser, G., Atagündüz, P., Tabak, F., Kaygusuz Atagündüz, I., & Kayhan, S. (2020). Cytokine storm in COVID-19: Pathogenesis and overview of anti-inflammatory agents used in treatment. *Clinical Rheumatology, 39*(7), 2085–2094. https://doi.org/10.1007/s10067-020-05190-5.

37. Thomford, N. E., Senthebane, D. A., Rowe, A., Munro, D., Seele, P. P., Maroyi, A., & Dzobo, K. (2018). Natural products for drug discovery in the 21st century: Innovations for novel drug discovery. *International Journal of Molecular Sciences, 19*(6), 1578. https://doi.org/10.3390/ijms19061578.

38. Uwimana, A., Legrand, E., Stokes, B. H., Ndikumana, J. L. M., Warsame, M., Umulisa, N., Ngamije, D., et al. (2020). Emergence and clonal expansion of *in vitro* artemisinin-resistant *Plasmodium falciparum* kelch13 R561H mutant *parasites* in Rwanda. *Nature Medicine, 26*(10), 1602–1608. https://doi.org/10.1038/s41591-020-1005-2.

39. van der Pluijm, R. W., Amaratunga, C., Dhorda, M., & Dondorp, A. M. (2020). Triple artemisinin-based combination therapies for malaria–A new paradigm? *Trends in Parasitology, 37*(1), 15–24. https://doi.org/10.1016/j.pt.2020.09.011.

40. Worm, M., Zidane, M., Eisert, L., Fischer-Betz, R., Foeldvari, I., Günther, C., Iking-Konert, C., et al. (2021). S2k guideline: Diagnosis and management of cutaneous lupus erythematosus–Part 2: Therapy, risk factors and other special topics. *JDDG Journal der Deutschen Dermatologischen Gesellschaft, 19*(10), 1371–1395. https://doi.org/10.1111/ddg.14491.

41. Zhang, Z., Zhou, L., Xie, N., Nice, E. C., Zhang, T., Cui, Y., & Huang, C. (2020). Overcoming cancer therapeutic bottleneck by drug repurposing. *Signal Transduction and Targeted Therapy, 5*(1), 213. https://doi.org/10.1038/s41392-020-00213-8.

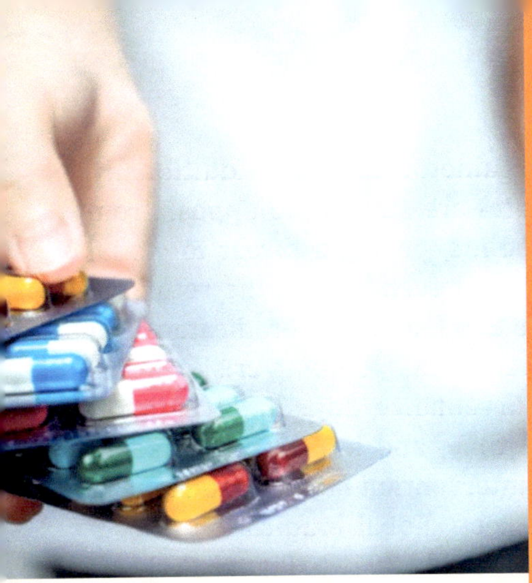

Chapter 8
DRUG RESISTANCE OF MALARIA

Contents

Introduction

Flight today makes it possible for diseases to take unexpected routes. Humans traveling around the globe in mere hours enable microbes to come out in unexpected places. Disease problems once stayed localized; today, sick travelers and microbe-carrying animals make what had been a local problem into a global one. This constant reshuffling not only stresses out outmoded public health infrastructure but also complicates diagnoses and containment. For most cases, the rapid spread calls for more monitoring efforts and concerted international response, especially considering that vector-borne diseases like malaria depend on both the pathogens and the roving carriers (Findlater et al., 2018). It's a challenging landscape in which global connectivity raises new challenges to the fight against drug-resistant strains. Malaria, whose primary cause is *Plasmodium falciparum*, remains an important global disease burden, particularly in the tropics where Anopheles mosquitoes seem to flourish. Even with all efforts to eliminate it, the disease remains recalcitrant and causes widespread illness and death.

What complicates matters is the emergence of resistance to drugs, which progressively weaken the effectiveness of our current treatments. For instance, resistance to artemisinin-based combination therapies (ACTs) is presently quite common in some parts of Southeast Asia, further taxing our treatment regimens. The biological details of the parasite itself, coupled with diagnosis delays, less-than-ideal healthcare systems, and heightened mobility among human populations, push all of these resistant strains into new grounds.

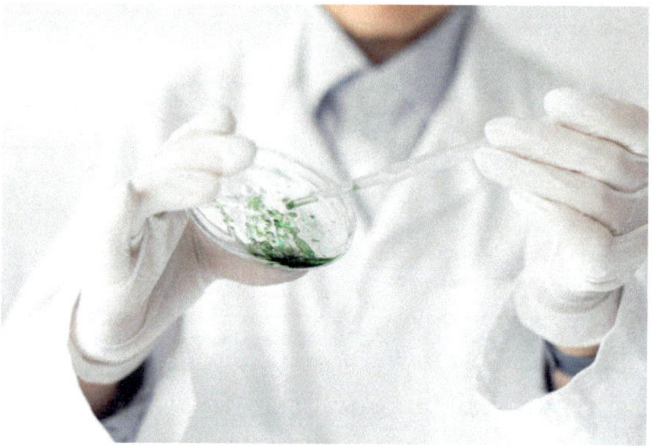

Figure 8.1. *Drug resistance and malaria.*

Source: MIT News. (2024). *Woman in Laboratory Doing Experiments.*

In many instances, a deeper understanding of how resistance occurs and looking for some outside-the-box, novel solutions simply appears to be crucial (Arjen et al., 2017). The development of drug resistance in malaria *parasites* is a multifaceted issue that erodes decades of progress in disease control. Resistance to artemisinin, which was first seen in Western Cambodia, demonstrates how quickly *Plasmodium falciparum* can evolve under drug stress. This adaptation takes the form of a decreased rate of parasite clearance from the blood; when combined with partner drug failure in ACTs, treatment efficacy plummets. These delays not only extend the duration of the infection but also increase its transmission by speeding up gametocyte levels. Additionally, resistant *parasites* are starting to appear from their starting points, posing a threat to global malaria control and even risking the return of malaria in areas that had nearly eradicated it. In total, a resolution to this looming crisis entails manipulating surveillance, adjusting treatment policies in real time, and implementing some out-of-the-box intervention methods to manage resistance and keep global eradication efforts on course (Arjen et al., 2017) (Figure 8.1).

Definition of Malaria and Its Global Impact

Malaria is a potentially life-threatening disease spread when an infected female Anopheles mosquito bites, carrying *Plasmodium parasites* that infect your body. You might experience symptoms like a sudden fever, chills, or even a flu-like feeling , and if not treated, it can quickly turn into serious complications or kill you. In spite of our step-by-step advances through prevention and treatments, malaria remains burdensome to tropical and subtropical regions. It not only affects personal health, but also the local economies, especially where the health care system is weak. In general, an understanding of how malaria works is most critical, since emerging issues like drug resistance increasingly erode our control efforts and further entrench the disease into the world (Christopher et al., 2022). Malaria has impacts extending far beyond the medical issues. It destabilizes the social and economic fabric of society in nations where it hits, systematically stopping development there in its tracks. Every year, millions of cases burden health systems and prevent economic growth, especially in regions like sub-Saharan Africa, where poverty and lack of medical resources constitute a tempestuous environment for the disease to flourish. It is picombining that children below five years and pregnant women, who are already at risk, are most impacted. This unequal burden is a testament to just how important it is to use efficacious interventions, despite the persistence of health care access disparities perpetuating the cycle of illness and poverty (Gregory et al., 2018). Over the last several years, the war on malaria has taken a setback with the discovery of drug-resistant forms of *Plasmodium*. Such resistant strains pose a threat to our traditional antimalarial medications, messing up treatment protocols and raising the likelihood of failures. So, all the hard-won achievements in lowering malaria-induced disease and death are now in the balance. Primarily, issues like inappropriate drug usage or simply a poor healthcare infrastructure—widespread in the most endemic areas—have a giant role to play. This resistance not only delays patients' easy recovery but also transmits further, complicating public health interventions. To address this problem holistically, we need a close examination of malaria biology, its transmission across the globe, and socio-economic determinants through which resistance is able to spread (Christopher et al., 2022; Gregory et al., 2018) (Figure 8.2).

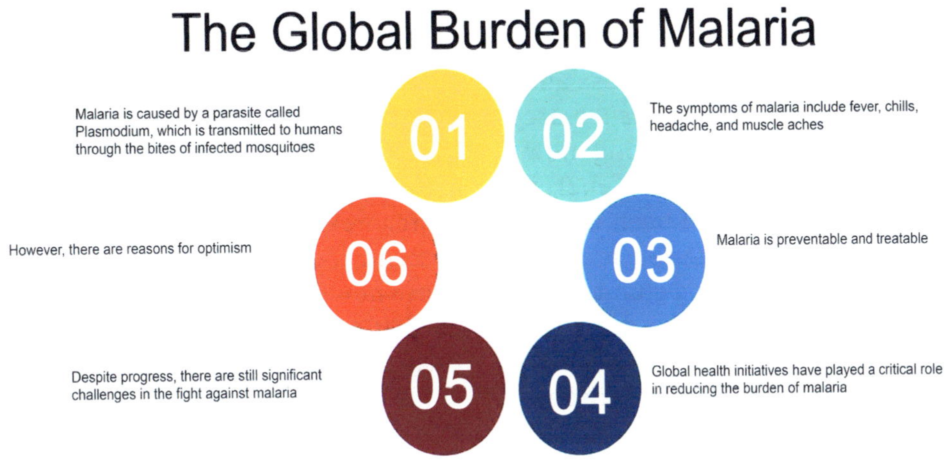

Figure 8.2. *Malaria and its global impact.*

Source: FasterCapital. (n.d.). *Malaria Control – Saving Lives Through Global Health Initiatives.*

Overview of Antimalarial Drugs

Antimalarial drugs have been a behemoth component of our fight against malaria—a disease caused by infected mosquito bites containing infinitesimal *Plasmodium parasites*. Over time, the drugs have shifted in ways you would not anticipate. The traditional standards like quinine and chloroquine used to be the best, but now we use artemisinin-based drugs in combination with others. All species of drugs target the parasite in different ways; chloroquine, for instance, interferes with the parasite's detoxification of heme to allow destructive accumulation to happen, whereas artemisinin somehow stirs up oxidative bedlam through the production of reactive oxygen species that destroy proteins and membranes. There will naturally come resistance as a consequence, though, which makes treatment on a global scale difficult. Generally, having a clear understanding of exactly how these drugs act is the most important step in getting past those barriers and directing next-generation drug development that can sidestep resistance problems. Artemisinin and its closest relatives, for the most part, lead the way among available options, because they are rapidly acting and effective even against multi-drug-resistant *Plasmodium*. These compounds disrupt the parasite's redox equilibrium, initiating free radicals that progressively kill the cells. Miraculously, this is not their destiny, there is growing hype over using them in viral infection, autoimmunity, and even cancer treatment. Their fungibility seems to be connected to that one endoperoxide scaffold, which can set off reactive species at iron-rich targets like the digestive vacuole of the parasite. Even despite their success, the detection of artemisinin resistance, mainly in Southeast Asia—suggests that combination therapies and new derivatives might be necessary. In most cases, ongoing investigations into how we can alter artemisinin's use could extend its effectiveness as an antimalarial and extend its clinical lifespan further (Guan et al., 2023). New discoveries regarding oxidative stress and controlled cell death in malaria *parasites* are generating some extremely interesting new research avenues. Mitochondria, the energy powerhouses in the parasite, have been linked to a process known as ferroptosis—a form of iron-dependent cell death involving glutathione depletion and quite critical lipid peroxidation. By targeting the parasite's own mitochondria to cause this form of cell death, scientists were able to bypass normal resistance mechanisms. This strategy interferes with the redox balance of the parasite and interferes with its main energy functions, making it vulnerable to oxidative damage. The control of ferroptosis in *Plasmodium* is complex and peculiarly specific, which means that drugs against this mitochondrial weakness would be able to maintain their action even after resistance has become widespread (Adegboro et al., 2024).

Importance of Studying Drug Resistance

Drug resistance to malaria is increasingly becoming an issue that takes a real toll on our achievements against the disease. Antimalarial drugs no longer hit as powerfully as they used to, and that means it's getting harder to keep the infection at bay—eradication seems to be an elusive mirage. Treatment failures are mounting, infections take longer to clear, and therefore the parasite is readily transmitted. Scientists investigate these patterns in part because they are interested in understanding how the parasite is evading our current drugs; that discovery spurs new concepts for treatment. Sometimes this kind of study also inspires policymakers to design interventions that are tailored to local patterns of resistance, so public health programs can become a bit more local. Without more careful study of these mechanisms of resistance, our efforts could quite readily fail, endangering already strained communities. Social and behavioral factors add a further degree of complexity to the issue. Throughout most of the globe, people have muddled ideas about the cause and best treatment of malaria. In most cases, such confusion leads to improper use of drugs, a condition that only serves to hasten resistance. For example, some studies in Benin reveal that when individuals do not know how malaria is transmitted or should be treated, they end up abusing antimalarial drugs, such abuse undermines the overall effectiveness of the drugs (Padonou et al., 2018). Educational efforts, even small ones, may make individuals follow correct treatments and adopt habits that quietly dampen the selection pressure against resistant organisms. And so, learning to resist is not only a lab experiment, it's making contact with individuals and applying science to the necessities of actual life. And finally, there is the issue of fewer new antibiotics being identified nowadays, and this makes our reliance on available treatments even more critical. In broad terms, pharma slump in innovation means firms largely reproducing older medicines rather than creating new ones (Coukell et al., 2016). This scenario may translate into, over time, resistance outpacing our medicine supply, paving the way for increased levels of illness and even mortality, particularly in malaria-endemic regions. Having a clear understanding of how resistance patterns develop can be used to maximize current drug regimens, giving us more time and slowing down the process to prolong their useful life. Ultimately, investigating these mechanisms is not just about solving short-term problems, it's about safeguarding a long-term bulwark against perils in the future (Figure 8.3).

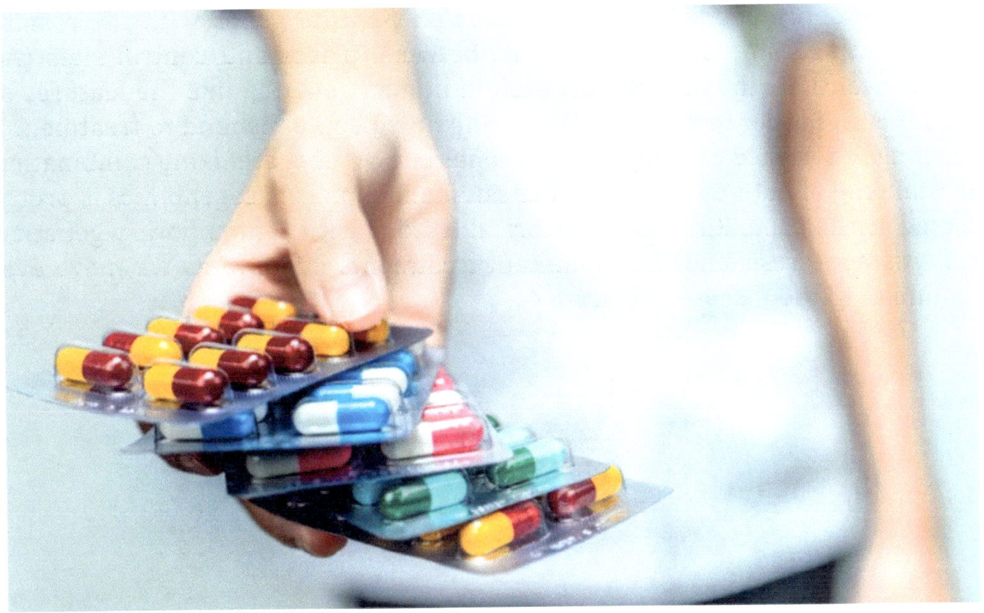

Figure 8.3. *Studying drug resistance.*

Source: The Conversation. (2022). *File-20220120-9679-1jg02yy.* https://images.theconversation.com/files/441722/original/file-20220120-9679-1jg02yy.jpg?ixlib=rb-4.1.0&rect=0%2C0%2C5991%2C3673&q=45&auto=format&w=926&fit=clip.

8.1. History of Malaria Treatment

Malaria treatment first started with nature's own medicines. During the 17th century, individuals discovered that quinine, which was extracted from cinchona tree bark, would soften the symptoms, and natural alkaloids became the primary treatment for an awfully long period of time. Man-made drugs arrived in the mid-20th century in the form of chloroquine, promising wider and more effective treatment. However, using these drugs so intensively over time forced *Plasmodium falciparum* to adapt, and drug-resistant strains developed. Combination regimens and polymorphic local practice in Southeast Asia have created Southeast Asia-specific mutations that are beneficial for parasites since studies revealed when comparing drug resistance changes to neutral genetic markers (Anderson et al., 2005). In retrospect, those early gains just so unintentionally laid the groundwork for some fairly daunting challenges down the line. As resistance mounted, treatment approaches started moving toward using combination therapies, especially artemisinin-based treatments, to overall decrease the potential for additional resistance and improve patient outcomes. In most instances, differences in how patients metabolize drugs can make the situation a little challenging. Genetic variation, particularly in drug-metabolizing enzymes like cytochrome P450 2B6 (CYP2B6)—means that patients often do not metabolize these medications in the same way. Evidence from places like Botswana, where multiple haplotype patterns exist in the presence of convergent metabolic phenotypes, indicates that adaptive pressures have balanced detoxification with drug response

(Dongho et al., 2018). This shows how host genetics should be taken into account when dose adjustment is being made and treatment failures are being prevented. Think of the fight against malaria as an ongoing tug-of-war between parasite evolution and human effort. Early reliance on monotherapy placed enormous selection pressures on parasite genes with the result that there were very clear contrasts in resistance patterns between places and control sites (Anderson et al., 2005). In the meantime, the natural variation in human genetics, like the features observed in CYP2B6, makes it even harder to treat by influencing how people respond to treatment (Dongho et al., 2018). The long experience of fighting malaria has shown us that mixing combination therapies with an understanding of both parasite genetics and human pharmacogenomics is pretty much our best bet. In some sense, combining these historical lessons with contemporary genetic knowledge may very well postpone resistance and maintain treatments effective as we move ever closer to the goal of eliminating the disease (Figure 8.4).

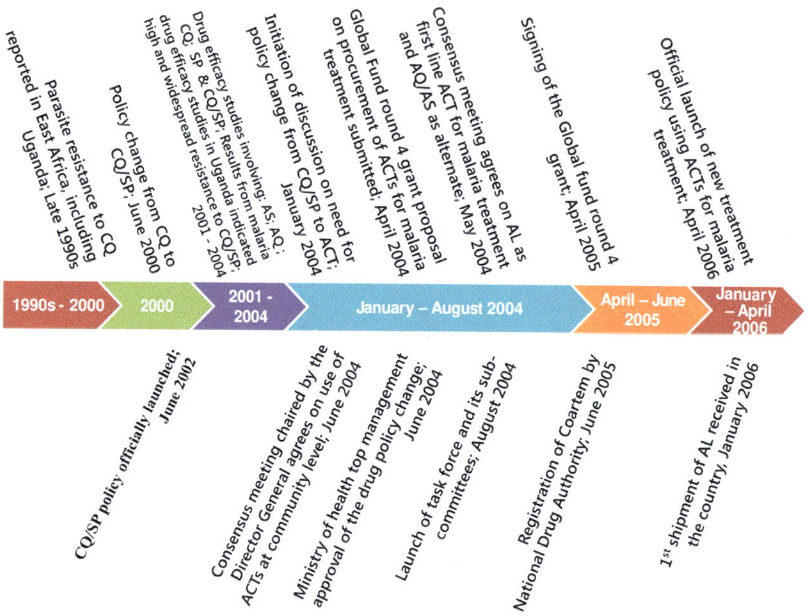

Figure 8.4. *Timeline of key events in changing the malaria treatment policy.*

Source: Nabyonga-Orem, J. (2014). *Timeline of Key Events in Changing the Malaria Treatment Policy.* ResearchGate.

8.1.1. Traditional Remedies and Early Treatments

Well before today's drugs became the focus, residents in endemic regions looked to ancient remedies with family histories. Local communities brewed herbal concoctions from indigenous plants they thought would combat the fever, and the natural remedies provided some measure of relief in areas where formal medical care was scarce. In certain African cultures, some felt even when the disease was caused by the sun or just due to a general weakness in the body (Abebe et al., 2019). Such beliefs meant that such interventions not only healed but also gave a sense of cultural identity, but sometimes ultimately ended up delaying the use of more effective, guaranteed drugs. Traditional healing's grip on the treatment of malaria teaches us that neighborhood ideas and gaps in well-being understanding play a role. Research, like analyzing web search trends for natural remedies and signs (Abebe et al., 2019)—serves to illustrate that patients still turn to these non-conventional sources alongside modern medicine. Most often, myths and stigma around the illness cloud judgment, and patients turn to herbalism when good medication is unavailable or too expensive. This uneven treatment, as it would later prove, sometimes left only the partial expulsion of parasites, and in most cases, that incompleteness permitted drug-resistant populations to develop. Studying the ancient techniques of malaria treatment is crucial in the fight against the new foe of drug resistance. The primitive approaches, not always used correctly, created sporadic doses that put only sufficient pressure on parasites to develop. While many communities embraced these herbal remedies culturally, even in implementing them without scientific proof, it made it all the more challenging to institute standard treatment regimens. It is challenging for national malaria programs today to bow to local tradition while encouraging individuals to implement a direction toward evidence-based treatment. Programs that demystify persisting myths regarding malaria and outline what works are likely to relieve this dilemma (Padonou et al., 2018). By interweaving the history of ancient remedies with modern medicinal advances, we can better confront the complicated issues behind drug resistance.

8.1.2. Development of Synthetic Antimalarial Drugs

Malaria has been a recurring headache that keeps changing its game because the parasite gradually manages to avoid our older medicines. The fact that the parasite can become resistant gives us the task of constantly developing new synthetic antimalarial drugs. Researchers, noticing that the conventional therapies are losing their steam, began trying out new chemical entities and even redesigning current drugs to maximize their benefits without their side effects. A tidy concept that's entered the scene is recycling established pharmacophores such as quinacrine—yes, that old synthetic antimalarial famed for its potent blood-stage activity, even though it has its own share of rough response. The past 20 years have seen activity that's been somewhat fragmented optimizing such compounds, and trying to create safer, more potent drugs that are able to avoid resistance. This strategy leverages the by-now-familiar antimalarial scaffold, which, in most cases, speeds up development and lowers costs—a tactical move especially as artemisinin-based treatments start to fail in regions where resistance is on the rise (Mélanie Fonte et al., 2021). The challenge gets even tougher when you add the way drug potency and parasite evolvability constantly compete with each other. Artemisinin resistance and that of its derivatives, especially in the Greater Mekong sub-region—shows us precisely how quickly the parasite can turn the tables on our first-line treatments, making it all but necessary to look for other synthetic drugs. New compounds are not only being targeted against other stages of the *Plasmodium* life cycle; they are being developed to act in modes that simply don't give the parasite an easy way out. These slight changes at the molecular level are aimed at optimizing bioavailability and minimizing toxicity so that the treatments are not just effective but also manageable, even in resource-scarce settings. Scientists, hopeful but cautious and attempting various modifications, are banking that by optimizing these synthetic antimalarials, they can maximize the drugs' therapeutic shelf life and keep malaria transmission firmly in check, which is a high-level global health security imperative (Mélanie Fonte et al., 2021). Another encouraging strategy is coupling conventional drugs with plant extracts—a synthesis that appears almost too good to be true. For the majority of malaria-endemic regions, herbal medicines have long been the recourse, and now research shows that they may supplement synthetic agents for a more effective overall efficacy, perhaps even slowing the rate of development of resistance through a type of multi-faceted attack. A number of studies, investigating herb-drug interactions, have instead hinted at a predominantly synergistic effect; the use of herbal medicines combined with man-made medicines can, in fact, enhance treatment outcomes in unexpected ways. Such biochemical collaboration not only opens up new avenues for the standardization of combination therapies but also brings in new concepts for treatment that can alleviate the immense burden of drug resistance. Successfully, these hybrid approaches provide a valuable complement to purely synthetic techniques, leveraging the age-old benefits of natural products alongside the tried-and-tested reliability of established drugs (Figure 8.5).

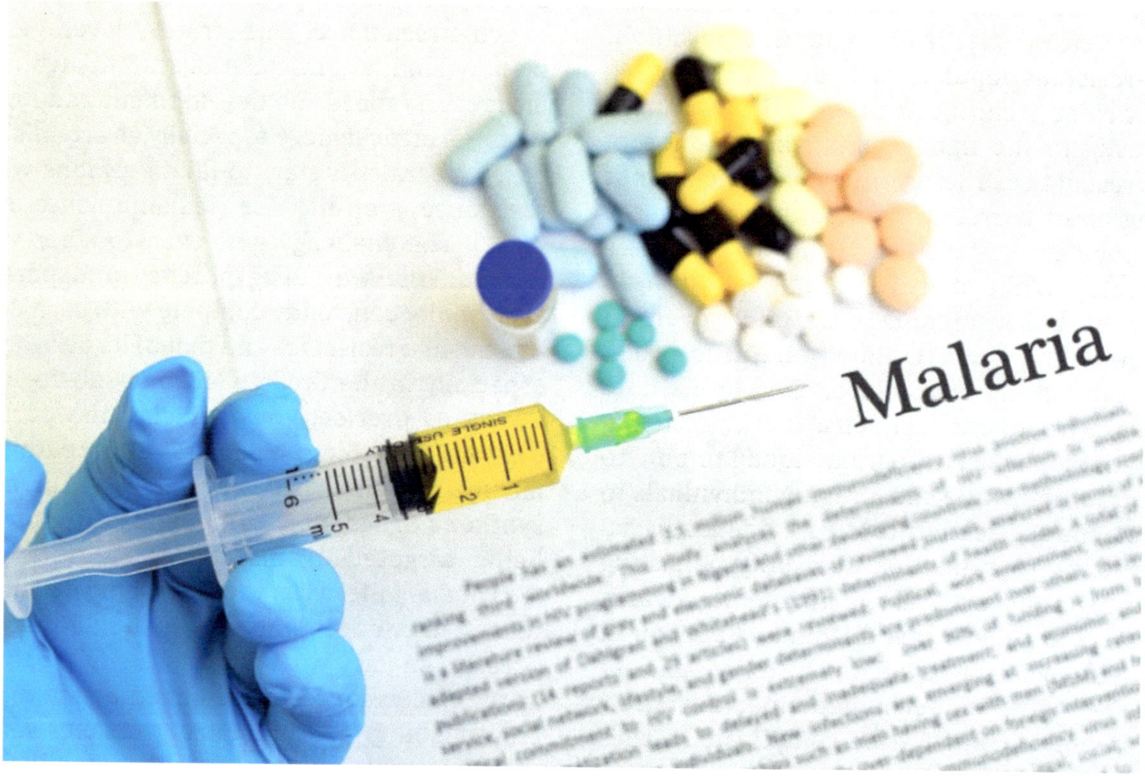

Figure 8.5. *Development of synthetic antimalarial drugs.*

Source: D1g9yur4m4naub.cloudfront.net. (n.d.). *Development of Synthetic Antimalarial Drugs.*

8.1.3. Emergence of Drug Resistance in Historical Context

Malaria control was ever a tough nut to crack, merely because the parasite evolves mechanisms fast enough to beat our drugs. During the mid-1900s, when chloroquine started being made available, it rattled treatment to its foundations, cutting mortality rates overnight. However, after chloroquine was being used here and there, left and right some *Plasmodium falciparum* strains, especially over in Southeast Asia and South America, began showing that they could outwit the cure. This game of cat and mouse between our drugs and the parasite's fast evolution shows how therapy can inadvertently drive evolution. If we look back at this whole saga, it's clear that despite antimalarial drugs bringing hope, they're also brought with gigantic limitations, and that's why we keep looking for newer solutions. In all cases, these learnings push us towards marrying nature cures with newer, newer molecules to bypass resistance (Zhou & Yue, 2022). It has not been a cakewalk learning about malaria, either. The ethical and practical issues involved in studying human infection slowed our comprehension of how the parasite infects and evades drugs. Thus, researchers had recourse to animal models, which turned out to be a handy stand-in to examine the challenging association of pathogen and host and to experiment with how drugs resist development at both the microscopic molecular level and the systemic level. Still, translating animal results to what goes on in humans is still less than perfect—our biology can be stubbornly so. Vaccines walk a thin tightrope, too; while the release of the RTS,S vaccine is a positive move, the devious parasite life cycle and ever-changing antigens keep it challenging. These recurring traps are a challenging reminder that fighting malaria resistance is a synthesis of concepts from biology, medicine, and how our immune systems resist (Nelson et al., 2022). Looking at the history of drug-resistant malaria, it's clear that how we consume drugs, what kind of parasite we're dealing with, and the surroundings around us all contribute to the equation. Resistance did not have long to wait—very soon it reared its head after drugs like chloroquine, sulfadoxine-pyrimethamine, and soon even those hopeful artemisinin-based ones arrived. Problems like administering too-low doses, sticking to mono-drug regimens, and irregular treatment schedules paved the way for resistant strains to develop. Prudence from those mistakes has guided current strategies that are largely based on combination regimens and compliant treatment protocols to prevent resistance. And, with *Plasmodium* being such a wretchedly adaptable parasite and mixed with socioeconomic and public health issues in so many endemic areas, resistance just keeps popping up. In a sense, history cautions us to remain vigilant and continue to drive the development of novel drugs, while similarly getting our heads around resistance as both a biologic surprise and a social issue (Nelson et al., 2022; Zhou & Yue, 2022).

8.2. Mechanisms of Drug Resistance

The evolution of resistance to malaria drugs is not a neat, linear process but a complex evolution under many different biological and environmental pressures. In infected hosts, while each parasite mutates infrequently on its own, the vast number of such organisms makes it more likely that one will change in a way that makes it less drug-sensitive. The parasite passes through several stages – from sporozoites to liver (hepatic) merozoites to the asexual blood stages , and each of these stages can be a chance for a mutation. Generally speaking, in the absence of drugs meddling in the process, the likelihood of resistance arising is near zero, but during treatment, especially when parasitemia is high—the likelihoods can increase exponentially, sometimes increasing as high as 100,000-fold (Adjuik et al., 2009). In effect, those parasite strains able to withstand the drug's attack tend to thrive, which ends up boosting the overall resistance and its spread. Grasping these dynamics is pretty essential if we're to design interventions that both delay resistance and prolong drug effectiveness. At the heart of malaria's resistance problem is how the parasite's own biological features mesh with the way antimalarial agents work. *Plasmodium falciparum*, largely responsible for the most serious cases of malaria, has developed resistance through primarily genetic adaptations and other physical changes. These adaptations can alter drug uptake, metabolism, or even how a drug binds to its target, often reducing the effectiveness of treatments. For example, when chloroquine was the frontline first-line drug, resistance developed because mutations in the parasite's transport proteins meant the drug did not build up inside the cells as needed. Frontline therapies now use artemisinin derivatives, which have another mode of action by acting on vital intracellular processes that deal with organic peroxide bonds. Though these newer drugs are frequently fast-acting and clinically effective, there is ongoing concern, and research—into how resistance will eventually catch up with them as well (Opsenica & Šolaja, 2012). Mostly, tracking these mechanisms advises more thoughtful drug design and combination therapies aimed at evading or at least delaying resistance. The development and transmission of drug-resistant malaria strains are due to many factors, including how drugs are taken and the diverse genetics of the parasite itself. Subtherapeutic dosing, abbreviated regimens, and even the extensive use of monotherapy medications all serve to select for resistant parasites. Furthermore, the patient's immune status differs; those with partial immunity alone can carry low-grade infections that, over a period of time, keep those resistant mutants alive. Artemisinin-based combination therapies (ACTs), which pair a fast-acting artemisinin with a slower-acting partner drug, try to hit the parasite at several stages and through several mechanisms. However, resistance to artemisinins has already started to emerge in some regions, highlighting the need for ongoing monitoring and policy revision in treatment. More recent, more complex mathematical models are still being developed, in most cases to more realistically predict the emergence of resistance and, more critically, to better inform policy decisions, all to protect the effectiveness of current antimalarial therapies (Adjuik et al., 2009) (Figure 8.6).

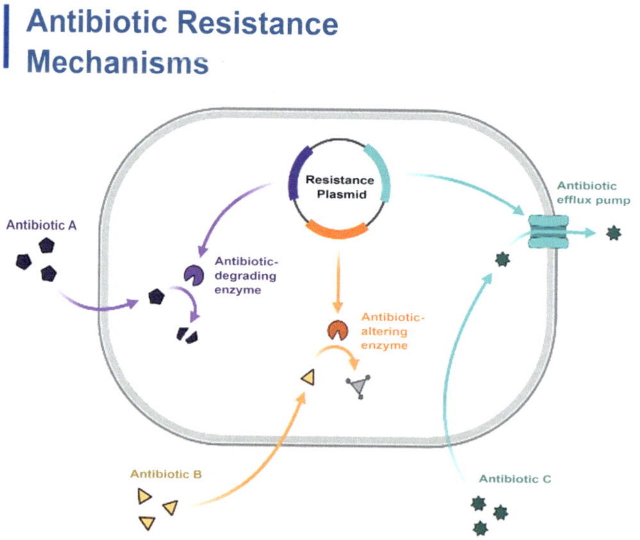

Figure 8.6. *Antibiotic resistance mechanisms.*

Source: Website Files. (n.d.). *Antibiotic Resistance Mechanisms.*

8.2.1. Genetic Mutations in Plasmodium Parasites

Malaria parasites can develop drug resistance in some relatively unexpected mechanisms. Genetic mutations – more specifically, those within the PfK13 locus of *Plasmodium falciparum* – modify the way these flies respond to treatment. In Uganda, for instance, a combination of 469Y, 675V, and 441L mutations have developed in different districts, typically where malaria control efforts have disintegrated or transmission has been sporadic. Such in-country, almost on-the-fly evolution suggests that resistance may naturally be occurring, without needing strains to travel from regions such as Southeast Asia (Melissa et al., 2023). In Papua New Guinea, on the other hand, it is a similar but different scenario. The notorious PfK13 C580Y mutation – perhaps most famously linked with resistance in Southeast Asia – appears to have emerged independently there. Genomic analyses reveal that the parasites possess a characteristic patchwork of mutations in genes such as mdr1, ferredoxin, atg18, and pnp; a type of incremental build-up of change that progressively stabilizes their survival against artemisinin. With such mutation linked to robust artemisinin survival, the findings necessitate a closer—if not more urgent—exploration of the molecular details in local parasite populations (Miotto et al., 2020). Studying these genetic mutations in detail makes one realize why the parasites are beating our drugs. Protein changes related to how the drug works or is metabolized, like in the PfK13 gene and alterations in mdr1 and ferredoxin—make treatments less effective. Mostly, these individual but successive mutations enable the parasites to live longer after treatment, which means a remarkable flexibility. This type of adaptive flexibility implies that integrating genomic surveillance into malaria-control initiatives isn't only clever, it's essential to identify new resistances early on and adapt treatments to prevent broad therapeutic setbacks (Melissa et al., 2023; Miotto et al., 2020) (Figure 8.7).

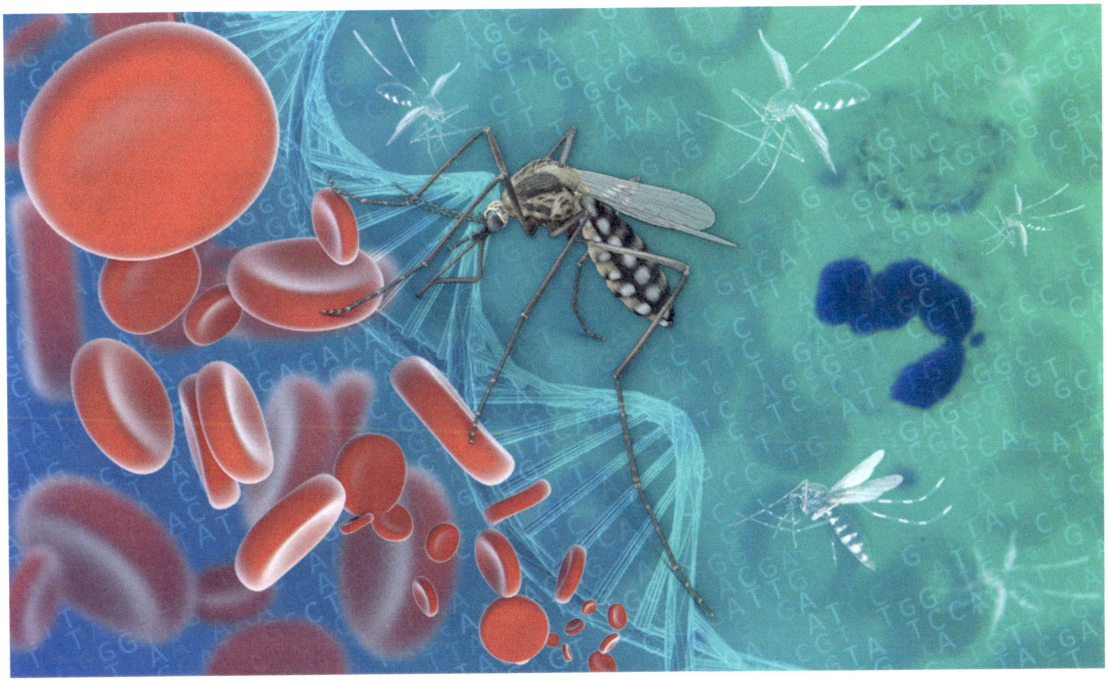

Figure 8.7. *Genetic mutations in Plasmodium parasites.*

Source: EMBL. (2024). *Malaria and Genetic Mutations.*

8.2.2. Pharmacokinetic Factors Affecting Drug Efficacy

How our bodies handle antimalarial medications—, whether and how they uptake, distribute, metabolize, and excrete them—is what governs the success of treatments. For the most part, the process isn't fixed; occasionally the pH of the gut, the gut's motility, or even whether you've just eaten will change how much medicine gets absorbed into the blood. When the absorption is less than ideal, the drug levels drop low enough that the malaria parasites have a chance to persist and even become resistant. When the drug arrives at the site, if it is not distributed uniformly throughout the tissues, there are small, isolated pockets in which the parasites wait for the treatment. Then there is the liver that breaks down the drugs primarily into forms that can either increase their effect or, conversely, repress them—so effectiveness is altered. Excretion should not be forgotten; if the body excretes the drug too quickly, it cannot stay around long enough to get rid of the infection.

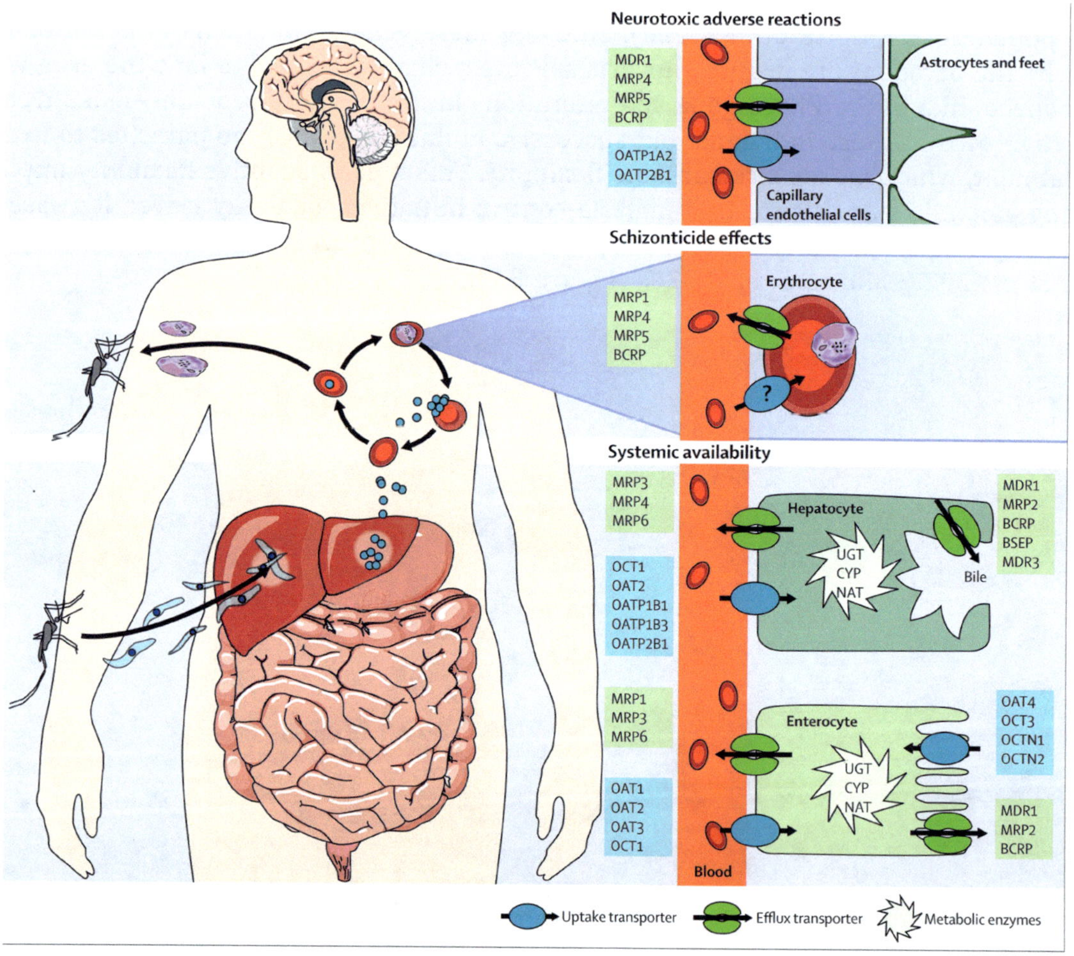

Figure 8.8. *Pharmacogenetics of antimalarial drugs.*

Source: The Lancet. (n.d.). *Pharmacogenetics of Antimalarial Drugs.*

Together, these processes in the body decide if there is still an adequate dose to kill the malaria parasite. Besides simply absorbing and metabolizing the drug, there is also the activity of transporter proteins and enzymes to contend with, further clouding the issue. Take efflux pumps like P-glycoprotein, which actively force the drug back into the bile or intestine, lowering the fraction that reaches the target cells. Additionally, genetic differences, like variations in cytochrome P450 enzymes—can speed up or slow down the way a person metabolizes these medications, so one's experience will be quite different from another's. In most cases, these genetic features will reduce the drug concentration below a therapeutic level or yield fewer effective metabolites, which both can enhance the survival of the parasite. This is why dosage titration on a case-by-case basis occasionally becomes unavoidable, and why finding a treatment that suits all is impossible. Understanding these multi-layered mechanisms, such as the sometimes complicated signaling mechanisms within cells—is relatively crucial for developing better treatment regimens (Hu et al., 2021). Drug interactions provide yet another problem by making the effect of these drugs shift subtly over time. When administered with other drugs, they can either stimulate or inhibit the enzymes involved in antimalarial metabolism, which changes the plasma level of the drug. This causes levels too low to treat malaria sub-therapeutically, or high enough to induce side-effects—both cases giving malaria parasites room to persist and eventually become resistant. Recent studies into repurposing drugs are hopeful in being able to counteract such mechanisms; by using established drugs in new ways, scientists are trying to act on multiple locations at once, thereby increasing the impact of antimalarial medications (Zhang et al., 2020). Of course, the success of such efforts relies in large measure on detailed, advanced understanding of how drugs interact with the body. Most commonly, dose adjusting and the design of carefully thought-out combination regimens are the key interventions against drug-resistant malaria parasites (Figure 8.8).

8.2.3. Environmental Influences on Resistance Development

Environmental conditions and the ability of the malaria parasite to evade drugs are closely related. Low transmission in most of the globe is likely to result in people typically building less natural immunity, in the course of which they tend to depend even more on antimalarial drugs, which in effect contributes to the convenience with which drug-resistant strains propagate more than in high-transmission situations. Timing also matters. When drugs like ACTs are rolled out quickly and widely, they tend to postpone the emergence of resistance; delay or poor cover, respectively, push it forward. Economic limitations, such as costly medications, only make it more difficult, global support may be all it takes to halt resistance development (Dondorp et al., 2008). It's not just biology here. Broad determinants of political will, legislation, and the general level of the economy tend to influence how well interventions perform. For example, underfunding, a dispersed health infrastructure, and complex regulation protocols for getting medicines manufactured and distributed all help to weaken surveillance and control. These defects create a type of breeding ground where deviant drug consumption and even counterfeit drugs take root, placing further pressure on parasites to develop resistance. A failure to include meaningful technology and industry studies in antimicrobial resistance planning only creates additional complexity, and it is a marker of why additional mixed, cross-disciplinary thinking is necessary (Ahmad et al., 2019). Overall, the combination of sound environmental studies with malaria control is the key to staying one step ahead of drug resistance danger. PESTELI tools, which take into account political, economic, social, technological, ecological, legislative, and industry variables—do offer some real inputs for on-the-spot decision-making. It so happens that resistance breaking is not only a scientific problem; it is a complex mix of social, economic, and supply problems with the inevitable dynamic interplay between hosts, vectors, and parasites. It is therefore that national and global health policy have to depend on adaptive, large-brush solutions underpinned by up-to-date evidence, stakeholder perceptions, and emergency preparedness plans. This approach, while not preferable, would render antimalarial drugs effective for a longer duration and help undermine the worldwide burden of malaria (Ahmad et al., 2019).

8.3. Current Antimalarial Drugs

The past ten years have witnessed a firm decline in the world's stranglehold on malaria due to newer drug therapies. More recent antimalarial drugs, particularly ACTs (short for artemisinin-based combination treatments), are now the preferred choice because they kill parasites quickly and reduce the spread—at least, this has been true. But here's the catch: resistant *Plasmodium* strains are on the rise, and clearly, we need new drugs. Researchers are now zeroing in on compounds like artefenomel, ferroquine, and cipargamin; these drugs have their own sleights of hand that might be able to evade the usual resistance mechanisms. The pursuit of new drug targets, such as proteases or transport proteins essential for survival—offers another promising avenue of attack. Overall, these efforts are a specific response to the intractable problem of multidrug resistance, all conspiring to control malaria and push us closer toward eradication goals (Matthews et al., 2018). Having good drug policies does make an enormous difference when it comes to making existing treatments effective.

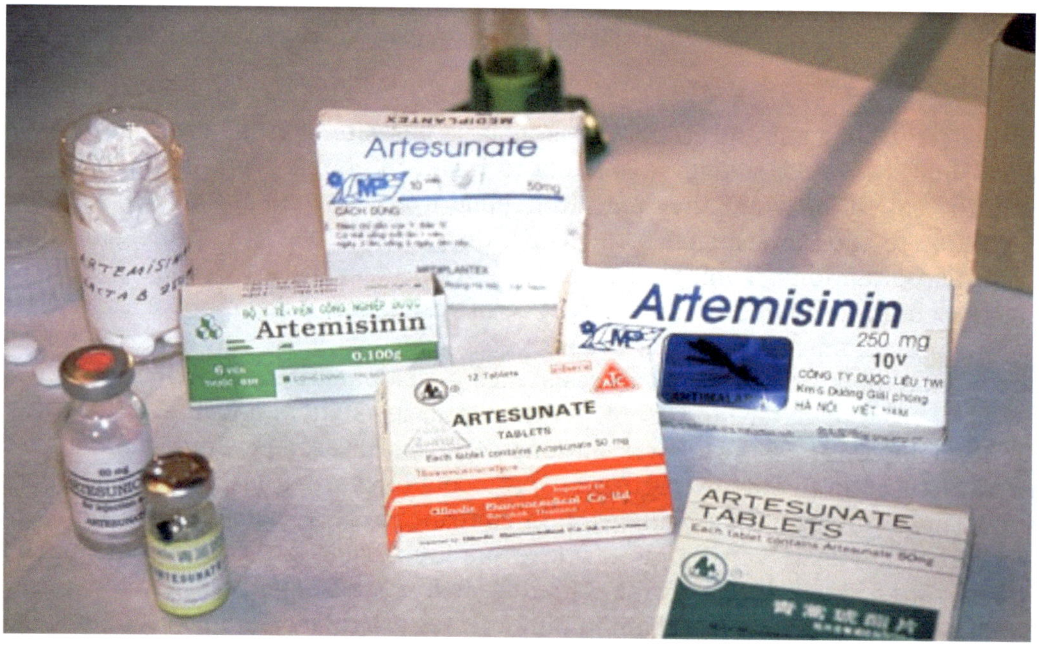

Figure 8.9. *Current antimalarial drugs.*

Source: Crump, A. & WHO/TDR. (n.d.). *Antimalarial Drugs from Artemisia Annua Plant*. Fine Art America.

A majority of nations affected by malaria have made ACTs their first line of medicine, just because the drugs truly are effective and have a greater inclination to avoid the evolution of resistance to them than would be the case with single-drug therapy. But as it happens, the rate at which the resistance emerges is a function of local levels of malaria transmission as well as actual application of the drugs—models even indicate that resistance develops earlier when the transmission is low. This makes it quite imperative to have high ACT coverage such that partner drugs stay on track. There have been a few instances when delays or limited access reduced the net benefit, and, frankly, the cost of ACTs still strangles some treatment programs. Global subsidies seem quite essential then to make these drugs accessible to everyone and bring their full public health potential (Dondorp et al., 2008). Despite the promise of today's antimalarials, however, the slippery target that is resistance to *Plasmodium* compels us continually to reinvent the wheel. Many groups are in the process of making next-generation antimalarials targeting new molecular targets—targets not previously occupied. Large resistance and genetic screens have even been key to finding these novel targets, with breakthroughs with drugs such as KAF156 and MMV048. A particularly interesting example is tafenoquine, which targets the hard-to-reach, liver-stage parasites, effectively extending treatment to cover all stages of the parasite's life cycle. Merging these new-fangled methods with good old-fashioned remedies may very well offer us a control strategy that's both more difficult and longer lasting. Wherever it is possible, the battle to ultimately eliminate malaria from the world will involve many discovery of new drugs, smart policy, and better access to medicine—each supporting the other in a grueling war (Matthews et al., 2018) (Figure 8.9).

8.3.1. Overview of Commonly Used Antimalarial Medications

Malaria drugs have come a long way. In the past, chloroquine and sulfadoxine-pyrimethamine were the initial choices as they were easy to give and potent enough in their day. But when parasites became adept at resisting them, we required something more effective. Nowadays, ACTs have been in the spotlight—welcomed for their fast action and ability for clearance of parasites efficiently. However, in the majority of cases, correct application of these drugs is the solution; misprescribed or dispensed carelessly, resistance gains speed, and that only implies it's not a case of finding new drugs but making both healthcare providers and patients comply with what works (Kamuhabwa & Silumbe, 2013). Different antimalarial drugs target the parasite differently, at different points in its life cycle. Take artemether-lumefantrine, for instance, it couples rapidly effective artemisinin with a longer-acting partner, which is likely to cure the infection and lower the risk of relapse. Other drugs like quinine and mefloquine are sometimes employed as stopgaps when resistance is an issue. Tourists, for example, are often issued with prophylactic prescriptions of doxycycline or atovaquone-proguanil, though these are less common where malaria is endemic. By chance, the success of such treatments is largely dependent on the dose as well as on compliance from the patient population, which is not always feasible, especially when physicians and patients themselves cannot have a clear grasp of everything there is to malaria transmission and even basic mosquito control methods (Ruberto et al., 2014).

Even with such a wide range of drugs available, there's an ongoing worry about emerging resistance patterns that affect treatment outcomes. Remember when chloroquine and sulfadoxine-pyrimethamine began to fail? That shift pushed the world toward relying more on ACTs. Yet, there are now signs, particularly in parts of Southeast Asia, which even artemisinin might be losing a bit of its edge, which calls for extra caution. In the majority of instances, this problem is worsened by not applying these drugs as they are supposed to; in some instances, doctors might not have all the information on how the drugs work and misprescribe, allowing resistant bacteria to survive

(Kamuhabwa & Silumbe, 2013). Meanwhile, public awareness of the prevention of malaria is poor, and that only highlights how important it is to pair effective drug use with education and vector control (Ruberto et al., 2014) (Figure 8.10).

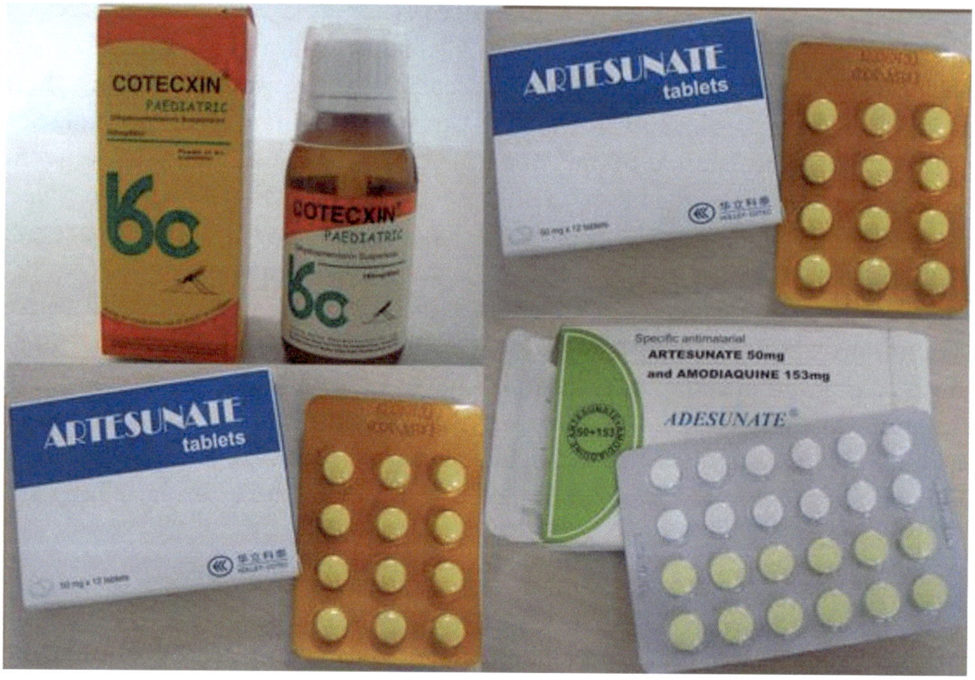

Figure 8.10. *Commonly used antimalarial medications.*

Source: EC21. (n.d.). *Sell Antimalarial Drugs and Generics.*

8.3.2. Mechanisms of Action of These Drugs

Malaria treatment remains a challenge, mostly because the *Plasmodium* parasites quickly develop means of resistance to our most common treatments. Learning about how those treatments work is at the heart of learning why resistance becomes an issue. Chloroquine, for example, once the standard treatment, targets the parasite's detoxification cycle in its digestive vacuole; it prevents the toxic heme from being converted to harmless hemozoin. This irritation leads to toxic heme to build up until the parasite eventually dies. Of course, parasite gene mutations, in particular those changing drug transport in the vacuole, cause chloroquine not to build up as it should and, therefore, not being as effective. Interestingly, the discovery of organic peroxides like artemisinins and their cousins changed the game; their special peroxide bond helps to initiate reactive oxygen species that kill key parasite proteins and membranes, offering a fast-acting, low-toxicity option with very few cases of resistance documented (Opsenica & Šolaja, 2012). Probing further, while chloroquine interferes with heme buildup, scientists have also uncovered the genetic subtleties driving resistance. The *pfcrt* gene, which encodes a vacuolar membrane transporter protein, is generally considered to be the prime culprit for chloroquine resistance in *Plasmodium falciparum*. Mutations in this area have been seen to change the expulsion of the drug from the vacuole of the parasite, the outcome being lower intracellular levels. Recent research, whole-genome resequencing and linkage analysis of the rodent malaria parasites, has shown a rather complex genetic setting in play with several gene loci. Unexpectedly, mutations in another gene, aat1 (an amino acid transporter), drive resistance even higher. The findings highlight the point that drug resistance is not due to one gene; it's an entire-genome effect that complicates treatment but also sheds light on the way to next-generation antimalarials (Modrzynska et al., 2012). Recently developed antimalarial drugs follow a broader approach in targeting a number of parasite processes simultaneously, which seems to minimize the opportunity to develop resistance. Overall, artemisinins and organic peroxide analogs differ in their mechanism compared to the traditional quinoline-type drugs. They cleave their peroxide bridges under intracellular iron, which leads to the generation of free radicals. These reactive species subsequently bind to and kill a number of parasite proteins and membranes, leading to the rapid killing of the parasite. Such broad, non-specific attacks could well be the reason why general resistance to these drugs has not developed. Synthetic derivatives and chimeric molecules carrying peroxide pharmacophores increase the structural diversity and stability of these molecules and thereby make them possible substitutes in fighting malaria. Research nowadays is still exploring such mechanisms, always refining our approach to circumvent resistance and enhance the potency of treatment against all forms of *Plasmodium* species (Opsenica & Šolaja, 2012).

8.3.3. Limitations and Challenges in Drug Effectiveness

Drug efficacy at treating malaria is riddled with obstacles both from the parasite itself and from issues with the greater system. *Plasmodium* has a tendency to alter its plan of action—small genetic adjustments allow it to shrug off drugs that once worked just fine, so medicines lose their effectiveness in short order. There isn't a one-size-fits-all vaccine either, leaving us relying on medications that in most instances work unevenly. Toxic side effects also appear and are troublesome to control the use of these drugs safely with high-risk patients. Treatment failures seem to be on the rise, i.e., in overall terms, our need for newer drugs is more than ever before, although it may cost big time and big money. In plain terms, drug resistance calls for fresh, creative approaches that are safety and affordability-first (Gujjari et al., 2022). The issue does not stop there. How the resistance piles up is as if seeing other infections to come back—repeated drug use puts pressure on the parasite, making it adapt faster. Others argue that drugs like parasite biofilms and other such defense mechanisms only make things more complicated by keeping the drugs from penetrating where they are needed. All this random adaptation leads to our supply of effective drugs being slowly depleted over time, chipping away at how long any one treatment will last. It's a reminder that we need to look for new therapeutic strategies and more efficient methods of drug delivery, perhaps combining molecular or genomic knowledge, even though our choices look woefully restricted on the public health front at the moment (Uddin et al., 2021). Considering the big picture, a number of recent studies are putting the spotlight on nanotech as a means of reimagining antimalarial therapies. These nanotechnology strategies can enhance the delivery of a drug in the body, target it to where it must go more precisely, and control its release so that toxicity will be reduced and efficacy will rise—although that's no magic pill. These new drugs might sidestep some of the previous barriers like resistance and cost, and with luck, better patient compliance. But shifting away from our traditional drug methodologies to ultra-miniature nanoparticle-based ones isn't straightforward; there are considerable development and regulatory obstacles along the way that could put the kibosh on. However, most see the promise of nanotech as an important new avenue in future drug development—a necessity given the numerous shortcomings of current therapies (Gujjari et al., 2022) (Figure 8.11).

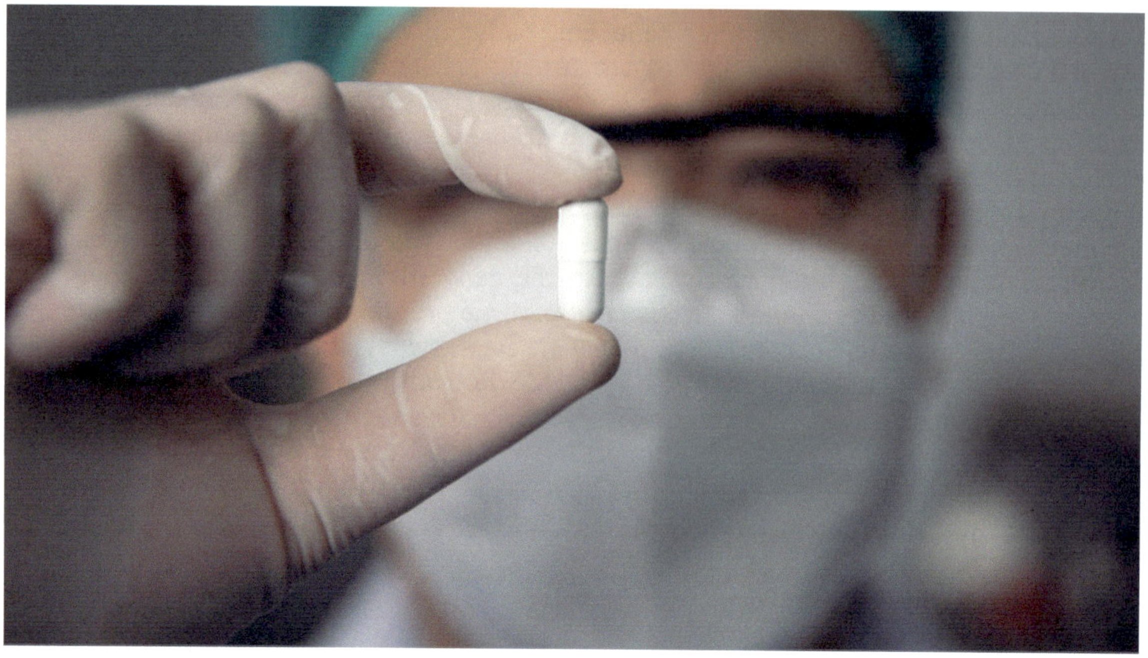

Figure 8.11. *Limitations and challenges in drug effectiveness.*

Source: CAS Insights. (n.d.). *Limitations in Drug Effectiveness.*

8.4. Case Studies of Drug Resistance

Scientists have also been tracking drug resistance to malaria quite a long time, following the progress of some *Plasmodium falciparum* strains seeming to skirt treatments. Take Ethiopia, for instance, genomic studies dug deep into parasite samples and found that approximately 8.0% of them carried the kelch13 622I mutation, which indicates partial artemisinin resistance. Curiously, parasites that lacked the pfhrp2/3 genes—the ones that interfere with diagnostic tests—did not bear this mutation as frequently. It is as though the drugs and the diagnostics are in a complex association of avoidance of each other. The commonalties genetically among such resistant strains, in most instances, point to relatively recent spread, i.e., multidrug-resistant malaria travels fast. This union of artemisinin resistance and diagnostic-evading features makes for a reasonably urgent call for increased alertness to guide treatments and control measures (Abebe et al., 2023). It's an unmistakable sign that trying to control malaria where it exists just keeps getting progressively harder and harder. Now, taking a glance over to the Sahel region, things fall into a bit of a different category with seasonal malaria chemoprevention (SMC) programs. Under the ACCESS-SMC project, across seven nations, the idea was simple: give under-fives a monthly sulfadoxine–pyrimethamine and amodiaquine injection during high malaria seasons. The large-scale tests had high coverage and a strong decline in both cases and deaths, with protection reaching more than 88% effectiveness. Nevertheless, although indicators of resistance generally remained at low levels, there was a slight increase in mutations associated with sulfadoxine–pyrimethamine resistance. As a rule, this informs us that even though SMC's benefits are apparently clear, it's important to monitor any resistance indicators to ensure the drugs remain effective. Having antimalarials within a controlled community setting sort of achieves a balancing act between short-term benefits and the risk of triggering resistance (Baba et al., 2020). Pitting these two against each other, you have two starkly different stories of drug resistance with malaria. The Ethiopian case clearly demonstrates how, without sharply targeted interventions, resistant parasite strains can emerge and rapidly spread, causing serious problems for treatment. Meanwhile, the Sahel SMC program suggests that if a well-planned prevention campaign is undertaken, it can harvest enormous health dividends without eliciting rapid large-scale resistance, provided coverage is high and molecular screening is underway. Overall, it simply boils down to the reality that local disease patterns and genetics have to be harmonized with malaria control efforts; you must forecast and deal with resistance as it happens. Sustained investment in genomic surveillance and nimble public health interventions remains critical in maintaining malaria in check in different regions (Baba et al., 2020; Abebe et al., 2023).

8.4.1. Resistance to Chloroquine in Southeast Asia

Drug-resistant malaria parasites have been the bane of global control attempts, and you wouldn't fault us for being aware that Southeast Asia—yes, that part of the world—is the hotbed for this debacle. Way back in the mid-1900s, everyone relied on chloroquine for the treatment of *Plasmodium falciparum* malaria until its effectiveness started fading away. The battle began in several locations, Cambodia being the most significant before resistance spread throughout the entire Greater Mekong Subregion. Overuse of chloroquine, often boosted by single-drug treatment and brief courses, finally gave these parasites that shove they required to survive. The consequences were hard to overlook higher treatment failure and higher rates of sickness and death, and eventually this resistant organism spread to Africa, causing a severe public health crisis and quite literally putting Southeast Asia in the spotlight of world drug resistance politics (Rob et al., 2020). All this previous history kind of sets the stage for the issues we now have with more recent antimalarial drugs. As chloroquine started to fail reasonably rapidly, alternative therapies like sulfadoxine-pyrimethamine (SP) entered the scene, only to be outgunned by resistance at virtually the same pace. This relentless march pushed a reversal toward ACTs as the first-line treatment. Southeast Asia remains, though, still on the cusp of building resistance. Instances of artemisinin resistance—traditionally linked to mutations in the *Plasmodium falciparum* Kelch 13 (K13) gene—are all part of the story. Some local studies suggest that even after chloroquine has been discontinued, remnants of its resistance seem to remain or change according to local drug fashions; it's like those resistant markers keep on surfacing at unexpected times. This strange resilience complicates the extinction of the resistant strains because it maintains a reservoir in the background which could, in most cases, disqualify even the novel combination therapies. More advanced molecular monitoring and tailored treatment regimens are clearly required to keep this barrier in line (Rob et al., 2020). New studies unearthing the genetic makeup of malaria parasites in Southeast Asia reveal a quite complex assemblage of mutations that make these insects resistant to a range of drugs, even chloroquine. Genotypic screenings across various disciplines have at times identified a wild-type version of the chloroquine resistance transporter gene (PfCRT), possibly reflecting that once the drug pressure was alleviated after chloroquine was put on the backburner, parasites had a temporary ability to regain some susceptibility. In the meantime, mutations in other genes implicated in partner drug resistance in the ACTs continue to perpetuate themselves, illustrating just how adaptable these parasites are. Essentially, pulling a drug off the list might allow for some short-term sensitivity, but new treatments bring in fresh pressures that lead to emerging resistance in other medications.

To summarize, a deep and nuanced grasp of these shifting molecular trends, and how they echo in treatment outcomes—is absolutely key if we're to craft sustainable strategies for countering malaria drug resistance in Southeast Asia (Figure 8.12).

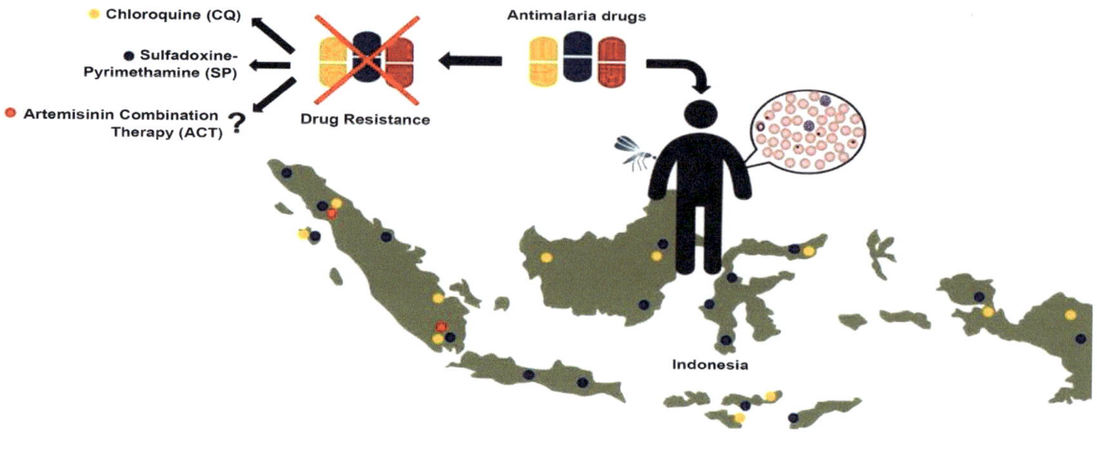

Figure 8.12. *Resistance to chloroquine in Southeast Asia.*

Source: Dove Medical Press. (n.d.). *Resistance to Chloroquine in Southeast Asia.*

8.4.2. Emergence of Artemisinin Resistance in Africa

Management of malaria in Africa for decades has largely relied on ACTs ; those artemisinin-based combination therapies that have been the go-to for uncomplicated *Plasmodium falciparum* infections all these years. But lately, though, something seems to be shifting in a direction that's hard to ignore. In several recent studies, for instance, researchers have indicated that these treatments are gradually but inevitably losing their potency. Look at Eritrea: rising numbers of patients are turning up with evidence of parasites being alive three days after standard ACT treatment has been initiated. Further examination shows that Pfkelch13 R622I mutation – a marker usually associated with one form of partial artemisinin resistance – is on the rise. This mutation is not only associated with higher day three parasite positivity rates but also, when subjected to laboratory testing, seems to lead to a measurable resistance. Additionally, the simultaneous hrp2 and hrp3 gene dropouts are throwing another wrench into the gears by making rapid diagnostic tests inaccurate, and this only serves to contribute to treatment and monitoring strategies (Mihreteab et al., 2023). Getting slightly more specific, though, the artemisinin resistance case is not so easy, one-size-fits-all. The relationship between K13 mutations and the malaria parasite's behavior seems to be very complex. Current genetics work demonstrates that all of these mutations, R561H, C580Y, and M579I, don't all do the same thing – they can change the sensitivity to the drug and general fitness of the parasite, subsequently that affects its ability to spread. Typically, in most parasite strains resident in Africa, the R561H mutation doesn't seem to have much of an effect, i.e., it doesn't inhibit the parasite. By contrast, mutations like C580Y and M579I typically have a readily apparent growth penalty, which could hamper their spread within heavily transmitting regions. Subsequently there is Southeast Asia, where these types of mutations place little to no growth burden on the parasite whatsoever.

This discrepancy emphasizes the importance of the parasite's genetic past when trying to forecast how resistance will evolve across Africa (Barbara et al., 2021). Overall, the development of partial artemisinin resistance in Africa – supported by an increase in K13 mutation rates and a decrease in drug efficacy – is sounding a clarion call for public health planners. The integration of molecular indicators with treatment outcomes from varying geographic locations shows that resistance is no longer a Southeast Asian story; nations like Eritrea and Rwanda are starting to see it take root. This kind of trend imperils the once-reliable ACTs with an aura of suspicion and the potential to undo progress in reducing malaria mortality and disease. In most cases, a rise in surveillance ; one that combines genomic data, phenotypic resistance tests, and good clinical follow-up – will be necessary to monitor the spread of resistance and adjust policy appropriately. Additionally, the diagnostic impacts of hrp2/hrp3 deletions mean new detection methods to ensure malaria control efficacy, despite challenges creeping in (Barbara et al., 2021; Mihreteab et al., 2023) (Figure 8.13).

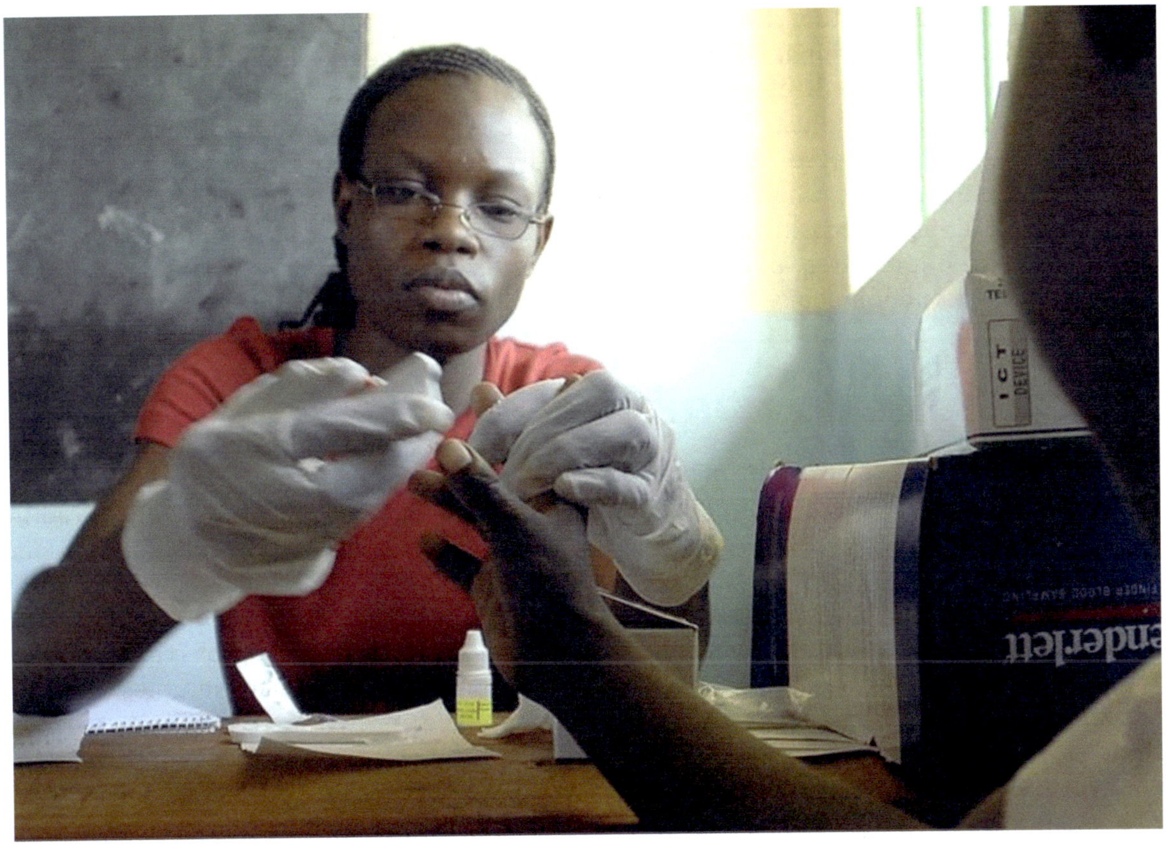

Figure 8.13. *Artemisinin-resistant malaria.*

Source: CIDRAP. (n.d.). *Malaria Testing by US Army Africa.*

8.4.3. Impact of Drug Resistance on Malaria Control Programs

Control of malaria had previously seen great triumphs, but all these successes are nowadays more and more under threat as drug resistance takes hold. Sizable investment in treatment and prevention has been sidetracked; *Plasmodium* strains now seem to push apart our favorite antimalarial drugs.

Such a shift typically means that people are in for a longer, harder fight when they fall ill, while the disease continues to spread silently among communities. It places further burden on already overburdened health systems coping with limited resources, making treatment both costlier and more complicated. The confluence of drug pressure and the parasite's resistance clearly calls for vigilant, on-the-ground monitoring and responsive strategies (Coukell et al., 2016). The impact of drug resistance goes far beyond mere treatment hiccups, it derails the whole public health apparatus set in place to contain malaria. Control programs, for the most part, are constantly having to re-hatch their plans to keep up with constantly shifting resistance patterns, occasionally even spending money on expensive new drug combinations or more sensitive diagnostic equipment to detect recalcitrant strains early. Too often, these financial burdens siphon money from other priority areas such as mosquito control or education outreach. Importantly, as the vast majority of drugs come from a handful of three-decade-old families of chemicals, our backup options dwindle as resistance arises (Coukell et al., 2016). In such circumstances, progress toward the eliminating malaria can all too easily be reversed. As the increasing burden of drug-resistant malaria confronts it, international efforts are gradually shifting gears. New developments, like the President's Malaria Initiative Strategy, highlight real-time tracking to identify building resistance patterns so policies can be adjusted as needed . There is also attempting to deploy ACTs, which cleverly mix drugs with diverse mechanisms to slow down resistance. However, keeping such treatments is an ongoing investment in research, training, and intersectoral collaboration. If we do not provide these all-encompassing measures, the international fight against malaria may weaken, highlighting the need for better, all-encompassing measures to protect treatment gains and drive long-term disease reduction goals.

8.5. Strategies to Combat Drug Resistance

There are always new drug-resistant malaria parasites arising, so we must consider alternatives beyond yesterday's chemo. Plenty of attention has been given in recent years to mixing in traditional herbal remedies. Indonesia, for instance, provides a veritable treasure trove of plants full of secondary metabolites—compounds like flavonoids, terpenoids, and alkaloids, which naturally fight malaria. Taking advantage of these natural extracts in combination with existing treatments might enhance their combined potency and, in most cases, even work despite the problem of resistance. It also helps to keep track of how drug resistance varies geographically and adjust therapies accordingly. Such a kind of methodology doesn't just try to slow parasite growth, it might even slow down resistance by diminishing our overreliance on one single class of drugs (Tobing et al., 2024). Public health measures are just as important as new pharmaceutical ideas in the struggle against malaria drug resistance. It's simple practices like the use of insecticide-treated bednets and indoor residual spraying that will decrease infection, which in turn equals fewer drugs needed and less pressure on the parasite to adapt. And, as communities are educated on following the correct treatment protocols—averting those all-too-familiar dosing mistakes, it also reduces further the potential for resistance to catch fire. Better healthcare infrastructure, especially in devastated regions, ensures correct diagnoses and appropriate case management, allowing treatments to be more effectively customized and resistance trends to be tracked. All these combined efforts set a strong basis to make our current drugs worthwhile, even as vaccine research is a vital complementary goal (Tonna, 2006). Above this, new vaccine technologies and novel drug combinations add further possibilities to our arsenal against drug-resistant malaria. Yes, vaccines have lowered disease loads previously, but the complex life cycle of malaria and its constantly shifting antigens make it more complicated. Researchers are now experimenting with multi-stage vaccines that could mitigate the severity of infections and parasite transmission and hence reduce drug treatments and slow resistance. At the same time, combining drugs with different mechanisms of action might hit the parasite on several fronts at once. Promisingly, global efforts to enhance research capability and integrate environmental, medicinal, and social intervention are offering us a balanced pathway towards diminishing drug resistance and eventually eliminating malaria altogether (Tonna, 2006) (Figure 8.14).

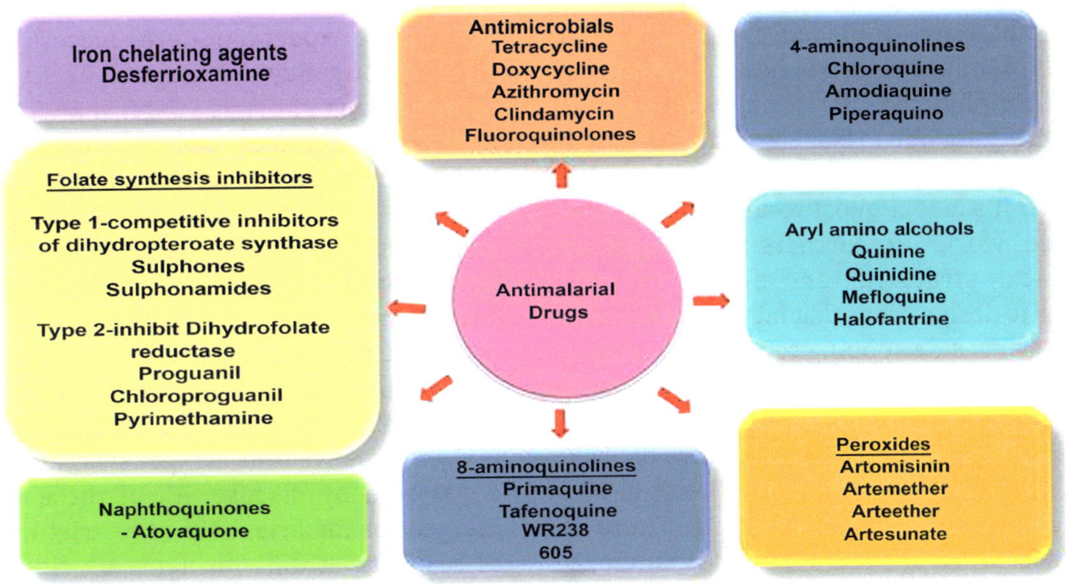

Figure 8.14. *Combat drug resistance.*

Source: Kumi RO, Oti B, Abo-Dya NE, Alahmdi MI, Soliman MES. Bridging the Gap in Malaria Parasite Resistance, Current Interventions, and the Way Forward from in Silico Perspective: A Review. *Molecules*. 2022; 27(22):7915. https://doi.org/10.3390/molecules27227915

8.5.1. Development of New Antimalarial Drugs

Malaria parasites just keep finding ways to evolve and outsmart our medicines, so finding new ways to fight them is more crucial than ever before. Scientists have moved past mere attempts at drugs for what they see happening and now use wily methods to attack particular molecules that are vital to the parasite's survival. One very interesting approach attacks lysyl tRNA synthetase (PfKRS). This isn't a one-string plan, it combines parasite strains that have become drug-resistant through evolution, introduces hybrid proteins for detailed structural study, and has chemical probes to verify that the drug hits the target in living cells. All these strategies combined allow us to understand how drugs interact with the parasite and with the host and tend to set the stage for smarter and more effective compound alters, a thrilling leap forward in our fight against rising drug resistance (Milne et al., 2022). Even with these state-of-the-art advances, nature's own medicines still make their mark. For centuries, natural products have served as the model for antimalarial drugs—take quinine from Cinchona bark or artemisinin from Artemisia annua. But when drug-resistant strains spread, the dependable artemisinin-based combinations sometimes fail, so a new option is an urgent requirement. Now scientists have targeted over 90 different plant species, including many in the African, Asian, and South American continents. Although few of the compounds that have been isolated have shown clear-cut benefits or known mechanisms of action, the range of bioactive molecules that have been identified to date indicates that delving further into phytochemicals may well provide the next step forward (Isabela et al., 2021). In the meantime, the search isn't just for novel chemicals; it's also a quest to understand how resistance works. Researchers are integrating biochemical, structural, and even proteomic strategies to design drugs that hit critical parasite enzymes while sidestepping common resistance mechanisms. Thermal proteome profiling, used to catch a glimpse of interactions in the living parasite, offers an unprejudiced view of drug targets, which goes on to influence better design and better resistance management. There is also more work in verification of ancient-world medical wisdom; indigenous species like *Ampelozyzyphus amazonicus*, for example, add to a growing list of possibilities that show protective as well as curative potential. In most cases, these convergent strategies might just give antimalarial drug development a lease of life, helping counter resistant strains and supporting malaria control efforts worldwide (Isabela et al., 2021; Milne et al., 2022).

8.5.2. Importance of Combination Therapies

Malaria remains such a long-standing enemy largely because the parasite quickly learns to outsmart our drugs. Single drugs can be effective at first, but when resistant strains emerge, they become useless almost overnight. This fact in general forces us to look for more resilient treatment strategies. Doctors have turned to using combinations of drugs—ACTs, for example, pair an artemisinin derivative with a second drug from another class. This pairing minimizes the risk of the parasite developing resistance to both at the same time. Interestingly, according to studies, under normal conditions, the artemisinin compound doesn't do much of the contribution; its partner drug clears out most of the parasites. That means we need to make sure we take care of these partner drugs if we expect long-term success (Hastings et al., 2016). Beyond malaria by itself, using combinations of drugs suggests a wider public health counterattack against diseases that tend to become resistant to treatment. You can get the same outcomes when treating diseases like visceral leishmaniasis—using different drugs in combination not only saves money but also lasts longer in the field. By attacking the parasite with different drugs that use different modes of attack, the likelihood of resistance developing slows down dramatically. This approach has proven effective and inexpensive in poor areas devastated by disease. All of these elements, merged for malaria, help to restrict the spread of resistant strains, bringing us closer to the eliminating diseases. Combination therapies thus serve a twofold purpose: they improve patient recuperation and preserve the viability of our existing drugs when the pipeline for the creation of new medications is virtually dry (Meheus et al., 2010). At the same time, maintaining the effectiveness of partner drugs in these combinations demands a new approach to public health policy—one that puts equal priority on saving artemisinin and its partner drugs. For if we let resistance to partner drugs get out of hand, our entire antimalarial approach falls apart. That takes vigilant surveillance, smart drug use, and agile response in changing treatment regimens. Furthermore, countrywide application of these methods requires increased focus on access issues, patient adherence, and clinician training appropriately. The real benefits in the field in terms of relapse rate reduction and overall reduction in disease transmission show why these techniques are so essential in our fight against malaria. Finally, rendering our current arsenal more efficacious through the utilization of such combinations is imperative to tipping the scales towards malaria elimination and evading the dire ramifications of drug resistance (Hastings et al., 2016) (Figure 8.15).

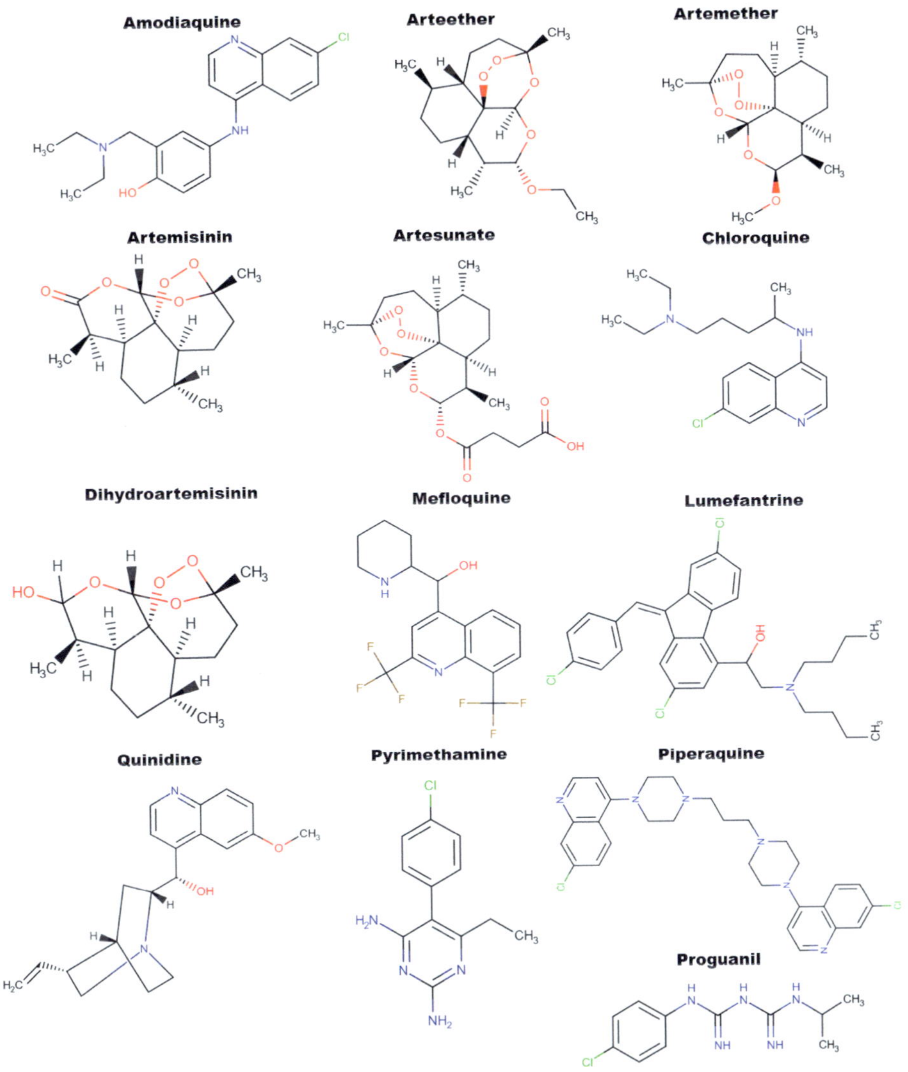

Figure 8.15. *Combination therapies in malaria.*

Source: Kumi RO, Oti B, Abo-Dya NE, Alahmdi MI, Soliman MES. Bridging the Gap in Malaria Parasite Resistance, Current Interventions, and the Way Forward from in Silico Perspective: A Review. *Molecules*. 2022; 27(22):7915. https://doi.org/10.3390/molecules27227915

8.5.3. Role of Public Health Initiatives in Prevention

Public health measures make an enormous difference in holding back drug-resistant malaria. In past outbreaks, coordinated responses have revealed that by strengthening local surveillance networks, spreading simple health information, and making sure that everyone receives the treatment they need, communities can cut disease transmission. Take Africa, for example, past experiences of infectious outbreaks show that it does make a difference to have strong, quick-responding health systems in place. If we strengthen health facilities in whole regions and countries, they can pick up early indications of resistance and institute workable measures. Local production of tests and medicines is also indispensable; it makes us less reliant on external sources and generally means that we get what we require when we require it. All these combination therapies, formulated in a strict health paradigm, come together to fight the stubborn menace of multi-drug-resistant strains of malaria (John et al., 2020). Investment in a well-trained public health workforce is absolutely vital to prevent this kind of malaria. Training epidemiologists, nurses, and community health workers—among other front-line workers—raises our general ability to track trends, supply targeted treatment, and help individuals stick to their antimalarial injections. Too frequently, when enough trained workers are not available, delays crop up and resistant parasites get loose to infect, which can severely undermine control efforts. Most frequently, leadership programs that develop many competencies translate upper-level science into lower-level policies, so prevention initiatives are both relevant to local demands and backed by solid information. Furthermore, bridging governments with local communities and global partners facilitates better knowledge transfer and pooling of resources. These joint activities make public health responses more robust against the spread of drug resistance (John et al., 2020). At a larger level, efforts towards increasing public awareness and guiding correct use of medicines play an important role in preventing drug-resistant malaria from worsening. Misuse of antimalarial drugs has hastened resistance, and thus there is a need to run campaigns that explain in clear terms to both health practitioners and the general population how to use such drugs responsibly. Alongside global initiatives towards combating antimicrobial resistance, highlighting practices like strong surveillance, prudent use of diagnostic tools, and greater control over physician prescriptions effectively cuts down on the type of abuse that encourages resistance. It's also about deterring dosing that's too low or unneeded while keeping all persons on their full regimen. And even changing how agriculture handles analogous compounds falls under a One Health umbrella, understanding how humans, animals, and nature all interact with each other in this soup. Lessons from other resistance programs teach us that when education, tough policies, and cooperation among different sectors come together, even with a few bumps along the way, it does keep antimalarial drugs working.

8.6. Future Directions in Malaria Research

Recent developments in molecular biology have opened up new and unexpected possibilities for understanding malaria's resistance to medication. The latest research is concerned with how certain genes—K13, in particular the C580Y change—are indicators for *Plasmodium falciparum* resistance. These mutations can impair the parasite's ability to respond to oxidative stress caused by antimalarial medications. In most cases, going deeper into these genetic modifications seems to be the cornerstone in creating therapies that bypass or even inactivate the resistance mechanisms. And now that multidrug-resistant strains are starting to appear, what is needed is twofold: either devise new drug combinations or even whole new classes of antimalarials based on these genetic and biochemical insights (Azmi et al., 2023). By tipping into a molecular comprehension of these mechanisms, we can sometimes anticipate how the parasites are likely to evolve and preemptively modify our treatment methods. Taking a step beyond just the genetics, scientists are now trying to see how host and parasite interact on a cellular signaling level—a move that offers some novel fresh possibilities for therapy. Take the Janus kinase/signal transducer and activator of transcription (JAK/STAT) pathway; it's well known for its role in the regulation of immune responses and inflammation, and when it goes wrong, a variety of diseases are the outcome. Generally, manipulating this pathway might regulate the host's immune response to *Plasmodium* infection, thereby inhibiting parasite viability and resistance development. Follow-up studies can, for example, attempt the use of JAK/STAT inhibitors to give the body a better chance of clearing resistant parasites, thereby complementing the antimalarial drugs' direct action (Hu et al., 2021). This marriage of parasite molecular insights with host immune manipulation, while not necessarily flawless at every step, is certainly a sophisticated strategy to tackle drug resistance. As our knowledge expands, there's also an evident need for more precise diagnostic and surveillance capacities to rapidly signal markers of resistance in locations most affected by malaria. Emerging genomic methods and real-time molecular assays can enable health workers to detect resistance trends as they arise and adjust treatments before failures become entrenched. Likewise, investments in vaccines against resistant malaria need to be increased urgently—either by targeting parasite features that do not mutate frequently or by enhancing the body's own immune system. Coupling these approaches with public health initiatives like enhanced vector control and more patient-friendly education could be the key to halting the spread of resistant malaria. Overall, future malaria research will likely combine molecular findings, immune system engineering, and day-to-day health efforts to tackle the evolving drug resistance crisis directly (Hu et al., 2021; Azmi et al., 2023).

8.6.1. Innovations in Vaccine Development

Scientific progress and new technologies have ignited new enthusiasm for parasite vaccines like those against malaria now that medicines have a way of losing their potency. It seems that, in most cases, success with developing vaccines is a question of working against different stages of the life cycle of the parasite for malaria, trying to stop the spread while establishing long-term immunity. Instead of the usual chemical approaches that sometimes push resistance further, vaccines bring salvation without putting extra pressure on the survival of the fittest parasites. Modern methods, such as protein fragments, genetically modified viral delivery systems, and mRNA magic tricks—help guide the proper signals to our immune system, mobilizing our body's defenses in clever and underhanded ways. These approaches also open the door to multivalent vaccines, which aim at various forms of parasites at once, a consideration of significance when genetic variation tends to upset efficacy. This expenditure on this vaccine research is, given the circumstances, the smart move against drug-resistant malaria strains (Paul et al., 2020). Besides these cutting-edge developments, there's an emerging trend to pair vaccine releases with older, long-trusted parasite-fighting strategies. In fact, animal vaccines have shown promise to reduce infection, which implies they could be viable in addition to, if not in place of, traditional chemical treatments. This combination method is particularly apropos with the ongoing rise of drug resistance, which requires a disruption of that cycle that won't be unfriendly to the environment. The recent shift in focus by the global animal health market towards these parasitic vaccines reflects an understanding that immunization might help lower our reliance on standard drugs and, in most cases, slow down the resistance train. Plus, combining vaccines with newer chemicals like isoxazolines—used in vector control—could potentially boost overall effectiveness in ways we're just beginning to appreciate (Paul et al., 2020). The imperative to combat antimicrobial resistance broadly has also fueled a vaccine innovation boom. The COVID-19 pandemic experience, for instance, reinforced the value of swift vaccine design, production, and deployment, and showed how preparedness in one area can ultimately reward others solving difficult issues such as drug-resistant malaria. Lessons from that crisis have pushed many experts to adopt a One Health mindset, accepting that human, animal, and environmental health are all inextricably linked. In most cases, channeling funds into cutting-edge vaccine platforms and better diagnostics is vital if we're to stop resistant strains in their tracks and keep current treatments effective. Coordinated global effort, and ongoing policy and legislative backing, remains necessary to maintain momentum for innovation and ensure that these new technologies are accessible to all who require them. In the end, such frameworks prove vital in the fight against malaria, where vaccine advances need to keep step with ever-changing parasite resistance and complex patterns of transmission (Paul et al., 2020) (Figure 8.16).

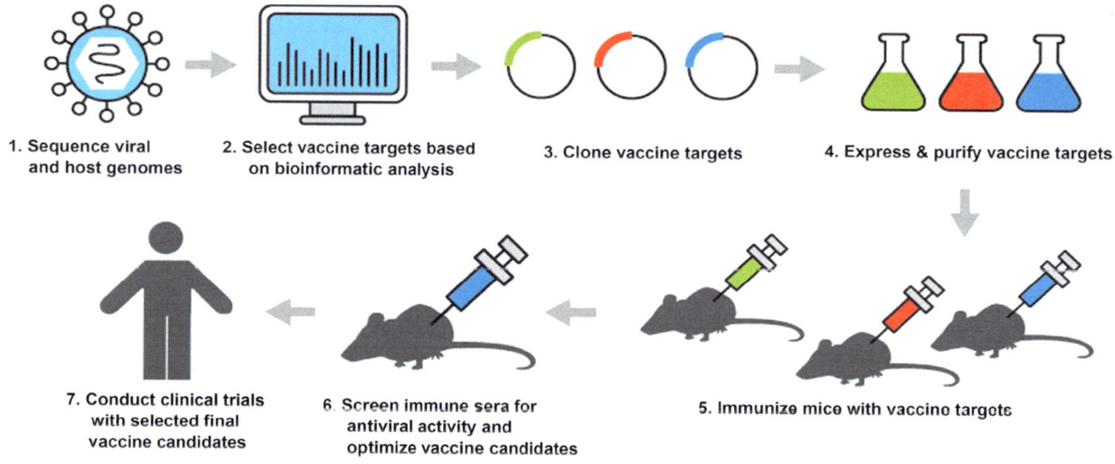

Figure 8.16. *Vaccine development.*

Source: Takara Bio. (n.d.). *Reverse Vaccinology.*

8.6.2. Genetic Engineering and Gene Editing Technologies

Combatting malaria that refuses to play by the old rules has led researchers to try their hand at some new, out-of-the-box approaches. Instead of turning to traditional drugs, many are now taking the leap into genetic manipulation—using gene editing tools like CRISPR-Cas9 to mess around in both the parasite's DNA and the DNA of the pathogens that spread it. Scientists aren't following a neat step-by-step recipe; they're mixing it up at the molecular level, altering single genes that allow the parasite to live or fend off drugs. By altering with the *Plasmodium* genome, scientists can have an idea of which genes are to blame for resistance, and such hands-on information opens doors for the discovery of new drug targets as well as breeding mosquitoes that just cannot pass on the parasite. It is a challenging, creative process aimed at reining in the expanding problem of drug resistance. Genetic engineering also promises a lot in terms of speeding up the discovery of novel vaccines and treatments. Others are using gene editing together with extensive omics studies to determine the molecular components that maintain the parasite—such a strategy, in most cases, gives rise to more specific treatment options. Targeting the problem at a genetic level can indirectly overcome the problem of parasite variability, along with its rapid capacity for developing drug resistance. Some even discuss releasing modified mosquitoes into the wild through gene drives, with the idea being that the insects would gradually replace the natural ones or be less likely to carry *Plasmodium* (Singh, 2020). In general, this is a move away from simply reacting to outbreaks and towards actively outwitting the parasite's defenses. However, even as these gene tools are so promising, there are several real-world challenges that remain. Foremost among them are the ethical, ecological, and regulatory issues attendant on releasing genetically modified organisms into the environment—they demand serious, even international, deliberation. Besides, the *Plasmodium* parasite is nothing if not resilient, so it may rapidly develop new mechanisms to avoid our genetic solutions, requiring us to continually monitor and adjust our strategy. As research continues at a slow pace, integrating these gene-based strategies with other developments such as artificial intelligence or even nanomedicine may iron out design and delivery wrinkles. All else being equal, gene editing is no silver bullet, although it is certainly a vital component of the multi-faceted fight to contain malaria's growing resistance and protect global health (Sohail et al., 2023) (Figure 8.17).

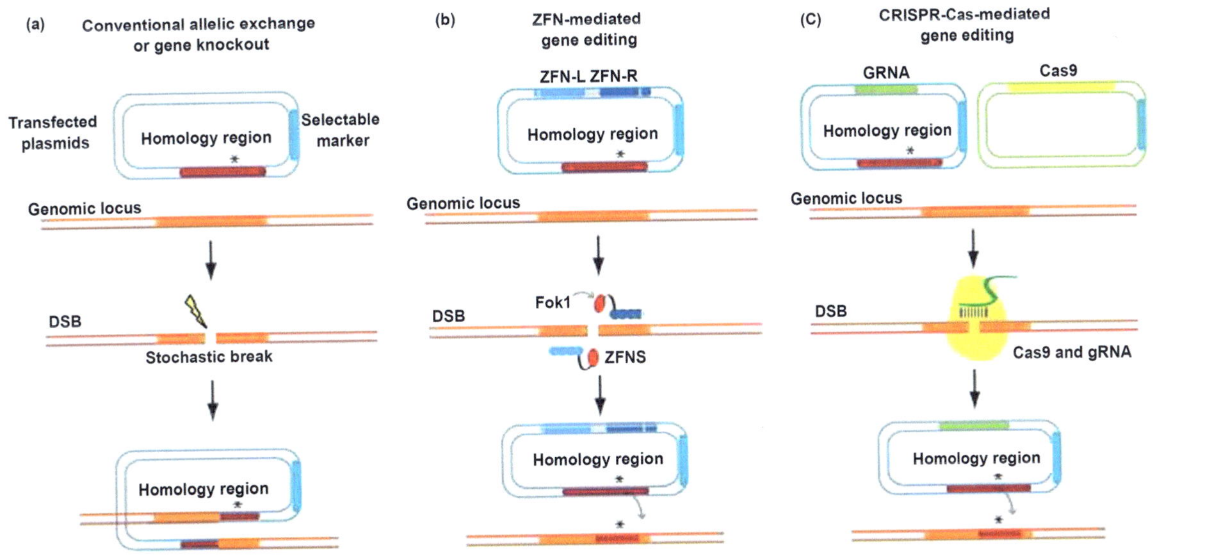

Figure 8.17. *Gene editing technologies battling malaria.*

Source: Lee, M.C., Fidock, D.A. CRISPR-mediated genome editing of *Plasmodium falciparum* malaria parasites. *Genome Med* **6**, 63 (2014). https://doi.org/10.1186/s13073-014-0063-9

8.6.3. Global Collaboration and Funding for Research

Fighting back against malaria's growing drug resistance is not all about new drugs, it's largely a case of global cooperation and smart money. Research initiatives that test new antimalarial drugs while adapting proven treatments take far more funding than any single country can muster, especially in the most affected places. For example, starting to switch to artemisinin-based combination therapies shows, in most cases, how global cooperation brings in smarter alternatives. Institutions like the Global Fund and the World Bank have been at the forefront of supporting funding for these treatments within nations like Tanzania. Sustained funding support not only enhances treatment success rates but also works to suppress the rate of accelerating resistance, which in turn underscores the extent to which international financial coordination is imperative in solving this public health issue (Derriennic & Wolf, 2005). Drug-resistant malaria in a way reflects the problems we have in developing antibiotics. Money concerns and scientific barriers long stood in the way of truly innovative drugs, giving us numerous treatments that were mere rehashes of the original compounds. This stagnation only contributes to more demand for collaborative funding of joint research, as government and industry are generally not willing to engage in the expensive and risky endeavor of finding new drugs independently. Pooling resources, skills, and knowledge in a multinational collaboration can result in drug discovery breakthroughs, even if sometimes advancement seems to be slow. At its essence, this form of cooperative framework is not merely fighting malaria; it is also a central component in fighting the broader threat of antimicrobial resistance (Coukell et al., 2016). Long-term success against drug-resistant malaria takes more than the initial burst of finance, it takes persistent financial planning and persistent political will from governments and institutions. Take initiatives like the Roll Back Malaria Partnership, where agencies, research institutions, and governments all come together to develop plans that integrate pieces like surveillance, drug procurement, and new research ideas. In order to keep the momentum going, often times medium- to long-term financial commitments are required, which in turn permit ongoing monitoring of drug efficacy and jumping into action right away when the resistance starts to occur. And, beyond that, such international action facilitates sharing of information and the building of capacity in regions of malaria endemicity, empowering local researchers and health sectors with a greater voice in the fight. All things considered, an extensive, concerted effort backed by sustained investments seems reasonably unavoidable to counter the dynamic obstacles posed by drug-resistant malaria (Derriennic & Wolf, 2005).

CLOSER LOOK

ARTEMISININ-BASED COMBINATION THERAPIES (ACTS)

ACTs are the treatment of choice for uncomplicated *Plasmodium falciparum* malaria, the deadliest form of human malaria. The treatments consist of the pairing of an artemisinin derivative and a longer-acting partner drug to enhance efficacy, reduce transmission, and forestall the emergence of drug resistance. ACTs are recommended by the World Health Organization (WHO) and have been the centerpiece of global malaria control and elimination campaigns since the early 2000s.

Artemisinin, derived from the sweet wormwood plant (*Artemisia annua*), is extremely effective at rapidly reducing the blood parasite load. It has a brief half-life, however, and when used alone is not capable of removing all the parasites, causing a recrudescence and resistance risk. To avert this, it is paired with a longer-acting antimalarial drug. This ensures that any persistent parasites are cleared out, thereby increasing cure rates in addition to delaying the development of resistance.

The most extensively used ACTs include artemether-lumefantrine (AL), artesunate-amodiaquine (AS-AQ), artesunate-mefloquine (AS-MQ), dihydroartemisinin-piperaquine (DHA-PPQ), and artesunate-sulfadoxine-pyrimethamine (AS-SP). ACT choice may be according to local malaria epidemiology, drug resistance patterns, and policy. For example, AL is widely used in Africa, while DHA-PPQ is more utilized in Southeast Asia.

ACTs are well-tolerated, with few side effects like nausea, vomiting, and dizziness. They have a rapid effect, causing fast relief from symptoms and high cure rates, typically over 95% if used correctly. It is crucial, however, to ensure complete adherence to the several-day treatment course to derive a complete therapeutic effect and to avoid resistance.

Among the threats to ACTs is the emergence of artemisinin and partner-drug resistance, particularly in Southeast Asia's Greater Mekong Subregion. The resistance is expressed as delayed parasite clearance times and reduced treatment efficacy. In response, surveillance systems and research on alternative regimens and triple-drug combinations (TACTs) have been initiated to preserve ACT efficacy.

ACTs have made a remarkable impact on malaria morbidity and mortality. Where ACTs are widely used and supplemented with vector control and diagnostic testing, the incidence of malaria and deaths due to malaria have declined significantly. Access remains an issue in some remote or resource-limited areas due to cost, logistical limitations, and counterfeit medications.

Continued investment in ACT distribution, drug resistance monitoring, and new drug development is required to sustain gains in malaria control. New artemisinin derivatives, new partner drugs, and combination therapies are in the pipeline to stay ahead of emerging resistance.

SUMMARY

Drug resistance in malaria is perhaps the most daunting challenge of global malaria control. New findings, in most cases, show that our current approach to signaling the "window of selection", the time at which drug levels favor resistant parasites, is incorrect. In fact, recent data show that we might be underestimating to what degree we have been, and continue to, slow resistance. Consider, for instance, the antimalarial combinations artemether-lumefantrine and artesunate-mefloquine; these compounds, persisting in the body for days on end, maybe providing resistant parasites with a few extra days to survive than have been reported through clinical trials. This minor fact tells us that we must adjust our pharmacokinetic-pharmacodynamic models to attain a better understanding of resistance timing. Lacking a more refined measuring rod, policy choices about the use of these medicines could inadvertently speed resistance, eliminating much of our progress in malaria control programs around the world (Kay & Hastings, 2015). Health programs need to tackle the money and organizational issues of putting new malaria medicines into practice, especially in the areas ravaged by the disease. Take Tanzania, where malaria rates are still alarmingly high—as an example. The shift to artemisinin-based combination therapies is an important policy change to address increased resistance to conventional drugs. But overall, this shift isn't simple: it involves steady, reliable funding to keep drug supplies flat and available. While international alliances and donors like the Global Fund and the World Bank supplement gaps to help out, long-term funding remains of greatest concern. If we don't sort out these finances, even a tried-and-true treatment such as Coartem® could come to a standstill, and resistant strains will take over (Derriennic & Wolf, 2005). If you step back and see the bigger picture, the war on malaria drug resistance isn't just a science problem, it's policy and finance. Greater accuracy in determining when the resistance is starting can lead to more intelligent treatment strategies, and intelligent fiscal decisions ensure treatments are available and used as they should be. Policymakers, in most cases, are required to marry new scientific knowledge with prudent funding methods for solving this emerging issue. Unless this is prevented, decades of success can be eradicated overnight, demonstrating that the fight against malaria drug resistance needs cautious, collective, and responsive action worldwide (Derriennic & Wolf, 2005; Kay & Hastings, 2015).

The drug resistance of malaria is a tricky problem—a combination of genetic features and day-to-day environmental pressures appears to drive this problem. Investigations find that multiple *Plasmodium* species, with *Plasmodium falciparum* at the center of attention, occasionally modify their inner mechanisms by adjusting the locations where drugs typically work or by boosting the mechanisms that expel drugs. This leaves our time-tested drugs rather ineffective. And also, when these drugs become overused or used too thoughtlessly, it only serves to make the issue worse, which ends up stumbling the efforts globally to control malaria. Exploring how these parasites modify themselves—whether through molecular transformations or broad genomic shifts—gives some important pointers for designing new drugs. The constraints of our current drugs, coupled with the adaptive defenses of the parasite, clearly make us mark to do things differently and to keep on watching in areas most impacted by malaria (Uddin et al., 2021). It gets even cloudier when you add multidrug resistance— the cloudiest of waters in malaria control. This form of resistance not only narrows down our medication options but also contributes to the financial burden on healthcare systems, especially in high-transmission regions. In all but a few cases, overcoming it requires an across-the-board strategy: mixing up combo drugs, improving test kits, and tightening up regulations in order to avoid abuse of drugs. It also matters a lot how well patients stick to their treatment plans and whether the drug quality is up to par. Some of the insights we've picked up from antibiotic resistance in bacteria give us a pretty good idea of what to expect and how to navigate these emerging hurdles (Uddin et al., 2021). Ultimately, more research and smarter public health initiatives are the crystal-clear requirement if we are to control drug-resistant malaria. Options like more vector control, more funding for drug development, and better community education all have a place as part of a good response. Addressing larger social determinants and making sure that everybody gets proper, effective treatment can slow the development of resistance. Global cooperation and sharing data, and every now subsequently even a bit of imperfect, off-the-cuff wisdom—are imperative to tracking trends and reacting swiftly. The whole fight against malaria drug resistance forces us to keep innovating and thinking outside the box on healthcare solutions, just as we are with other diseases such as dementia, where a multipronged strategy can indeed change the landscape.

KEY TERMS FROM THIS CHAPTER

- Chloroquine Resistance
- Mefloquine Resistance
- Multidrug Resistance (MDR)
- Plasmodium vivax Resistance
- PfCRT (Chloroquine Resistance Transporter)
- Molecular Markers
- In vivo Resistance
- Cross-Resistance
- Subtherapeutic Dosing
- Surveillance of Resistance
- Sulfadoxine-Pyrimethamine Resistance
- Artemisinin Resistance
- Plasmodium falciparum Resistance
- Kelch13 (K13) Mutation
- Copy Number Variation
- Therapeutic Efficacy Studies (TES)
- In vitro Resistance
- Drug Pressure
- Treatment Failure

References

1. Abebe, R., Hill, S., Schwartz, H. A., Small, D. S., et al. (2019). *Using Search Queries to Understand Health Information Needs in Africa*. http://arxiv.org/abs/1806.05740 (accessed on 13 May 2025).

2. Adegboro, A. G., & Afolabi, I. S. (2024). Molecular mechanisms of mitochondria-mediated ferroptosis: A potential target for antimalarial interventions. *Frontiers in Cell and Developmental Biology, 12*. https://doi.org/10.3389/fcell.2024.1374735.

3. Adjuik, M., Ashley, E., Barnes, K. I., Boni, M. F., Buckling, A., Cross, D. E., et al. (2009). Probability of emergence of antimalarial resistance in different stages of the parasite life cycle. https://core.ac.uk/download/pdf/8416178.pdf.

4. Germain Gil Padonou, Judith G. Gbenoudon, Razaki Osse, Albert Salako, Casimir Kpanou, Herman Sagbohan, Virgile Gnanguenon, Frederick Oke Agbo, Olivier Oussou, Martin Codjo Akogbeto Knowledge-attitudes-practices about malaria among communities in Southern Benin. International Journal of Public Health Science (IJPHS) Vol. 7, No. 3, September 2018, pp. 186~193 ISSN: 2252-8806, DOI: 10.11591/ijphs.v7i3.14395 (accessed on 13 May 2025).

5. Ahmad, R., Zhu, N. J., Leather, A. J. M., Holmes, A., Ferlie, E., & ASPIRES study co-investigators (2019). Strengthening strategic management approaches to address antimicrobial resistance in global human health: a scoping review. *BMJ global health*, *4*(5), e001730. https://doi.org/10.1136/bmjgh-2019-001730 (accessed on 13 May 2025).

6. Anderson, T. J., Nair, S., Sudimack, D., Williams, J. T., Mayxay, M., Newton, P. N., Guthmann, J. P., Smithuis, F. M., Tran, T. H., van den Broek, I. V., White, N. J., & Nosten, F. (2005). Geographical distribution of selected and putatively neutral SNPs in Southeast Asian malaria parasites. *Molecular biology and evolution*, *22*(12), 2362–2374. https://doi.org/10.1093/molbev/msi235(accessed on 13 May 2025).

7. Azmi, W. A. A., Rizki, A. F. M., Djuardi, Y., Artika, I. M., & Siregar, J. E. (2023). Molecular insights into artemisinin resistance in *Plasmodium falciparum*: An updated review. *Infection, Genetics and Evolution, 112*, 105460. https://doi.org/10.1016/j.meegid.2023.105460.

8. Baba, E., Hamade, P., Kivumbi, H., Marasciulo, M., Maxwell, K., Moroso, D., Roca-Feltrer, A., et al. (2020). Effectiveness of seasonal malaria chemoprevention at scale in West and Central Africa: An observational study. *The Lancet, 396*(10265), 1829–1840. https://doi.org/10.1016/S0140-6736(20)32227-3.

9. Ruberto, I., Camara, S., Banek, K., & Loua, M. K. (2014). Knowledge, attitudes and practices of malaria control among communities from the health district of Forécariah in the Republic of Guinea, West Africa. *Journal of vector borne diseases*, *51*(2), 119–127. (accessed on 13 May 2025).

10. Kinga Modrzynska, K., Creasey, A., Loewe, L., Cezard, T., Trindade Borges, S., Martinelli, A., Rodrigues, L., Cravo, P., Blaxter, M., Carter, R., & Hunt, P. (2012). Quantitative genome re-sequencing defines multiple mutations conferring chloroquine resistance in rodent malaria. *BMC genomics*, *13*, 106. https://doi.org/10.1186/1471-2164-13-106(accessed on 13 May 2025).

11. Meheus, F., Balasegaram, M., Olliaro, P., Sundar, S., Rijal, S., Faiz, M. A., & Boelaert, M. (2010). Cost-effectiveness analysis of combination therapies for visceral leishmaniasis in the Indian

subcontinent. *PLoS neglected tropical diseases, 4*(9), e818. https://doi.org/10.1371/journal.pntd.0000818

12. Bwire, G. M., Ngasala, B., Mikomangwa, W. P., Kilonzi, M., & Kamuhabwa, A. (2020). Detection of mutations associated with artemisinin resistance at k13-propeller gene and a near complete return of chloroquine susceptible *falciparum* malaria in Southeast of Tanzania. *Scientific Reports, 10,* Article 14201. https://doi.org/10.1038/s41598-020-60549-7.
13. Cerávolo, I. P., Aguiar, A. C. C., Adebayo, J. O., & Krettli, A. U. (2021). Studies on activities and chemical characterization of medicinal plants in search for new antimalarials: A ten-year review on ethnopharmacology. *Frontiers in Pharmacology, 12,* Article 734263. https://doi.org/10.3389/fphar.2021.734263.
14. Conrad, M. D., Asua, V., Garg, S., Giesbrecht, D., Niaré, K., Smith, S., Namuganga, J. F., et al. (2023). Evolution of partial resistance to artemisinin's in malaria parasites in Uganda. *New England Journal of Medicine, 389*(8), 722–732. https://doi.org/10.1056/NEJMoa2211803.
15. Coukell, A., Shore, C., Jungman, E., Talkington, K., Kothari, P., & Urahn, S. K. (2016). A scientific roadmap for antibiotic discovery: A sustained and robust pipeline of new antibacterial drugs and therapies is critical to preserve public health. https://core.ac.uk/download/75785719.pdf (accessed on 13 May 2025).
16. Derriennic, Y., & Wolf, K. (2005). Costing artemisinin-based combination therapy for malaria in Tanzania. https://core.ac.uk/download/pdf/11306999.pdf (accessed on 13 May 2025).
17. Tawe, L., Motshoge, T., Ramatlho, P. *et al.* Human *cytochrome P450 2B6* genetic variability in Botswana: a case of haplotype diversity and convergent phenotypes. *Sci Rep* **8**, 4912 (2018). https://doi.org/10.1038/s41598-018-23350-1 (accessed on 13 May 2025).
18. Dondorp, A. M., Smithuis, F., Woodrow, C. J., & von Seidlein, L. (2017). How to contain artemisinin- and multidrug-resistant *falciparum* malaria. *Trends in Parasitology, 33,* 353–363. https://doi.org/10.1016/j.pt.2017.01.004.
19. Dondorp, A., Hastings, I., Day, N., White, N., Yeung, S., & Pongtavornpinyo, W. (2008). The spread of antimalarial drug resistance: A mathematical model with practical implications for ACT drug policies. https://core.ac.uk/download/pdf/287665.pdf (accessed on 13 May 2025).
20. Erhirhie, E. O., Ikegbune, C., Okeke, A. I., Onwuzuligbo, C. C., Madubuogwu, N. U., Chukwudulue, U. M., & Okonkwo, O. B. (2021). Antimalarial herbal drugs: A review of their interactions with conventional antimalarial drugs. *Clinical Phyto Science, 7,* Article 8. https://doi.org/10.1186/s40816-020-00242-4.
21. Findlater, A., & Bogoch, I. I. (2018). Human mobility and the global spread of infectious diseases: A focus on air travel. *Trends in Parasitology, 34,* 772–783. https://doi.org/10.1016/j.pt.2018.07.004.
22. Fola, A. A., Feleke, S. M., Mohammed, H., Brhane, B. G., Hennelly, C. M., Assefa, A., Crudal, R. M., et al. (2023). *Plasmodium falciparum* resistant to artemisinin and diagnostics have emerged in Ethiopia. *Nature Microbiology, 8,* 1911–1919. https://doi.org/10.1038/s41564-023-01461-4.
23. Fonte, M., Tassi, N., Gomes, P., & Teixeira, C. (2021). Acridine-based antimalarials, from the very first synthetic antimalarial to recent developments. *Molecules, 26*(3), Article 600. https://doi.org/10.3390/molecules26030600.

24. Guan, L., Wang, H., Xu, X., & Fan, H. (2023). Therapeutical utilization and repurposing of artemisinin and its derivatives: A narrative review. *Advanced Biology, 7*(4), Article 2300086. https://doi.org/10.1002/adbi.202300086.

25. Gujjari, L., Kalani, H., Pindiprolu, S. K. S. S., Arakareddy, B. P., & Yadagiri, G. (2022). Current challenges and nanotechnology-based pharmaceutical strategies for the treatment and control of malaria. *Parasite Epidemiology and Control, 17*, e00244. https://doi.org/10.1016/j.parepi.2022.e00244.

26. Hastings, I., Tawe, E. & Kay, K. Quantifying the pharmacology of antimalarial drug combination therapy. *Sci Rep* **6**, 32762 (2016). https://doi.org/10.1038/srep32762(accessed on 13 May 2025).

27. Hu, X., Li, J., Fu, M., Zhao, X., & Wang, W. (2021). The JAK/STAT signaling pathway: From bench to clinic. *Signal Transduction and Targeted Therapy, 6*, Article 402. https://doi.org/10.1038/s41392-021-00791-1.

28. Kamuhabwa, A. A. R., & Silumbe, R. (2013). Knowledge among drug dispensers and antimalarial drug prescribing practices in public health facilities in Dar es Salaam. https://core.ac.uk/download/pdf/18174791.pdf (accessed on 13 May 2025).

29. Kay, K., & Hastings, I. M. (2015). Measuring windows of selection for anti-malarial drug treatments. *Malaria journal, 14*, 292. https://doi.org/10.1186/s12936-015-0810-4 (accessed on 13 May 2025).

30. Livingston, G., Huntley, J., Sommerlad, A., Ames, D., Ballard, C., Banerjee, S., Brayne, C., et al. (2020). Dementia prevention, intervention, and care: 2020 report of the Lancet Commission. *The Lancet, 396*(10248), 413–446. https://doi.org/10.1016/S0140-6736(20)30367-6.

31. Mathews, E. S., & Odom John, A. R. (2018). Tackling resistance: emerging antimalarials and new parasite targets in the era of elimination. *F1000Research, 7*, F1000 Faculty Rev-1170. https://doi.org/10.12688/f1000research.14874.1 (accessed on 13 May 2025).

32. Mihreteab, S., Platon, L., Berhane, A., Stokes, B. H., Warsame, M., Campagne, P., Criscuolo, A., et al. (2023). Increasing prevalence of artemisinin-resistant HRP2-negative malaria in Eritrea. *New England Journal of Medicine, 389*(13), 1191–1202. https://doi.org/10.1056/NEJMoa2210956.

33. Milne, R., Wiedemar, N., Corpas-López, V., Moynihan, E., Wall, R. J., Dawson, A., Robinson, D. A., et al. (2022). Toolkit of approaches to support target-focused drug discovery for *Plasmodium falciparum* lysyl tRNA synthetase. *ACS Infectious Diseases, 8*(9), 1962–1974. https://doi.org/10.1021/acsinfecdis.2c00364.

34. Miotto, O., Sekihara, M., Tachibana, S. I., Yamauchi, M., Pearson, R. D., Amato, R., Gonçalves, S., et al. (2020). Emergence of artemisinin-resistant *Plasmodium falciparum* with kelch13 C580Y mutations on the island of New Guinea. *PLoS Pathogens, 16*(12), e1009133. https://doi.org/10.1371/journal.ppat.1009133.

35. Murray, C. J. L., Ikuta, K. S., Sharara, F., Swetschinski, L. R., Robles Aguilar, G., Gray, A. P., Han, C., et al. (2022). Global burden of bacterial antimicrobial resistance in 2019: A systematic analysis. *The Lancet, 399*, 629–655. https://doi.org/10.1016/s0140-6736(21)02724-0.

36. Nkengasong, J. N., & Tessema, S. K. (2020). Africa needs a new public health order to tackle infectious disease threats. *Cell, 183*(2), 296–300. https://doi.org/10.1016/j.cell.2020.09.041.

37. Opsenica, D. M., & Šolaja, B. A. (2012). Artemisinins and synthetic peroxides as highly efficient antimalarials. *Macedonian Journal of Chemistry and Chemical Engineering, 31*(2), 137–182. https://doi.org/10.20450/mjcce.2012.50https://core.ac.uk/download/299290836.pdf

38. Roth, G. A., Abate, D., Abate, K. H., Abay, S. M., Abbafati, C., Abbasi, N., Abbastabar, H., et al. (2018). Global, regional, and national age-sex-specific mortality for 282 causes of death in 195 countries and territories, 1980–2017: A systematic analysis for the Global Burden of Disease Study 2017. *The Lancet, 392*(10159), 1736–1788. https://doi.org/10.1016/S0140-6736(18)32203-7.

39. Selzer, P. M., & Epe, C. (2020). Antiparasitic in animal health: Quo Vadis? *Trends in Parasitology, 37*(2), 77–89. https://doi.org/10.1016/j.pt.2020.09.004.

40. Simwela, N. V., & Waters, A. P. (2022). Current status of experimental models for the study of malaria. *Parasitology, 149*(6), 729–750. https://doi.org/10.1017/S0031182021002134.

41. Singh B. Molecular Medicines for Parasitic Diseases [Internet]. Methods in Molecular Medicine. IntechOpen; 2021. Available from: http://dx.doi.org/10.5772/intechopen.91956 (accessed on 13 May 2025).

42. Sohail, A., Noor, E., Fazal, I., Wahid, M., Tariq, M. N., Rana, M. S. F., Najmi, M. H., et al. (2023). Crisis averted: A world united against the menace of multiple drug-resistant superbugs—Pioneering anti-AMR vaccines, RNA interference, nanomedicine, CRISPR-based antimicrobials, bacteriophage therapies, and clinical artificial intelligence strategies to safeguard global antimicrobial arsenal. https://core.ac.uk/download/595463657.pdf (accessed on 13 May 2025).

43. Stokes, B. H., Dhingra, S. K., Rubiano, K., Mok, S., Straimer, J., Gnädig, N. F., Deni, I., et al. (2021). *Plasmodium falciparum* K13 mutations in Africa and Asia impact artemisinin resistance and parasite fitness. *eLife, 10*, e66277. https://doi.org/10.7554/elife.66277.

44. Strathdee, S. A., Davies, S. C., & Marcelin, J. R. (2020). Confronting antimicrobial resistance beyond the COVID-19 pandemic and the 2020 US election. *The Lancet, 396*(10257), 1050–1053. https://doi.org/10.1016/s0140-6736(20)32063-8.

45. Tonna, I. (2006). Is vaccination the only option for possible global malaria eradication? Malta Medical Journal Volume 18 Issue 02 July 2006. https://core.ac.uk/download/46602052.pdf (accessed on 13 May 2025).

46. U.S. President's Malaria Initiative. (2025). *President's Malaria Initiative Strategy 2015–2020.* https://core.ac.uk/download/144192566.pdf (accessed on 13 May 2025).

47. Uddin, T. M., Chakraborty, A., Khusro, A., Zidan, B. M. R. M., Mitra, S., Emran, T. B., Dhama, K., et al. (2021). Antibiotic resistance in microbes: History, mechanisms, therapeutic strategies and future prospects. *Journal of Infection and Public Health, 14*(12), 1750–1766. https://doi.org/10.1016/j.jiph.2021.10.020.

48. van der Pluijm, R. W., Amaratunga, C., Dhorda, M., & Dondorp, A. M. (2020). Triple artemisinin-based combination therapies for malaria–A new paradigm? *Trends in Parasitology, 37*(1), 15–24. https://doi.org/10.1016/j.pt.2020.09.011.

49. Tobing TCL, Wahrianto, Saputri E, Wafa NI, Zulfianti PD, Sihaloho LI, Husna AR, Salsabila D, Hotasi Silalahi FH, Sitohang AI, Sabrina A, Hasyati Harianja AD, Barus SA, Sabina S, Rahma AA, Velaro AJ, Khairunnnisa K, Salim E, Nurkolis F, Abdi Syahputra R (2024) Malaria in Indonesia:

current treatment approaches, future strategies, and potential herbal interventions. Pharmacia 71: 1-14. https://doi.org/10.3897/pharmacia.71.e116095 (accessed on 13 May 2025).

50. Zhang, Z., Zhou, L., Xie, N., Nice, E. C., Zhang, T., Cui, Y., & Huang, C. (2020). Overcoming cancer therapeutic bottleneck by drug repurposing. *Signal Transduction and Targeted Therapy, 5*, Article 113. https://doi.org/10.1038/s41392-020-00213-8.

51. Zhou, B., & Yue, J.-M. (2022). Natural products are the treasure pool for antimalarial agents. *National Science Review, 9*. https://doi.org/10.1093/nsr/nwac112.

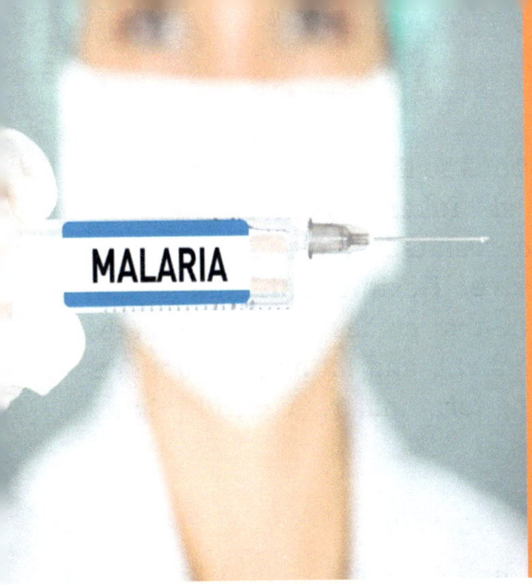

Chapter 9

EPIDEMIOLOGY OF MALARIA

Contents

Introduction

In much of the tropical and subtropical world, malaria continues to be a tenacious health threat. Malaria's spread is inextricably linked with the *Plasmodium* parasite, which is transmitted when an infected Anopheles mosquito bites a human being. In general, truly getting beneath the surface of how malaria travels—seeing its patterns, measuring its strength, and determining who bears the greatest burden—is central to the entire struggle. Such insight provides the opportunity for interventions to reduce cases and fatalities and more intelligent ways to allocate funds. Research monitoring malaria over time and across different geographic areas reveals both our achievement and the ongoing hurdles, prompting policymakers and scientists to make adjustments against challenges such as increasing drug resistance and even changes in mosquito habitats because of climate shifts (Alize et al., 2024). Examining the impact of malaria, you can observe a broad range of clinical consequences that vary with age, immunity, and resident locations. Generally, children under five and pregnant women in high-risk zones bear the brunt, although in other areas adults are not spared either. Surveillance system data; , ranging from incidence and prevalence to mortality, indicate hotspots where transmission gets out of hand and control follows at times. Urban expansion, migration, and other social transitions constantly shuffle these trends, so constant vigil is the key. By quantifying and situating the burden of malaria, the science of epidemiology not only makes public health interventions more robust, but it also enhances our overall perspective of the larger disease burden (Alize et al., 2024). Combining what we know about malaria with knowledge from the science of antimicrobial resistance provides another dimension to our perspective of the problem.

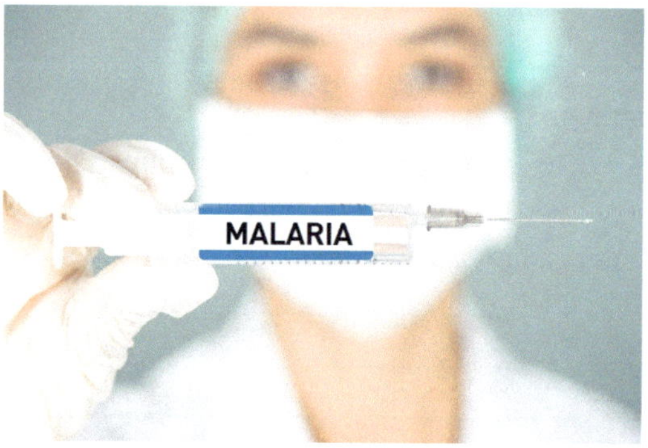

Figure 9.1. Epidemiology of malaria.

Source: Boca Biolistics. (n.d.). *Malaria*. Boca Biolistics.

Recently, drug resistance has insidiously begun creeping into malaria, making treatments more difficult and jeopardizing the hard-fought gains—much as with some bacterial infections elsewhere in the world. Some studies, which look at how pathogens evade medicines (and even correlate such profiles with mortality data), reinforce the necessity for constant, watchful monitoring in malaria-endemic regions. Increasing laboratory capacity and streamlining data collection processes are key steps; these activities allow for early detection of resistance trends so that treatment strategies can be adapted. Taken together, grappling with these interrelated challenges requires a comprehensive, flexible epidemiological framework—one that guides policy, stimulates vaccine development, and ultimately supports sustainable, long-term malaria control (Figure 9.1).

Definition of Malaria

Malaria is a complex disease caused by small protozoan parasites belonging to the *Plasmodium* family. The infection usually begins when an infected female Anopheles mosquito bites an individual, smuggling these creatures into the blood. The parasites infect the red blood cells, resulting in recurring episodes of fever, chills, and—when the situation worsens—severe complications that damage essential organs. Tropical and subtropical areas typically bear the brunt because of local environmental and social conditions that are conducive to the disease's transmission. To truly understand malaria, one has to look at it not only as a biological feature but also as a situation where host immunity is sometimes allied with mosquito behavior and changing weather conditions. Global initiatives to quantify the effect of malaria have increased our understanding of how infectious illnesses test health systems (Gregory et al., 2018). The way in which the disease appears in individuals can be quite diverse, in general. The species of *Plasmodium* involved makes a significant difference: *Plasmodium falciparum* is commonly associated with more serious illness and increased fatalities, but *Plasmodium vivax*, although typically less fatal, presents its own problems by remaining inactive in the liver and causing relapses. One of the telltale signs is the cyclical bursting of red blood cells, triggering bouts of fever, anemia, and various other symptoms that persist if not treated. There are also individuals who never develop obvious symptoms but continue to harbor the parasite, unknowingly contributing to further transmission. This combination of clinical presentations complicates pinpointing effective control and elimination strategies, which is why more explicit surveillance and detailed definitions are so frequently in demand (Spencer et al., 2018). Despite significant advancements in public health, malaria continues to be a persistent global phenomenon. Its own definition extends from a mere infection and captures how climate, economy, and regional health systems influence its occurrence. Incidence, prevalence, and mortality reports that combine these are a multifaceted description of the disease burden in various communities. Having a uniform perspective on the issue provides the ability to compare regions and inform intervention approaches designed to reduce transmission and enhance outcomes. Typically, international reviews call attention to how inequality in access to prevention and treatment increases disparities in disease and death, emphasizing the ongoing need for in-depth research and judicious resource deployment (Gregory et al., 2018; Spencer et al., 2018).

Historical Context of Malaria

Malaria's tale in the way we approach disease has changed a great deal over the years, as public health attention and the findings of new science have evolved. Years ago, particularly in the tropics and subtropics, malaria was the heavy burden, killing scores and making life difficult socially and economically. Initially, work was about managing patients rather than keeping the pathogen from spreading. Then, in general terms, the 20th century saw a twist: as nations observed chronic diseases taking over from infections, malaria still persisted as a principal threat. This peculiar resilience generated renewed interest in how infections function, distinguishing itself from chronic disease research. New study designs, alternate forms of crunching data, and new models for pathogens gradually mixed molecular and digital information into surveillance, all to build improved means of intervening (Lewnard & Reingold, 2019). Over the course of the last century, worldwide efforts to combat malaria oscillated between victory and defeat, frequently linked to political senses of humor and economic climates. A standout moment was the mid-1900s Global Malaria Eradication Program which boldly aimed to wipe out the disease worldwide through insect control and broad use of antimalarial meds. Although the plan was certainly ambitious, it soon bumped up against issues like growing insecticide resistance and challenging logistical hurdles—leading to results that were, at times, uneven. These early, mixed results remind us that no single fix can work everywhere. These days, plans tend to draw on those hard-fought lessons by mixing in with specially designed plans that are suited to a nation's own disease situation, surveillance, and even cross-border collaboration. More and more, as nations strive for elimination, they recognize that these multi-layered past experiences significantly influence malaria control efforts today (Feachem et al., 2009). Even today, the world's war against malaria is founded on understanding its long, complex past. Today, 39 countries are on the path to elimination with strategies that mirror their individual disease contexts.

This reinvigorated attention stems from a thoughtful, at times subtle, acknowledgment of both malaria's persistence over time and the numerous operational, technical, and funding barriers needed to maintain transmission at bay. In contrast to the old, blanket eradication attempts, contemporary approaches intermix close surveillance, local partnerships, and adaptive vector control strategies to address threats such as surprise reintroductions or outbreaks. Looking back, clearly, long-term control is based on political will, continuous altering of new approaches, and evidence-informed choices aligned with local circumstances. Through progression from far-reaching extermination programs to more flexible elimination strategies, we are able to see clearly how history guides us to a malaria-free future (Feachem et al., 2009).

Importance of Studying Malaria Epidemiology

Infectious disease dynamics have a major role in public health, particularly in regions where malaria is hard to miss. We can find out a lot by observing how malaria is—identifying routes of transmission, determining which groups are hardest hit, and even observing how the insects that transmit it tend to behave. Such observation is vital when attempting to create interventions that reduce the number of infections and prevent outbreaks from occurring. Unless we understand how malaria travels across rural and urban areas, our response as a nation may become disorganized or even misguided. Additionally, research that takes a glimpse at genetic changes in the parasite and its insects allows us to understand why certain medicines or pathogen sprays are not delivering as intended. Overall, exploring malaria's trends is quite critical to developing adaptive, evidence-based plans for handling this age-old global health problem (London School of Hygiene & Tropical Medicine, 2013).

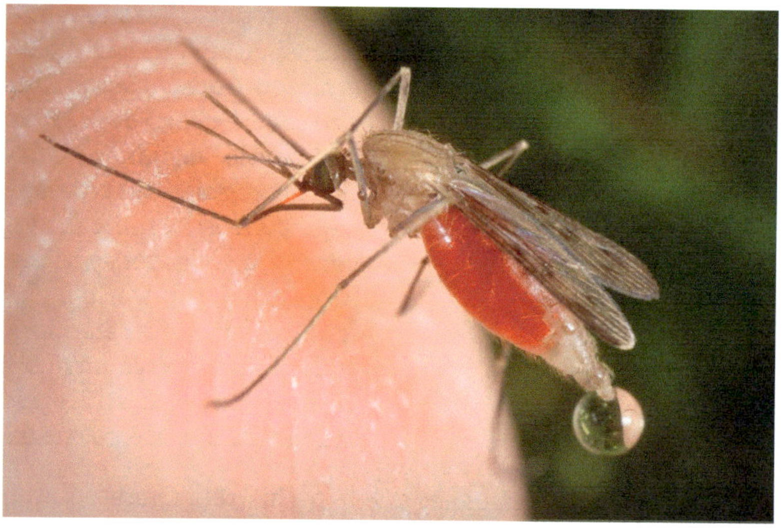

Figure 9.2. The importance of studying malaria epidemiology.

Source: Maine CDC. (n.d.). *Anopheles Freeborni Mosquito.* Maine Department of Health and Human Services.

Occasionally the turns and changes of how malaria spreads make it necessary to have constant fieldwork, as environmental and social forces have a tendency to redraw the landscape. Recently, a curious case caught researchers' eyes: *Anopheles stephensi*, a mosquito type we had mostly seen in South Asia, is now popping up in African cities. This unexpected arrival shakes up the usual story of malaria in urban areas, stirring new public health puzzles along the way. In most instances, looking at how much this mosquito is responsible for malaria's spread challenges us to revise existing mosquito control strategies and redirect our focus slightly. Scientists, for instance, combine field pathogen surveillance with cutting-edge molecular tools to trace where these vectors are congregating and what dangers they pose, which assists decision-makers in optimizing resource allocation and strategizing urban malaria protections (Alemayehu et al., 2024). Absent new epidemiological findings to capture these trends, our control interventions could readily fall short. Examining more closely the data also highlights how malaria cascades out to influence communities, not only in terms of health but socio-economically, too. The chronicity of malaria has a tendency to pull down work productivity and raise healthcare expense, generating a sort of downward spiral between disease and economic stress. When policymakers obtain a clear view of where and among whom the most harm is done, they can more effectively design education, prevention, and treatment initiatives for the most in-need populations, sometimes with some natural duplication of effort and emphasis. Also, by monitoring the effectiveness of such interventions over the long term, we obtain that all-important feedback to revise strategy when circumstances change or resistance develops. More often than not, learning about the spread of malaria is not necessarily about combating the disease but also directly relates to larger aspirations such as sustainable development and improving the overall quality of life within the affected areas (London School of Hygiene & Tropical Medicine, 2013) (Figure 9.2).

9.1. Life Cycle of the Malaria Parasite

Malaria does not spread so easily as some would imagine, it is all about the life cycle of the parasite that connects humans and mosquitoes in a most surprising way. The parasite, *Plasmodium spp.*, undergoes various transformations both within our bodies and within the mosquito. Most often, it begins when, quite by accident, an infected mosquito bites an individual, introducing sporozoites into the blood. These sporozoites race off to the liver where they infect liver cells and reproduce asexually to form schizonts. These schizonts, when mature, rupture, spilling merozoites into the bloodstream; these infect red blood cells and cause the cycles of fever with which we identify malaria, each cycle of ruptured red cells contributing to the increasing total of parasites (Nkrumah et al., 2024). But the parasite's shenanigans are not only reserved for humans. Once a mosquito feeds on the blood of an already infected person, it unwittingly feeds on gametocytes, the parasite in its sexual form. Normally, within the midgut of the mosquito the gametocytes disintegrate into what we can refer to as male and female components, which later on come into contact with each other and merge to become zygotes. These zygotes subsequently develop into motile ookinetes that thrust through the gut wall and begin to develop oocysts, each of which goes on to produce thousands of sporozoites. In a rather disorganized but critical process, the sporozoites eventually find themselves on their way to the salivary glands of the mosquito, ready to infect a new person. This stage of the mosquito not only remixes the parasite's genetic deck but also increases its overall diversity, hence making malaria control more difficult—intervention strategies simply have to address both ends of the story (Nkrumah et al., 2024). Mixing our knowledge of these life stages with information from genetics and epidemiology has provided some new insights into the fight against malaria. For example, coupling traditional models such as the Ross-Macdonald model with changing concepts of what goes on within the host can show, in most instances, a rapid change in parasite genetic diversity when infection levels shift, even if those changes appear subtle. And it turns out that tracking these life cycle checkpoints can be an effective measure for determining over the long haul how well interventions are succeeding. Overall, this hybrid strategy not only enhances our monitoring of malaria but also guides public health interventions in a more adaptive and responsive direction (Figure 9.3).

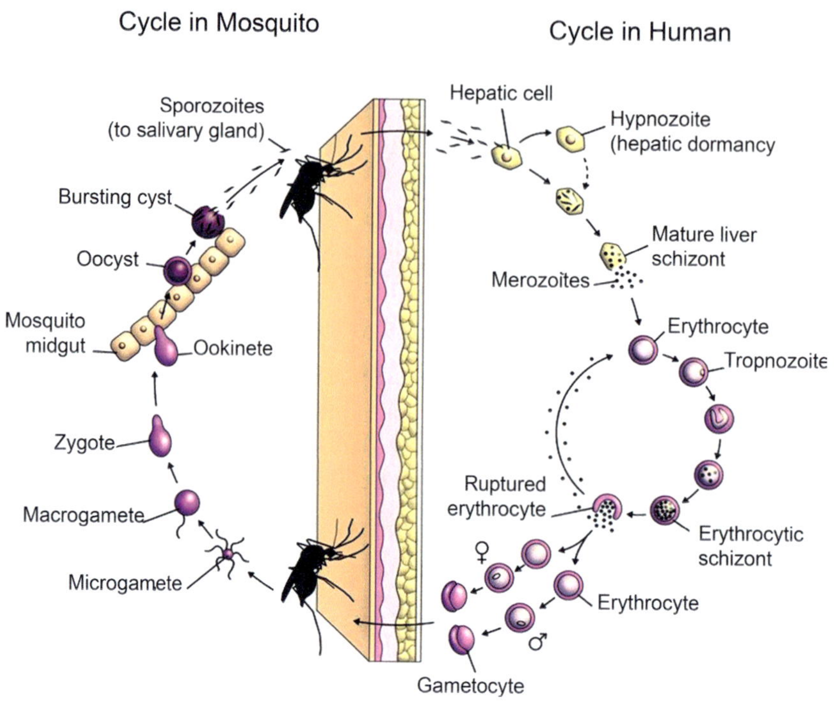

Figure 9.3. *Plasmodium* life cycle.

Source: Googleusercontent. (n.d.). *Untitled image.* https://lh3.googleusercontent.com/proxy/v4u_NxSmdgSSSwpahaHeLxPFFoPtIjuASg_qIDB3LIp6w3Xu6nQ5vN2EZLcwXFMUJFmoAfIZZ8wjHHhVYeYzSh5WPhisU8lxR7fPXS9ZIVIS49py.

9.1.1. Overview of Plasmodium Species

Malaria's transmission is linked directly into the biology of those small *Plasmodium* creatures – microscopic protozoan parasites that infect the disease. Their existence is a challenging highway between mosquitoes (primarily the *Anopheles* species) and humans, and that makes halting them a serious problem. Of many different species, five infect human beings: *Plasmodium falciparum, P. vivax, P. ovale, P. malariae*, and the zoonotic *P. knowlesi*. *P. falciparum* receives a lot of bad publicity, in the majority of cases, due to its acute virulence, particularly in sub-Saharan Africa, where it is responsible for the lion's share of malaria illness and mortality. Its ability to cause life-threatening complications , and, of course, its increasing resistance to most antimalarial medications – keeps the public health system on its toes. Knowing where each species likes to roam and how they work is central to constructing good models and intervention strategies, particularly when environmental and social disturbances are at hand (Daniel et al., 2020). In addition to *falciparum*, there's *P. vivax*, which casts its own epidemiological curveball. It is not just an African issue; this parasite is disseminated far and wide in Asia, South America, and elsewhere. In general, vivax can be latent in the liver as the hypnozoite, which on occasion causes relapses and complicates eradication attempts. It shares the world with human populations in parts of the globe where the bump and grind of diverse ecological and socioeconomic conditions provide an added complexity. Then there's *P. knowlesi*, a native of macaques, illustrating how lines of wildlife and human life become blurred , particularly when suspects such as deforestation and urbanization enter the frame, disrupting transmission patterns (Rebekah et al., 2020). This zoonotic complication serves as a reminder that environmental changes and altered land-use are key pieces of the malaria jigsaw. Various *Plasmodium* species require various strategies when it comes to public health reaction. It happens that there exist differences in incubation periods, symptoms, reaction to drugs, and how rapidly each one of them transmits not only render the disease unpredictable but also make the control even more challenging. Consider *P. ovale* and *P. malariae*: they may be less frequent and tend to produce milder disease, but they maintain a low-level transmission quietly that can keep malaria entrenched in some places. Control strategies must, thus, sweep the board, addressing both the stars and the lesser figures if the transmission is to ever be interrupted. Recent studies in modeling , and it is worth noting this fact – indicate that any hiccups in antimalarial treatments or vector-control measures risk an increase in infection rates and mortality in the different strains, highlighting the requirement for lasting, species-aggregated programs (Daniel et al., 2020) (Figure 9.4).

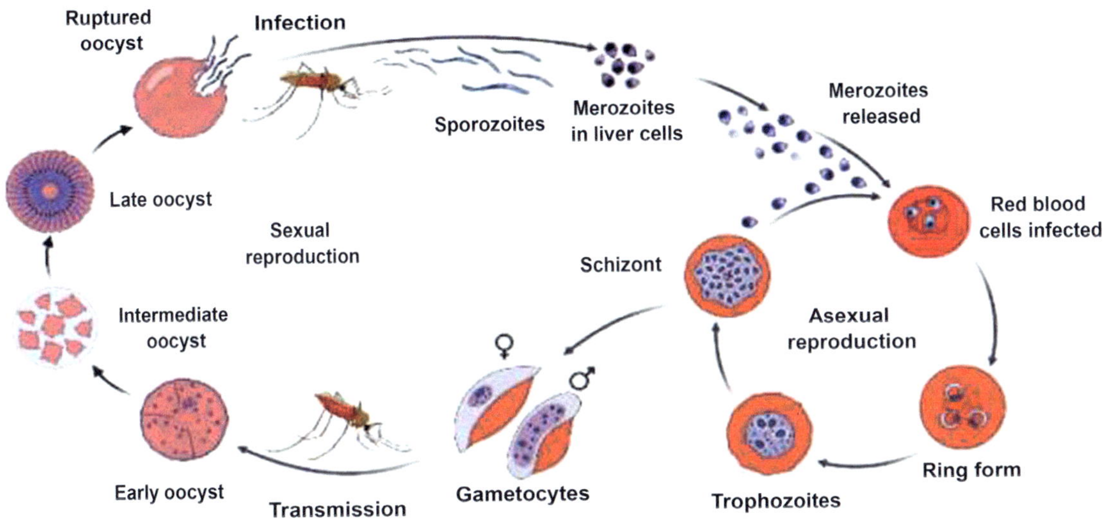

Figure 9.4. *Plasmodium* species.

Source: Elsevier. (n.d.). *Figure 1 from "Translational benefits of epithelial organoid culture for pediatric liver disease research.* https://ars.els-cdn.com/content/image/1-s2.0-S2667114X22000127-gr1.jpg.

9.1.2. Transmission Through Anopheles Mosquitoes

The spread of malaria is closely linked to Anopheles mosquitoes—those tiny creatures responsible for carrying the *Plasmodium* parasites behind malaria. In Southeast Asia, for instance, in regions of *Malaysian Borneo*, *Anopheles balabacensis* emerges as a key for *Plasmodium knowlesi*, a simian malaria parasite that has been infecting humans increasingly recently. Studies typically indicate that these mosquitoes peak in biting activity in early evening (about 1800–2000, or around 6–8 PM), which stretches our usual protection such as bed nets that people sleep under. In addition, mosquito populations and survival rates do not act in the same way: wooded forests and small-farm patches have times when infection rates are higher even when there are not as many mosquitoes present than there are in villages. And that means we require a relatively subtle examination of mosquito behavior and its environment to create effective malaria control policies (Chua et al.,

2015). Insecticide-treated nets, or ITNs, have been a success in reducing malaria cases in Africa, particularly when the most vulnerable individuals such as children and pregnant women are protected. Even so, evidence points to the fact that simply covering one individual's protection does not quite eliminate community transmission. Essentially, to truly break malaria spread, you must have wide ITN coverage—targeting about 80% or so of the community—so it compels that herd effect into play. This strategy provides both direct protection to individuals and an indirect reduction in overall vector counts and infection incidence. Therefore, knowledge of the intersection of mosquito behavior, human exposure, and numbers of people covered is still a key element in expanding malaria prevention (Killeen et al., 2007). However, malaria transmission tenaciously continues due to these resilient Anopheles mosquitoes. Take *Anopheles balabacensis* again—their tendency to bite outdoors, especially when people are active and not under any net protection, cuts against the grain of standard interventions like bed nets and indoor spraying. This outdoor biting, particularly in rural or forested spots, keeps humans and mosquitoes in close contact much more often than we would like. In order to create control programs that function, the need becomes paramount to combine learning on vector biology, human behavior, and environmental issues into a more holistic plan. Only by combining all these pieces of the puzzle—challenging as it may sometimes become—are malaria programs likely to challenge those persistent transmission clusters and move closer to elimination in endemic areas (Chua et al., 2015) (Figure 9.5).

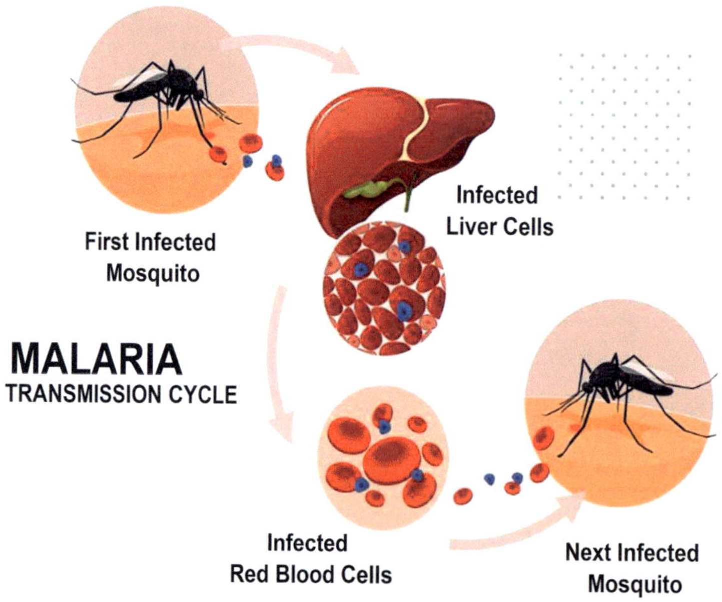

Figure 9.5. Transmission through anopheles mosquitoes.

Source: Noul Co. (2024). *Anopheles Mosquito.*

9.1.3. Human Infection Stages

Malaria in people does not happen along nice, orderly lines, it all starts when an infected Anopheles mosquito bites you. Almost immediately after the bite, small sporozoites enter your bloodstream and quickly make their way to the liver. There, they invade liver cells and begin to reproduce without creating any major commotion—a low-key beginning that very much lays the groundwork for everything else. With *Plasmodium vivax*, it gets even more complicated: some parasites enter a sort of suspended animation as hypnozoites, so they may re-emerge months or even years down the line, making it harder to eradicate them. This squishy, near-quiet liver phase is quite unlike the abrupt, all-out assault with *Plasmodium falciparum*—each one plays by its own script. In general terms, determining what takes place in the liver stage is most important, because that is the sole opportunity to intervene before the parasites overrun your red blood cells, when symptoms and danger peak. After the silent liver stage, all hell breaks loose to the blood stage. Merozoites explode out and infect red blood cells, doubling in a simple, asexual manner that triggers off the typical malaria symptoms such as fever, chills, and anemia.

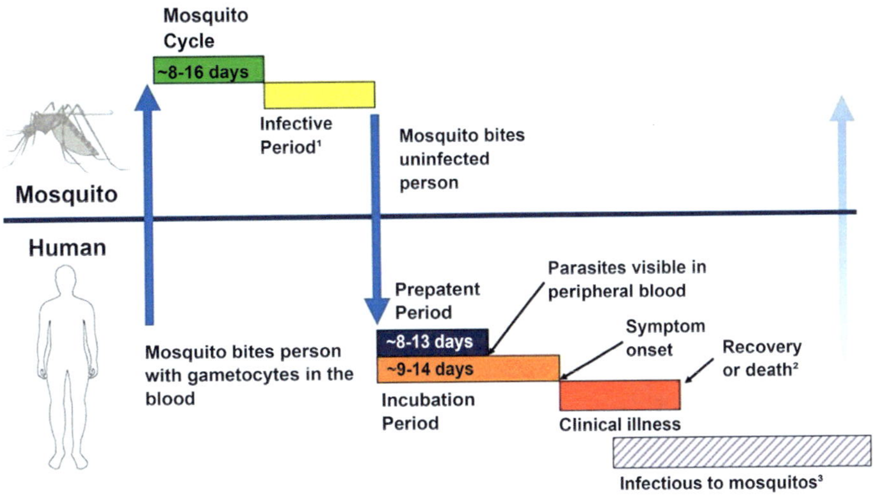

Figure 9.6. Human malaria infection stages.

Source: CDC. (2024). *Plasmodium falciparum*. Centers for Disease Control and Prevention.

The parasites even find a way to alter the appearance of red blood cells, allowing them to evade the immune system and secrete themselves away in tiny blood vessels—frequently setting off worse complications. In a surprise move, certain parasites shift gears to create sexual cells called gametocytes, which are central to transferring the disease back to mosquitoes. This combination of fast parasite growth and the body's sometimes clumsy effort at defense determines how severely malaria affects different populations. Due to this reason, most control measures target this blood stage in hopes of alleviating symptoms and ending the cycle of transmission. And there are the asymptomatic infections that add another monkey wrench to controlling malaria. Certain individuals, particularly when it comes to *P. vivax*, have low parasite burdens with no apparent symptoms, but they can still transmit the pathogen to mosquitoes—making it very difficult to follow the disease (Christopher et al., 2022). Additionally, increasing antimicrobial resistance and problems with bacterial co-infections complicate treatment strategies further (Christopher et al., 2022). All of these considerations combined emphasize learning each stage of the disease, from that quiet, silent liver phase to the aching blood stage and those latent asymptomatic instances, within the broader context of how malaria cycles through populations. In general, a fuller understanding of each phase contributes significantly towards developing intelligent interventions, better diagnostic tools, and ultimately reducing the global malaria burden (Figure 9.6).

9.2. Global Distribution of Malaria

Global campaigns all over the globe have worked tirelessly to combat infectious diseases, but still, malaria persists, particularly in warm, wet regions. It is no mystery why: nature is a large part of the issue here; the same ecological anomalies that allow Anopheles mosquitoes to survive in the first place ultimately drive the transmission of those annoying *Plasmodium* parasites. You can think it is all an African problem, and in a sense, it is—sub-Saharan Africa suffers the greatest loss due to weather that is conducive to mosquito survival, but the issue also rears its ugly head elsewhere. In regions of South and Southeast Asia, Central, and South America, even on a few Pacific Islands, malaria is present. Urbanization and the way humans travel further complicate this picture, changing where and when individuals become infected.

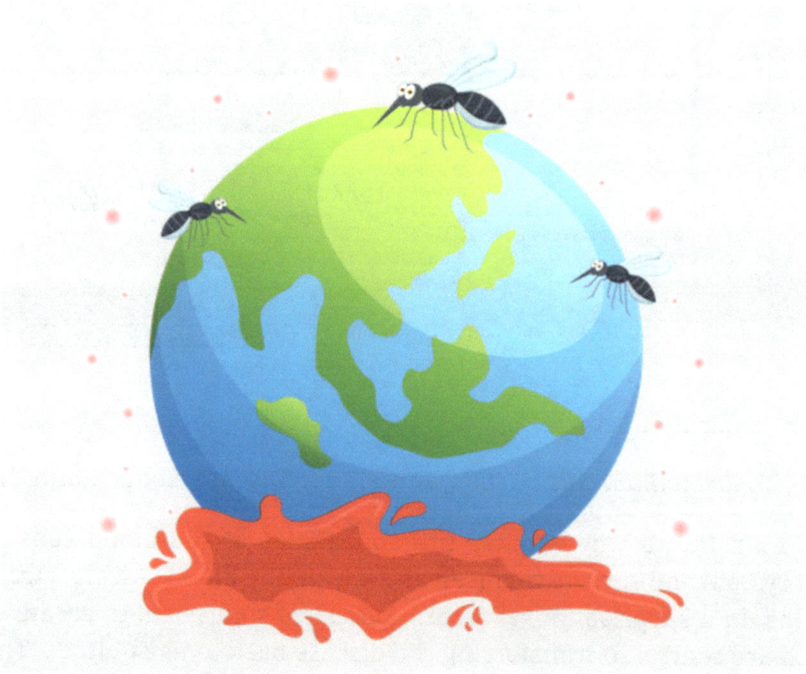

Figure 9.7. Global distribution of malaria.

Source: IconScout. (n.d.). *World Malaria Day Illustration.*

In the majority of instances, being able to identify these interlinked factors is central to crafting solutions that slice the transmission and relentlessly push toward a future free from malaria. Various types of *Plasmodium* parasites simply add fuel to the fire. *Plasmodium falciparum* is typically in the limelight for inducing the most perilous, if not lethal, cases, but do not forget the contributions of *P. ovale*, *P. malariae*, and *P. vivax*, which are also important, particularly in certain regions of Africa and Asia. Recent studies emerging from Kenya, for example, reveal an increase in non-*falciparum* cases among patients presenting symptoms; this development is indicative of a changing environment that may even threaten our existing methods of treatment and control of the disease. Infrequently, infections combine species, a phenomenon that disrupts treatment strategies due to variations in the response of each species to drugs. In general, these advances indicate an urgent need for improved diagnostic tests and surveillance systems capturing all forms of malaria—a necessity if public health interventions are to find the target (Hoseah et al., 2021). Wherever malaria's burden is greatest, there tend to be an entanglement of socioeconomic problems and failing healthcare systems. Citizens living in disadvantaged areas, with hospitals and prevention programs stretched to the limit, experience delays in treatment that translate to worse health outcomes and increased mortality. Subsequently there is the additional headache of drug resistance, which is not particular where it appears but strikes low-resource settings hardest, reducing the effectiveness of treatments and further elevating mortality rates. Broad assessments of this situation reveal that variations in resistance patterns demand an urgent boost in lab capacity, sharper data collection, and smarter antimicrobial management, particularly where the burden is most intense (Christopher et al., 2022). To summarize, a united and flexible approach seems essential if we are to lessen malaria's global impact over the long haul (Figure 9.7).

9.2.1. Regions Most Affected by Malaria

Globally, the disease has different impacts on different places, and researchers say that effects have a real influence on how infections such as malaria spread. Malaria once plagued almost every region of the world, but today its impact is largely concentrated in a few particular areas. Sub-Saharan Africa, for example, gets left carrying most of the cases and deaths, its environment is conducive to the Anopheles mosquito, and a combination of the presence of parasites, socioeconomic issues, and limited healthcare access are all contributing factors. In general terms, these chronically high rates indicate that targeted, local efforts are necessary. Even a study suggests that in most instances where there are limited health resources and it is difficult to implement vector control, mortality due to diseases such as malaria is still remarkably high (Naghavi et al., 2024). This uneven focus only contributes to the overall complexity of initiatives targeted at eliminating the disease worldwide. Outside of sub-Saharan Africa, regions of Southeast Asia and islands of Oceania struggle with significant malaria issues as well, although they do not witness as many deaths. There, malaria is a different entity—defined by an array of parasite species, changing drug resistance, and uneven transmission patterns. An assortment of conditions like regional climate, lifestyle, and the organization of health care all appear to sustain the persistence of the disease in the tropical and subtropical regions. At times, insecticides simply fail because mosquitoes mutate, and *Plasmodium* strains resist the cures—the outcome is an entwined battle against the disease. Recent evidence even suggests that antimicrobial resistance, which also suppresses malaria treatment, is ticking up as an issue (Christopher et al., 2022). Understanding such local nuances assists in customizing control efforts to respond to what fuels malaria's persistence. Although the worst malaria deaths are in low-resource locations, things are not all the same everywhere—differences appear even within tiny areas. Rain, temperature, and humidity can generate mini-hotspots where mosquitoes are breeding more intensively and transmission accumulates in brief bursts. Meanwhile, economic disparities and disproportionately distributed public health systems cause additional glitches at a very localized level. Urbanization, migration, and disparities of access to treatment further complicate the risk profiles. All of this concentrating of deaths in given places clearly highlights the reason why geographically targeted programs that intensify vector control, accelerate treatment, and get communities on board with the effort—are so critical. In most instances, such on-the-ground interventions alter local disease dynamics and even result in wider regional changes, as demonstrated in a number of epidemiologic studies (Naghavi et al., 2024). Better mapping of these differences continues to be crucial to perfecting plans for eliminating malaria.

9.2.2. Factors Influencing Geographical Spread

Conditions of nature affect so greatly how malaria appears in various regions. Hot weather, steamy humidity, and standing bodies of water create the type of place in which Anopheles mosquitoes—essentially the primary offenders for malaria transmission—can flourish. Rainfall, arriving in its own untimely fashion, has a tendency to alter mosquito infestation, so malaria surges or ebbs accordingly. And, more broadly, climate change is shaking things up by moving temperatures and rainfall patterns enough so that areas previously malaria-free may find it in their future.

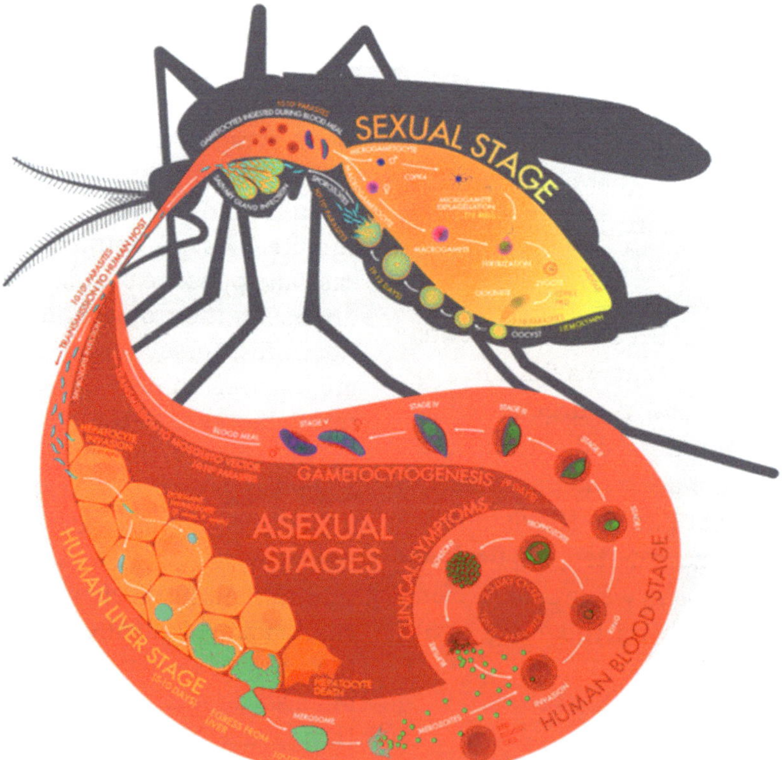

Figure 9.8. How malaria is spread.

Source: Choi R, Michaels SA, Onu EC, Hulverson MA, Saha A, Coker ME, Weeks JC, Van Voorhis WC, Ojo KK. Taming the Boys for Global Good: Contraceptive Strategy to Stop Malaria Transmission. *Molecules.* 2020; 25(12):2773. https://doi.org/10.3390/molecules25122773.

New locations, where individuals may not have developed immunity, become especially susceptible; more often than not, these areas also have economic troubles, which simply exacerbates the issue (Naghavi et al., 2024). In most instances, getting your head around these weather and ecological features is vital for designing interventions that find their target. Humans and the way that they live are big movers in terms of malaria's coverage. Flows such as migration or the flow of urban expansion can cause malaria parasites to spread into areas that never had the issue previously or just keep them circulating in areas that are already on the radar. Land changes, such as irrigation schemes or deforestation—tend to leave behind numerous small breeding sites for mosquitoes. Poverty also has a role; it is associated with poor housing, poor access to prevention materials, and poor healthcare. All of these factors are likely to exacerbate the malaria issue. The relationship between man and animals and sharing of space yet again presents a twist. For instance, close interaction with cattle has in certain instances been associated with changes in the flow of microbes (Asante et al., 2019). Addressing these economic and social determinants alongside healthcare and environmental policies is most likely the best option for reducing the spread of malaria. Subsequently there is the infrastructure of our healthcare systems. Where strong healthcare infrastructures and laboratories exist, cases of malaria get detected fairly quickly, so treatment is quick and mosquito control that prevents further transmission is enacted. But in places where healthcare is limited, particularly rural or war-torn areas—there are delays or underreporting, allowing disease to persist longer. Public health decisions are heavily dependent on good information regarding who is becoming ill or, unfortunately, dying (Naghavi et al., 2024), so having credible information typically helps make it simpler to effectively allocate resources. Adding a dash of One Health, one that considers humans, animals, and the environment as one holistic picture, can enhance efforts to control outbreaks, especially in regions where illnesses jump over from animals to humans (Asante et al., 2019). Strengthening this entire system arrangement is fairly key to maintaining malaria under control in the long term (Figure 9.8).

9.2.3. Trends in Malaria Prevalence Over Time

In recent decades, the infectious disease landscape of the world has indeed changed—largely due to increased antimicrobial resistance and evolving trends in how pathogens present. Consider malaria, for example. Caused by multiple *Plasmodium* species, its presence is no longer what it once was in most endemic countries. Long-term studies, if you consider the data over the years, reveal a decline in cases with a single species, particularly the infamous *Plasmodium falciparum*, while combined infections with other *Plasmodium* species appear to be increasing. This commingling suggests some untidy interactions occurring within hosts that may eventually fine-tune how bad an illness becomes or how efficacious treatments are. In most instances, monitoring this is that we just have to maintain routine surveillance and continue refining our molecular tests to get a grip on the changing malaria burden (Christopher et al., 2022). It does not end there, though. The entire picture only gets blurrier with antimicrobial resistance having its say, an element that now significantly negates standard treatment guidelines. Recent epidemiologic evaluations tend to highlight the fact that drug-resistant bacterial infections are taking an increasing percentage out of death statistics, particularly when they appear in conjunction with malaria. You are left with the problem of having to deal with opportunistic infections in malaria-endemic areas.

Signs/ symptoms	Definitions	1990	2000	2006	2010	2012	2014	2015
Severe anemia*,&	■ Hemoglobin (Hb) < 5 g/dL, or Hematocrit (Hct) < 15%	■						
	■ Hb < 5 g/dL, or Hct < 15% (Children) ■ Hb < 7 g/dL, or Hct < 20% (Adults)		■	■	■	■		
	■ Hb < 5 g/dL, or Hct < 15% (Children <12 years) with parasitemia >10,000 p/μL ■ Hb < 7 g/dL, or Hct < 20% (Adults) with parasitemia >10,000 p/μL						■	■
Severe renal impairment*	■ Urine output <12 mL/kg/24 h, or plasma creatinine concentration above the age-related normal values (Children)/Urine output <400 mL/kg/24 h, or/and a serum creatinine >3 mg/dL (Adult), and despite adequate volume repletion/rehydration	■	■	■				
	■ Serum creatinine concentration > 265 μmol/L (3 mg/dL)				■	■		
	■ Serum creatinine concentration > 265 μmol/L (3 mg/dL) or blood urea >20 mmol						■	■
Shock/Circulatory collapse*	■ Systolic blood pressure (SBP) < 70 mmHg (Adults) and < 50 mmHg (Children 1–5 years)	■	■	■	■			
	■ SBP < 80 mmHg (Adults) and < 50 mmHg (Children)					■		
	■ *Compensated shock*: capillary refill ≥3 s or temperature gradient on leg (mid to proximal limb), but no hypotension. *Decompensated shock*: SBP < 70 mmHg (Children) or < 80 mmHg (Adults) with confirmation of impaired perfusion (prolonged capillary refill or cool peripheries)						■	■
Abnormal bleeding*	■ Spontaneous bleeding from gums, nose, gastrointestinal tract, and venipuncture sites. Clinical evidence of bleeding using tests (e.g., prothrombin time, platelet)	■	■	■	■	■		
	■ Recurrent or prolonged bleeding from nose gums, gastro-intestinal tract, or venipuncture sites; hematemesis or melena						■	■
Disseminated intravascular coagulation (DIC)	■ Laboratory evidence (e.g., prothrombin time prolonged >3 s of the control)	■	■	■	■	■	■	■
Multiple convulsions	■ More than 2 convulsions observed within 24 h	■	■	■	■	■	■	■
Metabolic acidosis*	■ Plasma bicarbonate <15 mmol/L	■						
	■ Plasma bicarbonate <15 mmol/L or base excess (≥ 10 mmol/L)		■	■	■	■		
	■ A base deficit of >8 mEq/L or, if unavailable, a plasma bicarbonate of <15 mM or venous plasma lactate >5 mM						■	■

Hemoglobinuria*	■ Hemolysis not secondary to glucose-6-phosphate dehydrogenase deficiency
	■ Urine is dark or black, and urinalysis dipstick test is positive for Hb, associated with absence of microscopic hematuria (i.e., presence of blood in urine)
Impaired consciousness/ Cerebral malaria*,§	■ Rousable coma (impaired consciousness)/Unarousable come (cerebral malaria)
	■ A Glasgow coma Score < 9 (Adults), or a Blantyre coma score < 2 (Children)
	■ A Glasgow coma Score < 11 (Adults), or a Blantyre coma score < 3 (Children)
Prostration*	■ Weakness so that the patient cannot sit or walk, with no obvious neurological explanation
	■ The inability to sit upright or to drink (Children), Extreme weakness (Adults)
	■ Generalized weakness so that the patient is unable walk or sit up without assistance
Clinical jaundice*	■ Plasma/serum bilirubin concentration > 50 μmol/L (3 mg/dL)[a]
	■ Plasma/serum bilirubin concentration > 50 μmol/L (3 mg/dL)[b]
	■ Plasma/serum bilirubin concentration > 50 μmol/L (3 mg/dL) with parasite density > 20,000 parasites/μL[c]
	■ Plasma/serum bilirubin concentration > 50 μmol/L (3 mg/dL) with parasite density > 100,000 parasites/μL[a,c]
Multi-organ dysfunction	■ Clinical jaundice, and evidence of other vital organ dysfunction
Pulmonary oedema*	■ Diagnosed upon radiological examination
	■ Diagnosed upon radiological examination, or oxygen saturation < 92% on room air with a respiratory rate > 30/min, often with chest indrawing and crepitations on auscultation
Acidotic breathing	■ Deep breathing and respiratory distress
Hypoglycaemia	■ Whole blood glucose concentration < 2.2 mmol/L (40 mg/dL)
Hyperpyrexia	■ Core body temperature > 40°C
Hyperlactatemia*	■ Plasma lactate 5 mmol/L (Children) and > 6 mmol/L (Adults)
	■ Plasma lactate >5 mmol/L

Failure to feed	■ n.a (observable)							
Hyperparasitemia*	■ No parasitemia threshold defined[a]							
	■ Parasitemia >4% (unstable malaria endemicity), > 20% (stable malaria endemicity)[a]							
	■ Parasitemia >5% (low malaria endemicity), > 10% (high malaria endemicity)[a]							
	■ Parasitemia >2% (low malaria endemicity), > 5% (high malaria endemicity)[a]							
	■ Parasitemia >20% in any epidemiological context[a]							
	■ Parasitemia >10% in any epidemiological context[a]							
	■ Parasitemia >2%[c]							

DIC, Disseminated intravascular coagulation; Hb, Hemoglobin; Hct, Hematocrit; n.a, Not applicable; *Pf*, *Plasmodium falciparum*; *Pk*, *Plasmodium knowlesi*; *Pv*, *Plasmodium vivax*; SBP, Systolic blood pressure; WHO, World Health Organization. *These signs/symptoms have been revised by the WHO. [&]Defined as severe normocytic anemia in the previous guidelines (1990–2012). [$]Impaired consciousness (rousable coma) and cerebral malaria (unarousable coma) were clinically differentiated before advent of coma scales (16). *Pv* and *Pk* have been first mentioned as able to induce severe malaria in the 2006 and 2012 WHO guidelines, respectively. Manifestations of severe malaria due to *Pv* parasites may present to with some symptoms similar to severe *Pf* malaria. Manifestations of severe malaria due to *Pk* parasites are similar to those of severe *Pf* malaria with the exception of coma. [a]Used for *P. falciparum* severe malaria only. [b]Used for *P. vivax* severe malaria only. [c]Used for P. knowlesi severe malaria only. The color is related to linking the definition of a given sign/symptom to the period where this definition was retained in global WHO guidelines to diagnose severe malaria.

Figure 9.9. Trends in malaria prevalence over time.

Source: Kojom Foko LP and Singh V (2023) Malaria in pregnancy in India: a 50-year bird's eye. Front. Public Health. 11:1150466. doi: 10.3389/fpubh.2023.1150466.

Look at global maps of drug resistance and you will see quite a patchwork—a few areas, like sub-Saharan Africa, suffer the heaviest death toll despite already wrestling with malaria. This mix of resistance with malaria patterns clearly calls for better-integrated control measures and smarter policy moves (Christopher et al., 2022). Observe closely and you see a less obvious trend as well: with time, non-*falciparum* species such as *Plasmodium ovale curtisi* and even *Plasmodium ovale wallikeri* are appearing more frequently in cases that are symptomatic. There is a possibility that this increase is related to such as partially lower drug responses or even local ecological phenomena that promote these species. Such a shift poses a knock-on challenge for malaria programs that have traditionally zeroed in on *Plasmodium falciparum*—so, there is a risk that the less common infections might get overlooked. Add that to the steady, unchanged presence of *Plasmodium* malariae, and you have got a picture of evolving patterns that could shake up treatment guidelines, surveillance strategies, and even vaccine strategies. In the majority of instances, recognizing these nuanced yet critical trends is the secret to directing malaria intervention initiatives in the appropriate direction over a period (Hoseah et al., 2021) (Figure 9.9).

9.3. Risk Factors for Malaria Infection

Socioeconomic determinants heavily influence who bears the brunt of malaria. Not having money can mean going without such things as insecticide-treated bed nets (ITNs) or even a decent roof, and these are important to keep the mosquitoes away. Studies out in Western Kenya's highlands tend overall to indicate that poorer households experience more clinical malaria, poor incomes tend to have higher rates of infection. It is not only money, however; factors such as a mother's education and work history appear to be associated with reduced risks, likely because a working mother or one with more education knows a little more about keeping her family safe.

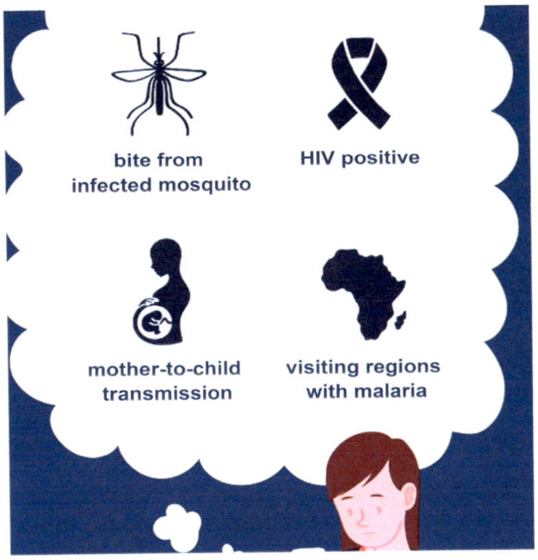

Figure 9.10. Risk factors for malaria infection.

Source: Verywell Health. (n.d.). *Causes of malaria.* https://external-content.duckduckgo.com/iu/?u=https%3A%2F%2Fwww.verywellhealth.com%2Fthmb%2Fbu_S0MMjA32dEs7r4LAob8Qj-GI%3D%2F1501x1001%2Ffilters%3Ano_upscale()%3Amax_bytes(150000)%3Astrip_icc()%2Fmalaria-causes-5ad755771f4e130038d953c9.png&f=1&nofb=1&ipt=90d08ad72d2b2a92b87801cd23b6e909c6d9d845d0e0e382e8c84162d4079052.

Home features such as open eaves allow mosquitoes to enter, increasing the likelihood of bites. Overall, the combination of money problems, social life, and even the construction of a home makes vulnerability to malaria quite complicated (Essendi et al., 2019). Individuals' behaviors and their occupations also combine into how susceptible they are to getting malaria. Consider, for instance, individuals whose occupation brings them nearer to where mosquitoes live; it formerly bothered a majority of epidemiologists. In one study done in Senegal, the researchers followed mosquito collectors, people who get bitten on a regular basis, and compared them with nearby neighbors who did not collect. To the surprise of the researchers, the figures did not reflect sharply increased malaria among the collectors, even in the time before chemoprophylaxis or long-lasting ITNs were the norm. By and large, this suggests that it is not necessarily about getting bitten more frequently, but perhaps about developing immunity or simply being that much more diligent while working. In effect, these findings refute the common perception that highly exposed jobs make you an automatic candidate for malaria, and they appear to support the safety of critical vector surveillance practices (Diagne et al., 2015).

Environmental surroundings and what occurs at home are also key factors in which malaria spreads. Mosquito numbers and breeding areas can genuinely tip the balance, but even easy measures such as the use of ITNs significantly reduce actual numbers. Families in Western Kenya that used the nets all the time ended up with significantly fewer malaria cases, despite the fact that the level of mosquito buzz was the same in all houses, it was the variation in net usage that created the difference. You could say personal habits and personal choices at homework their magic. And do not forget, open-eaved homes can be like welcome mats for mosquitoes, increasing the risk. To summarize, manipulating both environmental and household factors by improving housing and disseminating ITNs appears rather necessary to reducing transmission at a local level (Essendi et al., 2019) (Figure 9.10).

9.3.1. Socioeconomic Determinants

Populations' health typically has a connection to where and how individuals live; the quality of neighborhood and accessible resources determine how likely an individual is to contract diseases like malaria. Everyone does not have an equal chance at protection, many who are unable to afford items like insecticide-treated nets or consistent indoor spraying bear the highest burden of these infections. Living in crowded, substandard housing increases the likelihood of exposure to malaria-carrying mosquitoes, and tight finances usually translate into waits for appropriate diagnosis and treatment. All of these tribulations serve to place further odds against already struggling individuals. The resulting knock-on problems, such as anemia or productivity drops—can perpetuate a cycle of poverty and illness, which in turn further complicates halting malaria's spread. In general, the combination of health solutions with enhancements in living standards appears to be central to reducing risks and increasing health equity in malaria-affected regions (Camila et al., 2019). The relationship between malaria and wider social inequalities appears when you consider child mortality due to infection, including malaria. Socioeconomic status influences everything from what we eat to how we are being exposed to other diseases, let alone the chance to receive good healthcare—all of which are variables that adjust how severe the disease could get. Consider, for instance, children in poor households in malaria-endemic areas—who tend to develop increased rates of anemia that fuel the flames of an already brutal disease. Then there is the regional landscape: sub-Saharan Africa and southern Asia are where the largest malaria burdens occur, where poverty and poor healthcare systems converge.

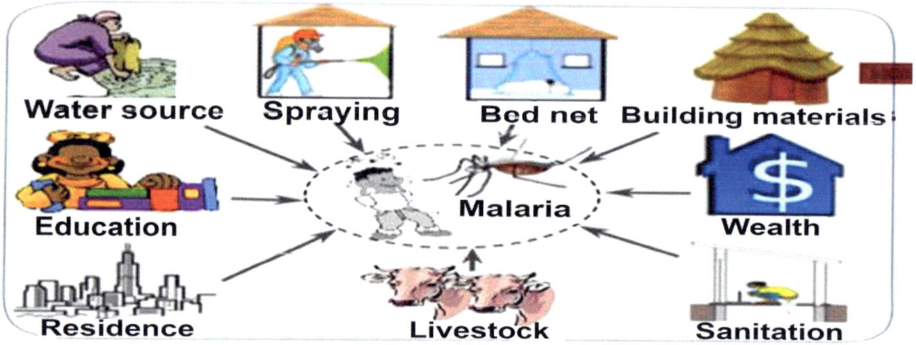

Figure 9.11. Determinants of human malaria.

Source: Semakula, H.M., Liang, S., Mukwaya, P.I. *et al.* Determinants of malaria infections among children in refugee settlements in Uganda during 2018–2019. *Infect Dis Poverty* **12**, 31 (2023). https://doi.org/10.1186/s40249-023-01090-3

The fact that previous global goals to reduce childhood mortality have been missed only serves to demonstrate that we require varied approaches targeting both the immediate illness and the broader day-to-day struggles. Actually, targeting policies at the most vulnerable and intensifying socioeconomic conditions might significantly reduce malaria illness and mortality and lay the groundwork for more equitable global health outcomes (Liu et al., 2016). Malaria control strategies need to place social and economic issues front and center if they are to make a real impact. Increasing education, alleviating poverty, and enhancing infrastructure not only promoted health awareness but also prompt people to access help early and reside in settings less hospitable to malaria vectors. As individuals attain a little more economic independence, they are in a position to better acquire preventative devices and high-quality care, which slows transmission and enhances follow-up with treatments. Understand that malaria does not affect every community equally allows us to direct interventions where they are most needed. Without addressing these larger, underlying challenges, even the most effective medical interventions may fall short, leaving fundamental vulnerabilities unaddressed. Evidently, an integration of public health measures that combines economic development and disease management is necessary for sustained declines in malaria and the persistent health disparities that accompany them (Liu et al., 2016; Camila et al., 2019) (Figure 9.11).

9.3.2. Environmental Factors

Environmental conditions play a significant role in the spread of malaria. Temperature, rain, and humidity combine to form the type of environment where Anopheles mosquitoes can breed, this then promotes disease levels. Chilly temperatures, for example, slow the growth of parasites within mosquitoes, but even a slight increase in night-time lows can accelerate both the insects' maturation and parasite growth. Rainfall plays its own puzzle: while it opens up breeding opportunities, prolonged periods with only light rain can concentrate those spots, inadvertently boosting mosquito numbers. In places like Burundi's highlands, these elements all add up; houses near these concentrated spots face a higher risk, perfectly illustrating how complex things can get (Protopopoff et al., 2009). Malaria does not strike each corner equally; various settings exhibit pretty high variation, thanks mainly to regional environmental adjustments. Seasonal fluctuations, such as variations in rain and temperature—play havoc with mosquito numbers and cause changes in the intensity of transmission over time. Subsequently there is the influence of land use and proximity to water in determining where mosquitoes do best, creating patterns of elevated infection levels. Actually, urban and rural environments appear to exert various pressures on insects such as *Anopheles stephensi*, both on numbers and timing of peaks, making one-size-fits-all control measures challenging. In general terms, understanding such local features is essential to developing malaria control strategies that suit the local context (Whittaker et al., 2022).

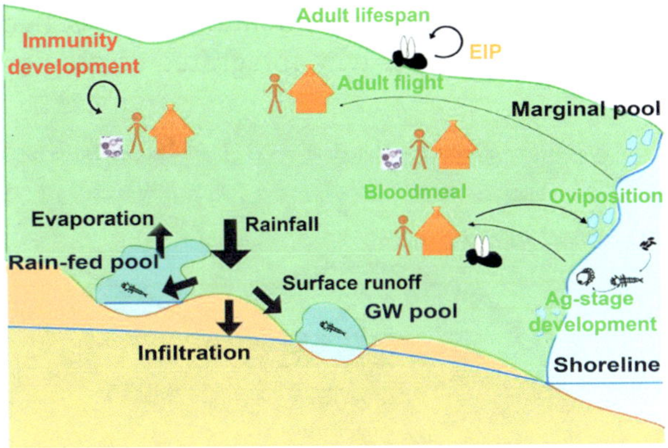

Figure 9.12. Environmental determinants of malaria transmission.

Source: AGU Publications. (n.d.). *Environmental Determinants of Malaria.*

Taking a closer look at malaria outbreak timing, seasonality truly is prominent. Temperature changes and rainfall variability have the tendency to drive mosquito cycles and parasite growth in a manner that produces recurring spikes and troughs in transmission. Time-series research even demonstrates clear seasonal trends that seem to be connected to land use or proximity to water, underscoring the importance of understanding local conditions comprehensively. Where seasons are strong, it is possible to have a significant effect by timing interventions, such as indoor spraying during peak mosquito periods. Finally, paying attention to both space and time is paramount in refining models and ensuring control measures are on target when seeking to alleviate malaria's burden on public health (Whittaker et al., 2022) (Figure 9.12).

9.3.3. Behavioral Aspects of Populations

Individuals' daily behavior greatly determines how malaria is spread. Migration, social patterns, and even where and how individuals sleep can influence the likelihood of receiving a mosquito bite when one is most active. For instance, utilizing bed nets ordinarily reduces bites, while travel and migration have the possibility of introducing malaria into regions where it was not prevalent previously. Failure to adhere to recommended practices, such as indoor spraying or prompt treatment, only exacerbates the situation. What one should be aware of is that how communities react to health education and practical interventions fits into this equation; in fact, when behavior comes into contact with environmental factors, it becomes a pretty complex task to predict the spreading of malaria, which is why integrated strategies are more and more in demand (Sadie et al., 2019).

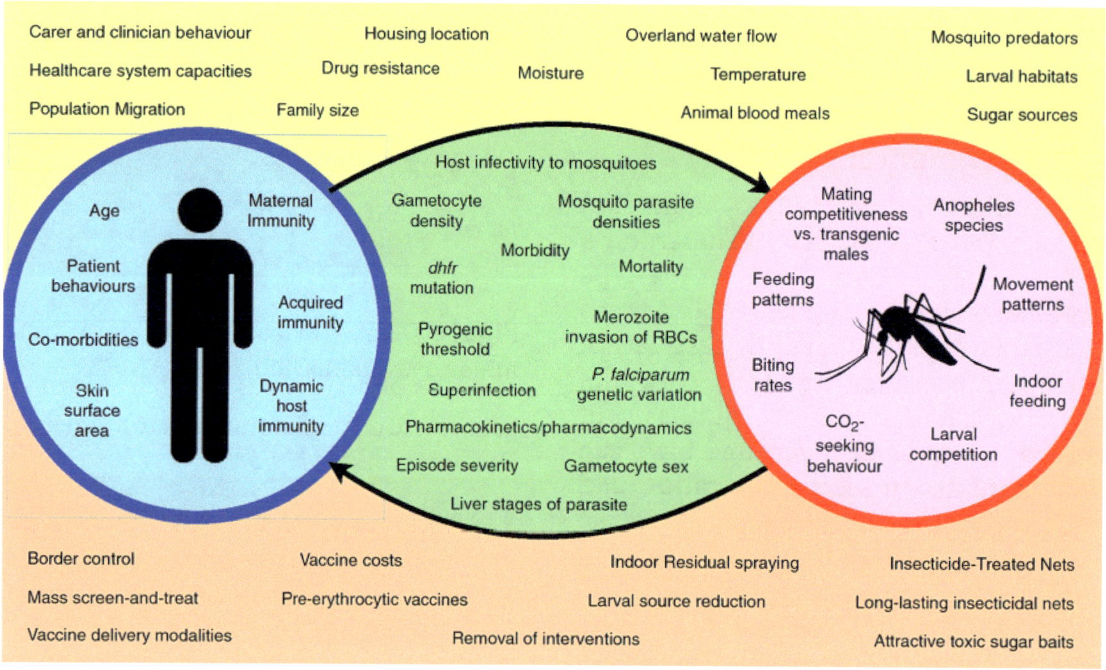

Figure 9.13. Behavioral aspects of populations on malaria spreads.

Source: ResearchGate. (n.d.). *Factors Influencing Malaria Transmission.*

Local practices and community culture also take center stage when issues of preventing malaria are concerned. In most of the areas severely affected by the disease, traditional treatments coexist with conventional medicine – the mix of the two can slow down diagnosis and treatment, maintaining parasite reservoirs for extended durations. Economic considerations, also, influence these decisions; if antimalarial medication or insecticide-treated nets are out of pocket or difficult to access, fewer use them. Subsequently there is a human factor: occasionally, when the public does not have confidence in health authorities or just misunderstands how malaria is transmitted, the conventional control measures fall flat. Seasonal activity, such as farming work or evening social collections—frequently results in individuals spending more time outdoors during the prime mosquito hours. We frequently notice that combining these sociocultural observations with disease models is able to enhance predictions and guide the development of specific interventions that work (Brauer, 2017). There is also the manner through which changes in behavior as a result of climatic changes impact malaria transmission as well. Global warming drives mosquitoes, such as not only Anopheles but also viruses such as Aedes—into new ranges, and human exposure risks are correspondingly altered in ways that are surprising. Changes in housing conditions, urban growth, and land use all adjust local mosquito breeding sites and human vector contact frequency. As risk perceptions change, public awareness and health-seeking behaviors will do likewise, even if slowly. Mathematically modeling this combination of changing human behavior with biological elements is no simple task—yet it continues to be important for predicting future situations (Brauer, 2017; Sadie et al., 2019). Finally, the incorporation of behavioral science into the research on malaria provides a critical dimension to our attempts at forecasting and containing the disease in a constantly changing environmental and social context (Figure 9.13).

9.4. Symptoms and Diagnosis of Malaria

Malaria is a latent disease that frequently does not make itself known immediately, particularly in regions where it is prevalent. It might begin with an assortment of flu-like symptoms, such as fever, chills, a nagging headache, and that persisting malaise sensation, which sometimes suddenly change into full-blown issues such as anemia, respiratory distress, or even neurological complications.

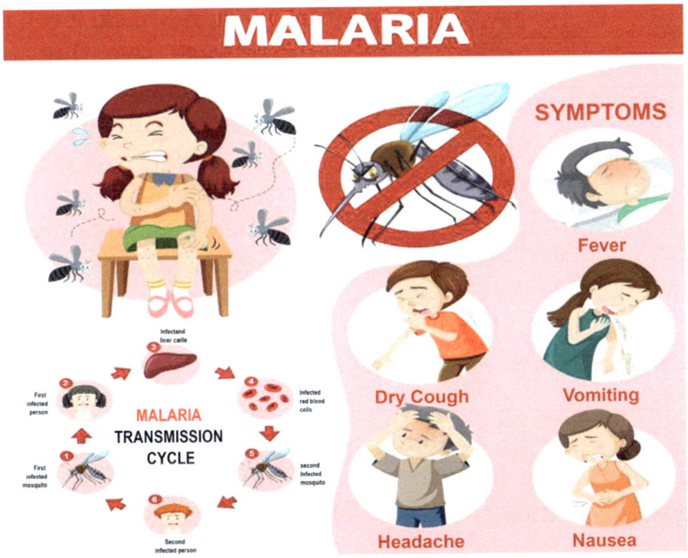

Figure 9.14. Symptoms and diagnosis of malaria.

Source: Being The Parent. (2022). *Symptoms of Malaria.*

Children under five, who are specifically vulnerable, may suddenly present disconcerting symptoms such as for a time losing consciousness, labored or spasmodic breathing, seizures, or serious anemia; all these may indicate that the disease has progressed to a point where immediate treatment is critical. Because symptoms occur in such vastly different ways, particularly where lab work is not consistently available, health practitioners have to fall back on both their clinical acumen and whichever tests are on hand—a reality highlighted by surveys that collected self-reported malaria symptoms among malaria-positive children (Taylor et al., 2021). The challenge is compounded when you factor in the diversity of *Plasmodium* species involved, each with its own spin. For example, *Plasmodium vivax*, which frequently presents in migrant cohorts like Eritrean asylum seekers, takes its sweet time to become symptomatic, sometimes appearing weeks after initial exposure. Such a delay can disrupt standard diagnostic timelines and compels medical personnel, even where the area is non-endemic, to remain vigilant at all times. Generally, physicians employ conventional tools, such as microscopy and rapid diagnostic tests (RDTs) and newer molecular techniques—all of which have their specific sensitivities and limitations.

It is also not surprising that imported cases are subject to further screening, such as glucose-6-phosphate dehydrogenase deficiency testing prior to primaquine administration, in an effort to prevent adverse reactions. Such experiences, especially among Eritrean migrants, remind us of the significance of interweaving a patient's history with laboratory results (Schlagenhauf et al., 2018). In general, getting the correct malaria diagnosis right matters not only for the salvation of individual lives but also to guide the efforts of public health. Most of the time, particularly when it comes to severe malaria in children, it is important to identify the correct symptoms and to verify them rapidly through the use of lab tests. At a larger level, estimates based on clinical presentations give us a glimpse of how the illness spreads within various regions and populations—data that public health measures are predicated upon. Despite that, similar symptoms to other febrile diseases and the resultant unequal access to diagnostic services introduce layers of complexity, so it is a little bit complex at times. Increasing tests' capacity by making them tests more tests accessible and sensitive to tests between infections such as *P. vivax* and *P. falciparum* is crucial. Not only do such advances enhance tests early detection and timely treatment but can also go a considerable way towards reducing malaria's total burden in both endemic and surprising non-endemic environments (Schlagenhauf et al., 2018; Taylor et al., 2021) (Figure 9.14).

9.4.1. Common Symptoms of Malaria

Malaria victims begin experiencing a combination of symptoms that arise from the body's response to the *Plasmodium* parasite. Initially, it may simply feel like a bout of the flu – you have a fever, chills, headaches, and muscle pains. Subsequently, as it all wears on, you may notice recurring spiking of the fever; this occurs when red blood cells explode simultaneously as the parasite completes its cycle. This cyclical fever, frequently accompanied by profuse sweating and extreme tiredness, indicates malaria, although the very sensation of it can vary depending on the type of parasite and the strength of your immune system. For the most part, identifying these symptoms is central to the early detection of the disease, particularly in areas where the same symptoms may arise from other diseases (Nakanjako et al., 2011). Other times, if the symptoms become worse or simply do not fade because treatment is not adequate, the complications set in. In general, serious malaria has additional, frightening symptoms – extreme fevers that just do not quit, life-threatening anemia due to an excess of red blood cells being broken down, respiratory problems, and even neurological problems such as confusion, convulsions, or coma. These red flags indicate the infection may be progressing to cerebral malaria or is damaging multiple organs simultaneously, and they are a large reason why malaria is so dangerous. Understanding these signs assists health workers in identifying high-risk groups and distributing appropriate treatments more quickly. Additionally, cases of individuals with few or no symptoms

, particularly if they have also diseases like HIV – make it even more difficult to depend only on what you can observe while taking an exam (Nakanjako et al., 2011). Beyond the clinical setting, public health evidence indicates that communities strongly desire accessible information regarding malaria. Individuals commonly engage in internet searching to gather information on early warning signs of the illness, how the sickness emerges, and what treatments or protective measures they can take.

The question stream reflects both individual concerns and community concerns. Such knowledge is crucial in informing education campaigns and intervention measures, especially in regions where misperception or stigma may deter people from seeking assistance promptly. By bridging such information gaps and encouraging individuals to seek care earlier, it is possible to minimize the overall burden of malaria, particularly in regions where the cases are more prevalent.

9.4.2. Diagnostic Methods Used

Improvements in how we make a diagnosis of malaria have quite genuinely transformed our struggle against the disease. The importance of an accurate diagnosis lies in it accelerating treatment and monitoring outbreaks. For many years now, clinicians have relied on looking at smears of blood under a microscope, a technique that illustrates, in a very obvious way, the variation among the *Plasmodium* species. But, as microscopy is dependent on skilled fingers and can be very time-consuming, it is not always the most suitable in low-resource environments or when quickly screening large numbers of individuals.

That is why RDTs emerged, providing a more rapid, less complex solution without the requirement for a proper laboratory setup. These tests have, for the most part, increased diagnosis access in areas most affected by malaria, resulting in more accurate data on disease transmission and enhanced control measures (Chen et al., 2012). Recently, novel testing methods have been compelled to provide further sensitivity and specificity while avoiding operational challenges encountered each day. Consider molecular techniques – polymerase chain reaction (PCR), say , which is typically capable of detecting low-level infection that both conventional microscopy and RDTs fail to detect; the latter becomes particularly critical in facilities working towards eradication of the disease. Other nucleic acid amplification techniques, similarly, detect minute parasitemia, even marking individuals showing no signs but harboring the infection. Naturally, such molecular diagnostics typically require well-equipped laboratories and trained personnel, which constrains their rapid use in the field. Nevertheless, research is continuing to simplify and adapt such methodologies for universal application by combining sophisticated tests with traditional screening techniques (Feachem et al., 2009). Malaria elimination being brought closer relies upon inserting diagnostic tools into responsive surveillance systems capable of rapidly detecting and responding to cases. Moving from simply controlling malaria to wiping it out means rethinking the entire diagnostic approach – there's now more focus on real-time data collection and on-the-ground case follow-ups. Enhanced capabilities like point-of-care testing and ultra-sensitive methods are essential if we are going to hit zero transmission. Surveillance systems, however, must adapt to the local environment by taking into account mosquito behavior, the intensity of transmission, and even local populations' immunity levels, to get interventions just right. Lessons from a number of countries suggest that combining routine testing with strong surveillance, and even some cross-border cooperation—underpins a genuinely sustainable elimination plan (Feachem et al., 2009; Chen et al., 2012) (Figure 9.15).

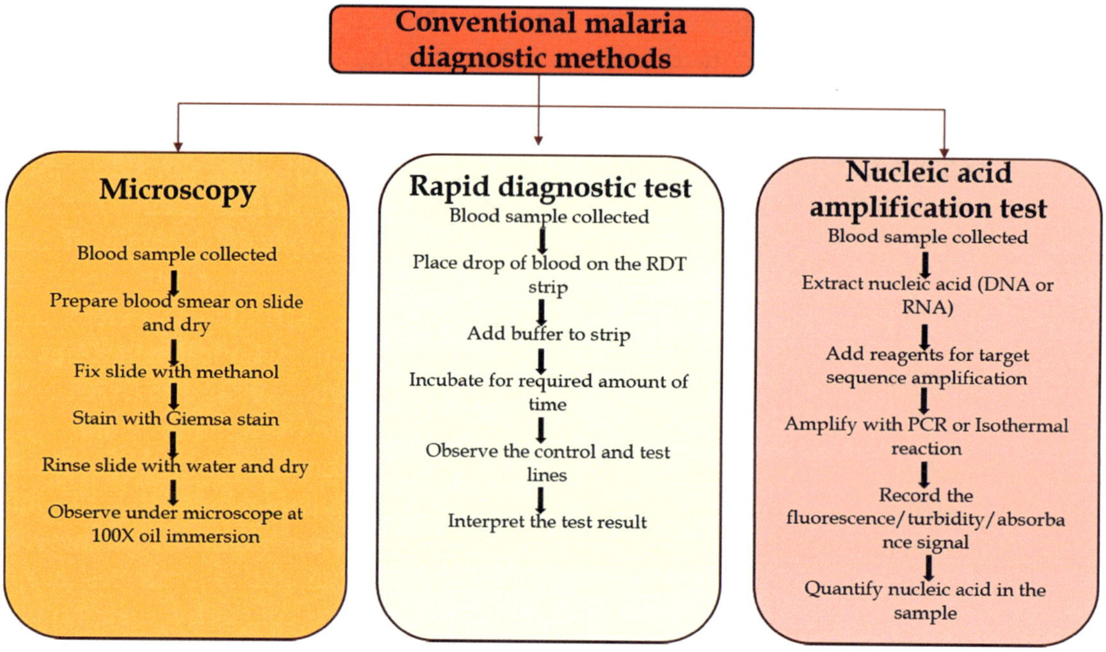

Figure 9.15. Diagnostic methods used on malaria spreads.

Source: Mbanefo A, Kumar N. Evaluation of Malaria Diagnostic Methods as a Key for Successful Control and Elimination Programs. *Tropical Medicine and Infectious Disease*. 2020; 5(2):102. https://doi.org/10.3390/tropicalmed5020102

9.4.3. Challenges in Accurate Diagnosis

Diagnosis of malaria faces a lot of obstacles today. The symptoms of malaria tend to resemble those of other illnesses—dengue, typhoid fever, and even some respiratory infections, which are all too prevalent in most of the affected areas. This similarity in symptoms can result in misdiagnosis or untimely treatment, which screws up proper care in a timely fashion. Where advanced laboratories are scarce, diagnostic tests such as microscopy or PCR may not be readily available, and so RDTs, which may be hit-or-miss in sensitivity and specificity, end up being used by healthcare workers. And in some cases, even frontline workers may lack proper training or appropriate protection, a situation made worse by health crises such as the COVID-19 pandemic. All of these contribute to distorting reported malaria data, which makes it difficult to get a grip on the disease's actual prevalence. Subsequently there's COVID-19—a problem that has just added more misery to the miseries for malaria control efforts worldwide. Both diseases typically come with fever in tow, which complicates their differentiation in settings where many fever-causing diseases are circulating simultaneously. Social distancing and changes in how individuals look for care have similarly constrained community health workers' access to patients for casual malaria testing and surveillance. The pressure to use personal protective gear and adhere to infection procedures, as required, is less effective than desired because of shortages and sporadic training, which only reinforces the bottleneck in diagnosing cases. This interruption postpones appropriate treatment and jeopardizes elimination goals. In the majority of instances, a clever combination of enhanced diagnostic techniques, such as multiplex tests and computerized decision-support systems—may prove to be the answer needed to differentiate malaria from other types of fever and stay ahead of surveillance during and in the aftermath of the pandemic. Below these short-term issues is a more profound issue of data collection and monitoring those obscurities the actual picture of malaria's advancement. In most endemic regions, particularly in low-resource settings, detailed microbiological data are not available, and this constrains estimates of infection rates and resistance patterns (Christopher et al., 2022). Besides this scarcity of detailed information making identification of resistant strains more difficult, it further restricts tracking of key trends required for public health planning that is sound. With limited laboratory capacity and patchy integration of surveillance and diagnosis systems, our grasp of malaria epidemiology is incomplete—frequently derailing prompt intervention strategies. In general, covering these gaps will necessitate substantial investments in laboratory facilities, improved training of healthcare workers, and deployment of new diagnostic technologies with the promise of improving accuracy and reliability, ultimately informing more robust malaria control policies (Christopher et al., 2022).

9.5. Treatment and Prevention Strategies

Malaria is not battled the same each day. Through the years, individuals have understood that having an early diagnosis and promptly taking the appropriate drugs matters. In most instances, artemisinin-based combination therapies (ACTs) are now at the center of treatment, particularly when tackling *Plasmodium falciparum*, as these medications tend to be effective and seldom result in the development of resistance. Travelers and individuals in regions where malaria persists are generally recommended to take preventive drug regimens to reduce their risk, as well. Rapid surveillance identifies cases in an instant and directs treatment efforts down the correct path – although, in all honesty, difficulties such as resistance to drugs and limited care access in less affluent areas mean that the hunt for new treatments never ceases (Androga et al., 2020). Prevention shares the same mix of measures that is a little hit-or-miss compared to strict scientific protocols. Rather than applying one uniform program, strategies now reach the mosquito itself as well as the individuals who may be bitten. For instance, spraying indoors (typically referred to as indoor residual spraying, or IRS) and distributing ITNs have each assisted in reducing the number of cases significantly. Long-lasting nets (LLINs) continue to provide protection year after year, which is quite impressive. There is also an effort being made to control the environment – such as reducing stagnant water where mosquitoes lay eggs or applying larvicides – that is part of a larger strategy. And, if communities know about it and feel engaged, they are more likely to utilize these tools more effectively, making the entire process more efficient. All this, of course, relies on good public health policy and stable finances to keep the wheels rolling (Dev et al., 2012). Looking around the world, some places demonstrate that doing it custom to a place makes a difference. Consider Bhutan, for example, their combination of targeted treatment and prevention has resulted in something approaching a 98.7% reduction in confirmed cases in 16 years. They supported their diagnosis and treatment, relying on ACT for difficult *Plasmodium* cases and intensified vector control through both IRS and ITNs. Nevertheless, there are also setbacks along the way , such as imported cases from neighboring regions that compel authorities to reconsider border checks and intensify surveillance on high-risk groups like migrant workers. Research Articles. This mix of immediate reaction and preventative effort, though not always flawless, demonstrates that being adaptable and mixing in fresh thinking is the solution. In the majority of instances, coping with shifting climates and changing socio-economic factors continues to be a perpetual challenge (Dev et al., 2012) as it also emphasizes the importance of constant innovation in our battle against malaria (Androga et al., 2020) (Figure 9.16).

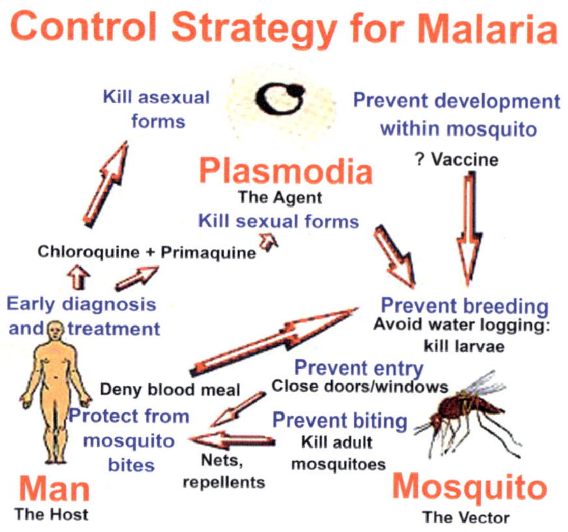

Figure 9.16. Treatment and prevention strategies on malaria.

Source: MalariaSite. (2015). *Malaria Control.*

9.5.1. Antimalarial Medications

Worldwide attempts to stem malaria have moved ahead while the role of drugs—whether prevention or treatment—continues to move center stage. People traveling into malaria-prone countries depend on what has come to be known as chemoprophylaxis, i.e., they take medication to reduce their risk of infection. But taking these regimens consistently is not always simple; many individuals have a hard time swallowing a pill every day for extended periods.

New strategies are arising in most scenarios, such as taking a three-day course of atovaquone/proguanil prior to travel. Compliant rates of more than 97% have been demonstrated in studies (Lau et al., 2019)—a finding some attribute to the regimen's ease and lower total number of pills, which mitigate against the issues of missing doses or suffering side effects that, though relatively minor and transient, tend to disrupt the routine. It is also, if not more, crucial to learn about how patients comply with antimalarial regimens after they fall ill. For instance, the first-line therapy, ACTs, requires strict compliance to preclude treatment failures and forestall the emergence of drug resistance. In the majority of instances, the degree of compliance differs significantly on the basis of variables such as drug form, clarity of instructions, and even packaging differences, all of which can provide scope for inconsistent findings when comparing studies. In general, such non-compliance may undermine the effectiveness of ACTs and even pose a risk of a resurgence in malaria transmission, highlighting the importance of closer monitoring and more focused interventions (Banek et al., 2014). At a larger level, judicious use of antimalarial drugs goes far beyond the treatment of individuals and becomes related to broader public health concerns. When individuals adhere to prevention and treatment regimens in close manner, not only does the impact of the disease diminish, but we also reduce the possibility of drug resistance erupting on a universal scale. Public health policy is then charged with integrating evidence-based interventions, such as educational campaigns, enhanced access to care, and less complicated drug regimens—into its initiatives. Scientists continue to emphasize that more research is needed to confirm the advantages of new dosing regimens and closely scrutinize the social and behavioral determinants influencing how individuals take their medication. Particularly in resource-poor environments, optimizing the use of medications goes hand in hand with enhanced vector control and laboratory advances in maintaining malaria prevalence downward (Banek et al., 2014; Lau et al., 2019) (Figure 9.17).

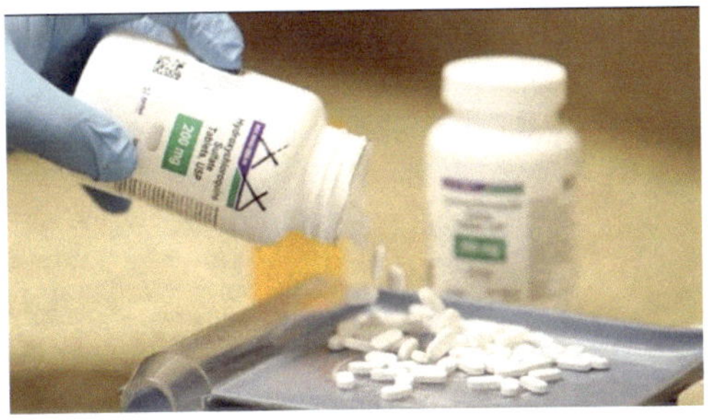

Figure 9.17. Antimalarial medications.

Source: RTÉ. (n.d.). *Antimalarial Medications.*

9.5.2. Preventive Measures (e.g., Bed Nets, Insecticides)

Prevention of malaria boils down to plain prevention where the disease is prevalent. Sharing easy health advice in communities counts—a good knowledge about the symptoms and mode of transmission of malaria tends to get more people to use ITNs. For instance, in Malawi in the south, when caretakers are aware of the symptoms and transmission of malaria, bed nets are more frequently used. Circumstances such as the amount of schooling people have, how close they live to a clinic, and what kind of local health care is available all affect net use. Although everyone can agree that bed nets can protect them, financial hardship usually stands in the way, combining economic problems with health hazards. It appears that when health workers in the local setting intervene to clarify facts and distribute nets at affordable prices to people, this concerted effort can reduce mosquito bites and instances of malaria (Masangwi et al., 2012). In the end, measures that complement community dynamics are responsible for prevention. Mosquito behavior plays a significant role in how effective interventions such as ITNs and indoor residual spraying (IRS) are. Research from across much of Africa usually indicates that malaria carriers bite during nighttime when humans are indoors—so the indoor controls can be quite effective. True, mosquitoes in the *Anopheles gambiae* complex and the *An. funestus* group do not adhere strictly to feeding indoors, but rather their biting patterns tend to fall into synchrony with human indoor activity, so nets and spraying are effective. However, should those behaviors change even slightly, the indoor measures can lose their potency, so monitoring the trends is essential. This combination of elements emphasizes why applying a combination of techniques—some of which address outdoor biting—is key to maintaining malaria control over the long term (Huho et al., 2013). Briefly, understanding these vectors' behavior is key to refining our prevention. In addition to keeping off bites, effective control of malaria requires controlling the environment and engaging the community. Simple home modifications, such as installing window screens and removing mosquito breeding areas, complement nets and pesticides in reducing both mosquitoes and opportunities for contact. Local health attendants and village councils are typically central places for mobilizing neighbors, identifying those at greater risk, and organizing larval control efforts. These diverse strategies address both the natural biology of the mosquito and the social aspect of disease transmission. As a general rule, when interventions are affordable and aligned with local tradition, individuals are more likely to maintain them even during economic hardships. Finally, linking individual tools with broader community and environmental measures develops a balanced strategy that gradually reduces transmission and enables malaria control programs to thrive in the long term (Masangwi et al., 2012).

9.5.3. Vaccination Efforts and Research

Vaccines have now become a big part of mitigating malaria's worldwide presence. Numerous groups now resort to creating and rolling them out, not only relying on the old treatments and insect control methods. In the past decade or so, the effort for malaria vaccines has accelerated—largely due to decreasing illness and death, particularly in sub-Saharan Africa, which simply feels so critical. The parasite's sly life cycle and its remarkable ability to evade our immune systems have always made vaccine development challenging. Nevertheless, certain promising new candidates such as RTS,S/AS01 have reported promising results in large trials, reducing clinical malaria cases in children, even if only somewhat. These measures suggest that more robust immunization campaigns could well be an important component in an overall approach to reduce malaria's burden and even achieve global health targets (Alize et al., 2024). Despite these developments, actual success for vaccination truly hinges on robust health systems able to spread, deliver, and maintain coverage consistently in high-risk areas. Governments, international organizations, and research institutions all end up performing roles that intersect in unanticipated manners. In most instances, obstacles like poor infrastructure, vaccine hesitancy pockets, and financial concerns make the entire scenario more challenging. Current research continuously attempts to increase the vaccine's potency and duration and address the parasite's genetic nuances which may alter how effectively a vaccine will function.

International cooperation among various sectors and investments in ground-based surveillance are important if we are to adjust immunization approaches to align with local patterns and develop resistance , all of which seriously highlight the need for coordinated global action (David et al., 2019). Alongside this, new research methods and technological developments are essential to accelerate vaccine production and enhance our knowledge of malaria's transmission. Genomics research combined with immunology research is gradually unraveling how the parasite leads to disease and how our immune systems respond back, thereby hinting at fresh targets for next-generation vaccines.

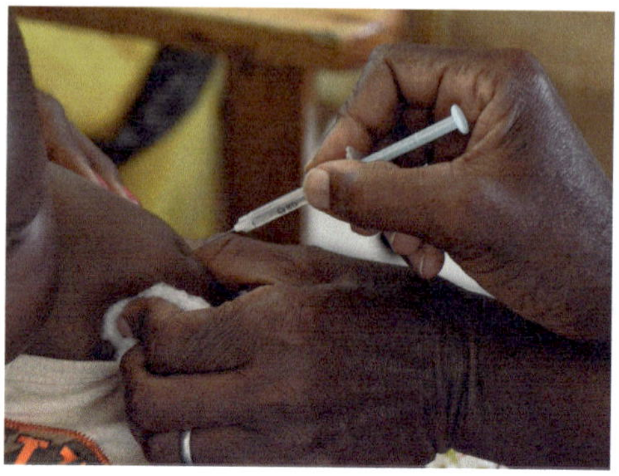

Figure 9.18. The vaccines have come to play a huge role in easing malaria's global impact.

Source: Getty Images. (2021). *Malaria Vaccine Shot*. Boston University.

And yes, the association of vaccination with other measures such as insecticide-treated nets and antimalarial drugs is continuously being reevaluated in order to achieve maximum collective effect. Overall, the worldwide health community needs to support these endeavors with robust financing and wise policies to take lab findings to application in everyday life. By collaborating across industries and geographies, vaccine development could quite possibly level the playing field on malaria, ultimately reducing disease incidence and saving lives in the long run (David et al., 2019; Alize et al., 2024) (Figure 9.18).

9.6. Impact of Malaria on Public Health

Malaria does not only injure individuals on a personal basis, it also messily strains public health systems, particularly in poorer areas. In most instances, the disease tests medical services to breaking point while exacerbating poverty traps through lost employment and increased medical costs. Its behavior is constantly evolving, with transmission patterns shifting erratically and resistance that continues to appear, so approaches must keep pace, by and large. Researchers explained that conditions such as the native habitat, slight alterations in human lifestyle, and even the genetic change of the parasite all come together to make this vector-borne and zoonotic disease hard to control (de Lope et al., 2016). Clever public health actions often mix ecological clues, biological specifics, and social factors in approaches that attempt to get to the various faces of malaria. From the economic perspective, the cost of malaria extends well past healthcare expenditure, it cascades through society and holds back long-term progress. Estimates in some analyses indicate that short-term calculations may overlook the heavy long-term expenses due to changing transmission and interruptions to overall health services. Complete models of malaria transmission, combined with cost-effectiveness analyses of interventions such as vaccines, assist in illuminating how resources can be utilized more effectively in endemic regions. For example, focused interventions such as vaccination campaigns integrated into well-established immunization systems can reduce both illness and mortality, though the reduction in actual transmission varies somewhat by local conditions (Tediosi et al., 2010). By combining health system variables with economic information, these models provide policymakers with a more complete, and occasionally imperfect—picture for creating plans that attempt to balance efficacy and budgetary issues. In the long term, combating malaria relies on new, innovative research that combines epidemiological models with real-world health system realities. Repeated testing of various vaccine types and delivery strategies illustrates that local factor, such as transmission intensity and availability of healthcare, influence to what extent an intervention is cost effective. For instance, early-stage (pre-erythrocytic) vaccines may perform more favorably where the disease is less intense in its spread, while blood-stage vaccines appear more promising where transmission is intensive. Moreover, mixing various vaccine types and pairing mass campaigns with routine immunizations may boost results without driving costs sky high. Overall, these active, evidence-driven strategies underscore the ongoing need for comprehensive models that adapt to changing disease patterns and system capabilities—models that ultimately help tailor control programs to regional realities and ease malaria's global public health impact (Tediosi et al., 2010) (Figure 9.19).

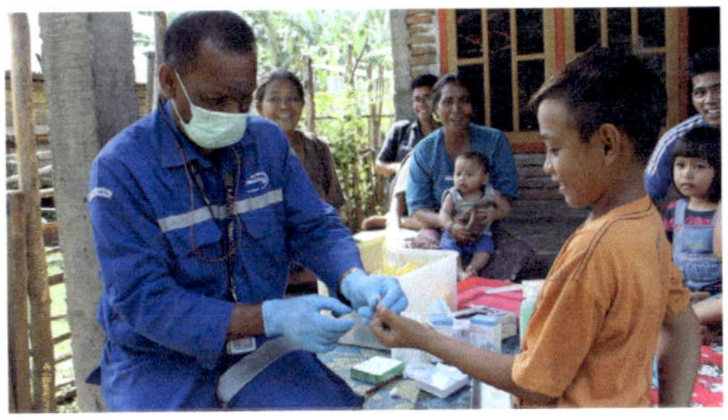

Figure 9.19. The impact of malaria on public health.

Source: International SOS. (n.d.). *Malaria Control.*

9.6.1. Burden on Healthcare Systems

Malaria continues to place a massive burden on healthcare services in much of the world where resources are already tight. There, the disease tends to afflict young children and pregnant women, populations that require extended, frequently high-level care. Hospitals and clinics may become clogged during high-transmission seasons when spikes in patient volume fill wards and deplete medical supplies. By and large, the stampede for expeditious diagnosis and effective treatment taxes local pharmacies and labs to capacity. Ongoing episodes of the disease frequently produce residual problems such as long-term anemia, so patients return repeatedly for more treatment as providers struggle with an apparently never-ending round of treatment. All of these elements, combined, slowly erode the overall effectiveness of healthcare provision in areas where malaria is an ongoing risk. At its worst, down in sub-Saharan Africa where malaria is most widespread, there is another complication added to the burden: antimicrobial resistance.

More often than not, the development of drug-resistant strains turns treatment on its head, compelling clinicians to rely on more expensive, and frequently less available—drugs. This not only prolongs hospitalization but also increases overall expense and utilization of resources. A fragile network of laboratories and uneven surveillance systems also make it even more difficult to detect and respond in a timely manner to these resistant bacteria. It should be noted that this issue reflects a larger global issue with antimicrobial resistance, which kills millions annually (Christopher et al., 2022). In essence, the complicated problems of controlling malaria with fighting resistance reflect a pressing demand for healthcare systems that can evolve to meet changing challenges. In addition to the immediate health effects, malaria's socioeconomic consequences stifle investments in both labor and infrastructure development. In most African countries, endemic diseases drain economic productivity by hundreds of billions of dollars every year, constraining government capacity to improve and upgrade health facilities (John et al., 2020). The COVID-19 pandemic, for instance, further revealed long-standing weaknesses, including weaknesses in disease surveillance, diagnostic capacity, and even public health leadership. Strengthening regional institutions such as the Africa CDC and enhancing local manufacturing of diagnostics, vaccines, and treatments appear like critical measures to decongest the system. Through improved training of health workers and increased international cooperation, resources could be better deployed and outbreaks resolved earlier. Generally, inclusive capacity building is central to easing the undue healthcare burden caused by malaria and other infectious diseases (John et al., 2020).

9.6.2. Economic Implications of Malaria

Developing countries also have an enormous economic cost associated with malaria that is far more than simply treating it. In most farming and rural communities where malaria is widespread, individuals become ill too frequently to work at maximum capacity. This frequent blow not only reduces daily labor but also devastates crop yields precisely when they are needed most. Local food economies suffer as a consequence, and overall growth suffers as well. Families then wind up moving what little money they do have towards prevention and treatments, usually leaving less for school or other investments in the future. Most often, this cost-swap exacerbates poverty and reverses social mobility, a strong indicator that far-reaching control measures are required (Naik et al., 2023). For a great number of high-risk areas, malaria compels healthcare systems to focus the majority of their efforts on the disease, and quite often, this leaves other essential public health priorities behind. Governments must then contend with increasing costs for diagnostics, ongoing treatments, and large-scale public campaigns, which often divert funds from endeavors such as infrastructure improvements or wider health programs. Even as investment in malaria control is required, it often overwhelms tight health budgets and exacerbates gaps in access and quality. Even more damaging, the indirect costs, caregiver lost time and children missing school due to repeated illness, drive communities deeper into underdevelopment cycles. As a general rule, integrating cost-saving prevention and intervention strategies is central to unloading the burden on health systems while increasing economic stability (Naik et al., 2023). In addition to that, malaria's effect waves over into global trade and tourism. Regions that are known to be malaria-endemic can acquire a reputation for health hazards that deter investors and tourists alike. Such a bad reputation can strangle foreign direct investment and inhibit industrial innovation, which is desperately required for development. The international network of commerce and tourism implies additional health and border controls, which come with their own substantial price tags for local as well as foreign partners. Despite these obstacles, more effective disease monitoring and wiser control measures can serve a dual purpose—guarding public health and stabilizing labor markets, reducing healthcare costs, and keeping economic transactions alive in the global arena (Naik et al., 2023) (Figure 9.20).

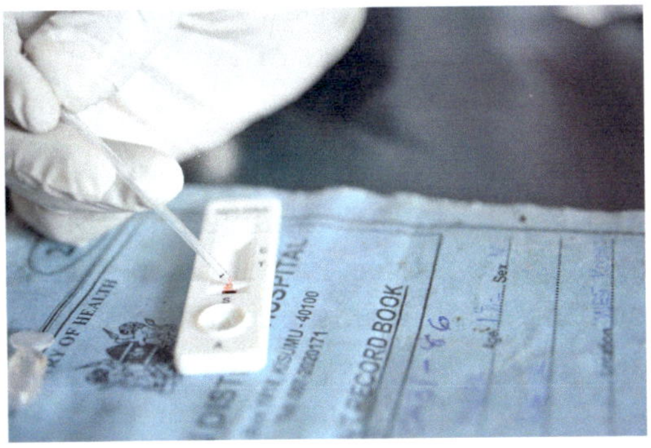

Figure 9.20. The economic benefits of malaria.

Source: Malaria Consortium. (n.d.). *Malaria rapid diagnostic test.* https://cdn.sanity.io/images/4rsg7ofo/production/6c4a42dabdaef2c3a81019ca4eced7aba092ac5b-1600x1065.jpg/images.ctfassets.net-dhpcfh1bs3p6-nrUDs5QP6gkYI0SAiwu6G-8f7f13fa932d129c5a936df468cf425c-Malaria_rapid_diagnostic_test_3.jpg?w=3840&q=75&fit=clip&auto=format.

9.6.3. Malaria's Effect on Community Health and Development

In most communities, local growth and disease come together in surprising combinations. Malaria recurs again and again—a parasitic disease that strikes hard, particularly where resources are limited. Individuals typically find themselves trapped in a cycle: frequent illness depletes their strength, increases medical expenses, and eats into workdays, which in most instances keeps poverty going. Families lose expensive treatment fees and productive time as well. Children and pregnant women suffer disproportionately, and this ripple effect disrupts overall social advance. In general, addressing malaria is not solely an issue of health, it affects education and the local economy as well, making it central to enhancing community resilience and driving sustainable development in malaria-endemic areas (Rob et al., 2020). And now that drug-resistant *Plasmodium falciparum* strains begin to appear, everything becomes more complicated. ACTs; artemisinin-based combination therapies—are what have been the solution of choice for cutting down on illness and death for quite some time. But in regions such as the Greater Mekong Subregion, developing resistance is undercutting these gains, threatening not only a resurgence of the disease but longer illness episodes. As this drug resistance seeps past its early pockets, infection treatment becomes more difficult, subjecting communities to longer recoveries and more opportunities for the disease to spread. This situation, strangely enough, enlarges health disparities, overwhelms local medical facilities, and erodes public confidence in treatments. School days and work hours are lost as well, burdening economic development. Scientists are now exploring new possibilities, such as triple ACTs; to maintain treatments active and hope to outwit the emergent resistance (Rob et al., 2020). Meanwhile, malaria is not only about the disease itself, it also comes with serious complications such as sepsis that add further pressure to communities. If malaria treatment is delayed or omitted altogether, sepsis can strike forcefully, frequently initiating life-threatening organ failures that overwhelm even the busiest, resource-constrained healthcare environments. Areas like sub-Saharan Africa and areas of Asia, where sepsis is all too prevalent, have added challenges that can weigh down community longevity and damage economic production. These concerns often reach far beyond personal hardship and instead go on to impact daily life in general. Overall, sound monitoring of disease patterns along with more coordinated health policy appears necessary in order to reduce malaria-related sepsis and its consequences, allowing for improved long-term health and consistent growth among the hardest-stricken.

CLOSER LOOK

ANOPHELES STEPHENSI

Anopheles stephensi is one of the mosquito species that are important vectors of malaria, especially *Plasmodium falciparum* and *Plasmodium vivax*, the most prevalent and harmful malaria parasites of humans. Compared with most other vectors of malaria that are limited to rural habitats, *An. stephensi* has a high potential to adapt in urban habitats and thus is an emerging threat for malaria control, particularly in cities.

Historically, *An. stephensi* has been reported from South Asia and the Middle East. But since 2012, the mosquito has been reported from some Horn of Africa countries, namely Ethiopia, Sudan, Djibouti, and Somalia. Its rapid spread on the African continent is causing public health officials to sound the alarm because this mosquito is an exceptionally efficient vector of malaria and can adapt to living in urban environments—a habitat in which most African malaria vectors are less prevalent. The expansion of *An. stephensi* into Africa could potentially negate years of malaria control progress. Urban communities, which had historically been relatively low risk for malaria, could now be increasingly exposed, potentially placing millions more in jeopardy.

One of the most worrying traits of *An. stephensi* is that it is easily adaptable to urban settings. In contrast to other Anopheles species, which find clean, rural water bodies more suitable for breeding, *An. stephensi* breeds in dirty water and artificial receptacles like water storage tanks, overhead tanks, building sites, and household receptacles. This increases the difficulty of controlling its transmission and breeding, particularly in cities with inadequate water infrastructure.

Its artificial habitat preference reflects characteristics in such mosquitoes as *Aedes aegypti*, which is a vector for dengue and Zika, making it more complex to control vectors.

An. stephensi is a highly effective vector of both *P. falciparum* and *P. vivax*. It feeds nocturnally and is anthropophilic (human host preferring) and endophilic (indoor resting), thus a strong transmitter of malaria in rural as well as in urban areas. The species' high vector competence combined with its increasing geographical range is a significant challenge to malaria elimination in regions in which it becomes endemic. It is difficult to control *An. stephensi* because it has an urban adaptation and is resistant to some insecticides. Traditional vector control measures such as IRS and ITNs are useful but less effective in the urban environment where breeding sites are ubiquitous and hard to find. Integrated vector management (IVM) strategies are being encouraged, such as larval source management (LSM), better urban water storage practices, and environmental sanitation. These can only be done with very strong community participation and municipal coordination, though, which is hard to do on a consistent basis.

The shift of *An. stephensi* to becoming a major urban malaria vector has important implications for controlling malaria all over the world. Urban centers, which were till now thought to be lower-risk environments, might need to be subjected to focused surveillance and intervention programs. Its extension into Africa could expose hundreds of millions of people to malaria, especially in fast-growing cities.

SUMMARY

Malaria remains a recalcitrant issue globally, and getting it well understood is not as simple as one would have thought. It has spread is determined by anything from local biology and ecology to social and economic determinants, and even though there have been many promising steps such as intensified vector control and improved diagnosis, the disease still strikes hard, particularly in impoverished regions. Climate change heightened human mobility, and constantly evolving cityscapes all can mix transmission patterns in new and unpredictable ways, so responses must keep pace as well. It is impossible to deny that additional complexities, such as superimposed infections and other medical problems—can complicate the real picture of its effect. More often than not, a close watch on trends with consistent data collection and monitoring is necessary. As it happens, just having knowledge of how malaria works is not sufficient; a more robust health system and greater community engagement are also vital components of the equation. Taking a step back, it is evident that the overall health system is one of the big drivers of holding malaria back and filling gaps in treatment and prevention. Quality care, equitable access, and durable infrastructure all feed into each other to convert scientific knowledge into actual, tangible outcomes for patients. Without a strong and trusted health system, even the most excellent diagnostics, prompt treatment, and useful tools such as insecticide-treated nets may fall flat. Social and economic disparities too often determine who is most hit by malaria and who receives proper treatment, emphasizing that equity has to be at the center of any strategy. With so many pieces in motion, strengthening our surveillance systems and the ability of healthcare workers is not just recommended, it is essential. Community involvement in most instances helps detect problems early and keeps treatment on course. Assembling these strategies into national malaria control plans and even making them converge with larger universal health coverage strategies, can improve our best opportunities to reduce rates of sickness and death (Troeger et al., 2018). All things considered, the nature of malaria presents both obstacles and opportunities for the advance of global health. To successfully manage, and eventually eradicate, this disease, there needs to be a mixed approach: closely tracking its spread and, at the same time, constructing health infrastructures that consistently provide high-quality care to all. Ongoing investment in research must continue to be an important factor in deciphering the puzzles of mosquito habits, drug resistance, and the complexities of our immune systems; in turn, this enables us to modify our interventions to continually changing circumstances. Similarly, persevering with efforts that enhance public health—leadership, worker skills, and true community engagement—is crucially important (Troeger et al., 2018). The future is not only about technological progress; it requires genuine political commitment to ensure malaria is a priority on the overall health agenda so that services continue to be accessible, trusted, and effective. Finally, the connection of firm epidemiological evidence with strong healthcare and resolute political support is paramount to controlling malaria and ultimately eradicating it.

Malaria remains a concern for the health systems of the world, it is a heavy burden, particularly in developing countries. Malaria is responsible for a lot of sickness and death, and its transmission is influenced by factors such as mosquito behavior, pathogens adapting, and even finances and social determinants. Existing information tends to indicate that antimicrobial resistance makes it more difficult to treat additional infections associated with malaria, which can potentially increase mortality rates. Other estimates link even millions of annual fatalities with drug-resistant pests (Christopher et al., 2022). If you think about it, combining resistance tests with the standard malaria controls just seems inevitable, particularly in sub-Saharan Africa, where poor health infrastructure and environmental setbacks converge, adding additional dangers. Historically speaking, successful malaria control relied on understanding the mosquito behavior and transmission information well enough to create strategies that work in local settings. Today, however, there has been too much reliance on insecticide strategies without observing those complex mosquito behaviors or monitoring developing insecticide resistance (Anne et al., 2020). Such a "one-size-fits-all" strategy can be dangerous to all the gains achieved, as mosquitoes are capable of developing resistance, thus undermining these measures. For the most part, the impression seems to be that a balanced combination of chemical and non-chemical controls—supported by good local information about both mosquitoes and disease patterns—is the future, even if the strategy is not always implemented optimally. Bottom line, controlling malaria requires a combined strategy addressing drug and insecticide resistance, probing local mosquito biology, and improving basic health care. That requires keeping close watch on levels of resistance and modifying control programs to fit local requirements and increasing labs and information systems where they are most in demand. By integrating these concepts together-even if the process turns out to be a little complex-public health policies are more likely to be able to contend with the mutable nature of malaria (Anne et al., 2020; Christopher et al., 2022). Finally, this general, imperfect view is central to ensuring consistent progress towards the eradication of malaria and reducing its world influence.

KEY TERMS FROM THIS CHAPTER

Incidence	Prevalence	Endemicity
Holoendemic	Hyperendemic	Mesoendemic
Hypoendemic	Epidemic	Transmission Intensity
Seasonal Transmission	Stable Malaria	Unstable Malaria
Vector Distribution	Basic Reproduction Number	Human Reservoir
Asymptomatic Carriers	Geospatial Mapping	Climatic Factors
Socioeconomic Determinants		

References

1. Huho, B., Briët, O., Seyoum, A., Sikaala, C., Bayoh, N., Gimnig, J., Okumu, F., Diallo, D., Abdulla, S., Smith, T., & Killeen, G. (2013). Consistently high estimates for the proportion of human exposure to malaria vector populations occurring indoors in rural Africa. *International journal of epidemiology*, *42*(1), 235–247. https://doi.org/10.1093/ije/dys214 (accessed on 13 May 2025).
2. Abebe, R., Hill, S., Schwartz, H. A., Small, P., et al. (2019). *Using Search Queries to Understand Health Information Needs in Africa*. http://arxiv.org/abs/1806.05740 (accessed on 13 May 2025).
3. . Essendi, W. M., Vardo-Zalik, A. M., Lo, E., Machani, M. G., Zhou, G., Githeko, A. K., Yan, G., & Afrane, Y. A. (2019). Epidemiological risk factors for clinical malaria infection in the highlands of Western Kenya. *Malaria journal*, *18*(1), 211. https://doi.org/10.1186/s12936-019-2845-4
4. Akala, H. M., Watson, O. J., Mitei, K. K., Juma, D. W., Verity, R., Ingasia, L. A., Opot, B., et al. (2021). *Plasmodium* interspecies interactions during a period of increasing prevalence of *Plasmodium ovale* in symptomatic individuals seeking treatment: An observational study. *The Lancet Microbe, 2*, e141–e150. https://doi.org/10.1016/s2666-5247(21)00009-4.
5. Alemayehu, E., Ashine, T., Assefa, G., Bashir, A., et al. (2024). Investigating the association between household exposure to Anopheles Stephens and malaria in Sudan and Ethiopia: A case-control study protocol. https://core.ac.uk/download/617964683.pdf (accessed on 13 May 2025).
6. Androga, D. A. (2020). A literature review about the impact of climate change on malaria in South Sudan. https://core.ac.uk/download/478462836.pdf (accessed on 13 May 2025).
7. Angrisano, F., & Robinson, L. J. (2021). *Plasmodium vivax*–How hidden reservoirs hinder global malaria elimination. *Parasitology International, 87*, 102526. https://doi.org/10.1016/j.parint.2021.102526.
8. Asante, J., Noreddin, A., & El Zowalaty, M. E. (2019). Systematic review of important bacterial zoonoses in Africa in the last decade in light of the 'One Health' concept. *Pathogens, 8*(2), 50. https://doi.org/10.3390/pathogens8020050.
9. Protopopoff, N., Van Bortel, W., Speybroeck, N., Van Geertruyden, J. P., Baza, D., D'Alessandro, U., & Coosemans, M. (2009). Ranking malaria risk factors to guide malaria control efforts in African highlands. *PloS one*, *4*(11), e8022. https://doi.org/10.1371/journal.pone.0008022 (accessed on 13 May 2025).
10. Chen, J. H., Wang, H., Chen, J. X., Bergquist, R., Tanner, M., Utzinger, J., & Zhou, X. N. (2012). Frontiers of parasitology research in the People's Republic of China: infection, diagnosis, protection and surveillance. *Parasites & vectors*, *5*, 221. https://doi.org/10.1186/1756-3305-5-221
11. Bloom, D. E., & Cadarette, D. (2019). Infectious disease threats in the twenty-first century: Strengthening the global response. *Frontiers in Immunology, 10*, 549. https://doi.org/10.3389/fimmu.2019.00549.
12. Banek, K., Lalani, M., Staedke, S. G., & Chandramohan, D. (2014). Adherence to artemisinin-based combination therapy for the treatment of malaria: a systematic review of the evidence. *Malaria journal*, *13*, 7. https://doi.org/10.1186/1475-2875-13-7(accessed on 13 May 2025).

13. Brauer, F. (2017). Mathematical epidemiology: Past, present, and future. *Infectious Disease Modelling, 2*, 113–127. https://doi.org/10.1016/j.idm.2017.02.001.

14. https://core.ac.uk/download/pdf/8550033.pdf. Nakanjako, D., Kiragga, A. N., Castelnuovo, B., Kyabayinze, D. J., & Kamya, M. R. (2011). Low prevalence of Plasmodium falciparum antigenaemia among asymptomatic HAART-treated adults in an urban cohort in Uganda. *Malaria journal, 10*, 66. https://doi.org/10.1186/1475-2875-10-66

15. Chaparro, C. M., & Suchdev, P. S. (2019). Anemia epidemiology, pathophysiology, and etiology in low- and middle-income countries. *Annals of the New York Academy of Sciences, 1450*, 15–31. https://doi.org/10.1111/nyas.14092.

16. Wong, M. L., Chua, T. H., Leong, C. S., Khaw, L. T., Fornace, K., Wan-Sulaiman, W. Y., William, T., Drakeley, C., Ferguson, H. M., & Vythilingam, I. (2015). Seasonal and Spatial Dynamics of the Primary Vector of Plasmodium knowlesi within a Major Transmission Focus in Sabah, Malaysia. *PLoS neglected tropical diseases, 9*(10), e0004135. https://doi.org/10.1371/journal.pntd.0004135

17. de Lope, F., García-Longoria, L., González-Blázquez, M., Magallanes, S., et al. (2016). *New Approaches for An Old Disease: Studies On Avian Malaria Parasites for The Twenty-First Century Challenges.* https://core.ac.uk/download/322428475.pdf (accessed on 13 May 2025).

18. Desmond, N., Nketia, R. I., Turkson, B. K., & Komlaga, G. (2024). *Malaria: Epidemiology, Life Cycle of Parasite, Control Strategies and Potential Drug Screening Techniques.* IntechOpen eBooks. https://doi.org/10.5772/intechopen.1007804.

19. Dev, V., Galappaththy, G. N. L., Gosling, R., Gueye, A., et al. (2012). Malaria control in Bhutan: Case study of a country embarking on elimination. https://core.ac.uk/download/pdf/8681713.pdf.

20. Diagne, N., Doucouré, S., Faye, N., Gaudart, J., et al. (2015). No difference in the incidence of malaria in human-landing mosquito catch collectors and non-collectors in a Senegalese village with endemic malaria. *PLoS ONE, 10*(5), e0126187. https://doi.org/10.1371/journal.pone.0126187.

21. Dittrich, S., Lamy, M., Acharya, S., Thu, H. K., Datta, R., Blacksell, S. D., Hein, P. S., et al. (2020). Diagnosing malaria and other febrile illnesses during the COVID-19 pandemic. *The Lancet Global Health, 8*(7), e879–e880. https://doi.org/10.1016/s2214-109x(20)30210-2.

22. Feachem, R.G.A., with A.A. Phillips and G.A. Targett (eds) (2009). Shrinking the Malaria Map: A Prospectus on Malaria Elimination. San Francisco: The Global Health Group, Global Health Sciences, University of California, San Francisco. Masangwi, S., Grimason, A., Morse, T., Ferguson, N., & Kazembe, L. (2012). Community knowledge variation, bed-net coverage and the role of a district healthcare system, and their implications for malaria control in southern Malawi. *Southern African Journal of Epidemiology and Infection, 27*(3), 116–125. https://doi.org/10.1080/10158782.2012.11441496 (accessed on 13 May 2025).

23. Ferrari, A. J., Santomauro, D., Aali, A., Abate, Y. H., Abbafati, C., Abbastabar, H., Abd ElHafeez, S., et al. (2024). Global incidence, prevalence, years lived with disability (YLDs), disability-adjusted life-years (DALYs), and healthy life expectancy (HALE) for 371 diseases and injuries in 204 countries and territories and 811 subnational locations, 1990–2021: A systematic analysis for the Global Burden of Disease Study 2021. *The Lancet, 403*, 2133–2161. https://doi.org/10.1016/s0140-6736(24)00757-8.

24. Lau, C. L., Ramsey, L., Mills, L. C., Furuya-Kanamori, L., & Mills, D. J. (2019). Drug-free Holidays: Compliance, Tolerability, and Acceptability of a 3-Day Atovaquone/Proguanil Schedule for Pretravel Malaria Chemoprophylaxis in Australian Travelers. *Clinical infectious diseases : an official publication of the Infectious Diseases Society of America, 69*(1), 137–143. https://doi.org/10.1093/cid/ciy854

25. Hendry, J. A., Kwiatkowski, D., & McVean, G. (2021). Elucidating relationships between *P. falciparum* prevalence and measures of genetic diversity with a combined genetic-epidemiological model of malaria. *PLoS Computational Biology, 17*, e1009287. https://doi.org/10.1371/journal.pcbi.1009287.

26. James, S. L., Abate, D., Abate, K. H., Abay, S. M., Abbafati, C., Abbasi, N., Abbastabar, H., et al. (2018). Global, regional, and national incidence, prevalence, and years lived with disability for 354 diseases and injuries for 195 countries and territories, 1990–2017: A systematic analysis for the Global Burden of Disease Study 2017. *The Lancet, 392*(10159), 1789–1858. https://doi.org/10.1016/s0140-6736(18)32279-7.

27. Kruk, M. E., Gage, A., Arsenault, C., Jordan, K., Leslie, H. H., Roder-DeWan, S., Adeyi, O., et al. (2018). High-quality health systems in the Sustainable Development Goals era: Time for a revolution. *The Lancet Global Health, 6*, e1196–e1252. https://doi.org/10.1016/s2214-109x(18)30386-3.

28. Killeen, G. F., Smith, T. A., Ferguson, H. M., Mshinda, H., Abdulla, S., Lengeler, C., & Kachur, S. P. (2007). Preventing childhood malaria in Africa by protecting adults from mosquitoes with insecticide-treated nets. *PLoS medicine, 4*(7), e229. https://doi.org/10.1371/journal.pmed.0040229 Lewnard, J. A., & Reingold, A. L. (2019). Emerging Challenges and Opportunities in Infectious Disease Epidemiology. *American journal of epidemiology, 188*(5), 873–882. https://doi.org/10.1093/aje/kwy264

29. Liu, L., Oza, S., Hogan, D., Chu, Y., Perin, J., Zhu, J., Lawn, J. E., et al. (2016). Global, regional, and national causes of under-5 mortality in 2000–15: An updated systematic analysis with implications for the Sustainable Development Goals. *The Lancet, 388*, 3027–3035. https://doi.org/10.1016/s0140-6736(16)31593-8.

30. London School of Hygiene & Tropical Medicine. (2013). Annual report 2013. https://core.ac.uk/download/19452766.pdf (accessed on 13 May 2025).

31. Murray, C. J. L., Ikuta, K. S., Sharara, F., Swetschinski, L. R., Robles Aguilar, G., Gray, A. P., Han, C., et al. (2022). Global burden of bacterial antimicrobial resistance in 2019: A systematic analysis. *The Lancet, 399*, 629–655. https://doi.org/10.1016/s0140-6736(21)02724-0.

32. Naghavi, M., Ong, K. L., Aali, A., Ababneh, H., Abate, Y. H., Abbafati, C., Abbasgholizadeh, R., et al. (2024). Global burden of 288 causes of death and life expectancy decomposition in 204 countries and territories and 811 subnational locations, 1990–2021: A systematic analysis for the Global Burden of Disease Study 2021. *The Lancet, 403*, 2100–2132. https://doi.org/10.1016/s0140-6736(24)00367-2.

33. Naik, B. R., Tyagi, B. K., & Xue, R. D. (2023). Mosquito-borne diseases in India over the past 50 years and their global public health implications: A systematic review. *Journal of the American Mosquito Control Association, 39*(4), 258–277. https://www.semanticscholar.org/paper/337c327ead0743eceaff42bc9ac1e62216fc360f (accessed on 13 May 2025).

34. Nkengasong, J. N., & Tessema, S. K. (2020). Africa needs a new public health order to tackle infectious disease threats. *Cell, 183*, 296–300. https://doi.org/10.1016/j.cell.2020.09.041.

35. Roth, G. A., Abate, D., Abate, K. H., Abay, S. M., Abbafati, C., Abbasi, N., Abbastabar, H., et al. (2018). Global, regional, and national age-sex-specific mortality for 282 causes of death in 195 countries and territories, 1980–2017: A systematic analysis for the Global Burden of Disease Study 2017. *The Lancet, 392*, 1736–1788. https://doi.org/10.1016/s0140-6736(18)32203-7.

36. Rudd, K. E., Johnson, S. C., Agesa, K. M., Shackelford, K. A., Tsoi, D., Kievlan, D., Colombara, D. V., et al. (2020). Global, regional, and national sepsis incidence and mortality, 1990–2017: Analysis for the Global Burden of Disease Study. *The Lancet, 395*, 200–211. https://doi.org/10.1016/s0140-6736(19)32989-7.

37. Ryan, S. J., Carlson, C. J., Mordecai, E. A., & Johnson, L. R. (2019). Global expansion and redistribution of Aedes-borne virus transmission risk with climate change. *PLoS Neglected Tropical Diseases, 13*(3), e0007213. https://doi.org/10.1371/journal.pntd.0007213.

38. Schlagenhauf, P., Grobusch, M. P., Hamer, D. H., Ásgeirsson, H., Jensenius, M., Éperon, G., Rothe, C., et al. (2018). Area of exposure and treatment challenges of malaria in Eritrean migrants: A GeoSentinel analysis. *Malaria Journal, 17*, Article 356. https://doi.org/10.1186/s12936-018-2586-9.

39. Taylor, C., Namasté, S., Lowell, J., Useem, J., & Yé, Y. (2021). Estimating the fraction of severe malaria among malaria-positive children: Analysis of household surveys in 19 malaria-endemic countries in Africa. *American Journal of Tropical Medicine and Hygiene, 104*(4), 1375–1382. https://doi.org/10.4269/ajtmh.20-1351.

40. Tediosi, F. (2010). Simulation of the costs and consequences of potential vaccines for *Plasmodium falciparum* malaria. https://core.ac.uk/download/18234515.pdf (accessed on 13 May 2025).

41. Torres, T., Filipe, P., Menezes Brandão, F., Figueiredo, A., Pinto Soares, A., Sousa Basto, A., Rebelo, C., et al. (2023). Epidemiology of psoriasis in Portugal: A population-based study. *Acta Médica Portuguesa*. https://www.semanticscholar.org/paper/2212b929e6450009dba9de42612fb8b74f852eb1 (accessed on 13 May 2025).

42. Troeger, C., Blacker, B. F., Rahim, F., Rao, P. C., Cao, J., Zimsen, S. R. M., Albertson, S. B., et al. (2018). Estimates of the global, regional, and national morbidity, mortality, and aetiologias of lower respiratory infections in 195 countries, 1990–2016: A systematic analysis. *The Lancet Infectious Diseases, 18*(11), 1191–1210. https://doi.org/10.1016/s1473-3099(18)30310-4.

43. van der Pluijm, R. W., Amaratunga, C., Dhorda, M., & Dondorp, A. M. (2020). Triple artemisinin-based combination therapies for malaria–A new paradigm? *Trends in Parasitology, 37*(1), 15–24. https://doi.org/10.1016/j.pt.2020.09.011.

44. Weiss, D. J., Bertozzi-Villa, A., Rumisha, S. F., Amratia, P., Arambepola, R., Battle, K. E., Cameron, E., et al. (2020). Indirect effects of the COVID-19 pandemic on malaria intervention coverage, morbidity, and mortality in Africa: A geospatial modelling analysis. *The Lancet Infectious Diseases, 21*(1), 59–69. https://doi.org/10.1016/s1473-3099(20)30700-3.

45. White, R. J., & Razgour, O. (2020). Emerging zoonotic diseases originating in mammals: A systematic review of effects of anthropogenic land-use change. *Mammal Review, 50*(4), 336–352. https://doi.org/10.1111/mam.12201.

46. Whittaker, C. F. (2022). Quantifying the impacts of variation in entomological and epidemiological determinants of malaria transmission. https://core.ac.uk/download/533450122.pdf (accessed on 13 May 2025).

47. Wilson, A. L., Courtenay, O., Kelly-Hope, L. A., Scott, T. W., Takken, W., Torr, S. J., & Lindsay, S. W. (2020). The importance of vector control for the control and elimination of vector-borne diseases. *PLoS Neglected Tropical Diseases, 14*, e0007831. https://doi.org/10.1371/journal.pntd.0007831.

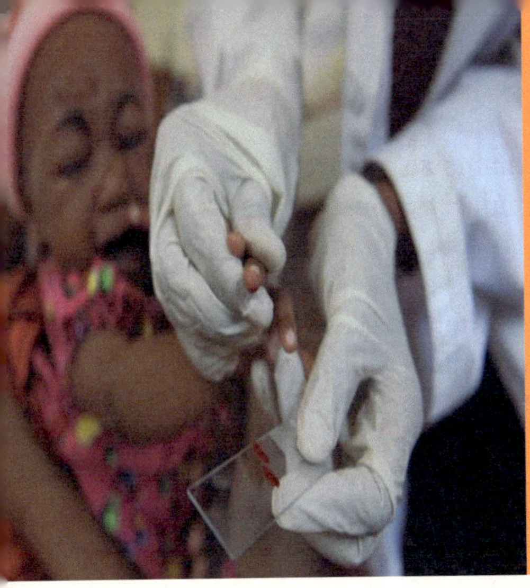

Chapter 10

SURVEILLANCE SYSTEMS OF MALARIA

Contents

Introduction

Global connections influence our health in ways we do not always see. Infectious diseases still strike hard throughout the world, even as we become increasingly connected, problems persist. Malaria is a prime example, an ongoing serious threat particularly in regions where healthcare lacks, and addressing it is not simply a matter of individual treatments. In a majority of instances, however, we must be thinking bigger: hospitals, prevention in the community, even some smart new technology all coalesces in our struggle. Monitoring outbreaks via malaria surveillance, allowing us to identify problems early and watch for spread, is one of those vital steps. It truly indicates that conquering malaria is not merely a matter of medicine, it is a matter of combining various disciplines, collection good data, and establishing networks that strengthen communities most vulnerable (Juvekar & Hegde, 2024). Global health initiatives have revolutionized the way we address disease tracking such as for malaria. The World Health Organization (WHO) began way back in 1948 and has long combined skills in monitoring outbreaks with strategies for containing epidemics and adapting health systems. In general, the WHO's leadership and push for international collaboration helped initiate major malaria programs—remember those mid-20th century eradication efforts? Despite some bumps and even criticism along the way, the agency's broader drive for disease control has politicized surveillance beyond mere counting of cases; it is a vital component of an overarching policy-driven response based on global governance (Cueto et al., 2019). Malaria surveillance in the present day combines emerging technology with health policy and international cooperation in a manner that incorporates both historical lessons and contemporary challenges. New diagnostics, intelligent data management, and better channels of communication now enable us to catch cases rapidly and track transmission patterns more accurately. That allows health officials to redelegate resources on the fly and roll out targeted interventions for the hardest-hit areas. Although high-tech solutions are valuable, addressing routine problems like poverty and scarce sanitation still accounts for a huge majority of making these systems function. Embedding malaria tracking within wider global disease and infrastructure planning is important to reduce disease rates, and, eventually, one hopes to eradicate it completely (Juvekar & Hegde, 2024) (Figure 10.1).

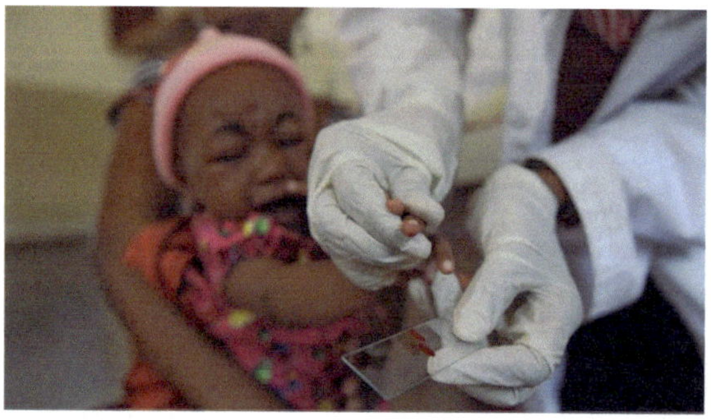

Figure 10.1. Surveillance systems of malaria.

Source: The Radio Community. (n.d.). *Surveillance Systems of Malaria.*

Malaria remains a significant public health concern, particularly where there is limited availability of resources and the complexity of the disease leads to high mortality rates. It begins with an infected Anopheles mosquito that bites an individual, dropping *Plasmodium* parasites directly into the blood. After the parasites find a place to settle, they reproduce inside liver cells before jumping into red blood cells, which induces fever, chills, and occasionally even anemia. The issues are not limited to short-term sickness; the long-term social and economic cost may be equally as harmful. To control malaria means gaining a solid handle on how malaria operates biologically, how it is transmitted, and what types of symptoms occur, so health interventions can be designed in response accordingly. Mostly, establishing systems to detect, forecast, and react to such infections hinges on having a good understanding of the spread of the disease (Christopher et al., 2022). As far as observing malaria through the eyes of surveillance is concerned, one cannot overlook the way its patterns change from one region to another. Various regions of the globe exhibit surprise in types of parasites, habits of mosquitoes, and even levels of natural immunity of the population in the area. That requires surveillance tools to function with laboratory-confirmed tests and clinical cases, as well, because the image tends to shift too rapidly to accommodate a one-size-fits-all strategy. Subsequently there is the complicating factor of drug-resistant *Plasmodium* strains, which requires additional work to monitor resistance markers in addition to straightforward case counts. Detail like this enables health officials to detect outbreaks earlier, assess how effective interventions are being, and even predict impending case spikes. Coordinating pieces of demographic, environmental, and clinical information in these environments proves to be quite important (Morgan et al., 2021). Attaining a solid, unshakeable definition of malaria is the foundation for public health surveillance system design worldwide. Successful monitoring depends on the capacity to distinguish malaria from other diseases that induce fever, oftentimes using laboratory methods such as microscopy or rapid diagnostic tests, particularly in areas where it is prevalent. The requirement for reliable laboratory infrastructure is difficult to exaggerate, actually. Measuring malaria by its direct effect, such as the number of cases resulting in severe illness or death—also allows us to estimate the overall burden and make the best allocation of scarce resources. When epidemiologists are operating on surveillance data that quantify these, they can more accurately model disease transmission and evaluate how well the control measures are maintained. Maintaining consistent definitions and procedures not only ensures transparency in the process but also allows for comparison of data globally (Morgan et al., 2021; Christopher et al., 2022).

Importance of Surveillance in Malaria Control

Timely, reliable information is at the center of good public health action, particularly in the case of malaria. Information gets collected, analyzed, and molded into intelligence day in and day out, as if it were a constant dialogue on the risk of outbreaks and how malaria transmits. The constant supply of information not only guides spending on resources but also informs responses that are tailored to local health contexts, often lending them much-needed bite. You may see that instruments such as machine learning, which combine information on climate, social aspects, and health figures, wind up refining projections on the number of individuals who may fall ill. In the majority of instances, such predictions allow the health officials to identify possible outbreaks and respond in advance, reducing sickness and fatalities. A study from Indonesia illustrates, for instance, that combining diverse data in smart surveillance systems provides malaria control with a strong kick, and it most definitely indicates just how important these systems are for adaptive, evidence-based public health interventions (Syabrina et al., 2024). Shifting from simply containing malaria to eliminating it entirely requires a new type of attention altogether. When governments embark on the journey to elimination, surveillance is no longer a mere exercise in number-crunching but begins to follow every infection and small transmission event. This new way of working requires tools that collect data quickly, report almost in real time, and even necessitate a bit of collaboration across sectors to get the details right. Generally speaking, reliable monitoring also helps in figuring out the risks of outbreaks or even cases brought in from outside, which becomes key when you are trying to keep a malaria-free zone intact. The Malaria Elimination Group's prospectus, for instance, points out that quick detection and swift containment of new cases (along with some cross-border teamwork) are essential to holding the line on elimination (Feachem et al., 2009). Thus, surveillance becomes more than simply another measure of control, it becomes a key strategy on the path to zero malaria. Maintaining a malaria-free status hand in hand with connecting surveillance data intimately to policy decisions and funding options. Frequently, the results from such monitoring give a type of roadmap for interventions that are tailored to be specific in various local contexts. In addition, data-driven approaches can assist in verifying whether elimination is more cost-effective than continuous control, which is very important if funds are low. Secure, reliable financing, supported by good data, is crucial to keeping programs running and responding to novel challenges such as insecticide resistance or changes in mosquito behavior. With such quantitative support, policymakers are provided with an opportunity to gauge progress, identify gaps, and adjust strategies at the moment. Ultimately, a strong surveillance system is not merely a matter of preventing new cases; it is about preventing any resurgence and securing long-term health gains for the community (Feachem et al., 2009) (Figure 10.2).

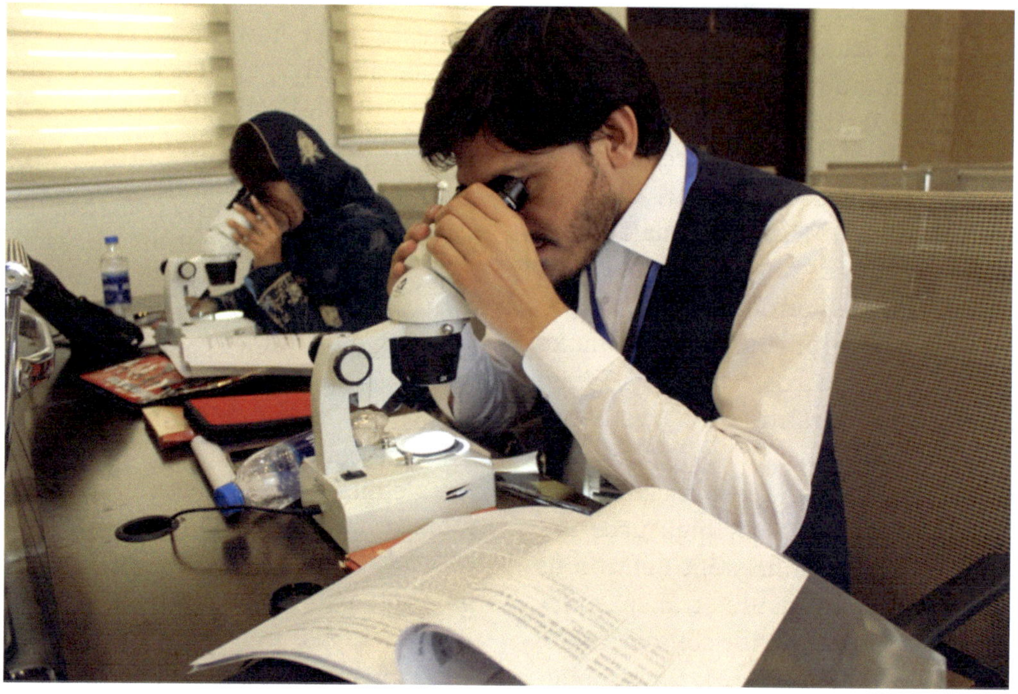

Figure 10.2. Surveillance in malaria control.

Source: Asia Pacific Malaria Elimination Network. (n.d.). *Surveillance in Malaria Control.*

10.1. Historical Context of Malaria Surveillance

Surveillance of malaria has advanced far since looking back at some of the previous public health challenges and how people reacted reactions that, indirectly, paved the way for current approaches. In the beginning of the 1900s, there was no proper system; collection of data was disorganized and coordination was thin, much like we experienced during COVID-19 when few diagnostic tools and severed data channels delayed response times. This chaotic arrangement made it absolutely clear that outbreaks could only be identified rapidly if systems were tighter and more interconnected. Ongoing population surveillance, work in the laboratory that could be scaled up, and electronic streams of data were regarded as crucial, and these concepts even inspired experts to work on finessing the technical aspects of standardizing and safeguarding information, while emphasizing the importance of national collaboration and some international openness. In general, it was even contended that only an investment of a moderate scale—approximately US $1 to 4 per capita annually—was required to establish surveillance structures robust enough to manage a range of health dangers (Morgan et al., 2021). Poring over historical epidemiological data provides some fascinating, if not somewhat unbalanced, information regarding malaria's evolution across time and geography. Consider early 20th-century Spain, for instance; statistics revealed that approximately

77% of malaria deaths among locals were concentrated in only 20% of the provinces, a highly disproportionate, nearly patchy pattern which highlighted the importance of geospatial technologies in disease transmission knowledge. Epidemic peaks during times such as 1917–1922 and once more in 1939–1944 were instigated by a combination of factors, such as wars and compelled populace migrations, which ensured that public health efforts broke down even as climate concerns, although a contributing factor, were not the dominant forces. Interestingly, anti-malarial dispensaries sprang up during these epochs, serving not just as treatment points but also as ad hoc surveillance sites, which provided a vital layer of epidemiological understanding. In general, this combination of Geographic Information Systems with other data sources indicates that tailoring surveillance to local circumstances is still a requirement (Sousa et al., 2020). By 1961, temperate Europe sections such as Spain had largely bid farewell to local malaria—a tremendous public health success. However, as soon as the 1970s came in, new issues arose with imported cases of malaria—these started to appear in manners that truly made the picture all complexed up. Abruptly, monitoring only local spread just was not sufficient; systems needed to also detect infections coming from somewhere else, particularly as individuals became increasingly mobile within our interconnected world. The history of malaria teaches us, as a general rule, that combining in-depth historical knowledge with current facts—whether pathogen genomic sequencing, clinical findings, or in-eruption-time reporting—is the best way to get ahead of outbreaks. To summarize, the take-home message is that robust, properly funded, and flexible surveillance systems are essential if we are going to tackle both old and new challenges in global health (Morgan et al., 2021; Sousa et al., 2020) (Figure 10.3).

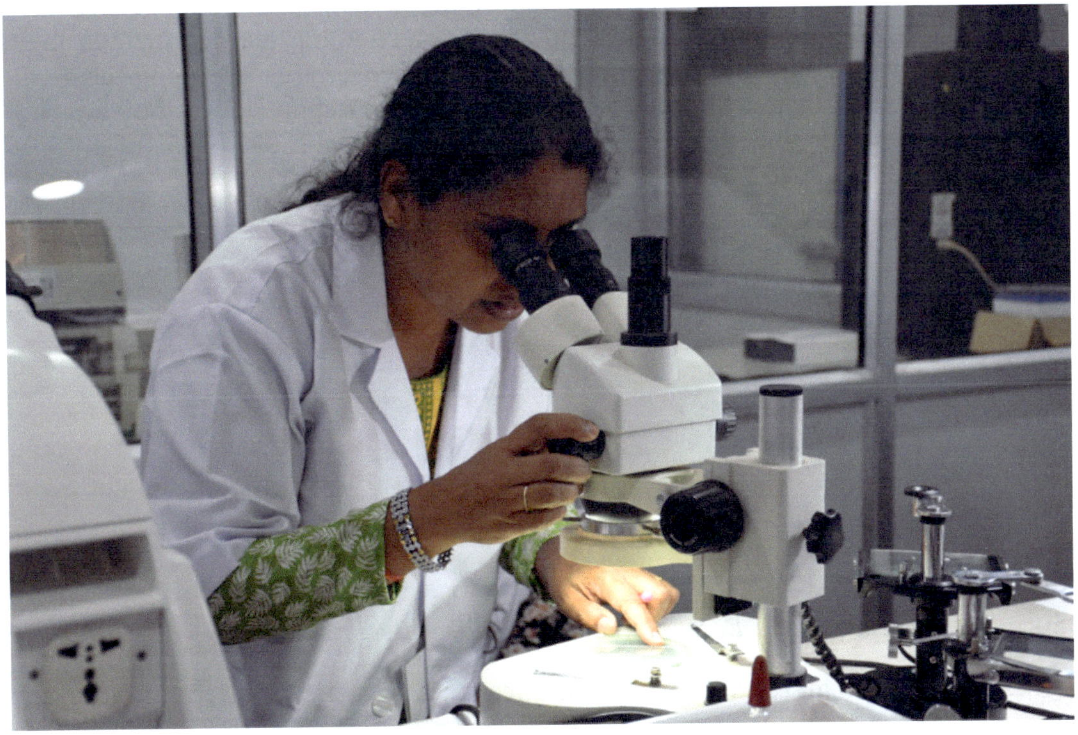

Figure 10.3. The historical context of malaria surveillance.

Source: Orene.org. (2022). *The Historical Context of Malaria Surveillance.*

10.1.1. Early Methods of Malaria Detection

Malaria surveillance began life employing fairly rudimentary techniques—health workers would scan for obvious signs and gaze at blood smears under a microscope. In areas most affected by malaria, specialists more or less relied on visually detecting *Plasmodium* parasites in red blood cells as the primary means of detecting the disease early on. Yes, this was tedious and required people with specialized training, but it did assist in confirming cases and influencing treatment decisions. Early detection of the disease was not merely about the care of any one patient; it was central to preventing outbreaks from occurring by making public health action timely. Unfortunately, these initial tests too often ran into a brick wall when laboratories were scarce, particularly out in rural or low-resource settings. All this essentially reinforced the necessity for intelligent tests that balance accuracy with what is possible in the field, leading the way to today's more sophisticated detection and monitoring systems. As more health information continued to accumulate, humans began combining computer-based approaches to detect malaria outbreaks earlier. Statistical sleight of hand, such as threshold models and outlier detection algorithms, were thrown into the mix to read case trends through time and pinpoint any unusual jumps. For example, in malaria hotspots such as the Amhara region of Ethiopia, such methods were helpful to catch renewed peaks of the disease. If you look at weekly threshold checks and the CDC's Early Aberration Reporting System (EARS), you notice that every approach has its own combination of strengths and features; accepting less sensitivity for fewer false alarms. Overall, applying these tools allowed public health staff to take the lead on transmission so that they could react faster, although it still was something of a high-wire act to get the ideal balance between identifying genuine cases and issuing false alarms (Christopher et al., 2022). Recent development in early detection has learned further on statistical models with capacity to address challenging factors like seasonality and long-term changes in malaria patterns. The Farrington improved method, say, has established itself as keeping a good balance between sensitivity and specificity allegedly detecting well over 70% of outbreaks with true positive rates rising above 70%.

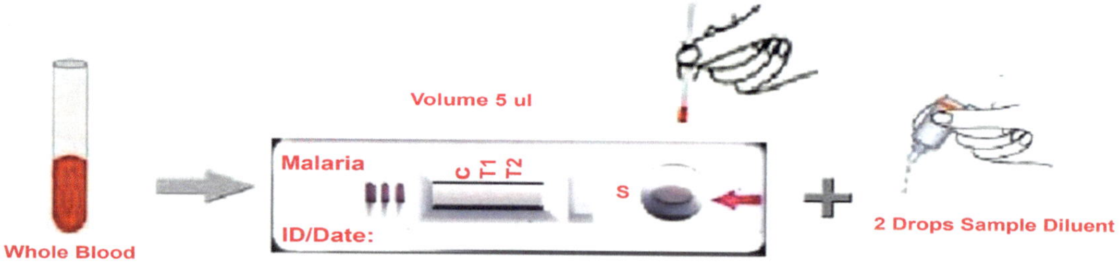

Figure 10.4. Early methods of malaria detection.

Source: Springer Nature. (2018). *Early Methods of Malaria Detection.*

This method, which marries past surveillance data into its predictions, is a significant improvement on the old, straightforward threshold-based tests, providing warnings that enable officials to act before it is too late. Such advancements are well aligned with international ambitions to track issues such as drug resistance and local patterns in the spread of malaria (Dawn et al., 2021; Christopher et al., 2022). Ultimately, these sophisticated methods have become an essential component of contemporary malaria surveillance, providing healthcare professionals with actionable knowledge they can use to reduce transmission and alleviate public health issues (Figure 10.4).

10.1.2. Evolution of Surveillance Techniques

Malaria reporting has evolved greatly over time, with the push being driven by technological advancements and the increasingly more complicated mechanisms the disease follows. In the past, the majority of reporting was done manually through traditional epidemiological practices that would take long and result in incomplete reports. Today, digital systems have taken up the mantle, largely improving the timeliness and accuracy of information in most instances. For instance, Brazil's National Surveillance System for Malaria (SIVEP-MALARIA) has been reporting cases for more than 15 years—a clear indication of how things have changed. Yet delays in reporting occur and can occasionally disrupt real-time estimates, so we must have methods that compensate for those delays. Methods like nowcasting—honed to work on huge data collections—have begun to bridge that gap (Mario et al., 2023). It is a case of balancing strengthening the systems with refining our approach. All the while, new technology is changing malaria surveillance from being a passive collection of data to something that nearly predicts outbreaks. Artificial intelligence and machine learning are among the key players, crunching environmental, climatic, and behavioral data into models that can predict outbreaks and identify vulnerable communities with remarkable precision. Natural language processing burrows into unstructured information, such as social media updates and public health announcements—to assist in identifying early warning signals in real time. When you pair these AI algorithms with pragmatic devices such as drones and mobile health applications, you have a digital evolution that personalizes public health actions for regional requirements (Krittanawong et al., 2021).

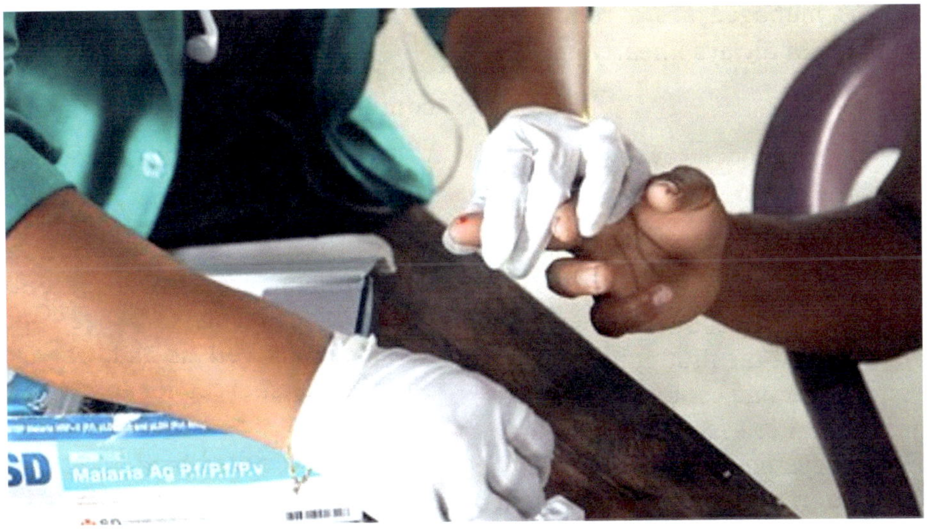

Figure 10.5. Early methods of malaria detection.

Source: Bing. (n.d.). *Microscopic view of malaria-infected blood cells.* https://external-content.duckduckgo.com/iu/?u=https%3A%2F%2Ftse3.mm.bing.net%2Fth%3Fid%3DOIP.vy_SQ_wKedc-uDT1KyqidwHaEK%26pid%3DApi&f=1&ipt=63aaeeb06429012152e5d745119147c3437d7b7fde1be8a6f6e15c294e487a2d.

In most instances, this combination of innovations makes the entire process slightly more proactive and refined. As a separate point, the development of surveillance practices now relies on combining different streams of data to tackle past limitations. Consider computer vision, for instance, it processes malaria diagnosis from microscopic images, eliminating human error and accelerating screenings where resources are low. Subsequently there is the fascinating mix of machine learning, blockchain, and cloud computing, which not only protects data integrity but also makes easier access available for analysis. Such developments not only increase case detection but also simplify logistics such as vaccine delivery and preventive outreach, particularly in distant or underserved areas. Ultimately, the integration of digital tools and clever analytics makes surveillance for malaria a dynamic system that responds to evolving trends and increasingly enhances global efforts at control (Krittanawong et al., 2021). Occasionally, those tiny, natural flaws in the way data is managed are a reminder that advancement is not always linearly perfect (Figure 10.5).

10.1.3. Impact of Historical Outbreaks on Surveillance Practices

Tracking disease has come a long way over the years—major outbreaks forced everyone's hand. When bubonic plague and yellow fever struck, people quickly organized the first public health organizations to monitor and contain the spread of disease. Those initial crises established that it was vital to have a system in place to identify outbreaks in order to reduce illness and death. Consider malaria, for instance; this tenacious disease taught us things that ultimately resulted in quicker data collection and reporting. The emergence of agencies such as the US Centers for Disease Control and Prevention, which initially began by specializing in malaria, illustrates how outbreak pressures can instigate enhancements in monitoring systems. Indeed, the introduction of the CDC's initial disease tracking program in 1949—spurred by those early alarms—continues to shape how we monitor malaria even today (John et al., 2020). Big epidemics tend to reveal fault lines in our public health infrastructure and remind us that collaboration locally and internationally is almost a necessity, overall. For example, the Ebola epidemics in the Democratic Republic of the Congo and West Africa uncovered gaps in case tracking and follow-up with contacts, ultimately pushing for more robust diagnostic labs and more effective networks. Those lean times also paved the way for the Africa Centers for Disease Control and Prevention, now responsible for coordinating responses in times of pandemic, like when malaria spikes. Investments in so-called Regional Integrated Surveillance and Laboratory Networks represent a genuine change of mindset; in most instances, strong systems must function autonomously while remaining networked across regions. Mixing field observations with laboratory findings and enhanced worker education has been a responsive action born of previous experience with outbreaks, facilitating the combat both of current malaria problems and future disease threats (John et al., 2020). In addition to remodeling large institutions, previous outbreaks have demonstrated once more that local production and capacity development are crucial for effective disease surveillance. The COVID-19 pandemic, for instance, showed us that relying too heavily on external sources for testing and treatments can delay critical responses and even allow an outbreak to worsen—a lesson applied as well to malaria control. Manufacturing diagnostics and medicines locally not only accelerates their delivery but also allows regions to develop solutions suited to their own particular health needs. Additionally, increasing training for field epidemiologists and community health workers is a top priority now, enabling early detection of cases at the very grassroots level. Overall, these mixed strategies—formed from hard-learned experience in previous epidemics and today's vulnerabilities—build a more dynamic, complex at times, but ultimately adaptive system to deal with the details of both malaria transmission and emerging infections (John et al., 2020).

10.2. Types of Surveillance Systems

Malaria tracking has evolved far beyond the old rituals. Today, new technology assists in collecting, examining, and interpreting data in ways ancient techniques never could. Clinics continue to report cases, this simple passive surveillance is fundamental, but it is not always timely or complete. That is why teams now venture out into communities for active surveillance, conducting focused screenings that detect outbreaks sooner. Some were chosen locations, or sentinel centers, monitoring change of trend as it happens. Subsequently there is the twist of employing AI, which combs through huge health records to identify trends beyond what traditional analysis could, providing predictive signals for rapid public action (Shuroug et al., 2023). In combining age-old approaches with new tech, we create a surprisingly robust foundation for combating malaria. A new generation of molecular surveillance is rewriting the book. Applying genomic information to examine parasite populations and transmission in detail provides information we could only dream of previously. Next-generation sequencing follows mutations associated with drug resistance and low-level genetic changes that may impact test validity. Targeting important markers within *Plasmodium falciparum*, these techniques identify new risks before symptoms appear, allowing treatment approaches to be refined. As an example, Mozambique research demonstrates how collection genetic information from varying areas is able to chart infection sources and transmission patterns. Merging this genetic information with epidemiology data makes our intervention sharper and enables more adaptive control procedures (Mayor et al., 2022). This genomic perspective is, in a sense, the added, important layer to our grand picture of malaria. Mixing cutting-edge innovations with old-school surveillance techniques truly opens up the field of malaria control. Artificial intelligence is increasingly automating diagnosis and informing clinical decision-making, lightening workloads for healthcare professionals and reducing errors. These AI systems rifle through everything, sometimes detailed clinical records, sometimes environmental conditions—to create treatment regimens that are nearly bespoke in feel while optimizing the use of resources. Implementing these innovative technologies, however, is not without its challenges. Issues like data privacy, ethical questions, and the need for human oversight to preserve clinical judgment emerge along the way (Shuroug et al., 2023). By fusing insights from molecular surveillance with AI's computational power, public health teams can forecast outbreaks, track how well interventions are performing, and fine-tune responses at both community and individual levels. Overall, this integrated strategy holds the promise of quicker, sharper, and more context-sensitive methods of marshaling malaria.

10.2.1. Passive Surveillance

Surveillance for disease usually draws its information from reports received at health facilities – what is commonly referred to as passive surveillance. Cases are reported by health care providers as they present in the course of their daily practice, but this will only capture instances when patients present themselves for treatment. In most rural communities that are severely affected by malaria and have limited access to health care, many cases pass undetected and unreported. Research tends to show that these systems are likely to miss a large proportion of infections due to geographical barriers and affordability constraints that prevent individuals from accessing care. Thus, even though passive surveillance is the default approach in most malaria-endemic areas, its figures must be interpreted with care, remembering issues of underreporting and spatial bias; adjustments for these weaknesses are necessary to obtain estimates that represent the true picture. Acknowledging these limitations, statisticians and epidemiologists have developed some rather creative modeling methods to enhance the precision and value of passive data. By combining information on how readily individuals can obtain health care with information on the availability of diagnostics, even recording when rapid diagnostic tests are depleted—technical experts refine reported data to give a richer picture of the effect of malaria. At times, statistical modeling that takes in pattern in children as well as adults even converts simple reports into high-resolution maps that bring out concealed hotspots of transmission. This kind of rich, detailed mapping can inform resource allocation and shape intervention strategies to actual local priorities. In all but a few instances, these approaches demonstrate that passive surveillance remains viable when paired with intelligent corrections (Christopher et al., 2022). With that being said, all it takes is some people not showing any symptoms or not making it to the clinic, and they are easily left out. This gap not only underestimates the aggregate burden of malaria but also inhibits attempts to monitor problems such as drug resistance and new strains, challenges that are important in the battle against the disease. The worldwide experience with antimicrobial resistance reminds us, quite forcefully, that larger, more extensive surveillance systems are required, particularly in low-resource environments where these gaps are most acute. Strengthening laboratory capabilities and building data collection facilities are essential measures. Otherwise, preventive, control, and eventual eradication efforts against malaria could lag behind since the underlying transmission patterns and resistance mechanisms may be miscalculated. Briefly, integrating passive surveillance data with broader activities is imperative to confront the multifaceted challenges posed by malaria and issues related to it (Christopher et al., 2022) (Figure 10.6).

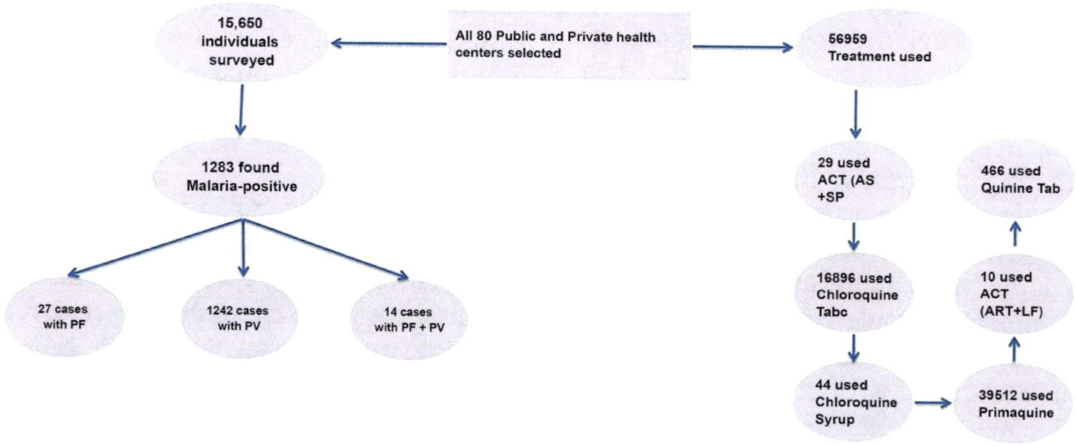

Figure 10.6. Passive malaria surveillance.

Source: Qureshi H, Khan MI, Ahmad A, Awan UA, Khattak AA, Khan AA and Sun Y (2021) Passive Surveillance of Malaria in Pregnant Women, Non-pregnant Women and Children Under 5 Years of Age in Bannu District, Khyber Pakhtunkhwa Pakistan. Front. Med. 8:751456. doi: 10.3389/fmed.2021.751456

10.2.2. Active Surveillance

Active surveillance comes into play when malaria begins to appear unexpectedly. Rather than sitting back and waiting for trickle-by reports from hospitals, teams spring into action—pursuing cases in the field with frequent outreach. This hands-on strategy, in some cases requiring routine home visits and systematic data collection, is effective at intercepting early evidence of an outbreak, particularly in areas where the spread changes rapidly. For instance, in a post-disaster environment, local teams would call in weekly to verify case numbers and even death, providing a continuous stream of new, real-time information. This active approach tends to capture what passive means miss, improving the health system's capacity for timely action (Polonsky et al., 2013). Nations trying to eradicate malaria are confronted with a different type of challenge. Overall, transitioning from basic control to outright eradication involves hunting for each case, even those with no clear signs. Active surveillance unearths more, collection information from every available source so that even suppressed transmission chains become apparent. It takes a fuller picture of the disease spread in different communities, informing directed efforts with a combination of practical methodology and technical expertise. In most strategic plans, such on-the-ground detection is considered an essential step to achieving that all-important zero-transmission target, supported by political momentum, inter-sector collaboration, and even enhanced logistics (Feachem et al., 2009). Staying malaria-free is not quite as simple as merely stopping transmission. When local cases fall, a system that merely waits for regular reports may overlook the rare case or imported infection that would rekindle an outbreak. That is where active surveillance on an ongoing basis steps, it serves to explore any abrupt alterations, initiates fast investigations, and initiates quick containment measures. This constant vigil is extended by data sharing across borders and regional cooperation, with the understanding that diseases are not concerned with political borders. It is all about achieving data precision, timely reporting, and ongoing community engagement. All these efforts, while not always ideally streamlined, are critical not only for initially conquering malaria but also for maintaining that malaria-free status in the long term (Feachem et al., 2009; Polonsky et al., 2013) (Figure 10.7).

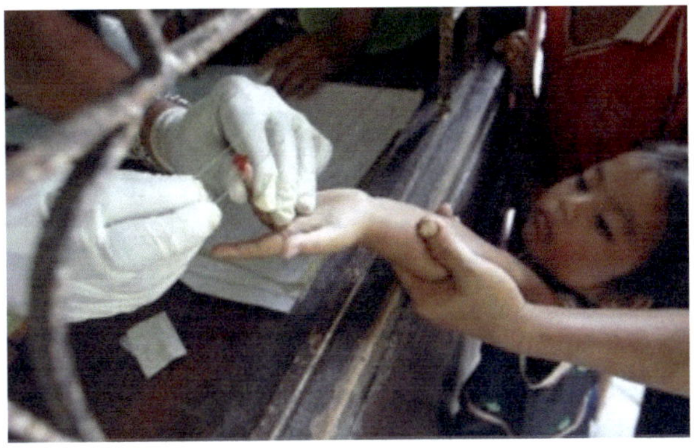

Figure 10.7. Active malaria surveillance.

Source: VOA News. (n.d.). *Active Malaria Surveillance.*

10.2.3. Sentinel Surveillance

Timely, good intel is the foundation of disease combat – it is what makes sentinel surveillance so stinking handy. These systems monitor a few health locations or defined populations for a continuous, real-time stream of information that guides public health decisions. In malaria, this approach is an intelligent means to monitor trends, verify whether interventions are on target, and even alert to emerging outbreaks. They tend to choose a few key locations, sort of combining amassing tons of information with making it achievable in reality. Health leaders subsequently are able to observe adjustments in malaria illness and death among various groups, allowing them to stir up responses that suit each case. It also provides a glimpse of the way that malaria numbers and deaths will fluctuate with the seasons, allowing people to drive resources into peak-transmission periods. Generally, relying on information like this is a cornerstone in fighting malaria's evolving guise and increasing the effectiveness of control programs wherever necessary. When such surveillance strategies are implemented in malaria-prone regions, they have a way of drawing the curtain back on disease management. The information coming from these regions usually indicates that testing is almost perfect and patients are being referred to the proper care paths ; as if every regulation is being followed just so. That being said, the data sometimes even raise red flags too: occasionally, a couple of critical test and treatment supplies dip below sufficient levels, particularly in the smaller, peripheral centers some months. Those supply blips disrupt speedy, efficient care, suggesting that the entire supply chain urgently could use a tune-up. The upside to these systems is that they post live data online (if properly maintained), so health teams can step in immediately and shift resources accordingly. Thus, sentinel surveillance is not simply about counts; it also indicates where the system may be failing (Christopher et al., 2022). Sentinel surveillance may be hailed for monitoring malaria on regional or national levels, but its application extends beyond. Widespread disease surveillance tends to rely on networks very similar to sentinel systems – they monitor infections and even resistance trends to guide specific actions. With antimicrobial resistance making it harder, including when malaria tags along for the ride, it appears essential to integrate these data into the larger picture of global health policy. In the majority of instances, these systems provide local, on-the-ground data that informs alters to infection prevention, stimulates intelligent use of antibiotics, and even indicates where new therapies may be necessary. They also identify how disease burdens and care resources vary significantly from site to site, disproportionately affecting low-resource sites. Briefly, strengthening these surveillance networks fits directly into wider efforts to reduce deaths due to resistant infections and ensure that vital medicines get put to use where they can save lives (Christopher et al., 2022) (Figure 10.8).

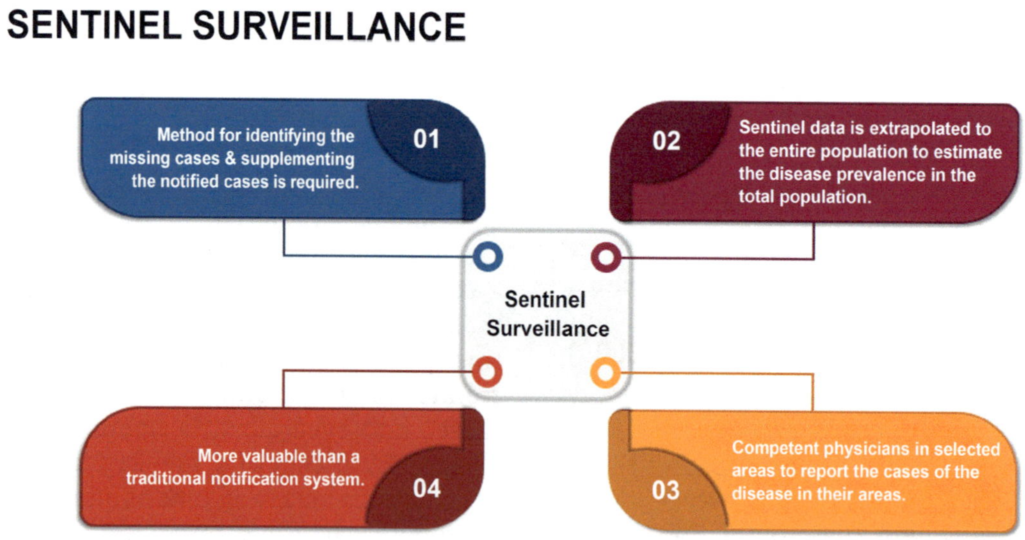

Figure 10.8. Sentinel surveillance.

Source: Collidu. (n.d.). *Sentinel Surveillance.*

10.3. Technological Advances in Surveillance

Advanced tools have consistently redefined how we monitor malaria. Previously, systems relied predominantly on manual data collection and scheduled reporting — practices that characteristically resulted in delayed responses. Currently, with real-time data collection and mapping technologies such as GIS, monitoring malaria has evolved significantly. One now collects detailed information from infection clusters and vector communities, which in most instances enables one to target interventions more effectively. Remote sensing, too, has its contribution in monitoring such environmental determinants as climate and land use; it can even suggest when an outbreak is likely to happen. This new, proactive way is not only intensifying surveillance but also making do with a more flexible allocation of resources, highlighting how new technology is flipping public health on its head (Alize et al., 2024). AI has also emerged as a mainstay in this new transformation. With its ability to process vast amounts of health data using machine learning algorithms, it provides means to identify issues early on, forecast trends, and inform decision-making. Such algorithms can detect subtle trends in disease transmission that may easily go unnoticed under human observation, which translates to risk evaluation and planning that are considerably more precise. Mobile apps driven by AI now enable people in far-flung or underserved communities to report cases in real time, avoiding the traditional setbacks such as a lack of enough qualified staff or adequate infrastructure. Naturally, implementing AI is not without difficulty; data quality, privacy, and human monitoring requirements still require attention. Overall, if AI is integrated into malaria surveillance responsibly, it can increase diagnostic accuracy and optimize resource use, eventually leading to more public health interventions that are slightly more specific to every situation (Shuroug et al., 2023). Apart from AI and mapping technologies, there has been some genuine surge in leveraging digital health platforms and cloud computing to reinforce surveillance at various levels. These virtual configurations allow local, national, and even global health organizations to swap information without hassle, triggering more cooperative reactions when outbreaks strike. Cloud-based tools allow huge quantities of data—everything from laboratory findings and vector control activities to epidemiological surveys—to be banked subsequently tapped into instantly for continuous analysis. This kind of tech mixing keeps monitoring robust and flexible, ready to pivot when faced with challenges like drug resistance or shifts in transmission driven by climate changes. Altogether, what we are seeing is a move from simply reacting to crises, towards anticipating them with data-driven insight, a shift that is steadily pushing global malaria eradication efforts forward (Shuroug et al., 2023; Alize et al., 2024).

10.3.1. Use of Geographic Information Systems (GIS)

Technology advancements have redefined public health surveillance, with new avenues for managing infections. GIS—Geographic Information Systems—was overnight turned into the standard equipment for tracking malaria trends, combining environmental signs, weather data, and crude disease statistics to highlight hotspots. By interweaving these various strands of information, it allows local units to identify malaria hotspots, so more wisely resources can be transferred around. This technique also suggests how malaria is spread by connecting mosquito breeding sites to increasing cases, and overall, it allows officials to leap into timely action with focused control measures. In addition, GIS's ability to play with live updates only enhances its importance in managing outbreaks for well-informed public health actions. GIS goes beyond mere mapping of malaria cases and gets down to the details of vector control and impact monitoring. In most instances, models based on GIS concepts model mosquito activity through the use of temperature, rainfall, and other variables that push mosquito survival and breeding. That forecasting advantage allows teams to sometimes predict when and where risk will spike—an action that tends to trigger proactive interventions. Subsequently there is the combination of environmental and social data, which superimposes data to identify communities at highest risk. This type of integrated detail is used to inform integrated control strategies that combine chemical, biological, and even environmental interventions, acting to combat challenges such as insecticide resistance or changing mosquito behavior.

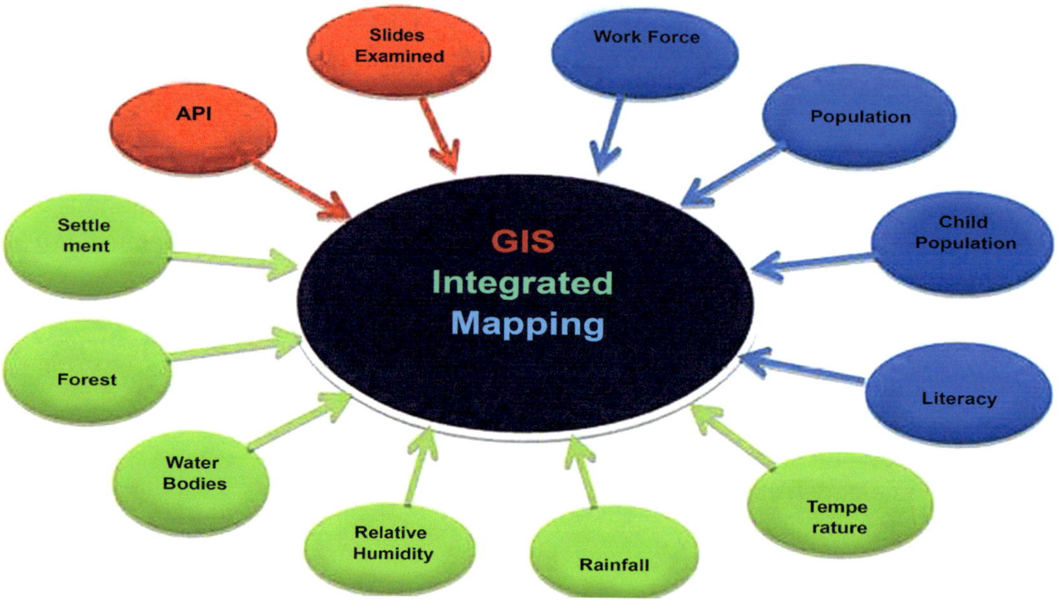

Figure 10.9. Spotting malaria use of geographic information systems (GIS).

Source: Springer Nature. (2015). *Spotting Malaria Use of Geographic Information Systems (GIS).*

Generally speaking, the capacity to track and even visually monitor intervention success is a large contributor to progressively enhanced malaria control programs, keeping gains in place and avoiding a rapid resurgence (Dyck et al., 2020). Nevertheless, nothing is smooth sailing with GIS. Its application to malaria surveillance is encountering obstacles—principal among them is data quality, accessibility issues, and a few privacy hiccups. Good, high-resolution data that is good at both spatial and temporal detail may be elusive, particularly in areas with limited resources. Additionally, combining diverse streams of data requires a few standard rules to avoid mismatches and to enhance the interoperability of how systems interact. As digital health information plays a growing part, patient data security is a top, albeit complex, priority. Overcoming these speed bumps involves enhancing local capacity in data collection and administration, along with policy adjustments that foster ethical use of geospatial information. Add to that newcomer technologies such as artificial intelligence and big data analysis, which could turbocharge what GIS can accomplish—providing more precise disease models and near real-time updates. In most instances, mixing these new methods with GIS could propel malaria control strategies further still, reinforcing its vital contribution to the public health landscape of the present day (Mbunge et al., 2020) (Figure 10.9).

10.3.2. Role of Mobile Health (mHealth) Technologies

Mobile health is disrupting the way we combat malaria. In countries such as Nigeria, where infrastructure is patchy and resources limited—the use of mobile phones ensures that data is captured and transmitted in real-time. Health workers are able to report cases quickly and, er, accurately, which ensures interventions are faster and more precise. These tools even serve to link various layers of the health system, from the local clinics all the way up through to the federal agencies, reinforcing that "one nation, one health" ideal. Where you digitize the records and improve data quality, you are left with more accountability and overall effectiveness in malaria programs (Abubakar et al., 2022).

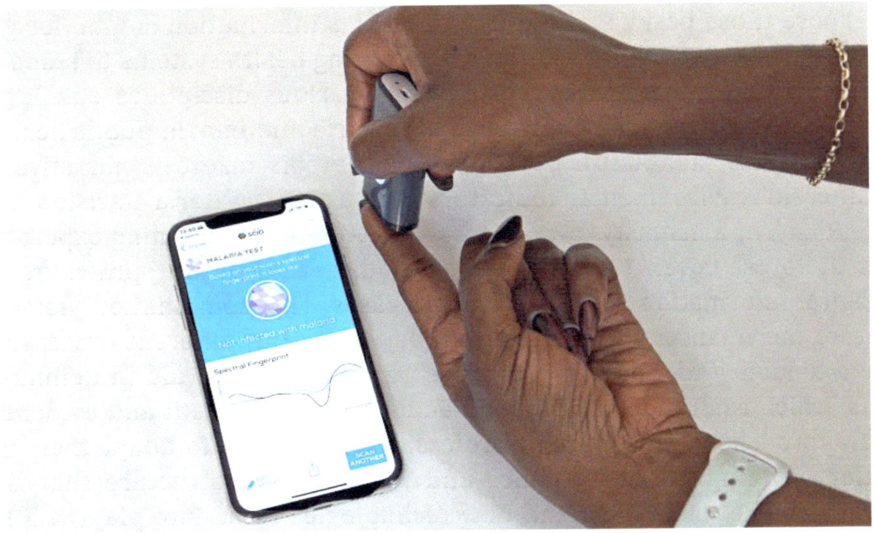

Figure 10.10. Role of mobile health (mHealth) technologies.

Source: SciDev.Net. (n.d.). *Role of Mobile Health (mHealth) Technologies.*

In some sense, mHealth not only raises the surveillance stakes but also strengthens governance and enhances health system resilience. Mobile health is not merely a matter of plugging in new devices, its true strength is its ability to integrate into the complex human edge of society and politics. On the whole, taking advantage of mHealth innovations involves grasping the complex nexus of social, political, and institutional determinants. It is not just about the tech; it requires conversation with community members, healthcare workers, and government officials. There are some case studies that indicate when there is local context and conditions included in the equation, people use and trust these systems more. Political will, and a team of experts, is required to sustain these platforms and ensure they sync with national health objectives. And beginning with interoperability built in is important to prevent fragmenting health data down the road (Huang et al., 2017). The hype around mHealth also relates to making health services more equitable and accessible. Many individuals who contract malaria reside in rural areas that are hard to reach for traditional monitoring. Mobile technology is able to bypass these geographic and resource barriers by providing constant surveillance and timely reporting of malaria cases, even in remote areas. That is, efforts can be targeted where malaria strikes most and budgets are limited. In addition, these technologies tend to disseminate health education, encouraging communities toward improved prevention and adherence to treatment regimens. When local health workers have better data and quicker feedback, they will be able to better manage resources, ultimately towards the larger goal of universal health coverage and disease control (Abubakar et al., 2022) (Figure 10.10).

10.3.3. Integration of Remote Sensing Data

Combating malaria is not a matter of following outdated playbooks. The old techniques of surveillance tend to capture the complex web of how our environment and conditions of society interact—so, by and large, we must think outside the box. Remote sensing information comes in here because it provides an abundance of spatial information about land use, vegetation, water features, and human population density. By merging satellite imagery with GIS technology, scientists can design risk maps that expose those pesky malaria hotspots. This information is vital for guiding targeted interventions, strategically deploying resources, and getting health systems to respond more rapidly to area outbreaks. Briefly, integrating expertise from various disciplines enables us to leverage environmental indicators to enhance knowledge of malaria and inform public health interventions in endemic areas (Zhao et al., 2020). Decision-support tools take this narrative a notch higher by combining different environmental indicators into a multi-criteria decision analysis (MCDA) framework. Essentially, in a majority of instances, MCDA entails combining expert-applied weights on factors such as forest cover, elevation, water bodies, and urban sprawl from satellite data with epidemiological information such as imported cases. This combination yields composite risk scores that capture the nuances of how malaria may spread in different areas. Informed models by experts have a tendency to enhance predictive performance and aid in defining priority areas for interventions, which can render elimination activities cost-efficient and evidence driven. Using these combined approaches, public health professionals are able to adapt their interventions to the local situation, refining the surveillance and response infrastructure that is critical to the control of malaria (Zhao et al., 2020). And new technologies come into play with remote sensing, particularly when worldwide health emergencies, such as COVID-19, put resources to the test. That pandemic served to demonstrate that embracing innovative technological solutions is vital for tracing disease under strained conditions. Such hardware as artificial intelligence, IoT sensors, and even UAVs (drones) sort through and disseminate remote sensing information near-real-time, assisting in monitoring mosquito breeding sites and tracing human movement. This dynamic spatial mapping is of paramount importance to forecasting outbreaks. As a result, combining remote sensing with advanced digital technology not only increases our situational awareness but also refines decision-making in complicated public health crises, ultimately strengthening the resilience of malaria surveillance systems.

10.4. Data Collection Methods

Surveillance for malaria relies on collection data that is not only accurate but also scalable when monitoring mosquito populations and disease transmission. Conventional methods such as human landing catches (HLC) have been the best way to count mosquitoes—a method that, although reliable, hits ethical and practical snags. Recently, new methods like the Ifakara Tent Trap (ITT-C) have emerged, allowing communities to participate with less risk to individuals. Granted, ITT-C may capture fewer mosquitoes on any given night than HLC, but it protects more territory for longer intervals. This wider coverage, combined with its affordability, renders it a good option for urban areas where transmission is low, providing crucial leads towards making malaria control programs. In the majority of instances, the appropriate balance between sensitivity, feasibility, and safety is fundamental (Chaki et al., 2012). Incorporating serological information into the equation provides malaria surveillance with an entirely different perspective, i.e., one centered on human exposure and immunity instead of the mosquitoes.

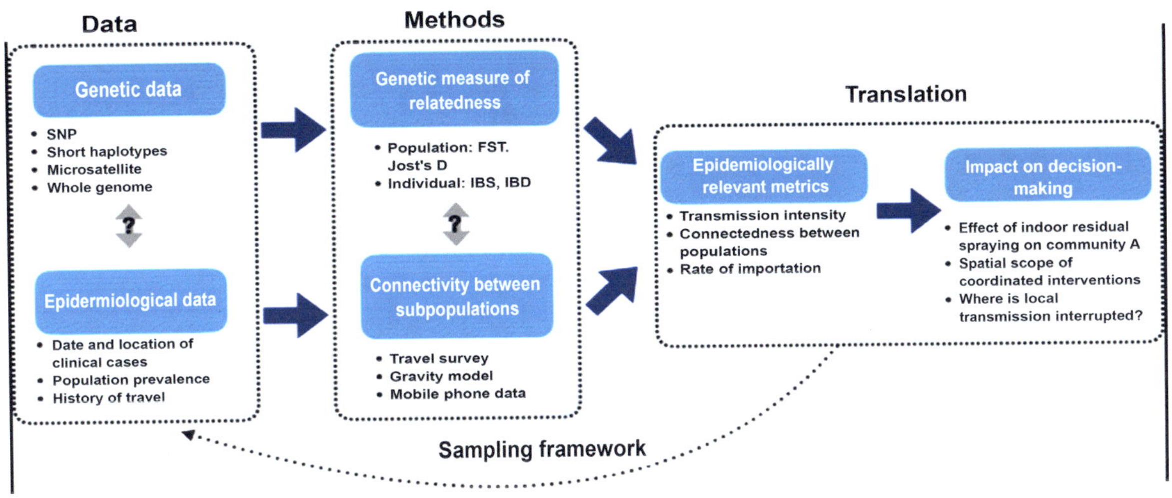

Figure 10.11. Malaria data collection methods.

Source: Springer Nature. (2018). *Malaria Data Collection Methods.*

Rather than relying exclusively on vector counts, antibody tests provide information about both recent and chronic infection, in reality a more complete picture. New breakthroughs in multiplex assays now enable testing for antibodies to several pathogens in one go, accelerating the entire process in combined platforms. The approach can assist authorities in identifying gaps in intervention coverage and detecting transmission patterns that mosquito data would not reveal. In general, incorporating antibody testing into regular monitoring increases the overall accuracy and effectiveness, closing the gap between exposure and active cases. In short, serological evidence has an important supportive role in any effective malaria control program (Arnold et al., 2018). It is still a challenging task to guarantee that the data is both excellent and representative, which is why sound sampling strategies and frequent checks are so vital. Community-based trap networks expand data collection but still require regular quality control—usually through comparisons against reference methods such as HLC or specialty traps—to level out variation caused by different trap sensitivities and environmental conditions. Connecting these results to health surveys, including those that quantify parasite prevalence, enhances our capacity to make inferences about how intense transmission of malaria is and what impact interventions could have. Coordinated procedures that synchronize the counts of mosquitoes with serological and epidemiologic data contribute to a multidimensional representation, one that is necessary for adaptive, well-informed decision-making. Ultimately, intelligent data-collection techniques underpin competent malaria surveillance and support focused vector control measures (Chaki et al., 2012; Arnold et al., 2018) (Figure 10.11).

10.4.1. Laboratory Diagnostics

Early detection of malaria is crucial – it essentially underpins the fight to keep disease outbreaks under control. Laboratory advances have raised the stakes in detecting such parasitic diseases more quickly and accurately. You tend to find that conventional microscopy, while still prevalent, is insensitive and relies on experienced technicians to consistently detect various *Plasmodium* species.

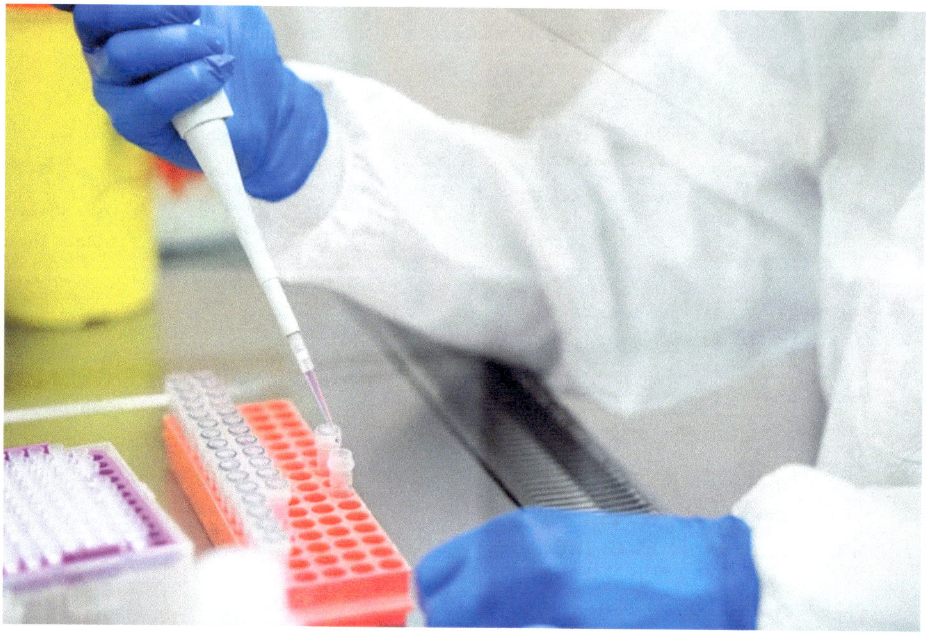

Figure 10.12. Malaria and its laboratory tests.

Source: Metropolis Healthcare. (2023). *Malaria and Its Laboratory Tests.*

Molecular and rapid diagnostic tests, however, have filled in the gap to reduce detection thresholds so that cases are signaled earlier. In most instances, these advances not only assist physicians in handling patients earlier but also increase the reliability of public health data, which is important while monitoring transmission changes and emerging drug resistance problems. Overall, today's lab systems now function as an important intermediary between routine clinical practice and real-time public health surveillance in malaria-endemic areas (Shuroug et al., 2023). Lab diagnostics technology is not merely about detecting infections, it is also about interpreting all that information. Artificial intelligence and machine learning, in general, are becoming smart helpers that can sense faint clues in lab tests and even assist in predicting outbreak patterns. These computer-based tools will likely automate tests, reduce human errors, and even customize treatment plans more to each patient's own needs. Occasionally, these systems will even integrate data from multiple health networks so that what emerges from the lab contributes to national and international malaria databases effectively. Certainly, issues such as data privacy and unequal resources still require solutions for these interventions to be maximally effective in practice (Shuroug et al., 2023). Ultimately, combining low-tech testing with high-tech analytics is gradually remaking the way we monitor and treat malaria. Despite all these technological advances, a lot of settings, particularly low-resource settings struggling with malaria—still have significant challenges with laboratory capacity and diagnostic access. Limited availability of good tests and proper know-how usually results in malaria being accurately and rapidly identified as a problem only, which again destabilizes the entire surveillance system. This creates even more difficulty in monitoring such areas as antimicrobial resistance, where evidence for resistant strains essentially relies on diligent lab work. Adding more strength to laboratory networks, investing in better machines (and training people too), appears to be a necessity. These measures would be able to nail down the actual spread of drug resistance and disease burden, allowing public health interventions and resource strategies to target on track. Thus, while laboratory tests are the foundation of detecting malaria, they are also important in influencing how we address drug resistance in hard-hit areas, even with periodic process glitches. These problems need to be addressed if we are to have surveillance systems that can keep up with changing patterns of disease (Figure 10.12).

10.4.2. Field Surveys and Community Engagement

High-quality malaria monitoring essentially boils down to collecting the appropriate type of general information – that is why getting out in the field is important. Field surveys allow researchers to scoop up critical pieces of information, such as how frequently malaria appears, how the nasty vectors act, and what of thc surrounding area would contribute to spreading the disease. Too often, local communities are brought in directly, providing high-granularity data that may be ignored by central systems. By doing so, the data is not only more reliable but also increases local awareness and provides an incentive for residents to have a stake in combating malaria. This type of community-based method can foster trust between residents and health officials, which can make aspects such as bed net usage and indoor spraying improve, ultimately making surveillance more resilient. Simply put, combining first-hand on-ground information with the latest technology for data collection keeps the system robust enough to deal with variations in disease trends (Tizifa et al., 2024). Linking raw numbers with firm malaria control requires genuine involvement from the community. Rather than simply serving as a passive reservoir of figures, community people get involved in educating, conversing, and even cooperating with local leaders and volunteers who serve as interfaces. Such layered participation extends interventions to greater depths and makes them persist from the grassroots level upwards. And in most instances, trained community volunteers visit homes, detect early signs, and assist in initiating on-time treatment—actions that greatly slow the transmission. Furthermore, when field surveys incorporate local perspectives, they tend to warn of social and cultural barriers that require customized solutions; ones that are sensitive to local traditions but still enhance health. The Global Technical Strategy of the World Health Organization (WHO) even identifies combining community involvement with governmental monitoring as central to getting long-term malaria elimination right (Tizifa et al., 2024). Technology is now making a significant difference by partnering with community involvement and field surveys. Digital platforms for recording data on the ground smoothed out information exchange, reducing errors and closing gaps in malaria data. Users like these systems a lot, particularly when good training and support are behind them – a tip of the hat to the value of combining human-centered design with technical expertise. All that being said, technology is not designed to operate in a vacuum; it performs optimally in conjunction with engaged community participation by offering real-time information required for making quick decisions. And further reviews of prevention strategies and information systems emphasize the necessity for transparency, evidence-based action, and consistent advocacy in order to sustain the momentum. To summarize, when these pieces come together, surveillance stays robust and adaptable—guiding targeted actions and smart resource allocation (Tizifa et al., 2024) (Figure 10.13).

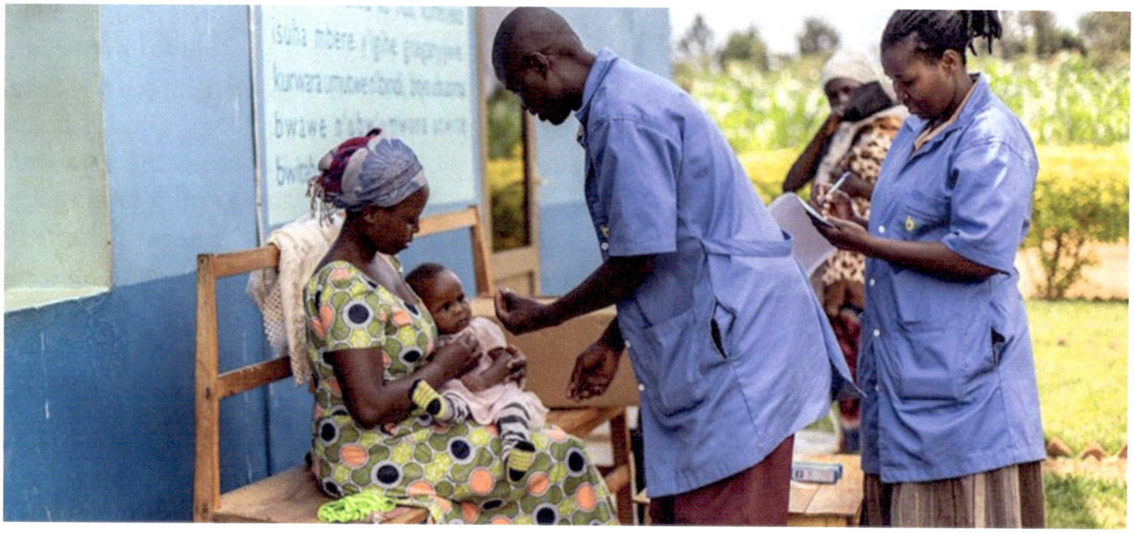

Figure 10.13. Field surveys and community engagement.

Source: India Blooms. (2025). *Field Surveys and Community Engagement.*

10.4.3. Use of Health Information Systems

Malaria surveillance relies on clever health information networks that collect huge volumes of information on how the sickness is transmitted. Such systems are not merely used to record cases—they enable administrators to easily view where outbreaks appear and how patterns shift. For instance, in the United States, information percolates in from laboratories, health care providers, and local public health groups, all of which channel into central repositories such as the National Malaria Surveillance System and the National Notifiable Diseases Surveillance System. Information from so many varied sources typically translates into greater accuracy and completeness, which is essential in identifying outbreaks, refining prevention plans, or even tailoring treatments. Having immediate access to these kinds of details equips public health officials to move quickly, and that usually is good for reducing sickness and deaths. They are also going beyond mere case counting with these data systems. They are now combining sophisticated lab techniques that track genetic tracers of drug resistance, a necessity since treatments occasionally encounter resistant forms. With lab-established resistance data thrown into the equation, authorities can monitor trends both domestically and internationally, typically culminating in wiser revisions in treatment protocols and chemoprophylaxis recommendations. This constant supply of molecular information also drives targeted research for new medications and vaccines, prodding policymakers and healthcare workers to rethink their strategies as the parasite evolves. Effectively merging conventional disease surveillance with resistance monitoring provides a vital link in the continuous battle to manage, and perhaps one day eradicate malaria. Although these health information systems are crucial, they do encounter a few very real challenges, particularly in low-resource settings where laboratory capacity and reporting infrastructure are not always state-of-the-art (Christopher et al., 2022). At other times, data gaps prevent us from obtaining a complete view of malaria's burden, making it more difficult to deploy effective control measures. In general, addressing these concerns involves strengthening laboratory networks, recruiting additional staff, and employing data platforms that integrate smoothly across regions and institutions. More modern digital technology such as cloud-based databases and mobile health apps has been assisting greatly by accelerating access to data and expanding it. Visualization dashboards, even some predictive models, now contribute to projecting outbreaks as well as informing resource allocation. Overall, proceeding with these technologies of enhancement is essential for overcoming surveillance challenges and sustaining malaria control programs on track globally, clearly correlating technology improvement with improved public health outcomes (Christopher et al., 2022) (Figure 10.14).

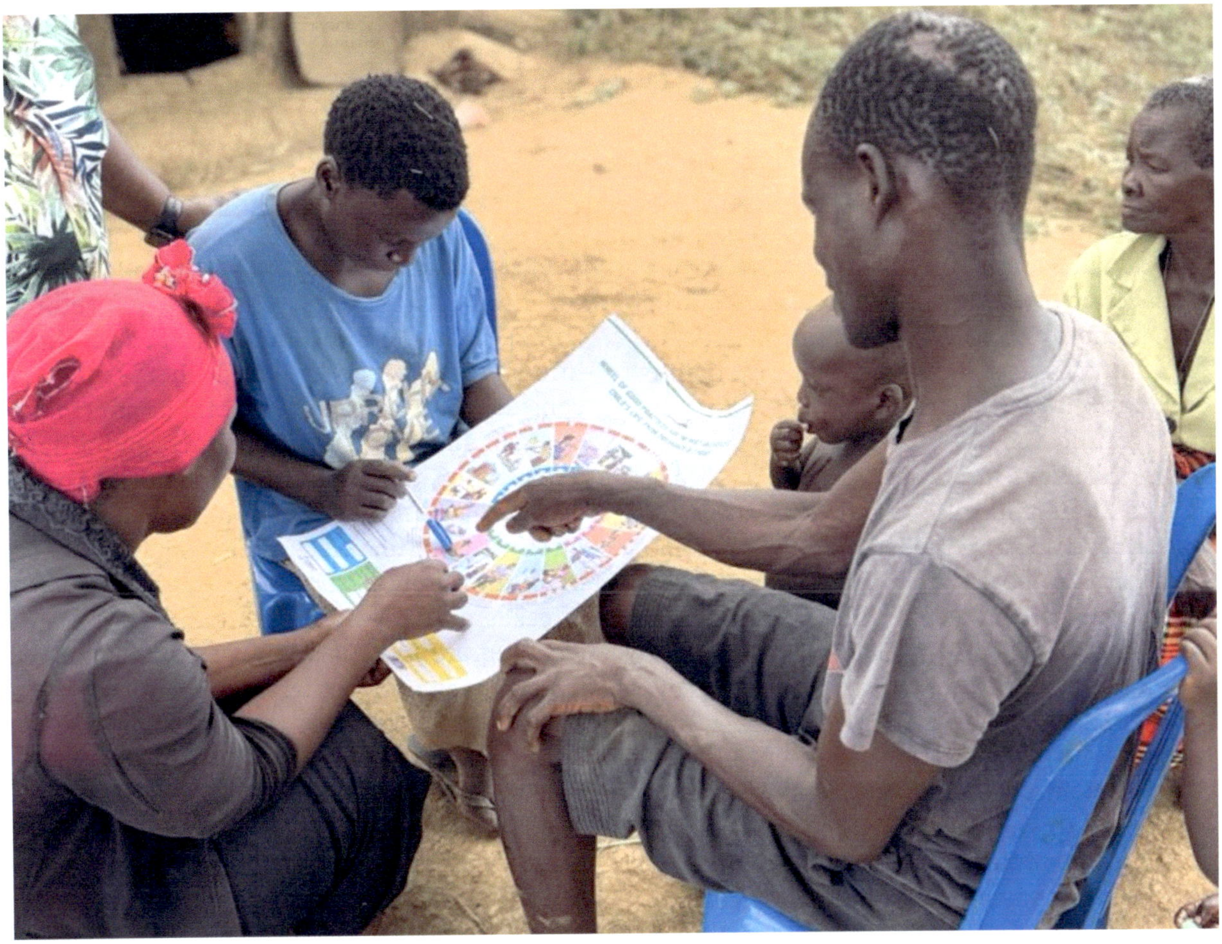

Figure 10.14. Use of health information systems.

Source: LinkedIn. (2024). *Use of Health Information Systems.*

10.5. Challenges in Malaria Surveillance

In most malaria-risk areas, surveillance efforts come to a standstill because basic infrastructure and day-to-day operations simply cannot keep pace with it. Some are plagued by labs that are inadequately equipped and struggle without reliable diagnostic equipment, so cases fall through the cracks with reduced accuracy and pace. Routine data collection takes a back seat, the foundation to understanding how malaria flows and whether control efforts are succeeding. Furthermore, there simply are not sufficient trained healthcare professionals to manage both the testing and complex business of managing data—rural areas bear the brunt. These challenges usually slow detection of outbreaks and muddy the opportunity to refine responses. In most cases, increasing lab services and adequate training for local personnel are key to repairing cracks and supporting strong malaria control measures (Christopher et al., 2022). Remote and economically disadvantaged groups introduce a further complication into the equation. Difficult-to-reach populations, where getting around is a hassle and health facilities fall short, hardly ever appear in official statistics. Underreporting produces a distorted picture that misleads where money and planning should strike hardest. Furthermore, local budget constraints tend to deter individuals from wanting quick diagnosis or treatment, and thus many cases fly under the radar. Throw into the mix of conflict or political unrest, and operating a secure, dependable surveillance system becomes all but impossible. Under these conditions, relying on community-based reporting and emerging technology such as mobile health solutions begins to appear as the only viable solution (John et al., 2020). The disease itself does not help. The disease's own vagaries, such as drug-resistant strains emerging and transmission patterns changing rapidly—are added to the difficulties. The emergence of strains that ignore first-line medications makes it harder to treat, so monitoring resistance becomes as critical as tracking new cases. Too often, existing systems are not designed to follow these resistance profiles regularly, stalling swift action when danger arises. In addition, natural seasonal patterns and transmission variation within small local areas require a degree of specificity that wide regional information simply is not able to provide. Without this kind of detailed, integrated data, public health officials are at a loss to identify where they need to act most successfully. Generally, overcoming these challenges requires more innovative, adaptive surveillance approaches that bring together knowledge from epidemiology, entomology, and even molecular research (John et al., 2020; Christopher et al., 2022).

10.5.1. Data Quality and Reliability Issues

Accurate malaria monitoring literally depends on having first-rate, reliable information. Unpredictable methods of accumulating information tend to cloud the issue quite considerably. Variations in methods of diagnosis, uneven laboratory infrastructure, and differing degrees of training among health workers across districts all serve to complicate matters, often leading to cases being underreported or inappropriately classified, which in the majority of cases delays response to outbreaks. Also, as we integrate artificial intelligence into medicine, it can streamline pattern detection and sort out discrepancies, but it has its own cross to bear such as fears about data privacy, prejudice, and over-reliance on machine watchfulness. All things considered, the unraveling of these issues is paramount if we hope that data responds to the way malaria spreads and can inform effective prevention (Shuroug et al., 2023). Health information systems are, in fact, complicated , and that complication tends to place more obstacles in the path of reliable malaria surveillance. Patchy information flows and variable site standards can make data comparability and completeness go haywire. Data stem from every kind of place: from verbal autopsies and vital registers to hospital records – each place with its own peculiarities in accuracy. Redistribution algorithms attempt to redistribute those loose or off-target cause-of-death codes, but ambiguities remain regarding attribution of death directly to malaria. And depending so much on population approximations and demographic adjustments provides a further layer of uncertainty that could simply obscure the true trends in malaria incidence. Evidently, these methodological issues require strong, sustained standardization and regular validation checks at both national and subnational levels (Gregory et al., 2018). Maintaining malaria surveillance in top condition requires ongoing investment in infrastructure, proper training, and new technology innovations. Spot-on data is essential to identify hotspots, monitor whether interventions are working, and best utilize resources on hand. But when reporting routines are random and complete datasets are difficult to access, real-time decision-making is a true challenge. On the bright side, innovative methods such as AI and machine learning may completely revolutionize the field by refining data analysis, highlighting early warning signs, and even assisting with clinical judgments. Nevertheless, implementing these technologies in a way that works effectively hinges on addressing recurring challenges such as data bias, ethical challenges, and the delicate process of integrating new systems with existing ones. In total, enhancing data reliability and quality requires a hybrid strategy that integrates technological innovations with tight regulation and that good old-fashioned human know-how (Gregory et al., 2018; Shuroug et al., 2023) (Figure 10.15).

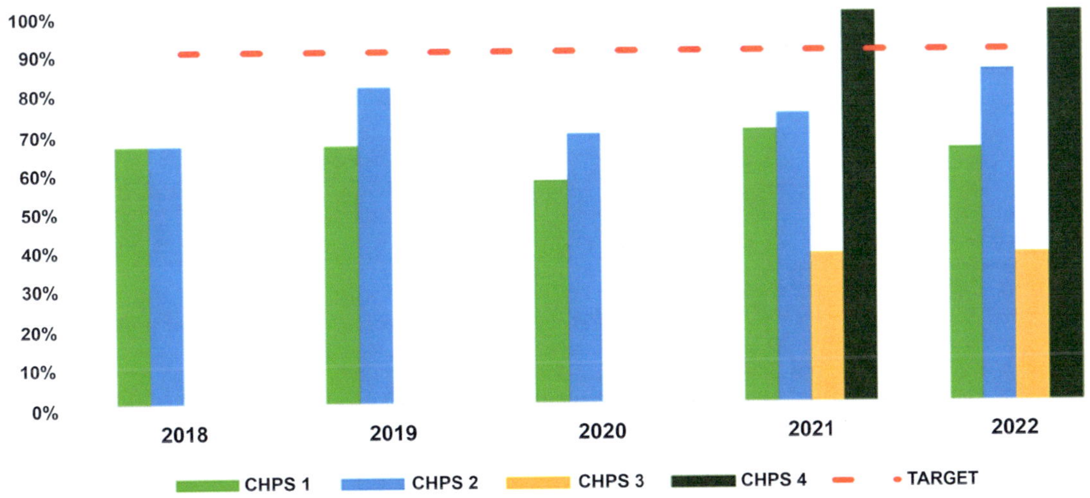

Figure 10.15. Quality of routine malaria data.

Source: Springer Nature. (2024). *Quality of Routine Malaria Data.*

10.5.2. Geographic and Socio-Economic Barriers

Surveillance for malaria becomes challenging in areas where the terrain is haphazard. Isolated, inaccessible areas with limited roads make it difficult to maintain an even surveillance. Poor road conditions and inclement weather inhibit the speed at which data are gathered, and what that means is that outbreaks are detected later than they ought to be. Isolation nearly always accompanies a deficit of healthcare facilities and erratic communication networks, which complicates the flow of data among agencies. Consequently, the problems result in isolated surveillance data and erode the capacity to effectively target interventions. In the majority of instances, addressing these geographic hitches requires innovative logistics and employing location-based technologies to assist in ironing out resource distribution (Piret & Boivin, 2021). On the other hand, economic and social considerations also go a long way in determining how effectively malaria is maintained under control. Individuals residing in poorer localities typically do not have stable access to primary healthcare, which disrupts consistent malaria reporting and treatment follow-up. Financing issues not only hold back establishing a strong surveillance system but also retaining well-trained health workers. Poor literacy and low health awareness could further decrease community participation, and individuals may be less responsive to detecting or preventing outbreaks. Often, these economic hurdles push malaria down the list of priorities when health emergencies compete for attention. That is why surveillance efforts need to take these social differences into account, using local community reports and native know-how to cover all bases fairly and thoroughly (Piret & Boivin, 2021). Despite all the hype surrounding emerging tech such as augmented reality and digital tools, the challenges of geography and lack of resources are still quite recalcitrant. New devices offer better data collection and better images of what is happening, but implementing these tools in regions with no basic infrastructure and little technology expertise is a problem of its own. Without complementing initiatives to improve socio-economic conditions, such innovations stand the risk of widening the chasm at the expense of more connected regions compared to those left behind. A cautious implementation of such technology must consider local constraints and involve measures to develop skills where needed most. Balancing is central to ensuring such advancements assist in controlling malaria rather than merely expanding gaps in surveillance (Figure 10.16).

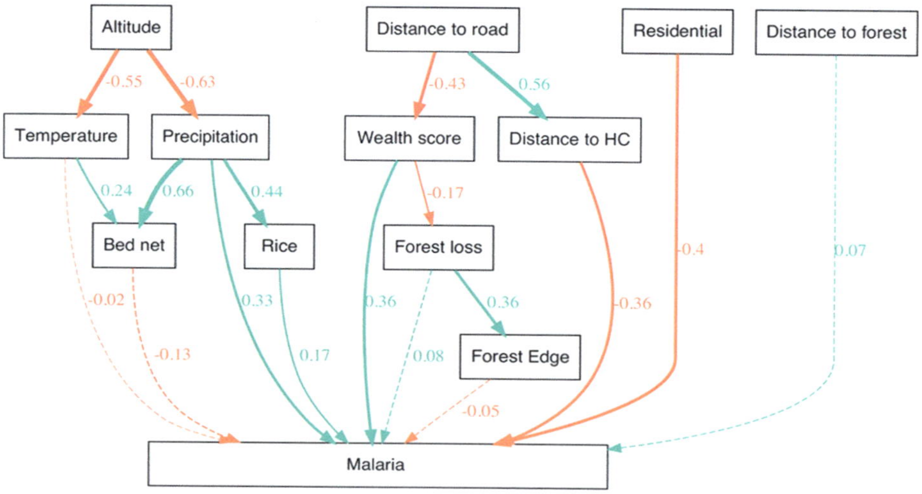

Figure 10.16. Geographic and socio-economic barriers in malaria surveillance.

Source: Pourtois JD, Tallam K, Jones I, Hyde E, Chamberlin AJ, Evans MV, et al. (2023) Climatic, land-use and socio-economic factors can predict malaria dynamics at fine spatial scales relevant to local health actors: Evidence from rural Madagascar. PLOS Glob Public Health 3(2): e0001607. https://doi.org/10.1371/journal.pgph.0001607.

10.5.3. Resistance to Surveillance Initiatives

Malaria control is not so much a battle of battling pathogens with high-tech wizardry, it is also wrapped up in complicated human and institutional unease about watching. Communities are concerned about privacy and fear of being labeled or judged, and these concerns appear repeatedly in the way data gets gathered. Such mistrust can readily derail the timely, solid data necessary to catch malaria's spread and to respond quickly. Too often, they look at these monitoring programs as off-the-shelf, top-down actions that simply do not resonate with local traditions. Lacking that genuine connection, local involvement plummets, and that makes any attempt to regulate malaria much less successful. Honest, open discussions that mix local agendas with monitoring objectives can serve to enhance both data quality as well as the long-term malaria battle (Okumu et al., 2022). Institutional barriers create yet another obstacle. Wherever the impact is felt, the local healthcare systems in most of these areas lack trained personnel, poorly developed infrastructure, and a mess of data handling that inhibits reporting and confuses analysis. Usually, overwhelmed personnel view surveillance as yet another added task—one without specific rewards or adequate feedback. It does not make things better when government institutions and global partners do not see eye to eye, resulting in a patchwork response that is as fractured as it is failing. Institutionalizing stronger commitment is more about integrating surveillance into routine health practice and establishing actual capacity-building prospects. In the majority of instances, emphasizing good-quality data not only maps malaria patterns but also informs focused, effective action (Okumu et al., 2022). The challenge becomes increasingly complicated with the emergence of antimicrobial resistance—a development that calls for heightened surveillance even as it provokes resistance due to its complexity itself. As drug and insecticide resistance mounts, surveillance systems need to shift gears swiftly to detect emerging risks and anticipate timely action, even if that entails tackling a raft of complications. This combination of drug resistance and malaria control highlights profound fissures in global health management and mismatched resource distributions. At times, anxieties about tech feasibility, budget constraints, and other acute health concerns contribute to the reluctance surrounding surveillance bolstering. A one-health approach, which unites understanding from human, animal, and environmental domains (even if that does sound like a mouthful)—might just be the way forward. Successful malaria surveillance, therefore, hinges as much on the collection of biological information as on penetrating the numerous layers of resistance to construct an adaptable, integrated monitoring system.

10.6. Case Studies of Successful Surveillance Systems

Surveillance for malaria is important for establishing targeted solutions and making sure resources land where they need to in disease-prone areas. Consider South Africa's KwaZulu-Natal, for instance – there, a malaria monitoring system utilizing the District Health Information System 2 (DHIS2) draws in case information and monitors trends nearly in real time. Despite how advanced the system is, it still falters somewhat: only around 61% of cases are reported within 24 hours of diagnosis. Nevertheless, the majority of users report it is easy to use and generally good enough for day-to-day operation, facilitating data flowing more freely. Subsequently, too, the very high overall data quality demonstrates its ability to enable malaria elimination by separating imported from locally acquired cases – a valuable distinction for informing response strategies that are targeted (Mabona et al., 2024). Overall, this example reminds us in the majority of cases that finding equilibrium between ease of use and stringent performance requirements is a continuous problem in malaria surveillance. Technology also has a large role to play. In Indonesia's Lahat District, for instance, there is an electronic Malaria Information System (eMIS) that relies on an android-based mobile platform to acquire case data entered into the system quickly and correctly – a definite improvement from older PC systems in terms of efficiency as well as real-time collaboration. Using the Framework for the Application of Systems Techniques (FAST), researchers in the main identified bottlenecks along the workflow and adjusted the system to improve performance serving health workers in endemic areas. The transition to mobile reporting, in addition to speeding up capture, also reduced errors, enhancing preparedness for rapid public health response. This case truly demonstrates the real utility of developing technology with a user-centered methodology in the process of upgrading surveillance infrastructures to achieve elimination objectives (Hasyim et al., 2024). Comparing both scenarios together highlights several important findings regarding what constitutes an effective surveillance system. Both illustrations emphasize that total data, prompt reporting, and engaged user participation are the cornerstone of success. While KwaZulu-Natal's eDHS2 system has good data quality and solid reporting habit in place, it continues to struggle with delivering notifications quickly enough to meet elimination goals. Conversely, Indonesia's eMIS demonstrates that mobile technology can streamline the process, although it requires careful local fit and additional user training. Collectively, these examples indicate that combining tech innovations with systems thinking and front-line engagement constructs a responsive configuration able to propel malaria elimination in epidemiologically heterogeneous areas (Hasyim et al., 2024; Mabona et al., 2024).

10.6.1. The Case of Rwanda's Malaria Control Program

Rwanda's anti-malaria effort begins with surveillance systems that can flip in an instant as circumstances change. They combine molecular monitoring with plain old epidemiological know-how – applying genomic tools to monitor parasite behavior and drug resistance in real time. It makes it simpler to identify emerging threats before they become large and facilitates the identification of local outbreaks in combination with cases originating elsewhere. Additionally, by combining biological laboratory results with day-to-day health records, their solution pushes policymaking in a data-based direction, an approach which tends to resonate with international trends in genomic surveillance present in some areas of sub-Saharan Africa and elsewhere (Clemente et al., 2024). Reducing malaria is not just a case of detecting cases early; it is the pace and planning of the response as well. Rwanda is heavily reliant on community participation plus facility screening, which of course increases how rapidly and accurately cases are detected and treatments implemented. They even customize various levels of intervention to correspond to the local transmission level—combining vector control and prophylactic medicine in ways that vary quite seasonally or with the onset of parasite resistance. More often than not, this sort of multi-layered, adaptive approach allows for rapid altering, keeping the entire endeavor strong and adaptive (Rotejanaprasert et al., 2024). Placing malaria surveillance within Rwanda's larger health system has ignited collaboration that develops both human talent and tech know-how. Education of health workers in data collection, molecular testing, and analysis has rendered the entire process more sustainable over time, with investments in digital infrastructure for real-time display of data generating rapid feedback loops to those on the ground and to policymakers. These feedback loops—albeit at times a little patchy—enable the operations to get continuously refined, which is critical when changing epidemiologic patterns and evolving drug resistance send curveballs. Rwanda's experience, which integrates genomic information, geographic data, and community-level observations, recalls us that a proper surveillance system is critical for consistent gains in the control of malaria and for moving towards elimination targets (Clemente et al., 2024; Rotejanaprasert et al., 2024) (Figure 10.17).

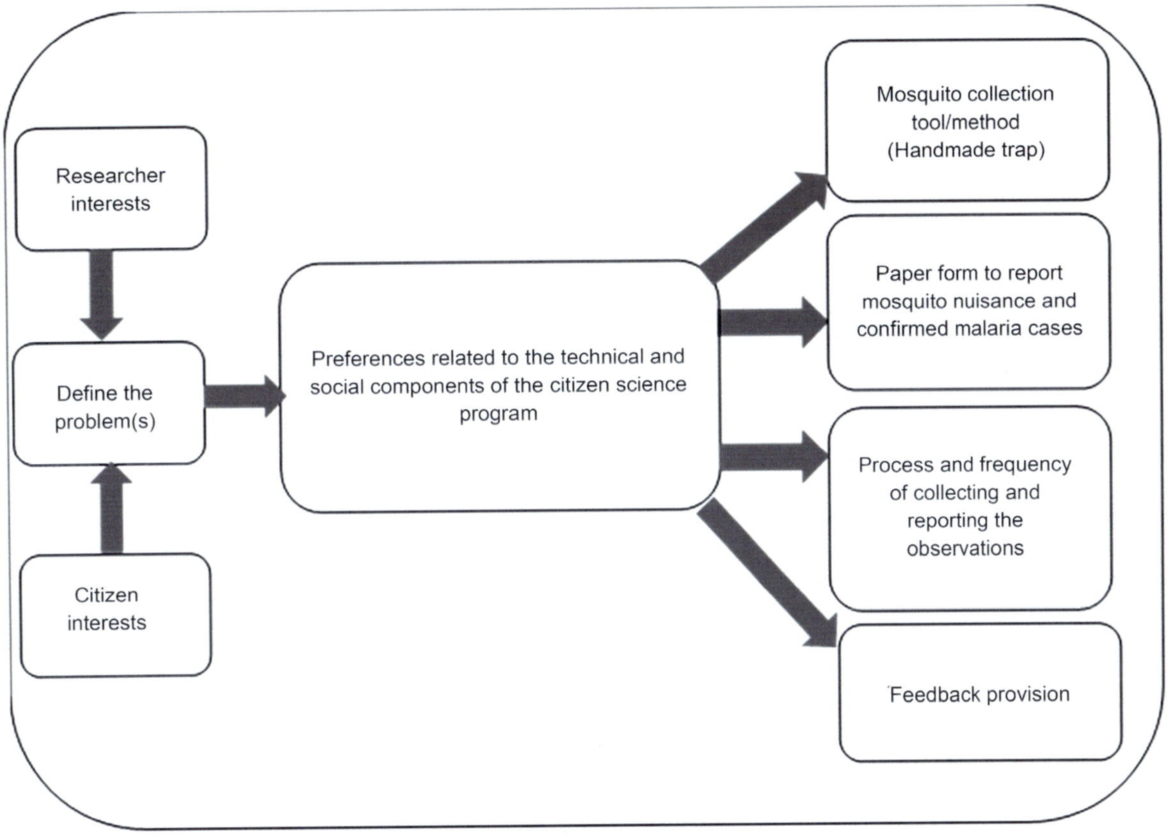

Figure 10.17. The case of Rwanda's malaria control program.

Source: Asingizwe D, Milumbu Murindahabi M, Koenraadt CJM, Poortvliet PM, van Vliet AJH, Ingabire CM, Hakizimana E, Mutesa L, Takken W, Leeuwis C. Co-Designing a Citizen Science Program for Malaria Control in Rwanda. *Sustainability*. 2019; 11(24):7012. https://doi.org/10.3390/su11247012

10.6.2. Lessons From the Amazon Basin

How disease and nature mix in the Amazon Basin can wake us up to new methods of monitoring malaria. Dense forests, varying river levels, and a chaotic combination of creatures have all made it difficult to identify cases of malaria. More often than not, these problems remind us that mixing what we do know about the environment with good old-fashioned health checks may well be the solution—not simply documenting cases when they occur, but potentially even predicting outbreaks by monitoring how habitats shift and how mosquitoes act. It is a push for developing tools that adapt to the environment, particularly where nature's disruption accelerates disease transmission, and that requires maintaining environmental vigilance alongside daily health practices. Add in the rich cultural matrix and practical barriers of the region, and the scenario is even more complex. Individuals in rural locations tend to have limited access to healthcare and may use indigenous local languages, further creating potholes in the way along which information travels. This forces us toward malaria monitoring systems that are not a universal fit; rather, they must interface with local epistemologies and discourses. Newer developments in machine intelligence that are specific to linguistic and cultural disparity have the potential to enhance network resilience by simplifying it for communities to engage even if how they disseminate information may differ slightly. When local voices help shape the data, it does not just improve accuracy; it builds trust and cooperation, all essential for keeping malaria in check in these diverse, isolated pockets (Tembin Hé et al., 2024). In a nutshell, it is clear that adding social and cultural layers to our health monitoring is a must. Referring to Amazon's case in particular, it can be seen that robust legal and institutional backing has a considerable role to play in both health and environmental monitoring. Poor enforcement of environmental legislation usually disrupts habitats, inadvertently altering breeding sites for mosquitoes and increasing the malaria threat. Achieving a stronger hold on these environmental laws serves to unify people to safeguard the very natural habitats that maintain low mosquito populations. When you mix information about how well the environment is being protected with classic health statistics, you have a richer, more detailed picture of malaria risk. This overall strategy-even when it occasionally comes off as a little scatterbrained-is backed by inclusive governance and intelligent policymaking, providing a sustainable foundation for tracking malaria in fragile settings. In the end, the Amazon's lessons go far beyond new technologies; they emphasize that partnerships among various sectors and good governance are equally important for successful disease control (Tembin Hé et al., 2024).

10.6.3. Innovations in Southeast Asia

Malaria control in certain regions of Southeast Asia has experienced some bumps in recent times, forcing the people on the ground to come up with new, nimble means of keeping track of outbreaks. Environmental changes have pushed the mosquitoes into new locations, so monitoring now must be nimble—as willing to change almost on a moment's notice. New molecular tests and complex mapping methods allow public health individuals to identify clusters of infections much more obviously, and data centers that combine information from pathogen studies, illness reports and regional climate are turning out to be a huge assist. Overall, these methods provide us with a better glimpse of how malaria manages to slip into communities and allow us to respond more quickly when outbreaks arise, all the while climate change and urbanization at breakneck speeds continue to shift the ground rules. In most instances, these technologies enhance the way resources are utilized and create a healthier, stronger malaria response as a whole. The combination of technology and community engagement is also proving to be a game changer. Mobile health applications—developed for frontline workers—allow reporting suspected cases, even sightings of the vector in real time, which hastens data collection. Combined with geotagging capabilities, such tools return useful location data, which assist in mapping hotspots, particularly in rural or inaccessible areas. Machine learning, meanwhile, peeks through surveillance data seeking out abnormal trends, usually flagging potential outbreaks well ahead of time. In most instances, when local health networks collaborate with these technological developments, they not only create local expertise but also foster a more direct approach to mosquito control. This local empowerment ensures that the surveillance system remains attuned to the region's specific disease patterns and cultural atmosphere, enhancing the general battle against malaria (Naghavi et al., 2024). Despite these advances, however, everything is not entirely smooth throughout Southeast Asia's varied terrain. Variations in how nations gather and report information sometimes obscure the true image of the malaria burden. To help iron out these wrinkles, regional groups have generally worked up standardized protocols and built data systems that allow for easy sharing and comparison. Plus, weaving climate data into these models has helped refine our grasp on mosquito behavior and disease timing—essential for planning early interventions. The continuing mix of traditional entomological screenings and advanced pathogen identification enhances our examination of malaria trends and death statistics, as reported in various world health research studies (Naghavi et al., 2024). Overall, these creative approaches, despite some unevenness here and there, are crucial to cutting-edge strategic planning and rapid responses required to move closer towards malaria elimination in the region.

CLOSER LOOK

SURVEILLANCE IN MALARIA CONTROL

Surveillance plays a critical role in malaria control and elimination efforts. It involves the systematic collection, analysis, and interpretation of malaria-related data to guide public health decisions and interventions. Effective surveillance helps identify areas of high transmission, detect outbreaks early, monitor the impact of control measures, and evaluate progress towards elimination goals. In malaria-endemic regions, surveillance systems are essential for tracking the number of cases and deaths, determining the distribution of malaria species, and understanding trends in disease transmission. This information enables health authorities to allocate resources efficiently, prioritize high-risk populations, and implement targeted interventions such as insecticide-treated bed nets (ITNs), indoor residual spraying (IRS), and prompt diagnosis and treatment with artemisinin-based combination therapies (ACTs).

As countries move towards malaria elimination, surveillance becomes even more important. It must evolve from simply tracking disease burden to actively detecting every infection, including asymptomatic cases. This requires robust diagnostic tools, active case detection strategies, and strong reporting systems at the community and national levels. Timely and accurate data collection allows for rapid response to emerging threats, such as drug or insecticide resistance. Digital technologies, such as mobile reporting tools, geographic information systems (GIS), and real-time dashboards, are increasingly being used to enhance malaria surveillance. These tools improve data accuracy, enable faster response times, and support more informed decision-making. In conclusion, surveillance is the backbone of effective malaria control and elimination strategies. By providing the evidence needed to guide interventions and measure their impact, strong surveillance systems help reduce malaria transmission, prevent deaths, and ultimately achieve a malaria-free world. Investing in surveillance capacity and technology is therefore vital to sustaining and accelerating progress against malaria.

SUMMARY

Malaria control has changed in leaps and bounds, and you can see how responsive strategies and contributions from a myriad of different groups have informed the fight against the disease. Look at Guangzhou, for instance – a case that, in most instances, illustrates how, if only methods are adjusted to suit the local health environment, local transmission can plummet, even disappear after a while. It began when health facilities leaped early into the fray, establishing a simple framework that was subsequently married up to what different community groups were trying to do. This combination of continuous monitoring with flexible, hands-on approaches appears to revolutionize disease control. Briefly put, such experiences suggest controlling malaria in the long run requires systems tailored to every setting but drawing upon assistance from a wide variety of community stakeholders (Chen et al., 2023). Meanwhile, breakthroughs in technology, particularly in artificial intelligence and data analysis—are leading to new opportunities for monitoring and combating malaria worldwide. AI is not all about flashy devices; it is assisting in accelerating diagnosis, personalizing treatment regimens, and even aiding more effective decision-making. The very same scaling tools also make real-time monitoring possible and enable forecasting outbreaks much easier, although, of course, ethical considerations and concern for data privacy still require some gentle balancing of good old human know-how. In general terms, the integration of high-tech understanding with proven public health practice provides a path to more responsive and accurate malaria surveillance (Shuroug et al., 2023). When you consider it all as a whole, combining varied control strategies with new technology appears to illuminate the way ahead for international malaria surveillance. It is not only about lessons learned from past programs but also about consistently evolving our methods and drawing on the latest scientific and technical insights. Consistent effort, careful data management, and ongoing community involvement are all essential if we are going to keep malaria at bay and prevent a comeback. The general strategy observed in Guangzhou provides a wide, practical design, recommending that sustainable malaria control is feasible through coordination, adaptability, and innovative imagination (Chen et al., 2023; Shuroug et al., 2023).

Medical care is changing in ways that most had not anticipated. New technology—data-crunching software and computer algorithms—is redefining the way we detect malaria and contain its spread, often in unexpected manners. Big stacks of data are digested and analyzed, revealing patterns older methods may only skip over, which can lead to improved outbreak forecasts and wiser deployment of resources. AI now even tailors interventions to match specific community requirements, providing some sort of bespoke public health kick. Naturally, all this progress takes its own puzzles—privacy concerns, moral tangles, and the ever-present requirement for specialists able to read and believe those AI findings. In the majority of instances, when our healthcare systems become more advanced, mixing in these more acute surveillance strategies proves to be the most important step towards reducing malaria cases and saving lives in the worst-affected regions (Shuroug et al., 2023). Considering malaria monitoring, there is nothing that surpasses collecting a wide array of data if we desire public health strategies that hit the spot. It is not merely a matter of case counts; it is seeing how frequently infections occur, charting where they spread, observing mosquitoes' behavior, and even monitoring drug resistance. All that diverse data—anything from clinical information to environmental indicators—allows for a more complete picture to be drawn, sometimes alerting before these areas blow up into full-scale outbreaks, so treatments like bed net drops or rapid spray treatments can be initiated. Nevertheless, maintaining high levels of data quality is not always a stroll in the open plains, particularly for regions where resources are limited, thus there is always a need for additional training and technology enhancements. Overall, systems that throw us actionable intel can significantly reduce malaria's impact by guiding decisions that are based on firm, hard evidence from the ground (Troeger et al., 2018). When you delve deeper into malaria surveillance, you realize that it does much more than just count cases. It moves beyond mere reporting to measure the effectiveness of health measures and even detects emerging problems, such as the development of insecticide resistance or changes in parasite character. AI-powered tools and bits of machine learning introduce yet another level by providing on-the-fly predictions and real-time updates, often turning the narrative from simply waiting around to proactively anticipating outbreaks. Long-term victories still hinge on ironing out infrastructure hiccups and social challenges such as establishing local health networks and bringing everyone along. All this underlines that malaria surveillance is not just a static checklist but a lively, evolving tool that is essential if we are ever going to outsmart malaria on a global scale (Shuroug et al., 2023; Troeger et al., 2018).

KEY TERMS FROM THIS CHAPTER

Case Detection	Passive Surveillance	Active Surveillance
Sentinel Surveillance	Case Notification	Malaria Information System
Early Warning System	Outbreak Detection	Case Investigation
Foci Investigation	Entomological Surveillance	Drug Resistance Monitoring
Rapid Reporting	Data Quality Assurance	Indicator-Based Surveillance
Surveillance-Response System	GIS Mapping	
Routine Health Facility Reporting	Community-Based Surveillance	

References

1. Abubakar, I., Dalglish, S. L., Angell, B., Sanuade, O. A., Abímbọ́lá, Ṣ., Adamu, A. L., Adetifa, I., et al. (2022). The Lancet Nigeria Commission: Investing in health and the future of the nation. *The Lancet, 399*, 1155–1200. https://doi.org/10.1016/s0140-6736(21)02488-0.
2. Alowais, S. A., Alghamdi, S. S., Alsuhebany, N., Alqahtani, T., Alshaya, A., Almohareb, S. N., Aldairem, A., et al. (2023). Revolutionizing healthcare: The role of artificial intelligence in clinical practice. *BMC Medical Education, 23*. https://doi.org/10.1186/s12909-023-04698-z.
3. Arnold, B. F., Scobie, H. M., Priest, J. W., & Lammie, P. J. (2018). Integrated Serologic Surveillance of Population Immunity and Disease Transmission. *Emerging infectious diseases, 24*(7), 1188–1194. https://doi.org/10.3201/eid2407.171928
4. Ayala, M. J. C., Valiati, N. C. M., Bastos, L. S., & Villela, D. A. M. (2023). Notification of malaria cases in the Brazilian Amazon Basin from 2010 to 2020: an analysis of the reporting times. *Malaria journal, 22*(1), 49. https://doi.org/10.1186/s12936-023-04464-y(accessed on 13 May 2025).
5. Chaki, P. P., Mlacha, Y., Msellemu, D., Muhili, A., Malishee, A. D., Mtema, Z. J., Kiware, S. S., Zhou, Y., Lobo, N. F., Russell, T. L., Dongus, S., Govella, N. J., & Killeen, G. F. (2012). An affordable, quality-assured community-based system for high-resolution entomological surveillance of vector mosquitoes that reflects human malaria infection risk patterns. *Malaria journal, 11*, 172. https://doi.org/10.1186/1475-2875-11-172 (accessed on 13 May 2025).
6. Polonsky, J., Luquero, F., Francois, G., Rousseau, C., Caleo, G., Ciglenecki, I., Delacre, C., Siddiqui, M. R., Terzian, M., Verhenne, L., Porten, K., & Checchi, F. (2013). Public health surveillance after the 2010 haiti earthquake: the experience of médecins sans frontières. *PLoS currents, 5*, ecurrents.dis.6aec18e84816c055b8c2a06456811c7a. https://doi.org/10.1371/currents.dis.6aec18e84816c055b8c2a06456811c7a (accessed on 13 May 2025).
7. Chamola, V., Hassija, V., Gupta, V., & Guizani, M. (2020). A comprehensive review of the COVID-19 pandemic and the role of IoT, drones, AI, blockchain, and 5G in managing its impact. *IEEE Access, 8*, 90225–90265. https://doi.org/10.1109/access.2020.2992341.
8. Chen, Y., Wang, Q., Chen, H., Song, X., Tang, H., & Tian, M. (2019). An overview of augmented reality technology. *Journal of Physics Conference Series, 1237*, 022082–022082. https://doi.org/10.1088/1742-6596/1237/2/022082.
9. Chen, Y., Zhang, H., Chen, H., Fan, L., Xu, C., Xu, J., & Chen, S. (2023). Malaria epidemiological characteristics and control in Guangzhou, China, 1950–2022. *Malaria Journal, 22*. https://doi.org/10.1186/s12936-023-04696-y.
10. Cueto, M., Brown, T., & Fee, E. (2019). Introduction: The World Health Organization and the dilemmas of the Cold War and the post–Cold War periods. *The World Health Organization*. https://www.semanticscholar.org/paper/48fff586e3c634de97e133f3c4adde31aa21266c (accessed on 13 May 2025).
11. da Silva, C., Matambisso, G., Boene, S., Rovira-Vallbona, E., Pujol, A., Komiche, K., Sanchez, A., et al. (2024). *Plasmodium falciparum* molecular surveillance to inform the Mozambican National Malaria Control Program strategy: Protocol. *VeriXiv*. https://www.semanticscholar.org/paper/407626c5e532c37b13ee9b0c8f6141ee86c9bd50 (accessed on 13 May 2025).

12. Dyck, V. A., Hendrichs, J., & Robinson, A. S. (2020). *Sterile Insect Technique*. CRC Press eBooks. https://doi.org/10.1201/9781003035572.

13. Feachem, R.G.A., with A.A. Phillips and G.A. Targett (eds) (2009). Shrinking the Malaria Map: A Prospectus on Malaria Elimination. San Francisco: The Global Health Group, Global Health Sciences, University of California, San Francisco.Ferrari, A. J., Santomauro, D., Aali, A., Abate, Y. H., Abbafati, C., Abbastabar, H., Abd ElHafeez, S., et al. (2024). Global incidence, prevalence, years lived with disability (YLDs), disability-adjusted life-years (DALYs), and healthy life expectancy (HALE) for 371 diseases and injuries in 204 countries and territories and 811 subnational locations, 1990–2021: A systematic analysis for the Global Burden of Disease Study 2021. *The Lancet, 403*, 2133–2161. https://doi.org/10.1016/S0140-6736(24)00757-8.

14. George, A. M., Ansumana, R., de Souza, D. K., Niyas, V. K. M., Zumla, A., & Bockarie, M. J. (2023). Climate change and the rising incidence of vector-borne diseases globally. *International Journal of Infectious Diseases, 139*, 143–145. https://doi.org/10.1016/j.ijid.2023.12.004.

15. Global HIV Prevention Working Group. (2010). *Global HIV Prevention Progress Report Card 2010*. https://core.ac.uk/download/71351545.pdf (accessed on 13 May 2025).

16. Hasyim, H., Heroza, R. I., Misnaniarti, M., Idris, H., Maharani, F. E., & Dale, P. (2024). Malaria surveillance information system using an Android mobile phone: A qualitative study in Lahat District, South Sumatra Province, Indonesia. *Malaysian Journal of Medicine and Health Sciences*. https://www.semanticscholar.org/paper/244eeb587349955cd0fb510959f7ff74422 78ae7 (accessed on 13 May 2025).

17. Huang, F., Blaschke, S., & Lucas, H. C. (2017). Beyond pilotitis: Taking digital health interventions to the national level in China and Uganda. *Globalization and Health, 13*, 1–7. https://doi.org/10.1186/s12992-017-0275-z.

18. Hyde, E., Bonds, M. H., Ihantamalala, F., Miller, A. C., Cordier, L., Razafinjato, B., Andriambolamanana, H., et al. (2021). Estimating the local spatio-temporal distribution of malaria from routine health information systems in areas of low healthcare access and reporting. *International Journal of Health Geographics, 20*. https://doi.org/10.1186/s12942-021-00262-4.

19. Inoue, H., & Minghui, R. (2017). Antimicrobial resistance: Translating political commitment into national action. *Bulletin of the World Health Organization, 95*, 242–242. https://www.semanticscholar.org/paper/481b9adfb1a15df3854dd630921451b67a615272 (accessed on 13 May 2025).

20. Juvekar, A., & Hegde, A. (2024). Persistent global health threats: The impact of infectious diseases in resource-limited regions. *Conduct Science Proceedings*. https://doi.org/10.55157/conductscience-proceedings.2024.1.52(accessed on 13 May 2025).

21. Krittanawong, C., & Kaplin, S. L. (2021). Artificial intelligence in global health. *European Heart Journal*. https://www.semanticscholar.org/paper/3d0fd9bf646f280b447e6dd9ffb299 93133b2a94 (accessed on 13 May 2025).

22. Mabona, M., Zwane, T., Raman, J., Kuonza, L., Mhlongo, B., & Phafane, P. (2024). Evaluation of the malaria case surveillance system in KwaZulu-Natal Province, South Africa, 2022: A focus on DHIS2. *Malaria Journal, 23*. https://www.semanticscholar.org/paper/d1f10492b1b860a2e43bbc844f0b89c0cf310eea (accessed on 13 May 2025).

23. Mace, K. E., Arguin, P. M., Lucchi, N. W., & Tan, K. R. (2019). Malaria surveillance–United States,

2016. *MMWR Surveillance Summaries, 68*, 1–35. https://doi.org/10.15585/mmwr.ss6805a1.

24. Mayor, A., da Silva, C., Rovira-Vallbona, E., Roca-Feltrer, A., Bonnington, C., Wharton–Smith, A., Greenhouse, B., et al. (2022). Prospective surveillance study to detect antimalarial drug resistance, gene deletions of diagnostic relevance and genetic diversity of *Plasmodium falciparum* in Mozambique: Protocol. *BMJ Open, 12*, e063456. https://doi.org/10.1136/bmjopen-2022-063456.

25. Mbunge, E., Akinnuwesi, B., Fashoto, S. G., Metfula, A., & Mashwama, P. (2020). A critical review of emerging technologies for tackling COVID-19 pandemic. *Human Behavior and Emerging Technologies, 3*(1), 25–39. https://doi.org/10.1002/hbe2.237.

26. Morgan, O., Aguilera, X., Ammon, A., Amuasi, J., Fall, I. S., Frieden, T. R., Heymann, D., et al. (2021). Disease surveillance for the COVID-19 era: Time for bold changes. *The Lancet, 397*, 2317–2319. https://doi.org/10.1016/s0140-6736(21)01096-5.

27. Murray, C. J. L., Ikuta, K. S., Sharara, F., Swetschinski, L. R., Robles Aguilar, G., Gray, A. P., Han, C., et al. (2022). Global burden of bacterial antimicrobial resistance in 2019: A systematic analysis. *The Lancet, 399*, 629–655. https://doi.org/10.1016/S0140-6736(21)02724-0.

28. Naghavi, M., Ong, K. L., Aali, A., Ababneh, H., Abate, Y. H., Abbafati, C., Abbasgholizadeh, R., et al. (2024). Global burden of 288 causes of death and life expectancy decomposition in 204 countries and territories and 811 subnational locations, 1990–2021: A systematic analysis for the Global Burden of Disease Study 2021. *The Lancet, 403*, 2100–2132. https://doi.org/10.1016/s0140-6736(24)00367-2.

29. Nekorchuk, D. M., Gebrehiwot, T., Lake, M., Awoke, W., Mihretie, A., & Wimberly, M. C. (2021). Comparing malaria early detection methods in a declining transmission setting in northwestern Ethiopia. *BMC Public Health, 21*. https://doi.org/10.1186/s12889-021-10850-5.

30. Nkengasong, J. N., & Mankoula, W. (2020). Looming threat of COVID-19 infection in Africa: Act collectively, and fast. *The Lancet, 395*, 841–842. https://doi.org/10.1016/s0140-6736(20)30464-5.

31. Nkengasong, J. N., & Tessema, S. K. (2020). Africa needs a new public health order to tackle infectious disease threats. *Cell, 183*, 296–300. https://doi.org/10.1016/j.cell.2020.09.041.

32. Okumu, F., Gyapong, M., Casamitjana, N., Castro, M. C., Itoe, M. A., Okonofua, F., & Tanner, M. (2022). What Africa can do to accelerate and sustain progress against malaria. *PLOS Global Public Health, 2*. https://www.semanticscholar.org/paper/4be9aaf8795726e71bfac78cbfe720620d5080c7 (accessed on 13 May 2025).

33. Piret, J., & Boivin, G. (2021). Pandemics throughout history. *Frontiers in Microbiology, 11*, 631736. https://doi.org/10.3389/fmicb.2020.631736.

34. Rotejanaprasert, C., Malaphone, V., Maysay, M., Chindavongsa, K., Banouvong, V., Khamlome, B., Vilay, P., et al. (2024). Malaria epidemiology, surveillance and response for elimination in Lao PDR. *Infectious Diseases of Poverty, 13*. https://www.semanticscholar.org/paper/78db852c3325b4ee7a034a08752413b4764dda81 (accessed on 13 May 2025).

35. Roth, G. A., Abate, D., Abate, K. H., Abay, S. M., Abbafati, C., Abbasi, N., Abbastabar, H., et al. (2018). Global, regional, and national age-sex-specific mortality for 282 causes of death in 195 countries and territories, 1980–2017: A systematic analysis for the Global Burden of Disease Study 2017. *The Lancet, 392*, 1736–1788. https://doi.org/10.1016/s0140-6736(18)32203-7.

36. Sousa, A., Alba, M. A., Vetter, M., García-Barrón, L., & Morales, J. (2020). Spatiotemporal distribution of malaria in Spain in a global change context. *Atmosphere, 11*(4), 346. https://doi.org/10.3390/atmos11040346.

37. Syabrina, Ratih, Wang, & Gunawan. (2024). Predictive analysis of malaria cases in Indonesia using machine learning. https://core.ac.uk/download/629198898.pdf (accessed on 13 May 2025).

38. Tembiné, H., Tapo, A. A., Danioko, S., & Traoré, A. (2024). Machine intelligence in Africa: A survey. https://doi.org/10.36227/techrxiv.170555182.20418305/v1.

39. Thomas, A., Bakaï, T. A., Atcha-Oubou, T., Tchadjobo, T., & Voirin, N. (2020). Implementation of a malaria sentinel surveillance system in Togo: A pilot study. *Malaria Journal, 19*. https://doi.org/10.1186/s12936-020-03399-y.

40. Tizifa, T. (2024). Exploring factors impacting the implementation of community-based malaria control, malaria burden, and surveillance in southern Malawi: Insights from the community and health system perspective. https://core.ac.uk/download/620593730.pdf (accessed on 13 May 2025).

41. Troeger, C., Blacker, B. F., Rahim, F., Rao, P. C., Cao, J., Zimsen, S. R. M., Albertson, S. B., et al. (2018). Estimates of the global, regional, and national morbidity, mortality, and aetiologies of lower respiratory infections in 195 countries, 1990–2016: A systematic analysis for the Global Burden of Disease Study 2016. *The Lancet Infectious Diseases, 18*, 1191–1210. https://doi.org/10.1016/S1473-3099(18)30310-4.

42. United Nations Environment Programme. (2023). *Environmental Rule of Law: Tracking Progress and Charting Future Directions*. https://doi.org/10.59117/20.500.11822/43943.

43. United Nations. (2016). *Millennium Development Goals Report*. https://doi.org/10.18356/98544aa9-en.

44. Zhao, X., Thanapongtharm, W., Lawawirojwong, S., Wei, C., Tang, Y., Zhou, Y. W., Sun, X., et al. (2020). Malaria risk map using spatial multi-criteria decision analysis along Yunnan border during the pre-elimination period. *American Journal of Tropical Medicine and Hygiene, 103*, 793–809. https://doi.org/10.4269/ajtmh.19-0854.

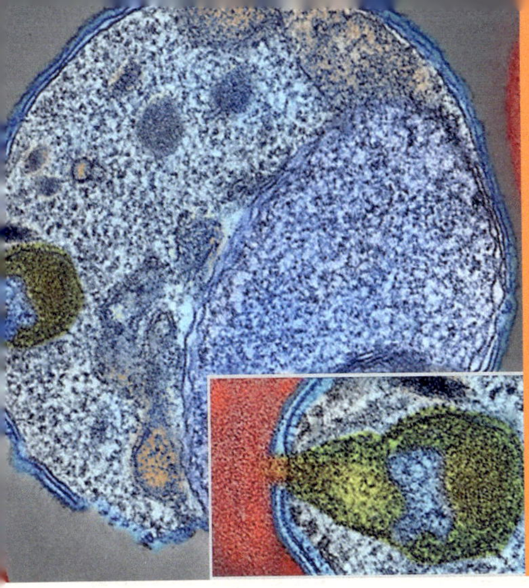

Chapter 11

OUTBREAK INVESTIGATION OF MALARIA

Contents

Introduction

Malaria remains a significant public health concern globally—periods of progress in control and elimination notwithstanding. The disease transmission isn't simple; it's a complicated interaction of individuals, mosquitoes, and the environment. In regions with loose borders, both human and insect travel allow malaria to leak through territories. Some recent research, for instance, discusses "border-spill malaria" as a term to describe what occurs when infected mosquitoes roam across country borders. Such spread can trigger fresh areas of infection even in areas that largely managed to keep it under wraps (Lin et al., 2022). Outbreak checks, therefore, must consider everything, ranging from broad case volume to mosquito and parasite specifics—to truly stay one step ahead of any outbreaks. Having a good system in place to detect and combat outbreaks is the important thing, and China's experience proves that in spades. Having initiated its National Malaria Elimination Action Plan in 2010, they promoted an approach called the "1–3–7" strategy. Essentially, a case is reported on day one, investigated in depth in three days, and if there is some potential source of trouble, it is tackled within seven days. Jiangsu Province is a case in point; during 2001–2020, its improved surveillance eliminated local cases by 2012, and the intelligent monitoring of imported cases prevented re-emergence (Cao et al., 2022). Such systems not only eliminate outbreaks promptly but also prevent malaria from occurring by remaining vigilant to risks from additional importation. Nevertheless, malaria has a habit of persistently existing in areas along borders, and combatting outbreaks there isn't necessarily easy. Research usually has to take into account such factors as how tightly individuals are settled along dangerous areas and how mobile the population is locally. For example, research along the China–Myanmar border revealed that worker shelters within 300 meters of internally displaced persons' camps experienced a significantly higher risk of *Plasmodium vivax* infection, presumably because infected Anopheles mosquitoes have a propensity to stray into these areas.

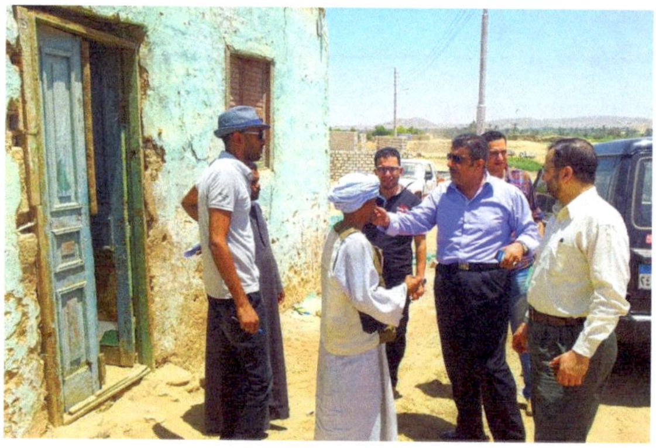

Figure 11.1. Malaria outbreak investigation.

Source: Picryl. (2015). *Malaria Outbreak Investigation, Egypt.*

In most instances, this indicates that both the hiding places of the parasite and the flight distances of the mosquitoes play a pivotal role in driving cross-border transmission (Lin et al., 2022). Overall, successful outbreak investigations must combine spatial analysis with intensive monitoring of vectors, a reminder that remaining malaria-free requires relentless, adaptive public health work (Figure 11.1).

Malaria is not only an illness, it's a complex combination of biology and social effect. Fundamentally, it's brought on by *Plasmodium* parasites that invade red blood cells, typically transmitted by female Anopheles mosquitoes. You may have realized that once they're inside, these parasites cause fever, chills, and anemia; in genuinely serious instances, they may even cause death. In general terms, the problem lies in the fact that malaria has a tendency to persist in so many varied settings, and that makes it difficult to control. Instead of just blaming it on one aspect, you are left having to determine precisely which parasite is involved, which mosquito is transmitting it, and how we are responding. This perspective – addressing malaria as a health problem and an ecological enigma – goes some way to account for why outbreak investigations regularly incorporate environmental, biological, and social screenings (Gregory et al., 2018). If you attempt to define malaria globally, it becomes even more complicated. Regions manage its burden in wildly disparate manners. Even with some reduction in death rates, in most low-income communities the disease continues to rage largely because infrastructure and resources for adequate treatment and prevention are lacking. Such vulnerable populations as small children and pregnant women are usually the ones most affected, further exacerbating pre-existing health disparities. There is also the reality that symptoms can differ quite significantly from individual to individual, due to variability in the exact *Plasmodium* species and how effective an individual's immune system is. All of this ultimately confuses diagnosis and reporting, which in turn distorts the data relied on when it comes to monitoring outbreaks. And in general, it requires that controlling malaria requires research approaches that are specific to the particular economic and environmental conditions in a region (Gregory et al., 2018). Attempting to pin down malaria in outbreak situations requires a fairly broad perspective on health in general. The One Health concept, for example, reminds us of that human, animal, and environmental health are all working together in complex ways. One moment, you're looking at how human behavior and mosquito bites interact; the next, you're considering climate patterns that shift where mosquitoes breed or how fast parasites develop. It turns out that mixing ecological studies, evolutionary insights, and clinical science, even if it sometimes feels a bit all over the place—gives a clearer picture of what's driving an outbreak. This integrated mode of thought, for all its eccentricities and inconsistency in punctuation, truly directs clever interventions into places where global health policy plans to intervene to eradicate developing infection dangers through thoroughgoing, ensemble style action (Destoumieux et al., 2018).

Importance of Outbreak Investigations

Outbreak investigations are an essential part of public health in that they identify where infection begins and how it is transmitted. In most instances, particularly in areas where malaria still poses gigantic health burdens, understanding the patterns of infection is quite literally crucial to informing targeted interventions. Malaria symptoms can masquerade as other feverish diseases; a challenge only exacerbated by illnesses like COVID-19, where fever, fatigue, and shortness of breath tend to accompany each other. In the majority of instances, this overlap renders it difficult to differentiate between illnesses, and minor errors in diagnosis can disrupt appropriate control efforts and treatment. Rapid laboratory tests, which typically verify the diagnosis, are essential not only for proper management of cases but also to check wider dissemination in the community. Using rapid diagnostics in areas with limited resources becomes a must-do step, helping to direct scarce health resources efficiently and reduce fatalities (Chanda et al., 2020). These investigations also yield a wealth of epidemiological details that ultimately shape policy decisions and resource allocation. Detailed mapping of malaria during outbreaks can unearth weak points in health systems and highlight which groups, often due to socio-demographic or environmental reasons, are at greater risk. That type of information, in general, enhances the effectiveness of prevention activities such as encouraging insecticide-treated nets, performing indoor spraying, and making antimalarial medicines available to those who urgently require them. Natural surveillance efforts at times even identify asymptomatic carriers who quietly spread the infection around. Mixing in such creative new tools as clinical metagenomic next-generation sequencing (mNGS) creates new avenues to take a closer eye to pathogens, identify co-infections or impending variants before they become full-blown, and even assist in mapping out resistance patterns and host immune response to an extent that informs treatment decisions and makes broader public health actions (Charles et al., 2019). At a wider scale, the influence of outbreak investigations extends far beyond direct patient treatment. They commonly expose inadequacies in diagnostic capability and case management—insights that spur investment necessary in laboratory infrastructure and staff training. Such an investigation by its very nature harmonizes various stakeholders and encourages cross-sector collaboration, which is necessary where malaria is coinciding with overlapping threats such as COVID-19. Routine surveillance and periodic re-assessments, guided by investigation findings, enable authorities to modify control interventions over time. By reducing transmission, and curtailing cases and deaths, these interventions help achieve sustainable malaria control and pave the way for eventual elimination. With new infections more frequently mixing with established health issues, maintaining effective, responsive outbreak investigation protocols proves to be an essential component in preserving global health gains and alleviating the overall disease burden (Charles et al., 2019; Chanda et al., 2020;) (Figure 11.2).

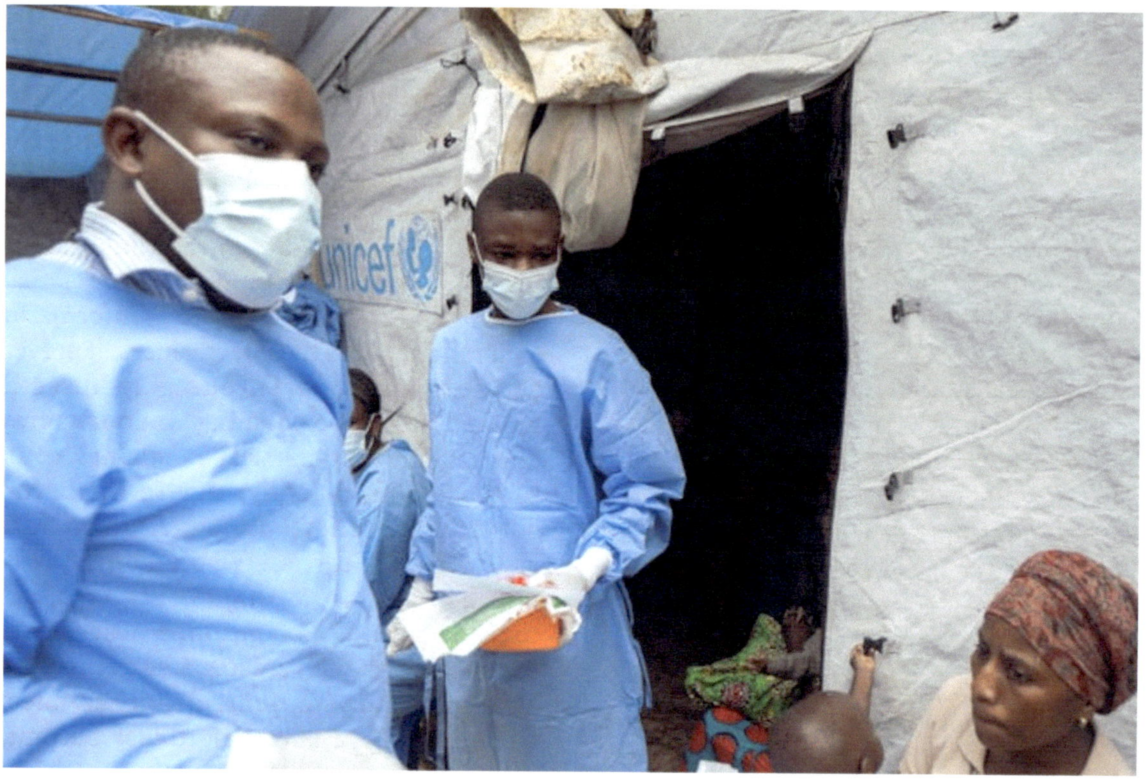

Figure 11.2. Outbreak investigations.

Source: USA Today. (2024). *Health Worker Responds to Outbreak in Congo.*

11.1. Background of Malaria

Malaria still poses a major global health worry, hitting tropical and subtropical areas especially hard. Female Anopheles mosquitoes bite people subsequently pass along the *Plasmodium* parasite that causes the disease. Sometimes, things like stagnating water near homes end up creating perfect little nurseries for these pathogens. It's not just the environment either—human routines play a part, too. For instance, one recent outbreak showed that being outdoors early in the morning or later in the evening bumped up infection risks even when measures like indoor residual spraying and public education campaigns had already been tried (Masango et al., 2020). Grasping these mixed factors is pretty key when trying to figure out how to tailor interventions to each unique outbreak—for many reasons, these details matter a lot. Looking back, malaria control usually relied on a combination of pathogen control, preventive drugs, and basic health messaging. Indoor residual spraying and insecticide-treated nets have certainly cut down transmission in many regions, yet these steps can only go so far if extra risk factors persist. People wearing protective clothing during high-risk times, for example, have shown noticeably lower rates of infection. Outdoor spaces that let mosquitoes breed freely, and even small design flaws in houses like open eaves—can let these insects in, which research has pointed out (Masango et al., 2020). In most cases, the fight against malaria is a complex challenge, one that mixes nature, everyday habits, and the homes we live in, underscoring the need for more integrated approaches. New diagnostic technologies have shifted the game in how we hunt down infectious diseases. Methods like clinical metagenomic next-generation sequencing (mNGS) are now catching a wide array of pathogens at once while also offering hints about how our bodies react. Sure, rapid diagnostic tests still play a central role when malaria outbreaks occur, but mNGS is showing promise by also detecting co-infections and even resistance patterns that could help adjust treatments. Mixing these cutting-edge tools with traditional outbreak tracking can boost our overall response, opening the door to smarter public health moves. Generally speaking, as the battle against malaria evolves, leaning on such innovative methods seems set to advance our surveillance and containment efforts in even the trickiest settings (Figure 11.3).

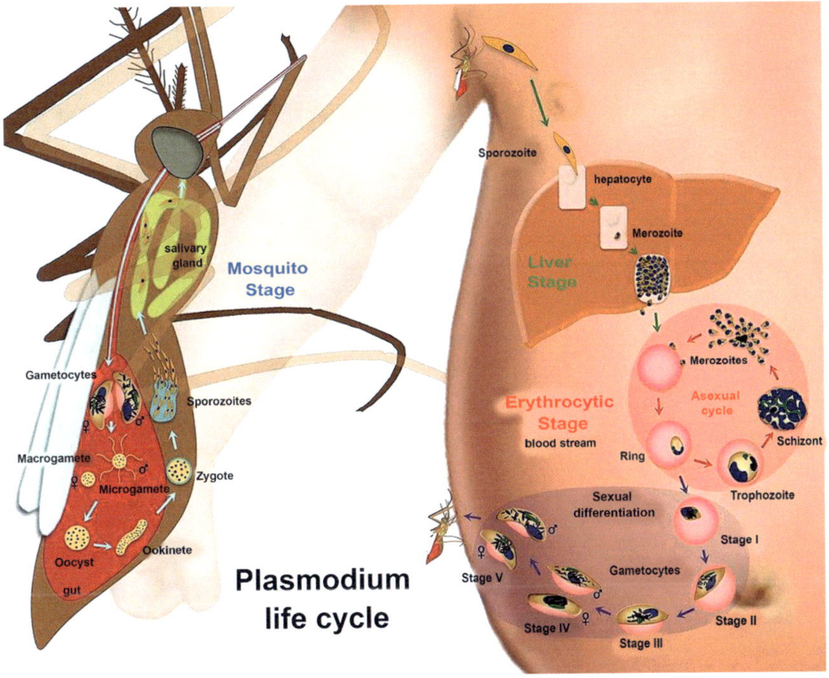

Figure 11.3. The background of malaria.

Source: By Le Roche Lab, UC Riverside - http://ucrtoday.ucr.edu/19520, CC BY 3.0, https://commons.wikimedia.org/w/index.php?curid=32649865

11.1.1. Historical Context of Malaria

Humans and infectious diseases have been complex up for ages—malaria, in particular, has long been a stubborn problem that reshaped public health in ways beyond just health issues. It wasn't merely a matter of sickness; the ripple effects touched economic productivity and even shifted population patterns across different regions. People long ago noticed bouts of fever in marshy areas and began speculating about foul air, eventually winding up with the idea that mosquitoes were the troublemakers. That insight, arriving after countless observations and gradual scientific refinement, wasn't a lone spark but rather part of a winding journey of understanding. Urban sprawl and increased travel eventually shuffled the spread of malaria, reminding us of that changes in the environment, social life, and even everyday human movement all play a part in the association of disease transmission. Fast-forward to the 20th century, and discoveries in parasitology and entomology reshaped our thinking on how outbreaks should be tackled. The identification of *Plasmodium* species as the culprits behind malaria prompted a deeper look into its life cycle and how it spreads; meanwhile, related research on other mosquito-borne viruses—arboviruses, for example, hinted that managing these insect populations wasn't as cut-and-dried as once thought. Africa's long history as a hotbed for mosquito-related illnesses, malaria included, underscored broader challenges for global health. With more people traveling, populations booming, and ecosystems fluctuating, new complications in containing outbreaks arose, generally speaking, and highlighted the need for a mixed, multidisciplinary approach that learns from past successes and setbacks (Braack et al., 2018).

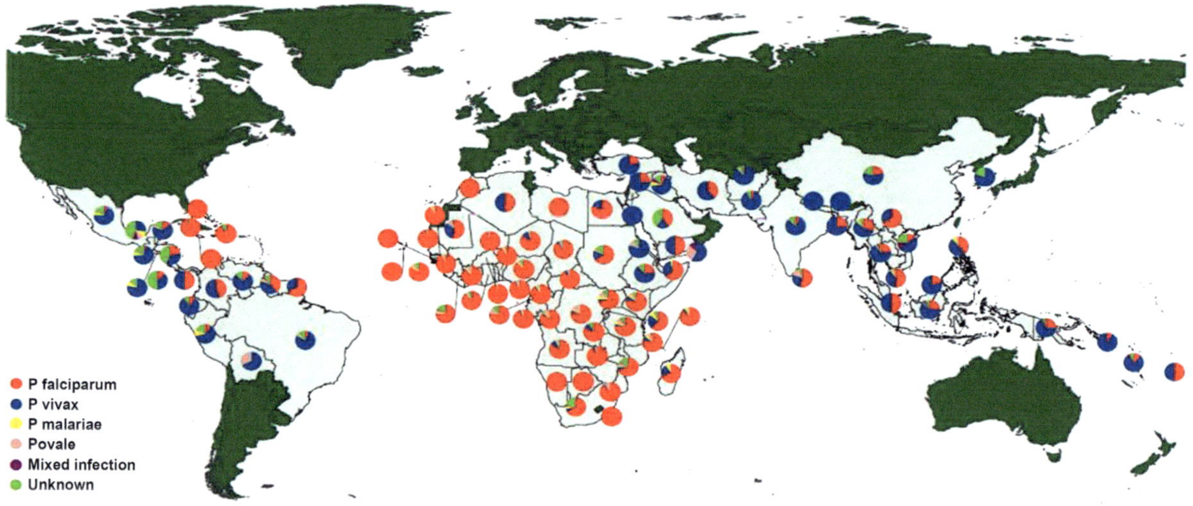

Figure 11.4. Historical context of malaria.

Source: By Tatem AJ, Jia P, Ordanovich D, Falkner M, Huang Z, Howes R - Tatem AJ, Jia P, Ordanovich D, Falkner M, Huang Z, Howes R (2017). "The geography of imported malaria to non-endemic countries: a meta-analysis of nationally reported statistics.". Lancet Infect Dis 17 (1): 98-107. DOI:10.1016/S1473-3099(16)30326-7. PMID 27777030. PMC: 5392593., CC BY 4.0, https://commons.wikimedia.org/w/index.php?curid=129748586

Looking back at how malaria has evolved helps set the stage for how we study modern outbreaks. Early breakthroughs in the 1900s, like Carlos Chagas' work on vector-borne diseases—demonstrated that even focused, single-disease studies could open up whole networks of epidemiological insight (Kárita et al., 2019). Over time, the persistent challenges in diagnosing, treating, and preventing malaria began to reveal themselves amid a backdrop of changing environments and shifting pathogen strains. In most cases, taking the historical context into account proves indispensable when designing interventions that address both the biological mysteries and social realities of these outbreaks. Mixing lessons from the past with today's surveillance and control techniques can ultimately lead to quicker, more effective responses that ease transmission and lessen malaria's heavy impact on communities worldwide (Figure 11.4).

11.1.2. Epidemiology and Global Distribution

Population growth and urban sprawl flip the script on how diseases like malaria show up and spread. Urban living is on the rise, especially in sub-Saharan Africa, where more than half the world's people already call cities home, a number that's predicted to hit about 68% by 2050. When individuals move into these buzzing cityscapes, it shakes up mosquito habitats, bumps up human–mosquito encounters, and alters the mix of environmental risks. City areas tend to have uneven malaria patterns, affected by things like migration, housing features, and crowding. So, plans to handle mosquitoes and public health need to stay on their toes. In most cases, getting a feel for how people and space interact in urban spots is key to keeping outbreaks at bay (Matthew et al., 2019).

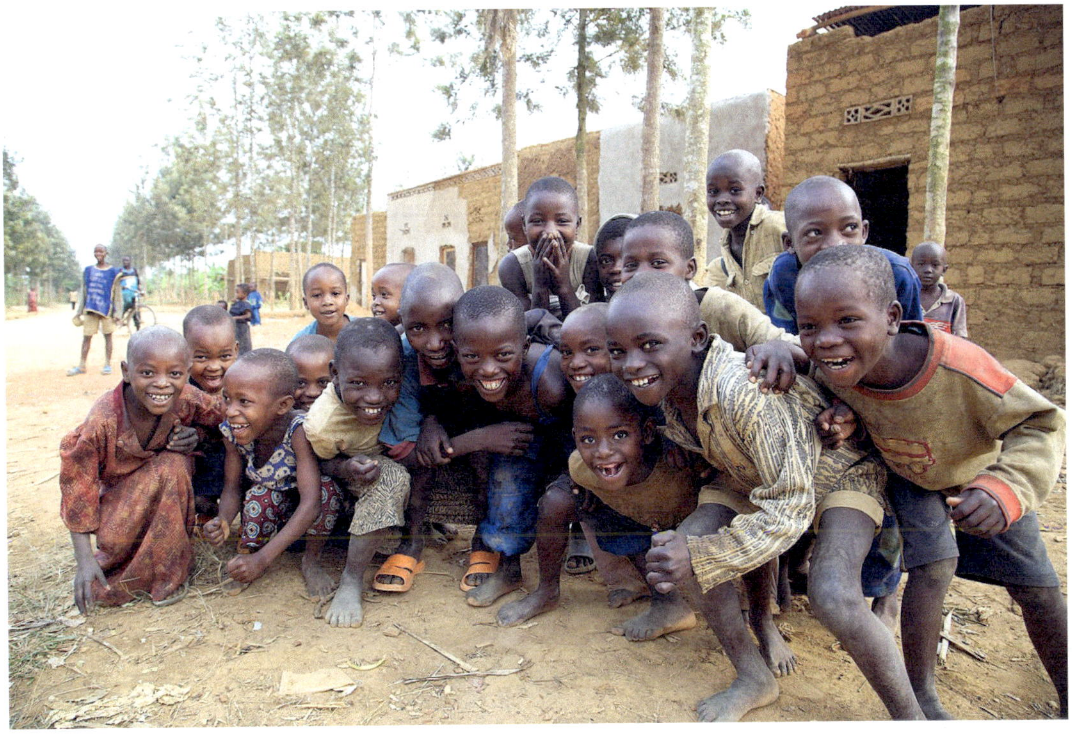

Figure 11.5. Global distribution of malaria.

Source: By President's Malaria Initiative - Credit: Brant Stewart, RTI, Public Domain, https://commons.wikimedia.org/w/index.php?curid=72085419

Looking at global death trends shows how malaria's weight shifts within the broader mix of diseases. Malaria still takes a toll in many endemic regions, but recent health numbers also point to fewer deaths from communicable, maternal, neonatal, and nutritional issues though the drop isn't even everywhere. Low-income countries, for instance, often see stubborn hotspots because their health systems can't always keep up. Generally speaking, having detailed, location-specific death data is pretty important for breaking down outbreaks and clearing up how to share resources. The Global Burden of Diseases Study even suggests that mixing in both overall death counts and cause-specific details can help fine-tune interventions to balance the impacts between city and country settings (Gregory et al., 2018). On a global level, malaria's spread winds up being complex with environmental, social, and demographic threads. Tropical and subtropical regions, like much of sub-Saharan Africa—bear the heaviest burden because conditions there naturally favor Anopheles mosquitoes and the transmission of the *Plasmodium* parasite. Poverty, limited access to healthcare, and patchy public health networks tend to fan the flames of outbreaks further. Plus, with climate change and cities expanding in unexpected ways, mosquito behavior and disease patterns get even trickier to predict. In most cases, digging into these local details is crucial for setting up surveillance, prevention, and treatment efforts that address all the unique challenges malaria throws at us (Gregory et al., 2018; Matthew et al., 2019) (Figure 11.5).

11.1.3. Life Cycle of the Malaria Parasite

Malaria isn't just a straightforward pathogen, it's a wild, multi-layered story starring the *Plasmodium* parasite, which flips between human bodies and mosquitoes. It generally starts when an infected Anopheles mosquito takes a blood meal and—almost without warning—injects sporozoites into the bloodstream. Those little invaders quickly hustle over to the liver where, without causing a fuss, they slip into liver cells and multiply over several days. When they're fully grown, they burst out as merozoites, setting off waves of red blood cell invasion, reproduction, and eventual rupture. In most cases, these repeated cycles spark the typical symptoms of malaria. This challenging, ever-changing life cycle is a big part of why controlling the disease remains so tough, especially in areas with conditions that naturally boost transmission and where healthcare resources are limited (Gregory et al., 2018). Once the parasite has replicated asexually in red blood cells, things take an interesting turn. A subset of merozoites shifts gears and turns into gametocytes—these are essentially the sexual forms that keep the cycle on track. When a mosquito feeds, it unwittingly picks up these gametocytes, which then kick off gametogenesis in its midgut. Soon enough, fertilization happens, forming a zygote that quickly changes into an ookinete. This form, almost boldly, penetrates through the mosquito's gut wall to settle as an oocyst. Inside that oocyst, through a process called sporogony, loads of sporozoites are produced; these eventually wander over to the mosquito's salivary glands, meaning the insect is set to infect another human. This looping process—complex and unpredictable—is what keeps malaria circulating in endemic populations, and it highlights why efforts to tackle outbreaks must address both the human and mosquito sides of the story (Gregory et al., 2018). Climate also has its say in malaria's spread. Temperature, humidity, and even rainfall patterns can reshape the breeding spots for Anopheles mosquitoes and even alter how fast the parasite develops inside its host. Generally speaking, rising global temperatures have been linked to shifts in mosquito ranges and longer transmission seasons, which can sometimes lead to outbreaks in places that had things under control before. At the same time, variable weather can mess with control measures by altering mosquito populations and changing parasite development rates, making outbreak investigations even more of a challenge. With drug and insecticide resistance on the rise, along with the curveballs thrown by climate change, ongoing research and flexible public health strategies become absolutely critical if we hope to lessen malaria's impact on global health.

11.2. Symptoms and Diagnosis

In many places battling malaria outbreaks, early detection often runs into trouble because the symptoms can be so similar to those of other infections. People usually mention fever, chills, headache, and a general sense of being unwell. These signs aren't unique to malaria at all – they emerge in other tropical illnesses too. It sometimes forces doctors to work hard at figuring out whether the patient has malaria or another feverish condition (AUFI).

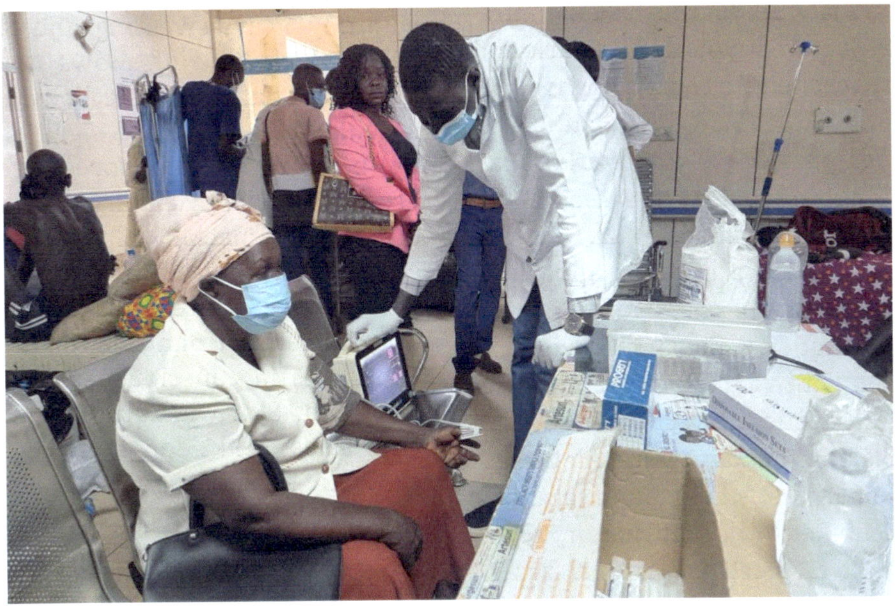

Figure 11.6. Diagnosis battling malaria outbreaks.

Source: Gavi. (2024). *Patient Undergoing Health Check During Malaria Outbreak.*

Things get even more complex when, say, respiratory infections are also making rounds at the same time. Getting a handle on the diagnosis quickly is vital since any delay not only risks more harm to the patient but also can lead to increased spread of the disease. In most cases, mixing a keen suspicion with a solid look at the patient's travel and exposure history becomes the key to understanding the symptoms well enough to jump into timely treatment and outbreak control. Diagnosing malaria during an outbreak comes down to mixing what you see in a patient with lab tests that back up the clinical findings. Microscopic checks of stained blood smears are still considered the gold standard because they let health workers spot the *Plasmodium* parasites and figure out the species and the parasite load. Still, this approach runs into a problem when experienced lab staff and resources are in short supply – a common issue in remote or low-resource settings. That's where rapid diagnostic tests (RDTs) step in; they deliver fast, fairly accurate results by detecting malaria antigens in blood samples. But one has to be careful with these tests, since they might confuse malaria with other febrile illnesses that show up similarly even though they call for different treatments. To summarize, careful laboratory confirmation is a must to clearly separate malaria cases from other infections and steer the right public health responses. Trouble often arises when outbreaks of other febrile illnesses mimic malaria – a situation that stresses the need for detailed differential diagnosis during epidemics. Diseases like dengue and certain viral respiratory infections can cause fever, muscle aches, and fatigue, yet they usually miss some of the key features typical of malaria. In most cases, early challenges came to light with newer pathogens like SARS-CoV-2; clinicians found themselves puzzled by the overlapping symptoms and not-so-specific lab results in tropical areas (Nunthavichitra et al., 2020). This overlap pushes for a broader approach where clinical judgment goes hand in hand with advanced lab techniques. A thorough review of symptoms, mixed with valuable epidemiologic data, can boost diagnostic accuracy when several infections are making rounds at once. All things considered, a sharp, on-the-ground clinical investigation combined with confirmatory tests helps ensure that targeted treatments reach the right patients and that disease containment measures hit their mark (Hu et al., 2020) (Figure 11.6).

11.2.1. Common Symptoms of Malaria

Malaria is a parasite-borne illness that shows up with many symptoms and catching it early, even though it can be challenging—is key to stopping outbreaks. At first, people often notice vague signs like fever, chills, or headaches that might easily be mixed up with other common illnesses. In most cases, these initial clues show up between a week and a month after an infected Anopheles mosquito bite, which is the main culprit handing over the *Plasmodium* parasite. A recurring fever, typically coming back every 48–72 hours, stands out as a classic sign that ties in with the parasite's activity in red blood cells. Fatigue and muscle aches usually follow along, adding to the overall feeling of being off. Spotting these signals early on is super important for getting treatment in time and nipping any outbreak in the bud—any delay might just make things worse or boost transmission. As the infection goes on, extra symptoms tend to appear and muddle the picture. Sometimes, patients start to experience vomiting, heavy sweating, and even abdominal pain, which kind of shows how broadly the infection is affecting the body. In many cases, an enlarged spleen and signs of anemia show up because of widespread red blood cell breakdown, clearly emphasizing the seriousness of malaria, especially in vulnerable groups like young children and pregnant women. In more severe instances, cerebral malaria can develop; this dangerous condition, marked by seizures and shifts in consciousness, demands urgent attention. Since malaria's signs can overlap with illnesses like dengue or COVID-19, doctors generally need to rely on a full clinical checkup together with lab tests (Hu et al., 2020; Pascarella et al., 2020) to get a sure diagnosis. Lab tests remain the top method for confirming malaria because leaning on symptoms alone often leaves room for confusion. Rapid diagnostic tests and looking at blood smears under a microscope are the go-to ways to detect the *Plasmodium* parasite and figure out how many parasites are present. This diagnostic step is crucial not only for treating the individual but also for tracking disease spread through epidemiological mapping. Keeping an eye on common symptoms along with lab results helps health officials pick up on outbreak patterns and roll out specific measures, like managing mosquito populations and even using preventive treatments. Plus, spreading awareness about what to look for in communities tends to prompt earlier medical visits, which is vital during an outbreak. To summarize, understanding everything from those early fever spikes to the more severe complications is essential for mounting a truly effective response against malaria.

11.2.2. Diagnostic Methods Used in Malaria Detection

Managing malaria outbreaks starts with spotting the parasite fast and correctly. People have long used the classic method—examining Giemsa-stained blood smears under a microscope—to identify which *Plasmodium* type is at play and even to count the parasites. That said, this microscope work relies on well-trained eyes and can sometimes miss infections, especially when parasite levels are very low. To get around these issues, RDTs were introduced; they detect unique parasite antigens using immunochromatographic techniques.

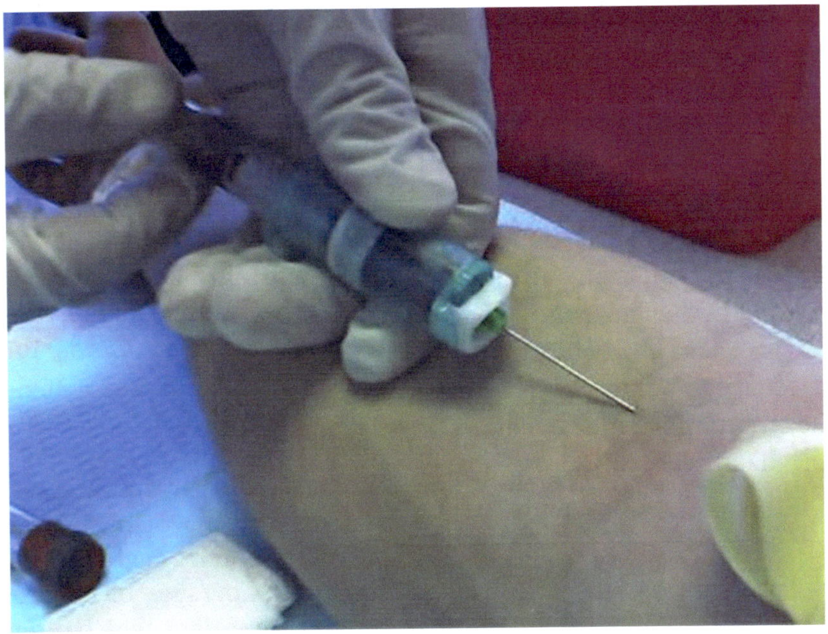

Figure 11.7. Diagnostic methods used in malaria detection.

Source: By Mad Max at the English-language Wikipedia, CC BY-SA 3.0, https://commons.wikimedia.org/w/index.php?curid=4128941

These tests deliver answers much quicker and can be easily used in the field without sprawling lab setups, although, in most cases, their sensitivity and specificity can fluctuate from one region to another, sometimes resulting in false negatives or positives. On a different note, modern molecular advances bring PCR-based methods into the mix as impressively sensitive tools. PCR works by amplifying tiny amounts of *Plasmodium* DNA from small blood samples, allowing detection of mixed infections and low-density parasitemia that might slip by unnoticed with microscopy or even RDTs. Generally speaking, this heightened sensitivity is crucial, particularly when asymptomatic carriers might be quietly fueling the spread, further complicating control efforts. Of course, PCR does come with its own set of hurdles; it requires sophisticated equipment, trained personnel, and stable lab conditions, which aren't always available in endemic or resource-limited settings. Newer innovations like loop-mediated isothermal amplification (LAMP) offer a practical compromise by combining high sensitivity with simpler gear. Together, these molecular methods can boost our accuracy in detecting cases and mapping outbreaks, ultimately guiding more targeted interventions. Yet, even as these diagnostic tools prove their worth, they need to be viewed within a broader epidemiological framework. Factors such as the local mix of *Plasmodium* types, the intensity of transmission, and the available resources all influence which method works best on the ground. Lately, the push for rapid, point-of-care testing—fueled in part by experiences with other outbreaks (Guo et al., 2020; Pascarella et al., 2020)—has underscored the importance of adaptable, scalable strategies. Sometimes mixing different approaches is the smartest move, since relying solely on one might miss parts of the picture. In the end, handling an outbreak effectively isn't just about having the latest diagnostics; it's also about applying them in a way that fits the outbreak's unique dynamics and the underlying healthcare infrastructure (Figure 11.7).

11.2.3. Challenges in Diagnosing Malaria

Accurate, speedy diagnosis is the cornerstone of outbreak investigations, even when dealing with malaria, which constantly complicates matters. Malaria's signs are pretty vague and can be easily mistaken for illnesses like dengue, typhoid, or various viral infections. The number of parasites in the blood can jump around depending on things like your body's defenses or the specific strain of the parasite, making it tough sometimes to spot them in a blood test. This means that a diagnosis might come too late or just might be wrong, which can then lead to treatments that don't hit the mark and more people getting sick. Microscopic examination still holds the title as the top test, but it relies on having both well-trained technicians and quality equipment—both of which can be in short supply in many areas. There's some buzz about using AI-based diagnostic aids too, and while they offer promise in boosting accuracy, they're still in the early days and have to overcome some ethical and technical bumps (Shuroug et al., 2023). On top of this, using many diagnostic tools adds another layer of uncertainty. In most cases, RDTs catch on for their simplicity and quick results, but even these can flounder when genetic mutations occur in the parasite or when there's just not enough parasite around to detect. The lack of a universally accepted test protocol also means that results can swing around from one region to the next, further muddling outbreak investigations. Subsequently there's the matter of serological tests—just as with diagnostics for emerging viruses, issues like cross-reactivity and the risk of false positives emerge and make antibody detection a bit of a mixed bag (Petherick, 2020). Generally speaking, these technical weak spots call for a deeper, more rigorous check of the diagnostics, so that the outbreak data truly reflects reality and helps to form an effective response. Beyond technical glitches, real-world, contextual hurdles can get in the way of a proper malaria diagnosis during outbreaks. Many regions battling malaria face constant shortages of diagnostic supplies and trained personnel, which often means cases slip through unnoticed.

The ever-changing pace of malaria transmission, swayed by environmental and socio-economic factors, makes it even more important to diagnose quickly so that targeted interventions can be applied. Yet, delays creep in when surveillance systems aren't up to speed or when health workers have to depend solely on clinical signs. Although the idea of incorporating new, AI-assisted interpretation methods looks promising for overcoming these barriers, it does require extra care to ensure that data privacy isn't compromised and that clinical oversight remains intact (Shuroug et al., 2023). In the end, wrestling with these layered challenges is key to boosting the accuracy of outbreak investigations and ultimately improving public health outcomes.

11.3. Transmission and Risk Factors

Anopheles mosquitoes carry the *Plasmodium* parasite and are at the center of how malaria spreads. They tend to settle in spots like stagnant water where egg laying and parasite growth naturally mix. Human activities—urban sprawl, certain farming methods, and the like, often end up creating extra breeding corners without anyone meaning to. Temperature changes, shifts in humidity, and even rainfall patterns can alter how many of these pathogens emerge and where they go, which in turn affects outbreak intensity. In most cases, figuring out how these natural cues mesh with our own actions is key. Merging what we know about mosquito behavior with local habit patterns might just help break the cycle and cut down disease in communities that are vulnerable. Travel also plays a big role in malaria's journey. Individuals moving between malaria-prone rural areas and urban centers, where immunity might not be as strong, can inadvertently carry the parasites farther than expected. Studies generally indicate that trips, especially ones to high-transmission zones or those involving little children, who tend to be even more at risk—increase the chance of infection by almost fourfold (Ahmed et al., 2020). This link is especially clear in parts of sub-Saharan Africa, where urban populations often face heightened vulnerability. Simple measures like better travel guidelines and targeted health education for mobile groups can help ease the spread. Recognizing that travel is just another way for parasites to hitch a ride deepens our overall grasp of containment strategies. Social and demographic factors add yet another twist to malaria's spread. In many poorer communities, access to things like insecticide-treated bed nets and prompt healthcare is limited, which not only ramps up exposure but can also slow down treatment. Groups such as pregnant women and immunologically naive children are hit even harder, partly because of these underlying gaps. Even local infrastructure, housing quality, sanitation, plays its part in how often humans come into contact with mosquitoes. All these elements need to be weighed together when laying out fair and effective intervention plans. Even though some studies zoom in on the transmission details of other diseases, keeping a sharp focus on malaria's own unique backdrop remains absolutely essential for public health responses that truly lower risks (Hu et al., 2020) (Figure 11.8).

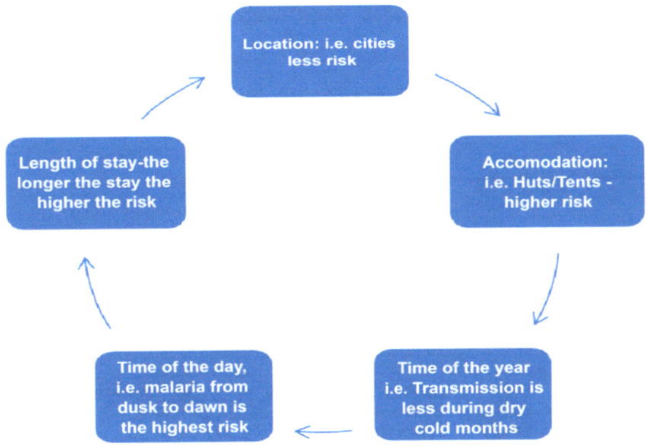

Figure 11.8. Malaria risk factors.

Source: Schellack, N. (n.d.). *Malaria Risk Factors*. ResearchGate.

11.3.1. Mosquito Vectors and Their Role

Mosquitoes and malaria have always been closely linked, almost like old partners in a association. Lately, shifting weather—warmer days and unexpected rains—has stirred things up, changing where these pathogens, especially those in the Anopheles group, tend to thrive. You get new mosquito hangouts emerging in places that once seemed safe, and when you factor in human travel and trade, the whole scene gets even messier. In most cases, getting a grip on both nature's features and our own impact is key to rethinking how we watch for and fight malaria outbreaks in different spots (George et al., 2023). Further, new mosquito types are starting to play a role in urban settings that traditionally didn't bear much malaria trouble. Take *Anopheles stephensi,* for example, it used to stick to South Asia and the Middle East but now shows up in several African areas where malaria is pretty common. Its quick spread into cities and nearby suburbs kind of flips the old script, because these places were once thought to be less welcoming to malaria pathogens. In Dire Dawa, Ethiopia, outbreaks have even pointed to a clear link between this mosquito and a spike in *Plasmodium falciparum* infections, reaffirming that it's now a player in urban transmission (Emiru et al., 2023). It's hard to ignore how this creature makes use of all sorts of breeding spots, including man-made containers, making it even more of a challenge in densely populated regions. Then there's the genetic twist—mosquito genes sometimes make them more open to *Plasmodium* parasites or more resistant to the chemicals we use against them. The joint appearance of *An. stephensi* and parasites marked with signs of drug and diagnostic resistance definitely sets off alarm bells for anyone counting on current treatments. Even our trusty tools like insecticide-treated nets and indoor sprays are taking a hit from populations of mosquitoes that have learned to dodge such measures. Generally speaking, this situation calls for a mix of control strategies, backed by a sharper look at mosquito genetics to spot emerging risks sooner rather than later. The bottom line is that ongoing research into mosquito behavior, breeding, and gene shifts, supported by enough funding, is absolutely essential if we're going to outsmart this ever-changing challenge (Emiru et al., 2023; George et al., 2023) (Figure 11.9).

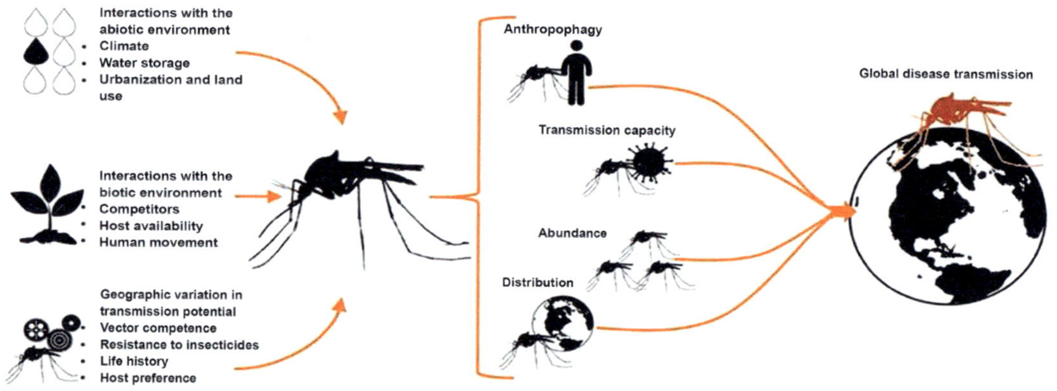

Figure 11.9. Mosquito vectors and their role.

Source: Murdock, C. (2017). *Mosquito-Pathogen-Host Interactions.* ResearchGate.

11.3.2. Environmental Factors Influencing Outbreaks

Environmental clues and malaria outbreaks mix in ways we're still piecing together. Temperature, moisture, and even how much it rains can mess with the mosquito life cycle—those Anopheles pathogens we all know play a major role. Warm days tend to speed up both how fast mosquitoes grow up and how quickly the parasite "cooks" inside them, often boosting the chance of disease spread. Then there's the flip side: wild weather events, like a sudden drought or a heavy downpour, might mess up old breeding spots or even accidentally set up new ones. Our own actions, too, like cutting down forests or changing the land—can shift local ecosystems and sometimes create better hideouts for these pathogens, upping the outbreak risk. To summarize, catching these subtle environmental twists lets researchers zero in on trouble spots and launch focused efforts to cut down mosquito numbers and break the cycle (Tudi et al., 2021). But it's not just Mother Nature at work—what we do matters as much. The factors behind malaria spread aren't only about natural climate swings; our agricultural habits play a big part as well. Pesticides, for example, are a mixed bag. Sure, they keep crop pests in check, but they can also stir up troubles with malaria transmission. In most cases, the runoff and persisting chemicals alter the natural balance, sometimes knocking down the numbers of creatures that usually keep mosquitoes in line—so the pathogens end up thriving even more. Also, because these chemicals hang around in soil and water, mosquitoes can eventually toughen up against insecticides. And, as our climate warms, changes in how we apply pesticides and rising pollution levels might further alter the very environments mosquitoes call home. In a way, all these complex issues call for a carefully mixed approach—one that takes agricultural development and mosquito control hand in hand—to curb malaria outbreaks (Tudi et al., 2021). New tools in spatial life course epidemiology are giving us fresh ways to get a grip on malaria's ebbs and flows. Scientists now use things like geographic mapping, remote sensing, and data crunching with spatial analytics to watch how shifts in weather and land changes affect both the pathogens and the people. These tools let researchers dive into data about temperature swings, rain patterns, land modifications, and even how individuals move around, helping them uncover when and where the risks spike. It seems that the environment, mosquito populations, and human behaviors are always on the move—a constantly evolving puzzle that makes malaria risk hard to pin down. Generally speaking, these innovative approaches boost our forecasts and readiness, paving the way for more spot-on public health moves (Jia et al., 2020).

11.3.3. Socioeconomic Factors Affecting Vulnerability

Socioeconomic struggles set the stage for malaria outbreaks in many communities. In areas where poverty keeps families struggling, living conditions often end up favoring mosquito breeding while proper healthcare remains out of reach. Low education levels and high unemployment further complicate the picture, making it tougher for people to learn about or adopt simple preventive measures. Factors like caste, religion, and whether you live in a bustling city or a quiet town mix in unexpected ways to produce uneven vulnerabilities, even in places that seem similar at first glance. Digging into detailed demographic data usually reveals clusters where these social and economic gaps align with higher disease transmission (Rai et al., 2024). This kind of insight is generally seen as essential for designing interventions that tackle both the health issues and the underlying social inequalities, aiming for a fairer distribution of care and resources. In border regions, where migratory trends and economic instability intersect—the risk of malaria spikes noticeably. Migrants, often jostling with uncertainty, tend to lack steady access to preventive tools like insecticide-treated nets and prompt treatment services; language barriers and limited health knowledge only add to the challenge. Certain ethnic groups, wrestling with their own set of socioeconomic hurdles, end up experiencing stronger exposure and less consistent use of available services. For instance, data generally reveal that individuals with lower incomes, older age, and specific ethnic backgrounds struggle a lot to access comprehensive malaria care (Sripoorote et al., 2024). These findings nudge us toward community-based healthcare models that are culturally sensitive and adjusted to the real-life challenges migrants face, ultimately boosting health literacy and trust. Addressing these deeper structural issues is a key step in reducing the unchecked spread of malaria among transient and marginalized groups. In many endemic regions, income gaps fuel malaria susceptibility by limiting what households can do in terms of prevention and treatment. Lower-income families often find themselves in homes without the basic protective features—missing things like window screens or even air conditioning, which only makes mosquito exposure worse. Economic constraints can also inhibit timely access to effective antimalarial medications, prolonging infections and letting the disease spread more widely. When larger families contend with tight budgets, scarce resources get stretched thin, further diluting the benefit of preventive measures. Generally speaking, successful malaria control strategies need to weave in socioeconomic supports like income aid and educational programs to empower those at risk. Besides, partnerships involving private sector players and ethnic health organizations have sometimes shown promise in broadening the reach of malaria services, underscoring the importance of multisector efforts in overcoming financial and social barriers (Sripoorote et al., 2024) (Figure 11.10).

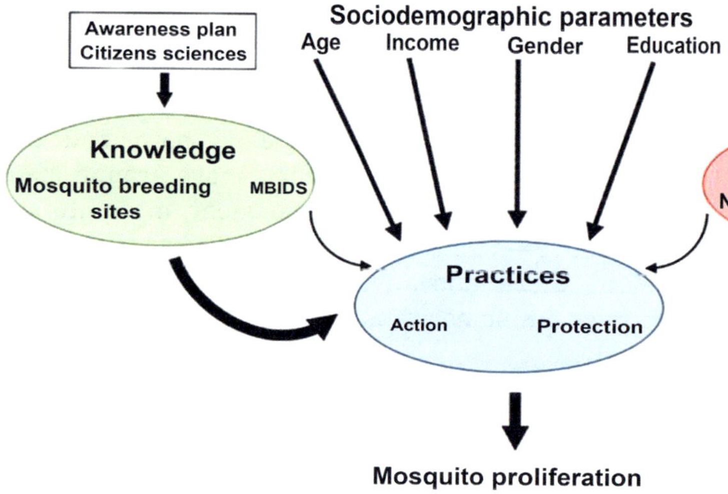

Figure 11.10. Mosquito socioeconomic factors affecting vulnerability.

Source: Duval P, Aschan-Leygonie C and Valiente Moro C (2023) A review of knowledge, attitudes and practices regarding mosquitoes and mosquito-borne infectious diseases in nonendemic regions. Front. Public Health. 11:1239874. doi: 10.3389/fpubh.2023.1239874

11.4. Outbreak Investigation Process

Noticing a sudden bump in the number of disease cases typically kicks off an outbreak investigation. Sometimes this jump is spotted through routine checks or even a tip from a healthcare provider. When it comes to malaria, that first alert is especially key because it sets a swift response into motion to stop further spread. In many cases, once there's a hunch that something's off, the next move is to compare current numbers with usual levels, this means double-checking diagnosed cases via lab tests and clinical reviews to be sure nothing's amiss. Then, a case definition gets put together to help decide who exactly is affected; having this kind of standard helps keep the data collection consistent. Collection comprehensive details. including who is getting sick, what symptoms they show, and where cases are popping up—builds the groundwork for getting a handle on the scope of the outbreak, and it gets everyone ready to target control measures.

Sampling characteristics	Number of studies			
	Urban	Periurban	Mixed	Total n(%)
Location				
Indoor	3	8	1	12 (11.9)
Outdoor	33	13	7	53 (52.5)
Both (indoor & outdoor)	25	8	7	40 (39.6)
Mosquito life stage				
Immatures (larvae, pupae & eggs)	23	5	6	34 (32.4)
Adult	22	21	7	50 (47.6)
Immatures & Adults	17	2	2	21(20.0)
Adult mosquitoes catch methods				
CDC light traps	9	11	5	25 (22.3)
Human landing catches	16	4	2	22 (19.6)
Bioagents-Sentinel traps	13	3	2	18 (16.1)
Pyrethrum spray catches	3	6	1	10 (8.9)
Prokopack aspirators	11	2	1	14 (12.5)
Other animal-baited methods [a]	10	1	3	14 (12.5)
Other unbaited methods [b]	8	2	0	10 (8.9)
Mosquito immature captures				
Ovitraps	13	2	2	17 (30.9)
Standard dippers	26	7	5	38 (69.1)
Mosquito identification techniques				
Morphological only	27	13	5	45 (58.4)
Molecular (PCR [c])	5	5	2	12 (15.6)
Morphological & Molecular methods (PCR)	11	7	2	16 (26.0)

(a) Includes animal odour- baited Mosquito Magnet Liberty Plus traps, odour baited suna traps and Ifakara tent trap,
(b) Includes Resting boxes, Mosquito electrocuting grids and pit traps,
(c) Polymerase Chain Reaction.

Figure 11.11. Outbreak investigation process.

Source: Joseph NK, Mumo E, Morlighem C, Macharia PM, Snow RW and Linard C (2024) Mosquito-borne diseases in urban East African Community region: a scoping review of urban typology research and mosquito genera overlap, 2000-2024. Front. Trop. Dis 5:1499520. doi: 10.3389/fitd.2024.1499520

After identifying cases, epidemiologists tend to dig deeper by analyzing the data around who, where, and when the disease is striking. Patterns start to emerge, like which age groups seem most vulnerable, where geographic hotspots might exist, and how trends change over time, guiding the next steps of an investigation. In the case of malaria, researchers look at many factors such as rainfall, temperature, and even the spots where mosquitoes breed, alongside how people behave in those areas, which all influence exposure. Checking the specific *Plasmodium* species in play and how the mosquito vectors operate is also crucial for shaping the right interventions. Generally speaking, drawing up a hypothesis from all that descriptive data helps investigators zero in on transmission routes, risk factors, and possible sources. Sometimes more detailed studies, like case-control or cohort studies—are pursued to prove cause and effect. This evidence-based way of work not only sketches out the outbreak but also backs up the public health actions needed to manage malaria outbreaks effectively (Hu et al., 2020). In the last stretch, the focus shifts to putting targeted control and prevention strategies into action while keeping tabs on the situation continuously. Quick steps like using insecticide-treated nets, performing indoor residual spraying, and managing the environment can cut down on malaria transmission. At the same time, getting the community informed about protective behaviors and encouraging speedy treatment rounds out the effort. There's usually a feedback loop with all the stakeholders, and sometimes public health policies get altered to lower future risks. In addition, surveillance systems are often ramped up to catch any new outbreaks sooner, which might involve bolstering lab capacities and streamlining data reporting. Carefully documenting every bit of the investigation not only adds to our scientific understanding but also guides how resources are allocated. While malaria outbreaks differ from something like COVID-19 in both causes and control details, the whole idea behind them—rapid detection, thorough analysis, and targeted, evidence-based interventions—remains a common thread in managing emerging infectious diseases (James et al., 2020) (Figure 11.11).

11.4.1. Initial Case Identification and Reporting

Catching the early signs of an outbreak is absolutely crucial. In the case of malaria, spotting the very first cases can change the course of how the disease spreads. Healthcare workers in places where malaria is common are on constant alert—they look for signs like periodic fevers and chills subsequently back those suspicions up with tests such as blood smears or rapid diagnostics. When a case is found quickly, treatment can start right away to cut down sickness and even death, and it kicks off extra measures like tracking down contacts and controlling mosquitoes. Sometimes, things get challenging, just as we saw with COVID-19, because symptoms might be vague or some individuals don't show them at all, which makes it all the more important to stay sharp with diagnoses and keep communities informed (Hu et al., 2020). Once someone is flagged as a malaria case, reporting becomes the next vital step. In most cases, getting accurate and quick reports together helps experts' piece together the bigger picture of an outbreak and figure out where to send help. The way the systems work is like a balancing act: they need to be sensitive enough to pick up new cases and yet smart enough to avoid mistaking harmless illnesses for malaria. New digital tools and platforms that share data in real time—tools that have been used during recent viral epidemics—show that improving communication and data clarity can boost outbreak investigations (Chamola et al., 2020). Better reporting also means local, national, and even international health bodies can work together more fluidly, forging a collaborative effort to keep outbreaks under control. There are definitely challenges when it comes to spotting subsequently reporting these initial cases, especially in areas with fewer resources where malaria is the worst. Generally speaking, strengthening community-based surveillance, training healthcare staff, and making sure reliable tests are on hand are all seen as key moves. A slight delay from when symptoms start to when a case is confirmed can hurt the speed of the overall response—a point underlined by recent experiences with COVID-19 (Chamola et al., 2020; Hu et al., 2020). Some experts now suggest leaning on technology, like mobile apps for reporting and geo-spatial mapping, to speed things up even more. In the end, the fight against malaria depends on how seamlessly we move from first noticing a case to getting accurate details reported out—a critical link in the global effort to keep this disease at bay (Figure 11.12).

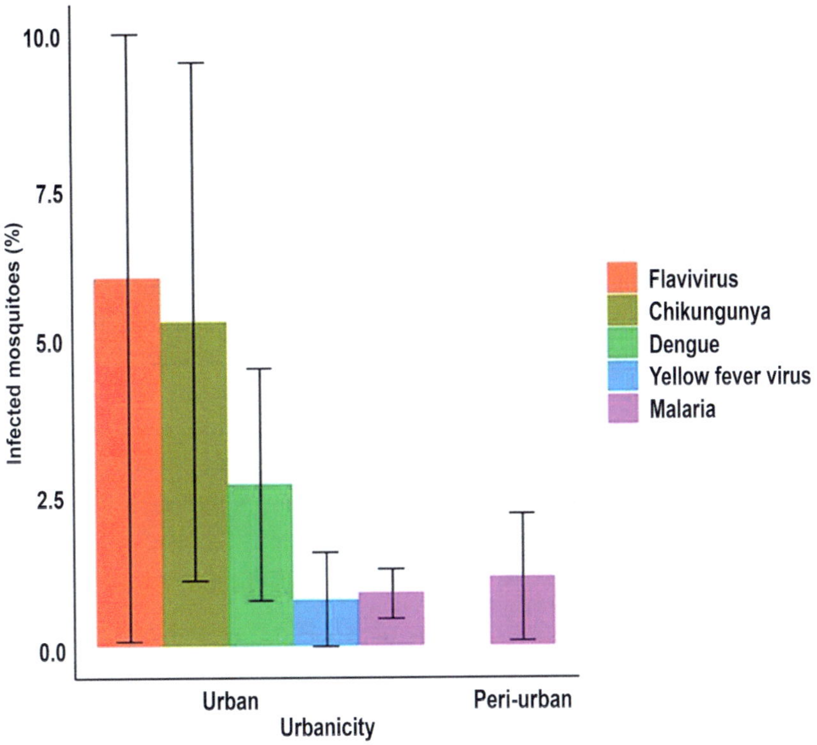

Figure 11.12. Initial case identification and reporting malaria spreads.

Source: Joseph NK, Mumo E, Morlighem C, Macharia PM, Snow RW and Linard C (2024) Mosquito-borne diseases in urban East African Community region: a scoping review of urban typology research and mosquito genera overlap, 2000-2024. Front. Trop. Dis 5:1499520. doi: 10.3389/fitd.2024.1499520

11.4.2. Data Collection and Analysis Methods

When an outbreak starts, getting prompt, accurate data is the cornerstone. It all kicks off with reaching out to people in affected areas and collecting details like case numbers, age groups, where individuals live, and even when symptoms first show up. In malaria situations, it's not just about spotting the sick—one has to consider the environment too, for example those mosquito breeding spots in the area. Data might come from quick surveys, records at health centers, or even active case hunts. Using standardized paper or digital forms boosts the chance that information stays complete and consistent. Also, lab tests on samples, sometimes using high-tech molecular techniques—can nail down which *Plasmodium* is causing trouble and flag any resistance markers. Tossing geospatial info into the mix can reveal hidden transmission paths, which helps in zeroing in on where to act. In most cases, the care taken to collect data sets the tone for later analysis and ultimately shapes how resources and responses are allocated. After collection this patchwork of details, analysts then dive into the numbers to unravel the mess of transmission and risk factors. A simple rundown of who got sick, what the issues are, where the cases fell, and when things happened can already paint a rough picture. Sometimes studies like case-control or cohort comparisons bring out particular risks that may be nudged to lower transmission. More complex statistical models and computer tools, adjusting for other confounding bits, help pick up on subtle patterns. Lately, there's been a turn towards using clinical mNGS for a deeper look at the microbes involved, the state of drug resistance, and even how the body is reacting (Charles et al., 2019). Usually, merging these advanced tests with conventional epidemiologic data makes the results a lot sturdier and puts policymakers in a better spot to decide which areas need focus. Looking at the situation on a global scale shakes things up with extra context. Big projects like the Global Burden of Diseases study compile huge sets of data, ranging from death records to verbal autopsies, which help set a baseline for malaria and gauge how interventions have fared over time (Gregory et al., 2018). This kind of data is drawn from many different sources subsequently run through models that, slightly imperfectly, reassign vague reasons for death to more relevant conditions. People studying local malaria outbreaks often use similar approaches to measure how fierce the spread is and how death rates change, keeping in mind demographic and socio-economic shifts. To summarize, using such wide-ranging data is crucial because it lets investigators decide if a surge in cases is just a short-term fluctuation or a sign of a growing public health threat that might need a bigger, faster response effort.

11.4.3. Establishing the Outbreak's Source and Transmission Dynamics

Tracing the origin of a malaria outbreak isn't a one-size-fits-all process. It usually kicks off with collecting detailed case histories that reveal shared factors, sometimes people have traveled to areas where malaria's common or been near spots teeming with mosquitoes. Mapping cases by place and time can suddenly show clusters where the disease might be spreading, and researchers often mix in samples from local mosquitoes to see which ones carry the parasite. Genetic tests on the *Plasmodium* taken from patients can then give clues about whether the infections stem from nearby transmission or were imported from elsewhere. All these bits of information, even if they seem oddly scattered at first, build a picture that helps sharpen efforts to target the outbreak and curb further spread. Understanding how malaria transmits is a matter of both nature and everyday life. Generally speaking, factors like temperature, humidity, and even rainfall affect mosquito breeding and survival, which in turn alters the chances of disease spreading. At the same time, the way people behave, like spending a lot of time outdoors during mosquito-active hours or living in houses that don't offer much protection—can raise the risk of exposure. There's also the odd twist that some farming practices, where pesticides are used, may inadvertently change how mosquitoes react to chemicals (Tudi et al., 2021). Looking at these elements all at once lets public health officials' piece together a rough model of transmission, helping them devise measures that can break the parasite's cycle. The details at the molecular and ecological levels add yet another twist to the story. Even small differences, like variations in how mosquito species feed, rest, or handle insecticides—can shape how an outbreak rolls out. By mixing data from vector monitoring with patient records, investigators can sometimes trace back transmission chains and spot trouble spots where the parasite seems to run rampant. In a way, it's a bit like what happened with the investigations into SARS-CoV-2, where knowing how the virus moved around was a crucial part of stopping it (Hu et al., 2020). All of these insights, taken together (and admittedly, sometimes with a bit of redundancy), underline how critical it is to nail down both the source and the spread of malaria in order to design control measures that truly fit the situation (Figure 11.13).

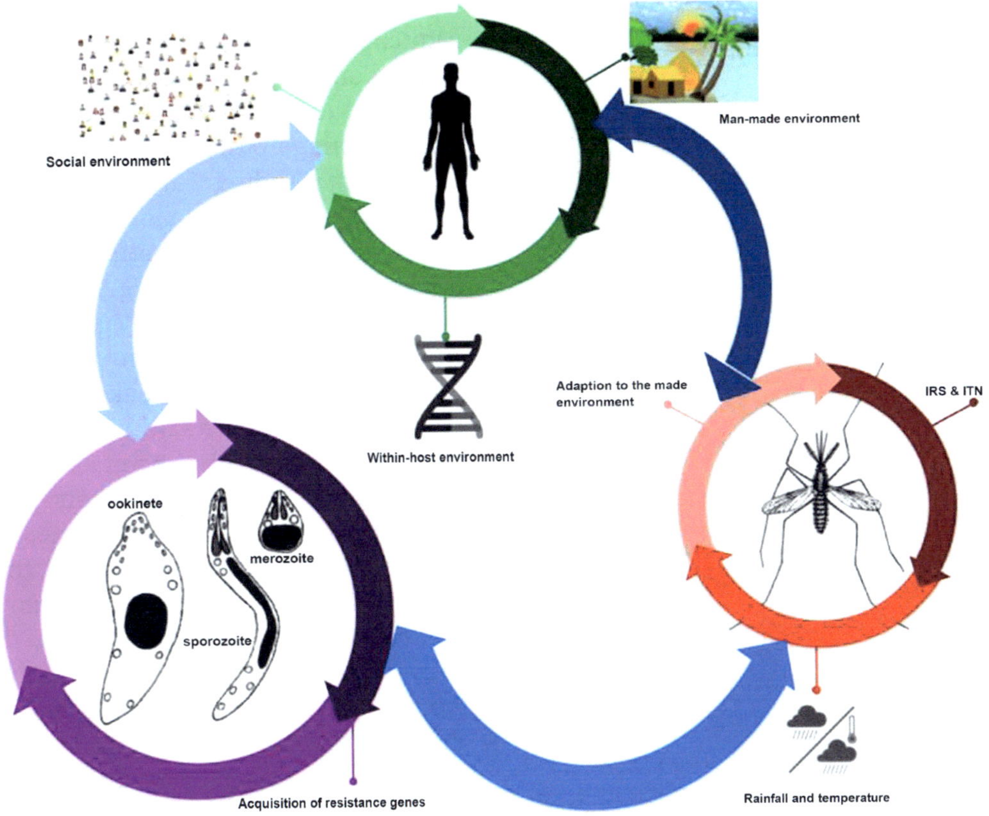

Figure 11.13. Outbreak's source and transmission dynamics.

Source: Savi, Merveille Koissi. 2023. "An Overview of Malaria Transmission Mechanisms, Control, and Modeling" *Medical Sciences* 11, no. 1: 3. https://doi.org/10.3390/medsci11010003

11.5. Control and Prevention Strategies

Malaria control isn't a one-trick pony, it calls for many nimble strategies that fit local vibes and lean on fast, on-point surveillance. Think about it this way: instead of sticking with broad efforts, some places have shifted gears toward pinpointed elimination. Take China, for example. Generally speaking, its move from wider control to a "1–3–7" strategy (where a case is reported in one day, looked into in three, and sorted within seven) shows a kind of dynamic planning that just clicks. Fueled by digital reporting in real time—so teams can jump into action quick, this method cuts down the chance of further spread. A boost in diagnostic skills through national labs along with some well-placed incentives for healthcare workers adds extra punch, making sure every case gets properly managed. At the end of the day, political drive, teamwork across different sectors, and guidelines altered from solid global evidence come together to create a replicable framework for managing malaria in a bunch of settings (Cao et al., 2021). But it isn't just about rapid replies; keeping mosquitoes at bay still tops the list. Indoor spraying and handing out insecticide-treated bed nets have both helped shrink mosquito numbers and limit risky bites. Still, with insecticide resistance creeping in, there's always a call for fresh research and innovative alters to make these tools work well. Simple steps like getting rid of stagnant water can add up, too, even if that sounds almost too straightforward. Plus, when communities get involved and health education rolls out naturally, people stick to these preventive measures better. In many cases, the lesson here is that mixing approaches to tackle both the parasite and the mosquito, with a steady dose of community input and ongoing checks, is crucial to breaking the transmission chain.

Then again, when you throw in other public health challenges—COVID-19 being a big one—the whole picture grows even more complex. The scramble for resources and the shakeup of normal health services means malaria control can easily take a back seat, risking a fresh surge. It becomes pretty clear that malaria programs need to fit snugly into the broader health system and emergency responses to keep things running smoothly. Even though COVID-19 is mostly about respiratory issues, its global fight reminds us that having a flexible disease surveillance setup—one that can juggle several threats at once—is no luxury at all. With a readiness to adapt and strategies that can pivot on the fly, health systems are better equipped to handle overlapping epidemics, ensuring that malaria control doesn't fall through the cracks (Hu et al., 2020).

11.5.1. Vector Control Measures

Controlling disease outbreaks, especially vector-borne ones like malaria, often means mixing a bunch of strategies rather than relying on a single fix. A key piece of the puzzle is getting how mosquitoes live and act, since these pathogens drive transmission. For example, reducing mosquito counts and cutting down on how often people come into contact with them can seriously help. Sometimes the plan starts with cleaning up the environment, like draining or treating standing water (those easy mosquito hangouts) and boosting local community efforts. Then there's the possibility of adding fresh strategies, such as using biological control agents or even genetically altered mosquitos, to give traditional methods an extra push. Looking at dengue outbreaks, where clusters of breeding sites near healthcare centers increase transmission risks (Haider et al., 2023), it makes sense to target high-risk spots and optimize resource allocation; overall, these combined moves help lower vector numbers and break the chain of transmission, keeping outbreaks under control. Another route to manage these issues is by putting physical and chemical methods to work, limiting how often people get bitten by infected pathogens. In many malaria-endemic areas, tools like insecticide-treated bed nets (ITNs) and indoor residual spraying (IRS) have cut down both cases and deaths. ITNs serve as a barrier against nocturnal Anopheles mosquitoes, while IRS—spraying long-lasting insecticides on indoor walls—helps by either killing or repelling them. Of course, challenges like insecticide resistance and economic hurdles can sometimes get in the way; plus, the timing and reach of these campaigns can make a big difference, as stepping in early during the transmission season might suppress a mosquito surge before it peaks. Generally speaking, lessons learned from other vector-borne disease outbreaks suggest that mixing biological, chemical, environmental, and personal protection measures creates a well-rounded plan for sustainable malaria control

(Haider et al., 2023). On top of the classic approaches, emerging vector control technologies are opening up some promising new paths to resist malaria outbreaks while backing up the existing strategies. One innovative method uses a Wolbachia-based approach—infecting mosquitoes with a symbiotic bacterium that makes them less capable of passing on pathogens; though first explored for dengue, this method might just work for malaria too. Genetic modification techniques, like gene drive systems, are also being tested to either shrink or alter mosquito populations in a significant way. These cutting-edge ideas underscore the constant need for careful, context-specific surveillance—both epidemiologically and entomologically—to fine-tune interventions. It also means that ongoing government and community support, along with efforts to build local capacity and infrastructure, are crucial for success. In short, fusing traditional methods with these innovative technologies, and bringing everyone into the loop—creates a robust strategy to curb malaria outbreaks and ease their toll on public health (Haider et al., 2023) (Figure 11.14).

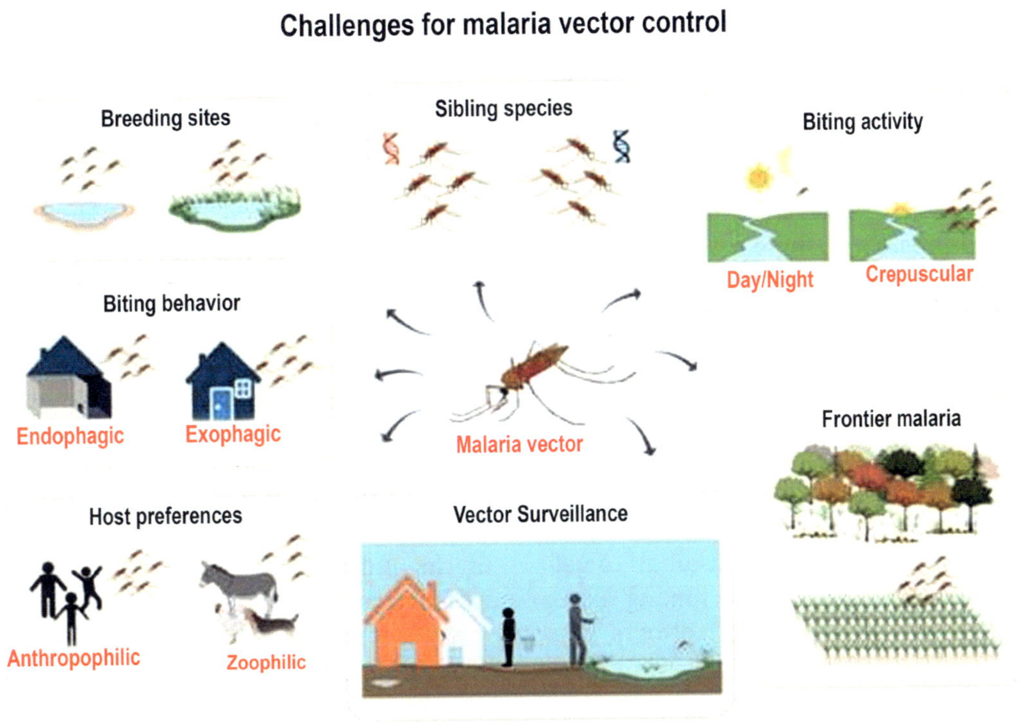

Figure 11.14. Malaria vector control.

Source: Rocha EM, Katak RdM, Campos de Oliveira J, Araujo MdS, Carlos BC, Galizi R, Tripet F, Marinotti O, Souza-Neto JA. Vector-Focused Approaches to Curb Malaria Transmission in the Brazilian Amazon: An Overview of Current and Future Challenges and Strategies. *Tropical Medicine and Infectious Disease*. 2020; 5(4):161. https://doi.org/10.3390/tropicalmed5040161

11.5.2. Use of Antimalarial Medications

Antimalarial drugs are the frontline when it comes to handling outbreaks; they're used both to treat people who are already sick and to keep at-risk individuals from getting infected. The choice of treatment often hinges on which *Plasmodium* type is causing the trouble and what kind of resistance is common in that area. In many places, artemisinin-based combos (ACTs) have earned their reputation because they work fast and well, yet emerging resistance, especially noticeable in Southeast Asia—forces us to keep an eye on the situation and look for different options. Giving these drugs at just the right time can cut the illness short while also knocking down the number of parasites around, which in turn helps slow community spread. Sometimes, when things get bad, authorities might roll out mass drug programs, though they have to weigh the risk of resistance and whether people will stick with the plan. Even with the progress made in antimalarial medicine, using these drugs perfectly during outbreaks is challenging. Drug resistance is a constant worry, often pushed by overuse, misuse, or simply poor-quality medications. This whole resistance thing means researchers are constantly experimenting with new ideas, ranging from synthetic biology to molecular tech—to either discover fresh compounds or boost the ones we have. Besides, sticking to the treatment plan is crucial if we want to prevent the parasites from staging a comeback. Further, factors like economic challenges, unreliable health services, and limited testing facilities can make it tough to get the drugs where they're needed. So, mixing these drug strategies with broader health efforts, like controlling disease-carrying insects and running community education programs—is pretty much essential for keeping outbreaks under control and pushing toward malaria elimination (Uddin et al., 2021). Antimalarial medications aren't only about curing; they also play a big part in prevention, especially for travelers or groups who face higher risks during outbreaks. Prophylactic use helps lower the chances of new infections and stands as a key piece of the puzzle when trying to contain an outbreak. Still, the type and length of preventive treatment must be chosen carefully, taking into account local disease trends and individual needs, so that protection is maximized and side effects are minimized. Regular checks through randomized clinical trials remain vital to proving the worth of new drugs and updated treatment plans. Reflecting on previous outbreaks, like those in viral pandemics where repurposing drugs and rigorous trials were critical—drives home the point that evidence-based strategies are key when using these medications. Ultimately, combining strong drug therapies with active surveillance and quick testing boosts our overall readiness to fight off malaria outbreaks (Pascarella et al., 2020).

11.5.3. Community Education and Awareness Programs

Managing malaria goes beyond just dishing out medicine, it's about giving everyday people the insights they need to change habits that let the disease spread. When individuals start to grasp how the parasite lives and how mosquitoes play into the mix, they naturally join in fighting back. Often, local efforts mix things up in unexpected ways: pamphlets in the mother tongue, radio bursts that feel lively, and hands-on workshops that bring home the message about prevention and treatment. Besides simply sharing facts, these initiatives slowly break down common myths and ease the stigma around the disease, which in turn opens the door for faster diagnoses and treatments. In many cases, this kind of grassroots outreach builds a spirit of communal care that noticeably lightens the load on tired healthcare systems (Shuroug et al., 2023). At the same time, it turns out that local education campaigns do best when they also pay attention to nature. People need to know that malaria isn't just about microbes, it's also about where those pesky mosquitoes find their homes. When communities understand that stagnant water and shoddy sanitation feed mosquito breeding, they're more likely to take simple steps like cleaning up puddles or fixing drainage systems. Such hands-on advice, woven into broader health moves like indoor spraying or dishing out treated nets, helps line up local actions with bigger public health plans. Generally speaking, coupling ecological clues with health tips gives a clearer picture of how changing weather and the environment can pump up malaria risks (Lio et al., 2023). Lately, tech is playing a bigger role in how these messages get out there. Digital tools, such as mobile apps and social media channels, now send out important health info fast and live, helping people keep up with preventive steps right when outbreaks flare. This modern twist isn't just about talking at people; it opens up a two-way chat where communities can share their thoughts and even help steer the strategy. Plus, these platforms work hard to squash bogus info while boosting trust in the guidelines, all while aligning with a broader shift in healthcare that sometimes even uses AI to tailor messages. Embracing these digital methods not only sharpens the malaria response but also helps communities get more comfortable with innovative, resilient health behaviors (Shuroug et al., 2023) (Figure 11.15).

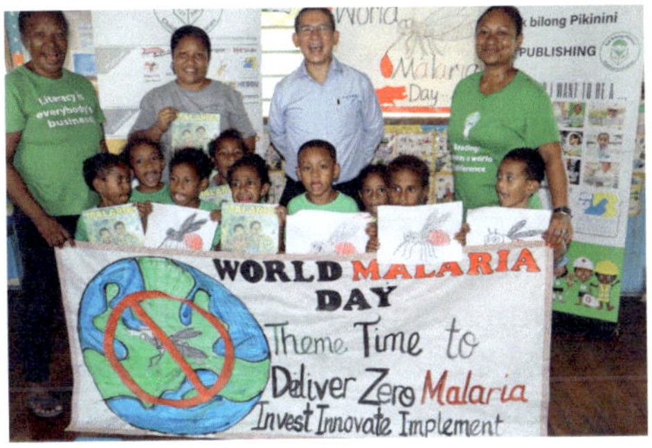

Figure 11.15. Community education and awareness programs.

Source: KOKI Foundation. (2023). *World Malaria Day Community Outreach.*

11.6. Case Studies of Malaria Outbreaks

Recent malaria rebounds show how transmission can suddenly change when mosquito habitats and expanding cities mix in unpredictable ways. Dire Dawa in Ethiopia, for example, had its own twist: *Anopheles stephensi*—a mosquito normally linked with Asia—started showing up in urban areas, shaking up traditional control plans. Research picked up that clusters of *Plasmodium falciparum* infections tended to form near households harboring these invasive pathogens, with sporozoite findings clearly indicating active transmission. Genetic work even hinted at clonal groupings of parasites resistant to core antimalarial drugs, which, in most cases, makes treatment tougher when new vectors and resistant strains meet (Emiru et al., 2023). All this underscores why keeping tabs on emerging mosquito populations in cities is so crucial. In another case, the Waghemra Zone in Northeast Ethiopia offered a vivid glimpse into how multifaceted malaria epidemics can be. A sudden surge in confirmed cases over just a short period pointed to weaknesses in both community knowledge and environmental upkeep. One study, looking into potential risk factors, noted that being close to artificial water pools and erratic streams—both great spots for mosquito breeding—played a significant role. Sleeping outdoors compounded these risks, especially for children under five who ended up facing much higher chances of infection. It also turned out that many locals simply weren't well-informed about how malaria spreads or how to prevent it, which suggests that it's not just about the presence of mosquitoes, but also about the mix of environmental, behavioral, and informational gaps that need addressing (Debash et al., 2023). Putting these cases together makes it clear that tackling malaria outbreaks isn't straightforward—ecological shifts and social challenges add layers of complexity. The appearance of an invasive vector like *An. stephensi* in urban locales throws routine surveillance off balance, calling for more focused entomological and molecular monitoring. Meanwhile, rural outbreaks like those seen in Waghemra remind us that natural factors and everyday behaviors both heavily influence epidemic outcomes. In most instances, managing such outbreaks calls for a multidisciplinary approach, one that weaves together insights on mosquito biology, parasite genetics, local environmental nuances, and even socio-cultural habits. Ultimately, these examples affirm the vital role of targeted health education and environmental management, showing that integrated strategies are essential to cut down transmission risks and protect vulnerable populations (Debash et al., 2023; Emiru et al., 2023).

11.6.1. Notable Historical Outbreaks

Tracking malaria's spread over the years wasn't straightforward. Old records tell us that slow case reporting and clunky surveillance setups only made outbreaks worse. In South Africa, before they tried mobile monitoring, getting real-time alerts was nearly impossible. Then came MalariaConnect—a mobile reporting system, which slashed the delay from over five days to under one day. This change, in most cases, meant outbreaks could be spotted quicker, which in turn spurred faster public health actions. Sure, the mobile method sometimes fell short in data completeness compared to old paper methods, but overall, that extra speed and accuracy proved vital for curbing outbreaks, showing that updating surveillance methods in malaria-hit areas is a must (Davies et al., 2019). Looking back, past responses to malaria also highlight how crucial controlling the mosquito vector is to slowing disease spread. Early mosquito control efforts, focusing mostly on anopheline mosquitoes, helped drop infection rates. Interestingly, experiences with other mosquito-borne illnesses, like when using IRS against Aedes mosquitoes for dengue, revealed both the upsides and the limits of such strategies. Generally speaking, extensive IRS campaigns before expected epidemic seasons could cut down early infections drastically; yet they might also erode natural immunity over time, leaving populations more vulnerable later. React too slowly—or stop these measures altogether, and you risk a huge comeback in cases. So, it seems mixing sustained mosquito control with additional steps like vaccination is key to securing long-term progress (Thomas et al., 2018). When you look at historical malaria outbreaks, it becomes clear that there's a complex association between tracking the disease, controlling the mosquitoes, and community immunity. South Africa's digital leap with early reporting is one clear example: quicker detection led to more focused, timely interventions. But while rapid responses help in the short term, sticking with mosquito control is essential to prevent immunity from fading and outbreaks from returning. What we learn from malaria, and even from similar mosquito-driven challenges—is that only many tech-savvy surveillance and ongoing vector management will set us up for lasting success. Grasping these interconnected lessons is pretty crucial for planning better outbreak investigations and crafting robust global malaria elimination strategies (Thomas et al., 2018; Davies et al., 2019).

11.6.2. Recent Outbreaks and Their Impact

Infectious disease outbreaks tend to emerge from a complex mix of nature, society, and biology. Take malaria, for instance, its recent flare-ups remind us of that weather factors like rain and temperature sway mosquito numbers and how parasites spread. In Nkomazi Municipality, research generally speaking shows that shifts in climate seem to line up with higher malaria cases. Mosquitoes, especially *Anopheles arabiensis*, often boom when conditions are just right, and there's usually a delay between those environmental triggers and a surge in cases, which kind of hints that acting early on vector control might be key (Gregory et al., 2018). It turns out that keeping an eye on nature and mixing in quick public health moves could help ease this recurring problem. Looking at the bigger picture, malaria fits into a story of progress mixed with ongoing challenges. While overall, deaths from communicable diseases have mostly dropped, outbreaks still hit the most vulnerable in low-resource areas pretty hard. Between 2007 and 2017, for example, younger populations enjoyed fewer deaths, yet older adults began showing more severe impacts, suggesting that age matters when it comes to disease vulnerability (Gbenga et al., 2018). This uneven spread of health improvements means that controlling malaria isn't solely about tracking shifts in weather or counting mosquitoes, it also involves addressing the unique struggles different communities face. In some epidemic hotspots, malaria's comeback throws even more complications into the mix. Environmental changes, political unrest, and even conflict seem to break down control efforts, making it tougher for communities to keep the disease at bay. Irregular rainfall patterns and unexpected temperature shifts in places like Southern Africa can lead to unpredictable mosquito booms, stretching out the transmission season and upping the risk of larger outbreaks (Gregory et al., 2018). By mixing health data with insights from environmental trends, experts can better forecast these surges and plan resource allocation more effectively—a crucial step to lessen the heavy toll on both people and economies (Gbenga et al., 2018) (Figure 11.16).

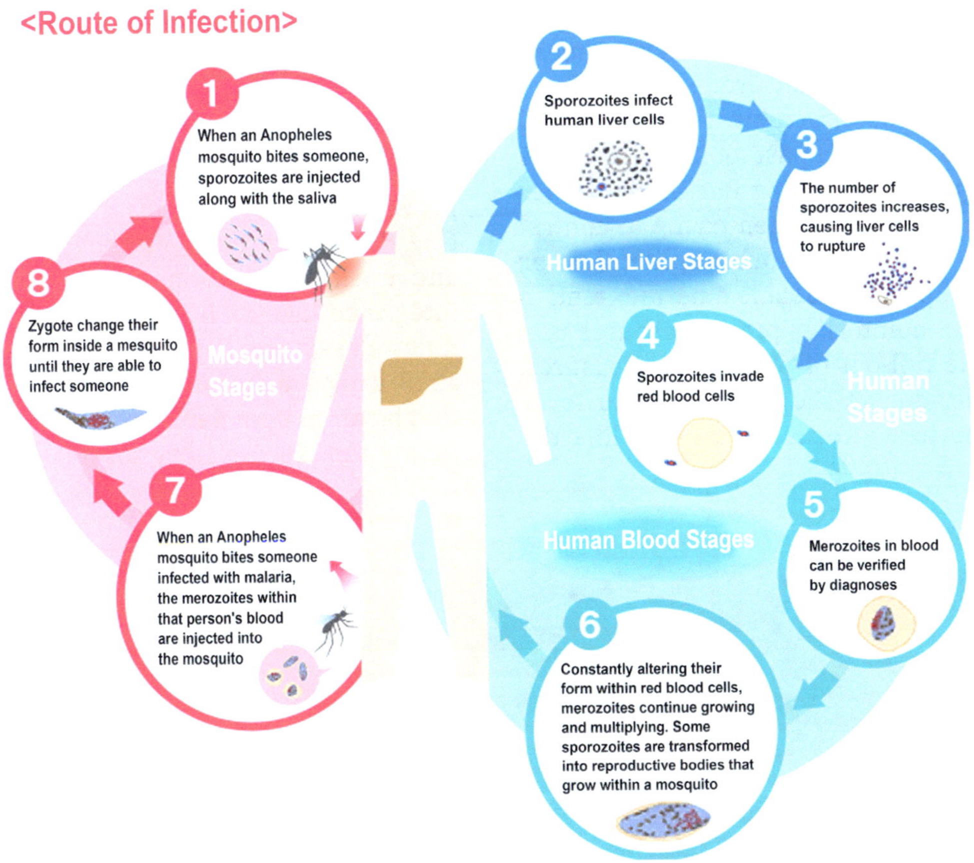

Figure 11.16. Infectious disease outbreaks of malaria.

Source: Eisai Co. Ltd. (n.d.). *Malaria Transmission Map.*

11.6.3. Lessons Learned from Past Investigations

Previous outbreak investigations have shown just how key a broad approach to data collection and surveillance is in getting a handle on how diseases behave. Detailed records about why people pass away, along with constant monitoring, help public health individuals spot trends and see the overall impact on communities over time. Some studies have mixed things up by drawing on everything from official vital records to informal autopsy interviews, which gives a stronger basis for decision-making (Naghavi et al., 2024). Using these same ideas in malaria outbreak checks can boost our ability to catch shifts in how the disease spreads, judge what works, and divide up resources in a smart way. It also points out, in most cases, that keeping an eye on different regions and groups is important so that help can be directed where it's needed most. A big lesson from past looks at infectious diseases is that overlapping health challenges can muddle the picture when trying to control outbreaks. When additional epidemics or pandemics crop up at the same time, they tend to derail careful monitoring, proper resource use, and even the roll-out of prevention measures. For example, during the African swine fever incident, the heavy focus on a crisis like the COVID-19 pandemic ended up shifting attention and resources away from other critical tasks, which then led to slower detection and lapses in biosecurity measures (Uwishema et al., 2021). In malaria investigations, it's vital to understand how these overlapping issues might come into play. Generally speaking, being prepared means building systems that can handle interruptions so that essential malaria control services keep chugging along during wider health emergencies. Looking back, there's also a clear message about how combining expertise from various fields and engaging local communities pays off in outbreak responses. Teaming up across the medical, environmental, and social arenas often leads to a more rounded view of what's driving disease spread and helps set up long-lasting control measures (Uwishema et al., 2021). In most cases, sharing health information with communities and getting them involved in monitoring efforts has been shown to speed up early detection and boost the use of simple prevention practices. Plus, the idea behind the One Health approach – linking human, animal, and environmental insights – offers a more integrated take on how diseases move through different settings. For malaria in particular, such a mix can pave the way for custom interventions that factor in both nature and society, ultimately easing the disease's overall toll.

CLOSER LOOK

SPOROZOITES

Sporozoites are a crucial stage in the life cycle of *Plasmodium* parasites, the causative agents of malaria. They are the infective form of the parasite transmitted to humans through the bite of an infected *Anopheles* mosquito. Understanding sporozoites is fundamental to comprehending how malaria is transmitted, how it spreads in the human body, and the key points for intervention in malaria prevention and treatment.

The malaria parasite's life cycle involves two hosts: the *Anopheles* mosquito and the human. Sporozoites are formed in the mosquito's gut and salivary glands after the mosquito feeds on an infected human's blood. This phase marks the start of the transmission cycle. When an infected mosquito bites a human, it injects sporozoites directly into the bloodstream via its saliva.

Once inside the bloodstream, the sporozoites rapidly travel to the liver, where they infect liver cells. The speed and efficiency of this initial infection are critical to the parasite's ability to establish malaria in the human host. The journey of sporozoites to the liver and their ability to infect hepatocytes (liver cells) is a defining characteristic of the early stages of malaria infection.

Sporozoites are slender, motile, and highly specialized for rapid movement through the bloodstream to reach the liver. They are equipped with a specialized structure called the *apical complex*, which allows them to penetrate host cells, such as liver cells, and initiate infection. The apical complex includes structures like micronemes and rhoptries, which release enzymes and proteins that facilitate the invasion of host cells.

Sporozoites are covered in a protective protein coat, which enables them to survive in the mosquito's saliva and travel through the human bloodstream without being easily detected or destroyed by the host's immune system. They are also very small and can travel quickly, making their journey from the skin to the liver efficient. In the liver, sporozoites mature into merozoites, which are the form of the parasite that later invades red blood cells and causes the symptoms of malaria.

Sporozoites are the initial agents of malaria infection. When a mosquito carrying the *Plasmodium* parasite bites a human, the sporozoites are injected directly into the bloodstream. They circulate through the bloodstream for a short period before heading to the liver. Once inside liver cells, the sporozoites mature into schizonts, which eventually rupture, releasing thousands of merozoites into the bloodstream. These merozoites then invade red blood cells, perpetuating the cycle of infection and causing the characteristic symptoms of malaria, such as fever, chills, and anemia.

The presence of sporozoites in the bloodstream of the host is not typically associated with the symptoms of malaria. Instead, the symptoms appear after the liver phase, once merozoites begin infecting red blood cells. However, the introduction of sporozoites marks the start of the disease process, as it begins the cycle of liver infection and blood-stage multiplication.

The sporozoite stage has garnered attention in the development of malaria vaccines. One of the most promising malaria vaccines, RTS,S (also known as Mosquirix), is designed to target sporozoites and prevent them from infecting liver cells. By focusing on the sporozoite stage, this vaccine aims to block the earliest and most critical step in the parasite's life cycle, reducing the number of parasites that reach the liver and, consequently, the number of merozoites that enter the bloodstream.

SUMMARY

Investigating malaria outbreaks shows just how urgently we need to get our surveillance systems working together and act fast to cut transmission and ease the disease burden. You can learn from similar crises, like those from Rift Valley fever virus cases, where spotting early cases and grasping how the infection spreads end up shifting control efforts in a big way. Outbreak studies don't just chart the spread; they also reveal environmental, biological, and sociocultural aspects that keep the problem alive. For malaria, which means dealing with mosquito breeding spots, making sure tests are spot-on, and boosting community awareness to break the cycle. In many cases, such hands-on, context-based actions ensure interventions are built on solid evidence and fit the local scene (Birungi et al., 2021). This layered insight is key for health officials to craft policies that are sustainable and ready to ward off future flare-ups. Looking at diseases that leap from animals to people, it becomes clear that working across fields matters a lot. Virologists, epidemiologists, and public health pros—when they join forces—can turn quick lab detections into steps that work on the ground. Just as rapid diagnostic tools, effective treatment plans, and strict vector control guide responses for epidemic-prone viruses, malaria control reaps benefits from a similar mix. Generally speaking, understanding zoonotic spillover in related viral scenarios offers clues about managing reservoirs and keeping an eye on environmental factors, thereby adding extra layers of precaution and scientific depth to malaria investigations (Hu et al., 2020). These mixed, cross-field efforts help sharpen overall readiness and bring a more relaxed, yet effective, approach to fighting both malaria and other infectious threats. At the end of the day, drawing broader lessons from outbreak probes stresses how vital solid public health setups and genuine community involvement are for malaria control. Successful containment isn't just about technical fixes, it depends on residents pitching in with prevention actions and timely reporting. The evidence suggests that outbreaks, regardless of what starts them, call for risk communication strategies tuned to local realities and continuous monitoring to keep up with evolving trends. Data-driven tips from detailed outbreak work can even kickstart global efforts aimed at malaria elimination. With ongoing investments in research, capacity-building, and resource management, public health systems can lessen malaria's toll while toughening defenses against future infectious surprises (Hu et al., 2020; Birungi et al., 2021).

The study into the malaria outbreak uncovered many vital insights that could shape both quick fixes and longer-term plans. It turns out that nailing a fast diagnosis is crucial to keeping the spread in check. Modern tech, like AI sifting through complex patient data, can up the accuracy of diagnoses and help manage cases more smoothly. In most cases, this is what we see today—doctors leaning on artificial intelligence for prompt, evidence-based choices that boost patient outcomes and cut down on mistakes and costs. Still, rolling out these smart tools isn't all smooth sailing; issues like data privacy and making sure the systems work reliably across different settings still need careful attention. So, mixing trusty epidemiological methods with these fresh tools seems key to better controlling malaria in affected communities (Shuroug et al., 2023). Another angle the research poked at was how vital smooth supply chain management is during outbreaks. Ensuring that medical supplies and antimalarial drugs get to where they're needed isn't just a side note, it's central to an effective response. Often, when supply channels break down at the worst times, crisis response can stumble. Analysis suggests that proactive planning in resource allocation, along with digitizing supply channels, might be the trick to easing these disruptions. Generally speaking, lessons drawn from global emergencies like the COVID-19 pandemic underline how necessary it is to have flexible, resilient systems that can quickly mobilize what's needed now and support long-term health system strength. In simple terms, a holistic view of supply chains is instrumental to ensuring treatments keep flowing and preventing further outbreak waves (Maciel et al., 2020). The investigation didn't stop there. It also pointed to how behavioral and environmental factors play a big role in shaping the outbreak's course. Local differences in mosquito control, community involvement, and conditions like still, stagnant water were shown to have a direct impact on malaria's spread. What this means is that simply focusing on vector control isn't enough—enhancing public education and boosting community participation are just as important to keeping up preventive behaviors. In most cases, integrating technology with solid supply chain mechanisms and community-centered approaches offers a promising blueprint for future outbreak management. Altogether, these intertwined findings highlight just how layered malaria control is and open up new avenues for integrated intervention models.

KEY TERMS FROM THIS CHAPTER

- Case Definition
- Active Case Finding
- Larval Breeding Sites
- Incubation Period
- Environmental Assessment
- Control Measures
- Outbreak Containment
- Epidemiological Curve
- Passive Case Reporting
- Vector Density
- Travel History
- Diagnostic Confirmation
- Mass Drug Administration
- Cluster Detection
- Entomological Survey
- Attack Rate
- Risk Factors
- Drug Resistance Testing
- Vector Control Interventions

References

1. Abiodun, G. J., Njabo, K. Y., Witbooi, P. J., Adeola, A. M., Fuller, T., Okosun, K. O., Makinde, O. S., et al. (2018). Exploring the influence of daily climate variables on malaria transmission and abundance of *Anopheles arabiensis* over Nkomazi Local Municipality, Mpumalanga Province, South Africa. *Journal of Environmental and Public Health, 2018*, 1–10. https://doi.org/10.1155/2018/3143950.
2. Ahmed, S. H., Reithinger, R., Kaptoge, S. K., & Ngondi, J. (2020). Travel is a key risk factor for malaria transmission in pre-elimination settings in Sub-Saharan Africa: A review of the literature and meta-analysis. *American Journal of Tropical Medicine and Hygiene, 103*(4), 1380–1387. https://doi.org/10.4269/ajtmh.18-0456.
3. Alowais, S. A., Alghamdi, S. S., Alsuhebany, N., Alqahtani, T., Alshaya, A., Almohareb, S. N., Aldairem, A., et al. (2023). Revolutionizing healthcare: The role of artificial intelligence in clinical practice. *BMC Medical Education, 23*. https://doi.org/10.1186/s12909-023-04698-z.
4. Birungi, D., Aceng, F. L., Bulage, L., Nkonwa, I. H., Mirembe, B. B., Biribawa, C., Okethwangu, D., et al. (2021). Sporadic Rift Valley Fever outbreaks in humans and animals in Uganda, October 2017–January 2018. *Journal of Environmental and Public Health, 2021*, 1–8. https://doi.org/10.1155/2021/8881191.
5. Boyce, M. R., Katz, R., & Standley, C. J. (2019). Risk factors for infectious diseases in urban environments of Sub-Saharan Africa: A systematic review and critical appraisal of evidence. *Tropical Medicine and Infectious Disease, 4*(4), 123. https://doi.org/10.3390/tropicalmed4040123.
6. Braack, L., de Almeida, A. P. G., Cornel, A. J., Swanepoel, R., & de Jager, C. (2018). Mosquito-borne arboviruses of African origin: Review of key viruses and vectors. *Parasites & Vectors, 11*. https://doi.org/10.1186/s13071-017-2559-9.
7. Caminade, C., McIntyre, K. M., & Jones, A. (2018). Impact of recent and future climate change on vector-borne diseases. *Annals of the New York Academy of Sciences, 1436*, 157–173. https://doi.org/10.1111/nyas.13950.
8. Cao, J., Newby, G., Cotter, C., Hsiang, M. S., Larson, E., Tatarsky, A., Gosling, R., et al. (2021). Achieving malaria elimination in China. *The Lancet Public Health, 6*, e871–e872. https://doi.org/10.1016/s2468-2667(21)00201-2.
9. Cao, Y., Lu, G., Cotter, C., Wang, W., Yang, M., Liu, Y., Liang, C., et al. (2022). Improving the surveillance and response system to achieve and maintain malaria elimination: A retrospective analysis in Jiangsu Province, China. *Infectious Diseases of Poverty, 11*. https://doi.org/10.1186/s40249-022-00939-3.
10. Chamola, V., Hassija, V., Gupta, V., & Guizani, M. (2020). A comprehensive review of the COVID-19 pandemic and the role of IoT, drones, AI, blockchain, and 5G in managing its impact. *IEEE Access, 8*, 90225–90265. https://doi.org/10.1109/access.2020.2992341.
11. Chanda-Kapata, P., Kapata, N., & Zumla, A. (2020). COVID-19 and malaria: A symptom screening challenge for malaria endemic countries. *International Journal of Infectious Diseases, 94*, 151–153. https://doi.org/10.1016/j.ijid.2020.04.007.
12. Chiu, C. Y., & Miller, S. A. (2019). Clinical metagenomics. *Nature Reviews Genetics, 20*, 341–355. https://doi.org/10.1038/s41576-019-0113-7.

13. Davies, C., Graffy, R., Shandukani, M., Baloyi, E., Gast, L., Kok, G., Mbokazi, F., et al. (2019). Effectiveness of 24-h mobile reporting tool during a malaria outbreak in Mpumalanga Province, South Africa. *Malaria Journal, 18.* https://doi.org/10.1186/s12936-019-2683-4.

14. Debash, H., Nigatie, M., Bisetegn, H., Feleke, D. G., Tesfaw, G., Amha, A., Abate, M. A., et al. (2023). Malaria surveillance, outbreak investigation, response and its determinant factors in Waghemra Zone, Northeast Ethiopia: Unmatched case–control study. *Scientific Reports, 13.* https://doi.org/10.1038/s41598-023-36918-3.

15. Destoumieux-Garzón, D., Mavingui, P., Boëtsch, G., Boissier, J., Darriet, F., Duboz, P., Fritsch, C., et al. (2018). The One Health concept: 10 years old and a long road ahead. *Frontiers in Veterinary Science, 5.* https://doi.org/10.3389/fvets.2018.00014.

16. Emiru, T., Getachew, D., Murphy, M., Sedda, L., Ejigu, L. A., Bulto, M. G., Byrne, I., et al. (2023). Evidence for a role of *Anopheles stephensi* in the spread of drug- and diagnosis-resistant malaria in Africa. *Nature Medicine, 29*, 3203–3211. https://doi.org/10.1038/s41591-023-02641-9.

17. George, A. M., Ansumana, R., de Souza, D. K., Niyas, V. K. M., Zumla, A., & Bockarie, M. J. (2023). Climate change and the rising incidence of vector-borne diseases globally. *International Journal of Infectious Diseases, 139*, 143–145. https://doi.org/10.1016/j.ijid.2023.12.004.

18. Guo, Y. R., Cao, Q. D., Hong, Z. S., Tan, Y. Y., Chen, S. D., Jin, H. J., Tan, K. S., et al. (2020). The origin, transmission and clinical therapies on coronavirus disease 2019 (COVID-19) outbreak–An update on the status. *Military Medical Research, 7.* https://doi.org/10.1186/s40779-020-00240-0.

19. Haider, N., Asaduzzaman, M., Hasan, M. N., Rahman, M., Sharif, A. R., Ashrafi, S. A. A., Lee, S. S., et al. (2023). Bangladesh's 2023 dengue outbreak–Age/gender-related disparity in morbidity and mortality and geographic variability of epidemic burdens. *International Journal of Infectious Diseases, 136*, 1–4. https://doi.org/10.1016/j.ijid.2023.08.026.

20. Hladish, T. J., Pearson, C. A. B., Rojas, D. P., Gómez-Dantés, H., Halloran, M. E., Vazquez-Prokopec, G. M., & Longini, I. M. (2018). Forecasting the effectiveness of indoor residual spraying for reducing dengue burden. *PLoS Neglected Tropical Diseases, 12*(8), e0006570. https://doi.org/10.1371/journal.pntd.0006570.

21. Hu, B., Guo, H., Zhou, P., & Shi, Z. L. (2020). Characteristics of SARS-CoV-2 and COVID-19. *Nature Reviews Microbiology, 19*, 141–154. https://doi.org/10.1038/s41579-020-00459-7.

22. Jia, P., Dong, W., Yang, S., Zhan, Z., Tu, L., & Lai, S. (2020). Spatial lifecourse epidemiology and infectious disease research. *Trends in Parasitology, 36*(3), 235–238. https://doi.org/10.1016/j.pt.2019.12.012.

23. Lidani, K. C. F., Andrade, F. A., Bavia, L., Damasceno, F. S., Beltrame, M. H., Messias-Reason, I., & Sandri, T. L. (2019). Chagas disease: From discovery to a worldwide health problem. *Frontiers in Public Health, 7.* https://doi.org/10.3389/fpubh.2019.00166.

24. Lin, Z., Yin, S., Yang, J., Guo, X., Dong, C. L., Lin, Y. K., Ding, C. L., et al. (2022). The public health response to an outbreak of border-spill malaria along China-Myanmar border. *PLoS ONE, 17*(12), e0275932. https://doi.org/10.1371/journal.pone.0275932.

25. Magnano San Lio, R., Favara, G., Maugeri, A., Barchitta, M., & Agodi, A. (2023). How antimicrobial resistance is linked to climate change: An overview of two intertwined global challenges. *International Journal of Environmental Research and Public Health, 20*(3), 1681. https://doi.org/10.3390/ijerph20031681.

26. Masango, T. T., Nyadzayo, T. K., Gombe, N. T., Juru, T., Shambira, G., Chiwanda, S., & Tshimanga, M. (2020). Factors associated with malaria infection in Mudzi District, Mashonaland East Zimbabwe, 2019: A case-control study. *BMC Public Health, 20*. https://doi.org/10.1186/s12889-020-09872-2.

27. Naghavi, M., Ong, K. L., Aali, A., Ababneh, H., Abate, Y. H., Abbafati, C., Abbasgholizadeh, R., et al. (2024). Global burden of 288 causes of death and life expectancy decomposition in 204 countries and territories and 811 subnational locations, 1990–2021: A systematic analysis for the Global Burden of Disease Study 2021. *The Lancet, 403*, 2100–2132. https://doi.org/10.1016/S0140-6736(24)00367-2.

28. Nunthavichitra, S., Prapaso, S., Luvira, V., Muangnoicharoen, S., Leaungwutiwong, P., & Piyaphanee, W. (2020). Case report: COVID-19 presenting as acute undifferentiated febrile illness—A tropical world threat. *American Journal of Tropical Medicine and Hygiene, 103*(1), 83–85. https://doi.org/10.4269/ajtmh.20-0440.

29. Pascarella, G., Strumia, A., Piliego, C., Bruno, F., Del Buono, R., Costa, F., Scarlata, S., et al. (2020). COVID-19 diagnosis and management: A comprehensive review. *Journal of Internal Medicine, 288*, 192–206. https://doi.org/10.1111/joim.13091.

30. Petherick, A. (2020). Developing antibody tests for SARS-CoV-2. *The Lancet, 395*, 1101–1102. https://doi.org/10.1016/s0140-6736(20)30788-1.

31. Queiroz, M. M., Ivanov, D., Dolgui, A., & Wamba, S. F. (2020). Impacts of epidemic outbreaks on supply chains: Mapping a research agenda amid the COVID-19 pandemic through a structured literature review. *Annals of Operations Research, 319*, 1159–1196. https://doi.org/10.1007/s10479-020-03685-7.

32. Rai, A., Routh, D., & Bhunia, G. S. (2024). Measuring social vulnerability indicators to COVID pandemic: A GIS based analysis in North 24 Parganas, West Bengal, India. *IOP Conference Series: Earth and Environmental Science*. https://www.semanticscholar.org/paper/f43425da21b52941b23f24c700c8826d5b23bce8 (accessed on 13 May 2025).

33. Roth, G. A., Abate, D., Abate, K. H., Abay, S. M., Abbafati, C., Abbasi, N., Abbastabar, H., et al. (2018). Global, regional, and national age-sex-specific mortality for 282 causes of death in 195 countries and territories, 1980–2017: A systematic analysis for the Global Burden of Disease Study 2017. *The Lancet, 392*, 1736–1788. https://doi.org/10.1016/s0140-6736(18)32203-7.

34. Sanders, J. M., Monogue, M. L., Jodlowski, T. Z., & Cutrell, J. B. (2020). Pharmacologic treatments for coronavirus disease 2019 (COVID-19). *JAMA*. https://doi.org/10.1001/jama.2020.6019.

35. Sripoorote, P., Wattanagoon, Y., Inthitanon, N., Petchvijit, P., Thongyod, W., Win, K. M., Anantjitsupha, A., et al. (2024). Demographic and socioeconomic obstacles to access to malaria services for Myanmar migrants in Thailand. *Malaria Journal, 23*. https://www.semanticscholar.org/paper/dc874aa3c0ec9f10905d521959c0bdef2dbd4bd6 (accessed on 13 May 2025).

36. Tudi, M., Ruan, H. D., Wang, L., Lyu, J., Sadler, R., Connell, D., Chu, C., et al. (2021). Agriculture development, pesticide application and its impact on the environment. *International Journal of Environmental Research and Public Health, 18*(3), 1112. https://doi.org/10.3390/ijerph18031112.

37. Uddin, T. M., Chakraborty, A., Khusro, A., Zidan, B. M. R. M., Mitra, S., Emran, T. B., Dhama, K., et al. (2021). Antibiotic resistance in microbes: History, mechanisms, therapeutic strategies

and future prospects. *Journal of Infection and Public Health, 14*(12), 1750–1766. https://doi.org/10.1016/j.jiph.2021.10.020.

38. Uwishema, O., Chalhoub, E., Zahabioun, A., David, S., Khoury, C., AlSaraireh, T. H., Bekele, B. K., et al. (2021). The rising incidence of African swine fever during the COVID-19 pandemic in Africa: Efforts, challenges and recommendations. *The International Journal of Health Planning and Management, 37*, 561–567. https://doi.org/10.1002/hpm.3357.

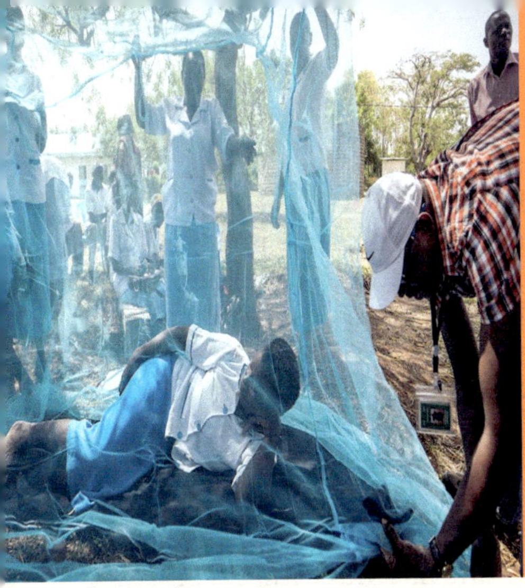

Chapter 12

VECTOR CONTROL STRATEGIES FOR MALARIA

Contents

Introduction

Malaria still poses a major public health challenge worldwide, hitting developing nations in tropical and subtropical regions especially hard. Even with notable strides in treatment and prevention, millions continue to suffer each year, leading, in most cases, to high rates of illness and death. The disease's spread isn't simple; it involves humans alongside Anopheles mosquitoes as vectors, so battling malaria means looking at both biological details and the environment. Controlling these mosquitoes is a key tactic, one that's growing even more crucial now as many countries near pre-elimination and find themselves juggling shifting disease patterns and rising parasite resistance (Feachem et al., 2009). Across the globe, the renewed push to wipe out malaria has spurred fresh ideas for mosquito control that suit varied local conditions. It isn't only about cutting down the number of mosquitoes; it's also about breaking the parasite's life cycle. In recent years, measures like insecticide-treated nets and indoor residual spraying have shown promising results in lowering case numbers. Still, these methods sometimes run into problems, such as insecticide resistance or patchy coverage, which means that innovative and more mixed approaches might be needed. Reaching high coverage, particularly among vulnerable groups, brings both direct protection and broader community benefits, making an expanded focus on vector control an essential part of public health strategy (Killeen et al., 2007). When planning effective malaria control, it helps to understand local disease dynamics, available resources, and operational capabilities—a process that can be somewhat complex. Generally speaking, assessing technical feasibility alongside financial limits is a challenge because every region and time period is different. Effective strategies need to fit snugly with surveillance efforts, cross-border collaborations, and supportive policies to keep transmission at zero and block any reintroduction. Plus, emerging technologies and a deeper grasp of mosquito behavior are opening up paths for more focused, flexible control measures. To summarize, vector control remains indispensable for eliminating malaria; it ties together scientific insights with the practical realities of on-the-ground implementation (Feachem et al., 2009) (Figure 12.1).

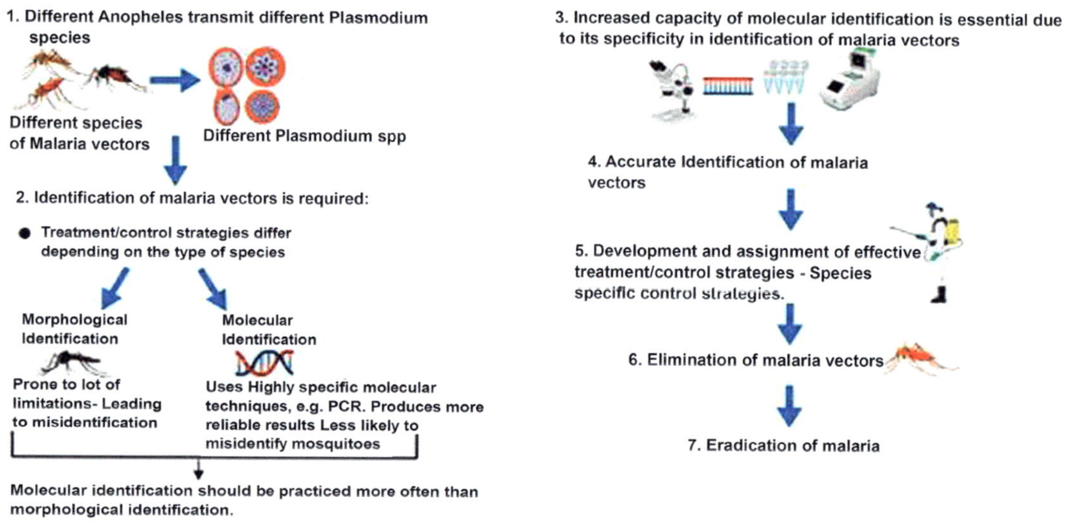

Figure 12.1. Vector control strategies for malaria.

Source: Hadebe MT, Malgwi SA, Okpeku M. Revolutionizing Malaria Vector Control: The Importance of Accurate Species Identification through Enhanced Molecular Capacity. *Microorganisms*. 2024; 12(1):82. https://doi.org/10.3390/microorganisms12010082

Definition of Malaria and Its Global Impact

Humans have been complex up with disease-spreading pathogens for ages, and this bond has shaped how infections emerge. Malaria, for instance, has stuck around as one of the most stubborn and harsh illnesses carried by these tiny pathogens. It happens when you get bitten by a female Anopheles mosquito carrying a *Plasmodium* parasite – little protozoans that cause all the trouble. The parasite's erratic journey between mosquito and human, well, it often throws a wrench in efforts to break its cycle. Millions suffer every year, especially in warm, humid areas where control measures run into major roadblocks. Figuring out the basic biological and ecological roots of this illness is essential if we're going to come up with new, creative ways to control these vectors and ease the socio-economic burdens they bring. Even with leaps in treatment and prevention, malaria still leaves a heavy imprint on public health, in sub-Saharan Africa, where *Plasmodium falciparum* tends to dominate. This nasty variant is behind most severe cases and deaths, which clearly shows its aggressiveness and underscores our urgent need to update control measures. Rising drug resistance and habits like self-medicating (which sometimes weaken treatment efficacy) only make things worse. In most cases, these overlapping issues point to the need for mixing vector control with medical care and community-based strategies. Strengthening our health systems along with these strategies remains pretty crucial if we hope to cut down malaria's far-reaching impact and eventually wipe it out (Bauer et al., 2023). Taking a step back, malaria's ripple effects extend well beyond immediate health problems—they also drag down economic productivity and slow development across many affected regions. A ton of effort and investment goes into research for everything from vector controls and new drugs to repellents and vaccines. Yet, current methods can fall short, sometimes proving less effective while stirring up unplanned ecological side effects. For example, the heavy reliance on insecticides has led to a drop in insect diversity, which, in turn, can upset local ecosystems and indirectly impact human well-being. These challenges push us to explore fresh, eco-friendly, and sustainable ways to manage disease carriers—approaches that try to balance illness prevention with keeping nature intact. Revisiting some ideas once overlooked, now backed by insights from fields like entomology and molecular biology, opens up promising paths for fighting malaria while keeping collateral damage to ecosystems in check (Bauer et al., 2023).

Importance of Vector Control in Malaria Prevention

Malaria still takes a heavy toll on public health, especially in areas where nature and climate let the female Anopheles mosquito flourish. In the African highlands, for instance, research has repeatedly found that when you see more of these mosquitoes around, malaria cases tend to rise too. Rain patterns, temperature shifts, and even how close people live to breeding spots all mix together to influence these mosquito numbers. And , when there aren't proper control measures in place, that risk just goes up. Analysts have used tools like classification and regression trees to show—quite clearly, which the number of mosquitoes plays a huge role in predicting outbreaks, which points to the need for smart, targeted control efforts (Protopopoff et al., 2009). For decades, progress in cutting down malaria cases and deaths has mostly depended on using vector control tools like ITNs. These nets work by lowering the chance people get bitten during peak mosquito hours, and in many parts of sub-Saharan Africa, they've helped reduce both cases and fatalities dramatically. Still, even though ITN coverage is high in many spots, progress has recently started to plateau. In most cases, this slowdown reveals that there are still gaps—whether from how effective the nets are or from certain human behaviors that still leave people exposed. This situation kind of pushes us to dig deeper into how human practices, mosquito habits, and the environment all interact, so we can tighten up our strategies. Also, adding in well-thought-out social and behavioral change campaigns might just boost the nets' impact over time (Monroe et al., 2020). When it comes to fighting malaria, it's clear that sticking only to traditional tools like ITNs and indoor spraying isn't enough. Sure, vector control remains the main way to lessen transmission, but things like the variety of mosquito species, emerging insecticide resistance, and shifting ecological conditions all call for a more flexible approach. In many cases, effective control doesn't just lower malaria rates right away, it also helps build longer-term systems for tracking outbreaks and predicting when things might flare up again. For example, keeping tabs on mosquito numbers together with climate data can sometimes offer just enough of an early warning to roll out targeted measures before an epidemic gets out of hand. To summarize, a solid grasp of mosquito ecology, mixed with adaptable control strategies, is absolutely key if we want to push forward with malaria prevention and, ultimately, aim for sustainable disease elimination (Protopopoff et al., 2009; Monroe et al., 2020) (Figure 12.2).

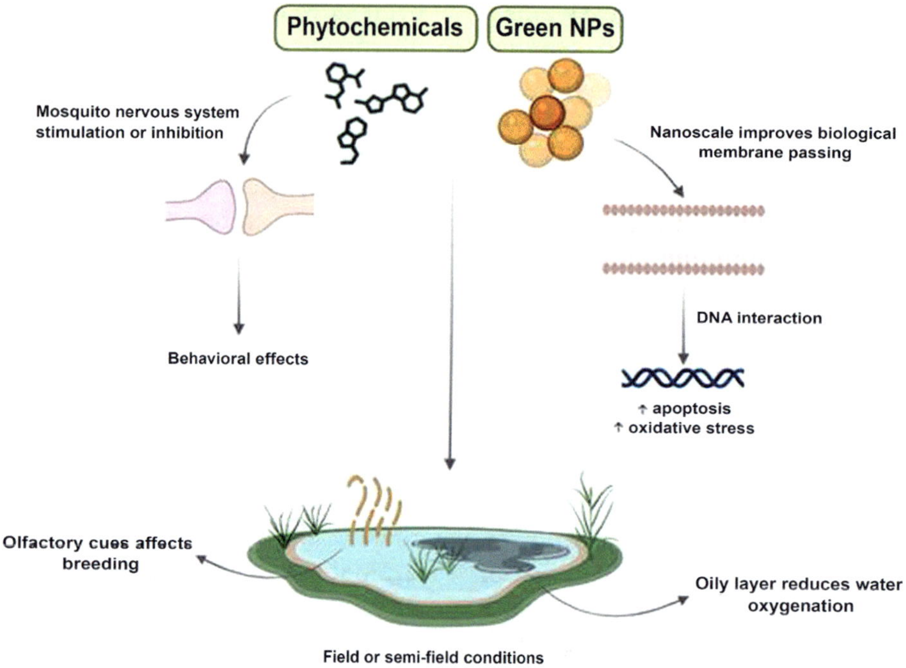

Figure 12.2. Vector control in malaria prevention.

Source: Moraes-de-Souza I, de Moraes BPT, Silva AR, Ferrarini SR, Gonçalves-de-Albuquerque CF. Tiny Green Army: Fighting Malaria with Plants and Nanotechnology. *Pharmaceutics*. 2024; 16(6):699. https://doi.org/10.3390/pharmaceutics16060699

12.1. Understanding Malaria Transmission

Malaria control hinges on knowing how our surroundings shape the spread of the disease. People and mosquitos get complex up in many climate and geography, which defines where the Anopheles mosquitos, those main carriers of malaria parasites, tend to thrive. Technology has stepped in here—tools like satellite images and geographic information systems now help spot potential mosquito hangouts by tracking wetlands and various land covers. Scientists even map out risk zones in sometimes unexpected ways, using these geospatial tools not just to count mosquitos but also to see how shifts in the environment sway transmission patterns. In most cases, mixing this data with national control plans helps fine-tune resource use and intervention plans, cutting down on both the sickness itself and its extra social and economic burdens (Bauwens et al., 2015). In parts of Southeast Asia, the story gets a bit twisty. Studies there reveal that *Anopheles balabacensis*, a key vector for *Plasmodium knowlesi*, tends to bite outdoors in the early evening; a habit that dodges the protection of indoor bednets. This behavior, along with changing vector densities and infection rates across villages, forests, and farms, shows how much local conditions matter. , if you don't get how these mosquito habits shift from place to place, it's tough to design interventions that pause transmission and also tackle the rising challenges from malaria parasites that jump from animals to people (Chua et al., 2015). Then there's the added layer of complexity from malaria parasites that don't stick to just one host. The emergence of *P. knowlesi* as a leading cause in some areas reminds us that looking only at human factors is too narrow. Instead, control strategies have to mull over the interactions of simian hosts, human carriers, and mosquito vectors across varied settings. This calls for long-running studies—both in the field of insects and disease spread—to work out how these cycles tick over time. When you stitch together the environmental, behavioral, and ecological pieces, you get a much sturdier framework for cutting down malaria and pushing closer to regional elimination goals (Bauwens et al., 2015; Chua et al., 2015) (Figure 12.3).

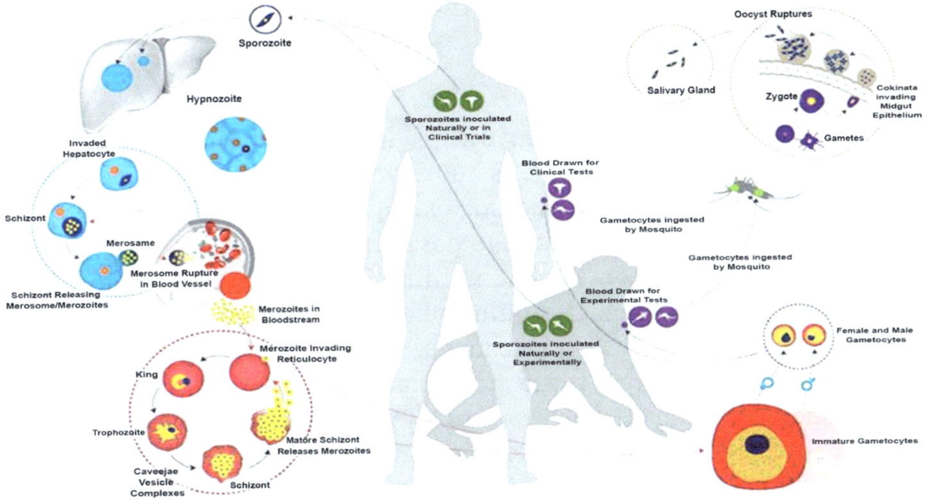

Figure 12.3. Understanding malaria transmission.

Source: CDN InTech. (n.d.). *Understanding Malaria Transmission.*

12.1.1. Life Cycle of the Malaria Parasite

Malaria's life cycle is complex and full of twists, swinging between humans and female Anopheles mosquitoes. After an infected mosquito bites someone, sporozoites jump quickly into the bloodstream and rush off to the liver, where they multiply in a burst of asexual reproduction. Soon enough, these parasites invade red blood cells—then, as the cells burst, more merozoites spill out to infect others. Interestingly, some of these parasites switch strategies and become gametocytes, the sexual forms needed to restart the cycle in a mosquito. Generally speaking, factors like how many parasites are present and the strength of the host's immune system play a huge role in determining whether these gametocytes stick around, directly influencing the spread of malaria (Maheu-Giroux & Castro, 2013). Inside the mosquito the scene shifts dramatically. When a mosquito takes a blood meal carrying gametocytes, the parasite embarks on a whole new journey. In a sort of spontaneous mating association, male and female gametes fuse to create zygotes that quickly evolve into motile ookinetes. These ookinetes then sneak through the midgut wall and settle into oocysts, which later fork out scores of sporozoites toward the salivary glands. The mosquito stage ends up being a bottleneck—a period when the parasite numbers shrink sharply, but it's also when genetic mixing happens, adding diversity that helps these organisms dodge immune responses and sometimes even resist drugs. Unfortunately, recreating this challenging mosquito environment in labs has been challenging, leaving us with only a patchy molecular understanding (Parres-Mercader et al., 2023). The parasite's ability to change its game based on its surroundings shapes malaria's overall impact, and our fight against it. For example, if a host becomes anemic or if parasite levels start to fluctuate unpredictably, the parasite may increase its gametocyte production to boost its transmission odds. This flexible, responsive strategy often muddles efforts aimed at blocking transmission because the parasite shifts its priorities on the fly (Maheu-Giroux & Castro, 2013). Plus, the genetic reshuffling inside the mosquito not only stirs up diversity but can also lead to drug-resistant strains, which is a big worry for current treatments. To summarize, any effective strategy to control malaria needs to factor in these ever-changing life cycle stages and adaptive behaviors to truly break the transmission cycle (Parres-Mercader et al., 2023).

12.1.2. Role of Anopheles Mosquitoes as Vectors

Anopheles mosquitoes are a curiosity in their own right – their biology is a big reason they're so effective at carrying malaria. These pathogens come with unique habits and built-in body traits that let the *Plasmodium* parasite hitch a ride; for example, females need a blood meal to develop eggs, which naturally creates an opening for the parasite to move between mosquito and human. Genetic alters, along with everyday environmental influences, weigh in on how well they do this job. In most cases, recent advances in mosquito genomics have peeled back the layers of these processes, showing us how genes shift and change, with regulatory pathways dancing along to boost their adaptability. Understanding these molecular details lays a kind of foundation for novel, targeted control methods; tailoring interventions to hit the mosquito's weak spots might be our best chance (Célia Lutrat et al., 2019). To summarize, mixing insights from genomics with the features of mosquito behavior seems pretty essential in the global fight against malaria. Control strategies targeting these mosquitoes demand a deep understanding of their population dynamics and how they reproduce. Techniques such as the sterile insect technique (SIT) are designed to impact mosquito reproduction by releasing sterilized males that compete with wild ones. Of course, during mass rearing one must be extra careful to correctly separate the sexes – even a few mis-identified females can keep disease transmission alive. Recently, improvements in sex separation (using tools like gene editing and approaches that explore Diptera's own sex-determination processes) have opened promising, cost-effective, and safer paths forward. By focusing on releasing only those sterile males, the natural cycle of reproduction gets disrupted and the malaria spread drops. Still, challenges remain—scaling up production, ensuring these males can hold their own in the wild, and winning community support for these genetic methods are all issues to tackle (Célia Lutrat et al., 2019). Looking deeper, the evolutionary twists within Anopheles populations bring both hurdles and new opportunities for control. These species show a complex mix of genetic diversity, adaptive shifts, and introgression events that color their ability as malaria vectors and their resistance to insecticides. Comparative genomic studies suggest that gene flow on autosomes alongside differences in sex chromosomes can speed up adaptation, making standard control measures less reliable than one might hope. Generally speaking, these findings advocate for the integration of evolutionary genomics into our management strategies if we're to anticipate and counter resistance as it develops. Researchers have even pointed out specific male-determining factors on the Y chromosome—marking novel targets for sex distortion or genetic suppression efforts. As mosquito populations continue to evolve, fine-tuning control methods with these genomic and evolutionary insights remains critical for keeping the push toward malaria eradication on track (Ruzzante et al., 2018) (Figure 12.4).

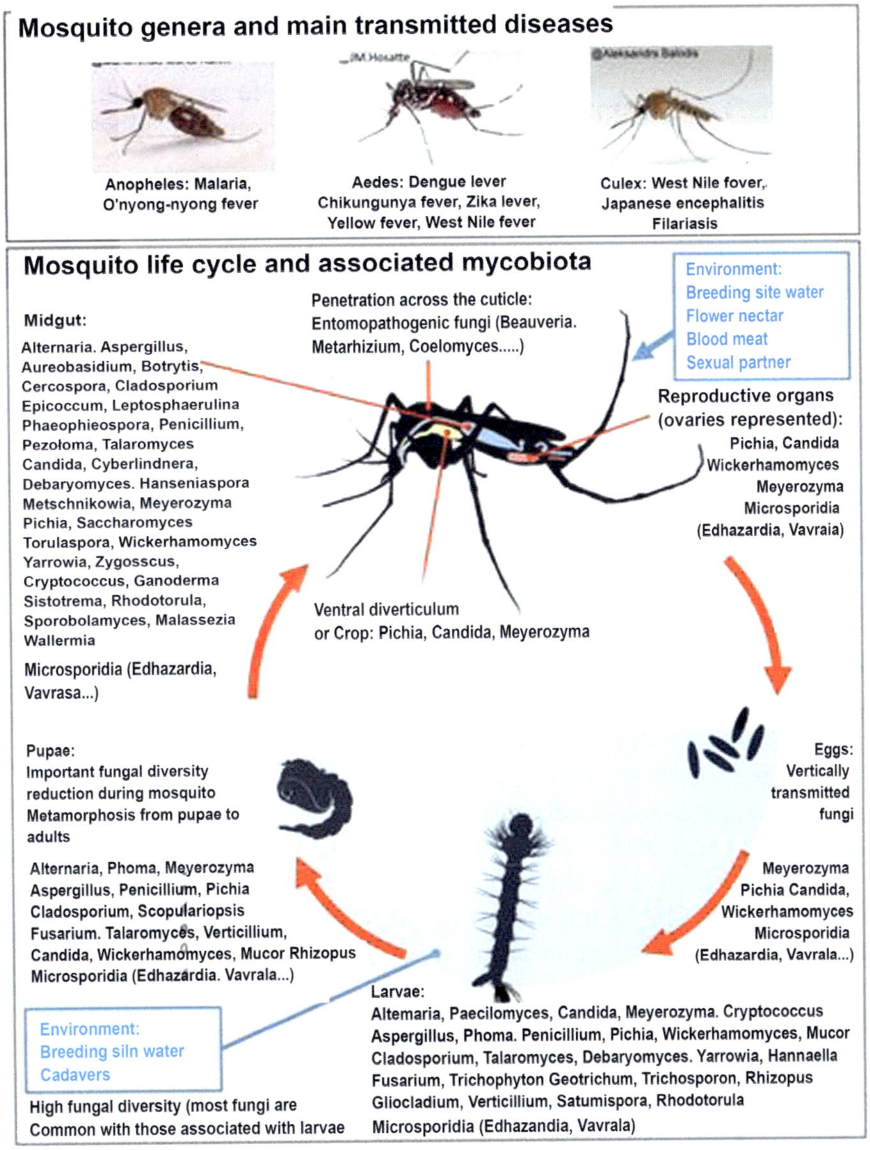

Figure 12.4. Role of Anopheles mosquitoes as vectors.

Source: Malassigné S, Valiente Moro C, Luis P. Mosquito Mycobiota: An Overview of Non-Entomopathogenic Fungal Interactions. *Pathogens*. 2020; 9(7):564. https://doi.org/10.3390/pathogens9070564

12.1.3. Factors Influencing Malaria Transmission Dynamics

Malaria's spread doesn't follow a single, tidy pattern, it's the outcome of many factors all complex together. Think first of the human host, the parasite itself, the mosquito that carries it, and even the features of the environment. In most cases, what we see now is as much a product of long-ago transmission patterns as it is of today's infection levels. You might notice, for example, that some infections slip past standard microscopy; these submicroscopic cases, though hard to spot, still keep the cycle going. They crop up unevenly across communities, even in places with similar overall transmission, and complicate efforts to home in on every infected group. To summarize, this complex mix of influences calls for vector control plans that are custom-made for each local patch (Whittaker et al., 2022). If you look deeper, the spatial side of things adds another twist. In many neighborhoods, particularly at the household level, malaria cases tend to cluster; interestingly, as the overall number of cases drops, these clusters become even more pronounced. It's almost as if the infection gets pickier about where it shows up. A community-wide approach might work well in some areas, while in others a door-to-door tactic might be the better play. Then there's time—mosquito numbers change with the seasons. Rainfall, temperature swings, how close people live to water, and shifts in land use all mix together to shape mosquito populations in unpredictable ways. Recognizing these ever-changing patterns helps pinpoint when methods like indoor residual spraying can be deployed most effectively (Whittaker et al., 2022). Local malaria trends aren't just about nature, either—they're deeply influenced by how people live and move. In Rwanda, for instance, some districts seem burdened by malaria far more persistently than others. These pockets of high incidence are often combined to the local climate's ups and downs, differences in how well control measures work, and even cross-border movements of people. Age, gender, and other demographic features further twist the risk, meaning that a one-size-fits-all strategy rarely cuts it. Plus, as the parasite and mosquitoes grow resistant to drugs and insecticides, traditional control methods hit unexpected roadblocks. All that said, weaving in detailed, spatio-temporal analyses into national malaria strategies can lead to nimbler, data-driven responses—ones that match local realities and make the most of every resource (Figure 12.5).

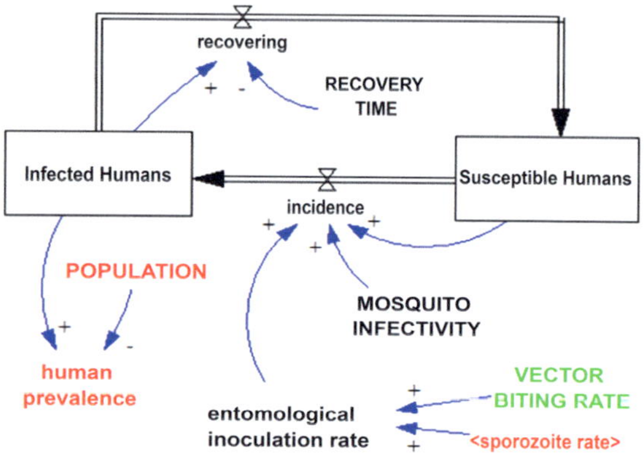

Figure 12.5. Factors influencing malaria transmission dynamics.

Source: Fortune Journals. (n.d.). *Statics and Dynamics of Malaria Transmission.*

12.2. Traditional Vector Control Methods

Malaria control has long leaned on reducing the chance that people and Anopheles mosquitoes come into contact. In many places where malaria is common, individuals tend to depend on things like insecticide-treated bed nets and indoor spraying, which aim mainly at mosquitoes that rest inside houses. These measures, generally speaking, work by damping down the adult mosquito population and cutting off the disease's spread. Still, their strength can waver; issues such as insects building resistance and nets not being used every night keep cropping up. In some communities, local views and knowledge even muddle things further. For instance, in southern Benin, a lack of clear understanding of mosquitoes' role leads people to adopt habits that don't fully protect them, underscoring why health education is so necessary (Padonou et al., 2018). Consequently, mixing these tools with efforts to change behavior seems to bring better results. Another angle of the challenge comes from the very homes people live in. It turns out that the quality of housing plays a big part in how well these traditional methods work. If houses are poorly built, with lots of cracks and flimsy barriers, mosquitoes can slip in easily, rendering bed nets and spraying less effective. A study in Swaziland, where transmission was relatively low, showed that those living in low- to medium-quality houses faced higher odds of malaria than those in sturdier dwellings (Dlamini et al., 2017). These findings highlight that even when control methods perform well on a personal level, environmental factors can limit their reach. Improving things like window screens, patching up walls, or even swapping thatched roofs for better alternatives can cut down mosquito access, and overall help traditional interventions do their job. At the same time, keeping these strategies going demands ongoing community support and resources. Regular use of bed nets and scheduled indoor spraying aren't just about having the materials available; they also rely on cultural acceptance and day-to-day habits. Without addressing local opinions and making sure people understand how malaria spreads—as seen in those Benin examples where misunderstandings hampered proper control practices—the benefits aren't fully realized (Padonou et al., 2018). Then there's the challenge of insecticide resistance, which means that careful monitoring and periodic rotation of chemicals are needed to keep efficacy up. Even with fresh ideas on the horizon, these traditional methods remain a big part of fighting malaria. So, a mixed approach that combines better housing, thoughtful education, and smart alters based on mosquito behavior appears to be key to making lasting progress against the disease (Figure 12.6).

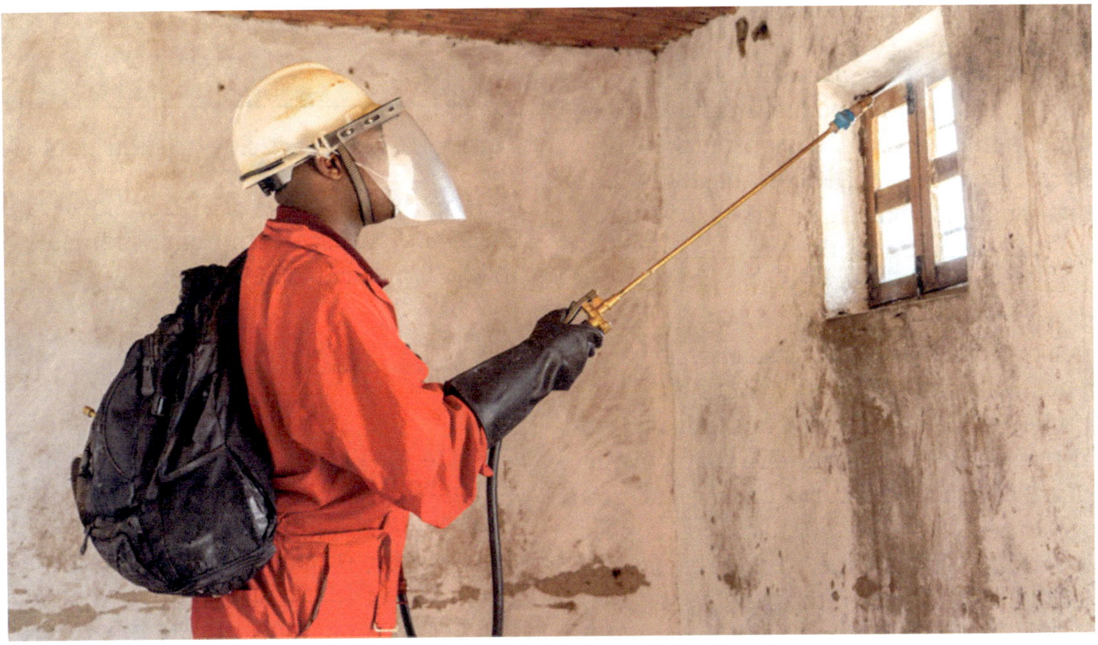

Figure 12.6. Traditional malaria vector control method.

Source: Science. (2021). *Mosquito Spraying for Malaria Control.*

12.2.1. Insecticide-Treated Nets (ITNs)

Malaria control relies on many methods, but mixing personal protection with direct vector measures seems especially effective. For example, using insecticide-treated nets isn't just about blocking mosquito bites; these nets also deliver a chemical punch that cuts down on mosquito numbers. Research out in parts of rural Sub-Saharan Africa generally shows that when these nets are spread around and used regularly, malaria cases and deaths fall noticeably, with kids under five often seeing the biggest benefits. In many cases, proper use can lower the number of malaria episodes by about half and trim mortality by some 20%. They work at night, when people are most vulnerable, and at the same time help reduce transmission on a community level. Still, issues like rising insecticide resistance and how carefully people use the nets can affect their long-term success (Zikayo, 2025). Even with all these advantages, several practical and local issues can muck up the nets' performance in everyday life. Things like how long the nets hold up, whether people maintain them properly, and simply using them consistently, make a difference—if individuals misuse them, the protection slips away. Socioeconomic challenges and turbulent situations, such as conflict or resource-scarce settings, can also get in the way. And, since most nets use pyrethroid insecticides, there's the ongoing worry that mosquitoes will build up resistance over time. For these reasons, research is now pushing next-generation nets that mix in new chemicals or synergists designed to outsmart resistance. It turns out that pairing these improvements with community education and engagement, even if the messages repeat the same points from time to time— boosts usage and the public health benefits overall (Zikayo, 2025). New ideas are also popping up as experts look at how to mix these nets with other emerging tools to fight malaria, especially in places where standard plans might not do the trick. Spatial repellents, for instance, have been getting some buzz, mainly because they might help in emergency or humanitarian setups where nets alone aren't enough. ITNs still stand as a solid option under regular conditions, but current studies are examining how spatial repellents, with or without nets—might better shield those at risk. The early findings should, in most cases, help steer policy choices and fine-tune how we roll out these interventions across different social and health landscapes. To summarize, a flexible, evidence-based strategy seems key if we're to edge closer to wiping out malaria (Figure 12.7).

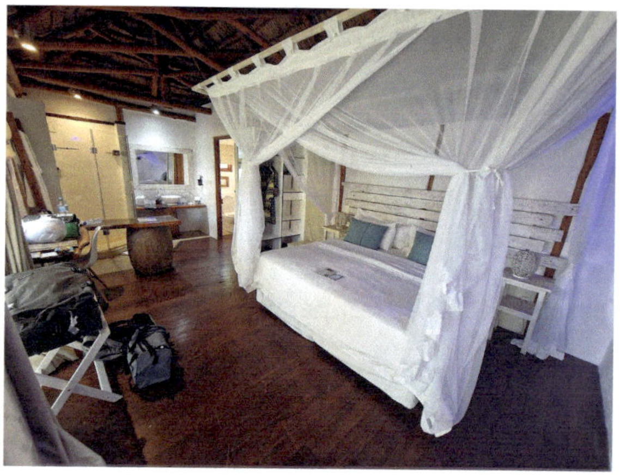

Figure 12.7. Insecticide-treated nets (ITNs).

Source: By FrogsLegs71 - The photographer, CC BY-SA 3.0, https://commons.wikimedia.org/w/index.php?curid=151708895

12.2.2. Indoor Residual Spraying (IRS)

Malaria still plagues many communities—in sub-Saharan Africa especially, even with all the control efforts tossed at it. IRS comes up as one of those key measures. , it means releaseing long-lasting insecticides on home walls and ceilings so that mosquitoes, once they've had their meal, end up resting on treated surfaces. This hit not only cuts down their lifespan but, in most cases, also limits the spread of parasites to people. Field observations from places like Kenya and Burkina Faso, using organophosphate chemicals, have shown—quite clearly, which IRS is a big deal for reducing malaria overall, and they even push the idea of mixing IRS into bigger vector control plans (Traore et al., 2019). Even with its track record, IRS isn't without its share of stumbling blocks. In many instances, mosquitoes develop resistance to the chemicals we use, which, frankly, weakens the spray's punch and forces the use of newer or alternative insecticides. Further, getting IRS applied correctly everywhere comes with its own set of headaches—logistical issues, cost challenges, you name it. And now there's the added twist of mosquitoes biting outdoors and the ongoing resistance problem, which generally nudges experts to think about integrating IRS into a wider, more balanced vector management setup (Beier et al., 2018). New strides in fighting malaria make it pretty clear that IRS alone might not cut it. Researchers are now betting on many fresh approaches to cover the gaps left by insecticide resistance and changing mosquito habits. Some ideas include managing larvae, with the help of genetically modified bacteria even—new insecticide combines, attractive toxic sugar baits, and eave tubes. Still, if you look at most national programs, IRS and long-lasting nets (LLINs) still steal the show, mostly because they've been around for a while and work out to be cost-effective. That said, to get a handle on malaria for good, it seems imperative to combine IRS with these emerging tools and beef up efforts to manage insecticide resistance, in most cases (Beier et al., 2018; Traore et al., 2019) (Figure 12.8).

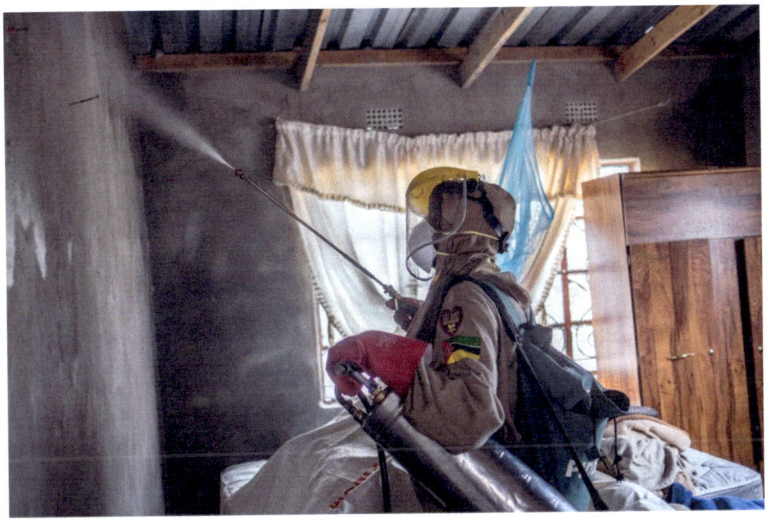

Figure 12.8. Indoor residual spraying (IRS).

Source: World Health Organization. (n.d.). *Indoor Residual Spraying.*

12.2.3. Environmental Management and Habitat Modification

Understanding how to tackle malaria essentially means getting a clear picture of how mosquitoes interact with their surroundings. Researchers have long noticed that shaking things up in the environment—by cutting off mosquito breeding spots and making it tougher for them to find the stuff they need—can put a dent in their numbers. Rather than treating mosquitoes as just targets for chemical sprays (which, in most cases, struggle with resistance problems), one can simply see their need to find water for larvae and blood meals as a matter of chance encounters. This way of looking at things lets us gauge how nature's shifts might alter malaria spread. It also calls attention to the need for local expertise and better infrastructure in areas like sub-Saharan Africa, where the know-how isn't always there yet. Mixing these environmental changes with health and clinical efforts might just breathe new life into long-term malaria control programs (Killeen et al., 2004). Larval source management stands out as one neat trick to break a mosquito's life cycle before they become pesky adults, especially in cities, where breeding spots are easier to pin down. Sometimes, community-led microbial larviciding—when done in a steady, organized fashion—has been shown to drive down malaria cases significantly. For example, in Dar es Salaam, Tanzania, such a push managed a 21% drop in the odds of getting infected, which highlights how changing mosquito habitats with biologically based larvicides can pay off. This method tends to work best during dry spells, when breeding sites shrink into more manageable patches. Plus, pairing larviciding with other tools like insecticide-treated nets and small-scale house modifications creates many defenses that seem to work better together (Maheu-Giroux & Castro, 2013). Keeping up with these environment-based alters isn't a walk in the park, especially in places where resources are tight. One big hurdle is rallying experts from all sides—entomologists, public health officials, environmental scientists, and even local community voices—so they can team up on interventions that genuinely stick. Further, mosquito habitats change all the time with the seasons and weather, so being adaptive and using real-time data becomes pretty crucial. When you mix habitat changes with regular check-ups, you can fine-tune the measures and get a better hold on malaria's spread. Investing in local talent and building up infrastructure, with a healthy dose of community involvement—turns what might be a quick fix into a lasting cornerstone of mosquito control (Killeen et al., 2004; Maheu-Giroux & Castro, 2013).

12.3. Biological Control Strategies

Malaria control today demands fresh approaches that step away from the usual chemical fixes. Mosquitoes are getting tougher—more resistant and quicker to adapt, and heavy insecticide use can hurt our surroundings. One neat idea is to let nature do some of the work. For instance, introducing fish that feast on larvae into ponds or ditches targets the mosquito's early life stage, effectively breaking their life cycle before it kicks in. This trick reduces the need for artificial larvicides and eases the impact on local ecosystems. Bacteria that zero in on mosquito larvae without disturbing other creatures add another layer of precision to this plan. All these nature-driven methods come together to support a broader, integrated vector management scheme that health experts often back (Shuguang et al., 2021). Knowing where and how mosquitoes breed turns out to be a game changer. Research from all over—be it highland stretches or busy peri-urban spots—shows that most breeding places spring up because of human habits. Focusing on the main culprits, *Anopheles gambiae* and *Anopheles arabiensis*, helps ensure that the biological strategies hit the mark at the right moments in these mosquitoes' growth. Sometimes, it even makes sense to fiddle with the environment itself, say by shading water bodies until they become too cool for larvae, mixing that with the use of predatory fish and biolarvicides. This kind of multi-pronged, almost patchwork approach not only slashes the number of mosquito young but also encourages locals to get hands-on with managing breeding grounds, which in most cases ends up lowering the risk of malaria spread (Imbahale et al., 2025). Getting communities involved is key to keeping these nature-based control ideas alive and kicking. Even though most locals see malaria as a serious problem, many still don't know about practical control measures, which clearly calls for more on-the-ground education along with the interventions. Local projects that mix in biological control methods tend to boost participation since people feel a sense of ownership, this, in turn, helps keep the control measures running consistently. And by altering strategies to fit the specific social and environmental flavors of each area, these approaches end up being both relevant and highly effective. Besides, when individuals start learning more about the issue, they naturally change habits, like clearing out makeshift water spots that serve as mosquito nurseries. In the end, mixing nature-based solutions with an engaged community builds a resilient foundation that chips away at mosquito populations and helps curb malaria transmission (Imbahale et al., 2025) (Figure 12.9).

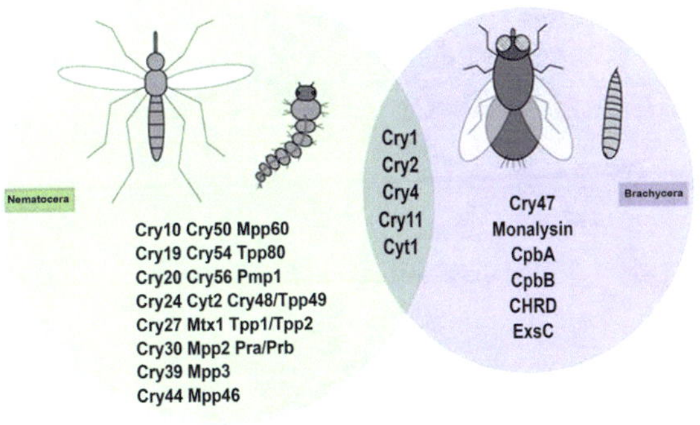

Figure 12.9. Biological control strategies for malaria.

Source: Valtierra-de-Luis D, Villanueva M, Berry C, Caballero P. Potential for *Bacillus thuringiensis* and Other Bacterial Toxins as Biological Control Agents to Combat Dipteran Pests of Medical and Agronomic Importance. *Toxins.* 2020; 12(12):773. https://doi.org/10.3390/toxins12120773

12.3.1. Use of Larvivorous Fish in Water Bodies

Malaria still poses a stubborn challenge, and nature-based fixes have started drawing attention instead of relying solely on chemicals. One idea that's been floated involves adding fish—ones that happily snack on mosquito larvae—to local water spots where Anopheles mosquitoes breed. These fish eat larvae and even the pupae, which might cut off the mosquito life cycle before they can take off. The World Health Organization (WHO), in most cases, backs this idea by recommending that water bodies near homes get stocked with these fish to slow down malaria's spread. But a closer look shows that there isn't strong, consistent proof that this trick lowers malaria cases or adult mosquito counts reliably (Adeel et al., 2013). Even though many regions have tried it, the mix of complicated ecosystems and study challenges makes it hard to claim that larvivorous fish offer a foolproof solution. When you dig into the actual evidence, the picture becomes even more complex. Some studies suggest that cramming a lot of these mosquito-eating fish into wells, ponds, or even rice paddies might briefly hold back the surge of young mosquitoes, yet these effects don't stick around or show up uniformly across different places (Adeel et al., 2017). Research sometimes points to fewer water spots hosting mosquito larvae overall, but the results jump around too much between different ecological settings to draw solid conclusions. In plain terms, no one has nailed down a strong, direct link between introducing these fish and a sustained drop in malaria or adult mosquito levels, which tells us we need more careful, controlled studies to figure out what's going on. Beyond whether these fish work as hoped, there's a fair bit of worry about what they might do to local ecosystems. The current research barely scratches the surface when it comes to understanding how these extra fish might impact native species or disturb the broader balance of local waters (Adeel et al., 2013). Also, the long-term success of this approach isn't only about how many larvae get eaten, it's also tangled up with whether communities can support the programs, how easy they are to run, and if they gel well with other mosquito control methods. Given the gaps and mixed findings in the evidence, most experts now suggest that incorporating larvivorous fish should be tried under controlled field trials rather than rolled out everywhere all at once. This careful path aims to balance the goal of controlling mosquitoes with the need to protect natural environments and manage resources wisely, a reminder of just how challenging it is to use biological methods for malaria control (Adeel et al., 2017) (Figure 12.10).

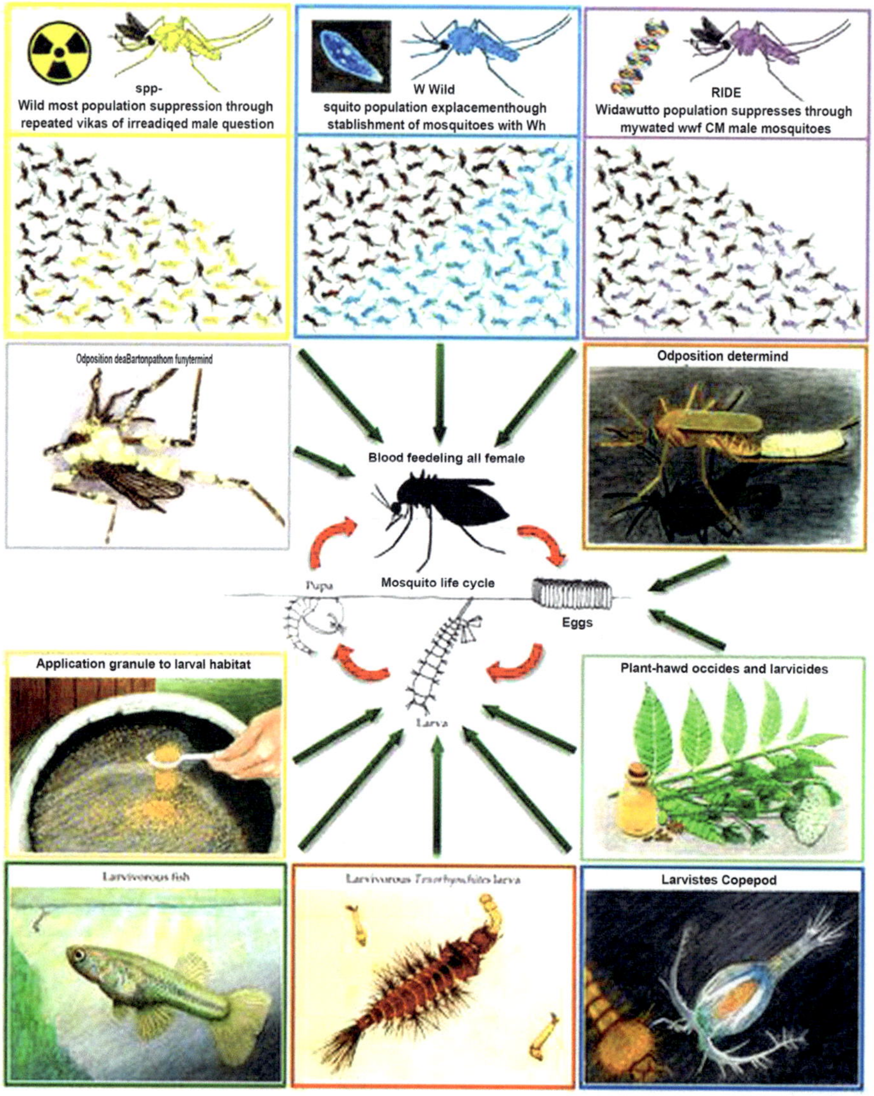

Figure 12.10. Use of larvivorous fish in water bodies.

Source: Benelli G, Jeffries CL, Walker T. Biological Control of Mosquito Vectors: Past, Present, and Future. *Insects*. 2016; 7(4):52. https://doi.org/10.3390/insects7040052

12.3.2. Introduction of Genetically Modified Mosquitoes

Global efforts to beat malaria have hit some obstacles. Bed nets treated with insecticides and sprays inside homes have helped drop the disease burden, but they're not a magic fix, especially in areas where transmission runs high. Mosquitoes seem to find ways around these measures—by building up resistance to chemicals or altering their behavior. One idea getting a lot of chatter is using genetically modified mosquitoes. In simple terms, these lab-altered insects would either bring down or replace the natural ones by altering their genes, aiming to cut down on their ability to spread malaria or simply lower their numbers in a way that lasts. It underscores the point that we need to look at mosquito life in a broader way—beyond just how they feed—to come up with lasting malaria control strategies (Schairer et al., 2019). There's no doubt that bringing genetically modified mosquitoes into the mix comes with a heap of social and ethical puzzles. When you start altering with nature like this, it's crucial to have individuals in the community and all kinds of stakeholders chatting openly about it.

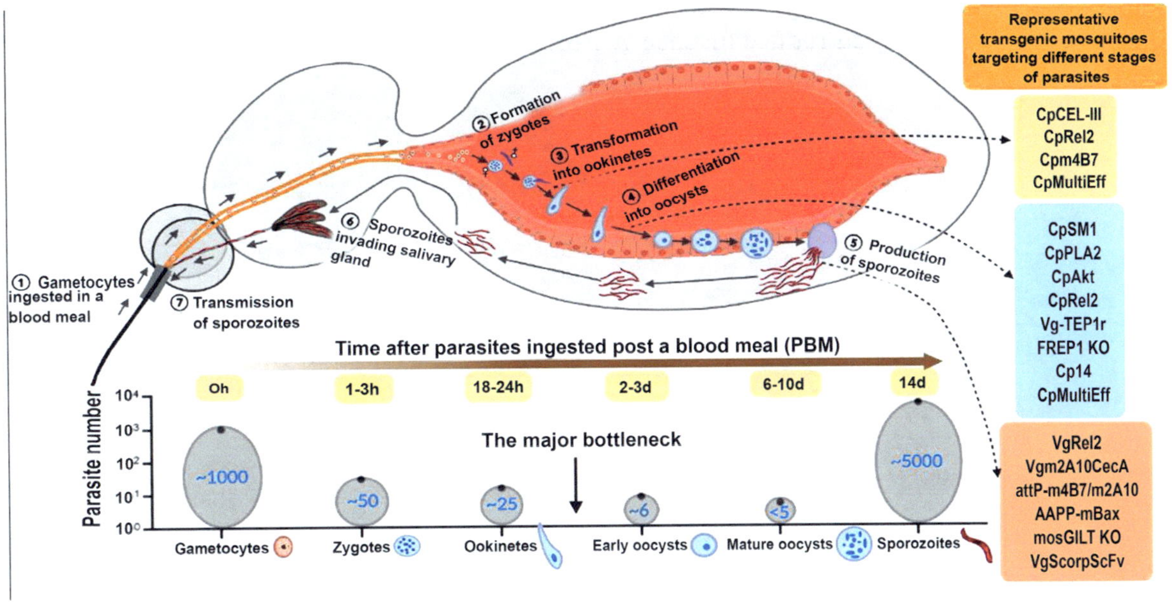

Figure 12.11. Mosquito transgenesis for malaria control.

Source: Cell Press. (2021). *Mosquito Transgenesis Approaches.*

Lately, research shows that ways to involve the public vary a lot, but you can usually break them down into approaches that ask, influence, or even invite deeper involvement. This kind of community engagement—not always perfectly neat in its execution—can build the trust we need, set realistic expectations, and ensure that people know what they're getting into. All of this becomes especially important when dealing with new genetic methods and their possible ripple effects on the environment (Schairer et al., 2019). Scientifically speaking, these genetically altered mosquitoes might be just what we need to sidestep the limits of chemical controls. By zeroing in on specific genes, they might block the malaria parasite from developing or cut down entire mosquito populations. But this strategy isn't just about swapping one idea for another; it calls for a complex, cross-disciplinary effort that mixes insights into how mosquitoes live, adapt, and interact with their surroundings. Generally speaking, the success of these genetic techniques will hinge on non-stop research, ongoing monitoring, and the ability to adjust plans as we learn more about the socio-ecological scene. In the end, nailing malaria control means betting not only on genetic fixes but also on deep, continuous study of the mosquito's world (Ferguson et al., 2010) (Figure 12.11).

12.3.3. Role of Natural Predators in Controlling Mosquito Populations

Vector control often works best when we have a good grip on the natural factors shaping mosquito numbers. Natural predators—fish, dragonfly nymphs, and even some amphibians—play a key role by eating both larvae and adult mosquitoes. You might find that ponds, marshes, and rice paddies (all common spots for Anopheles mosquitoes) turn into lively hubs where these predators flourish, which in turn keeps mosquito populations in check. In many cases, having these predators around cuts larval numbers enough to break the mosquito life cycle and lower the risk of malaria transmission. This kind of ecological alter fits in nicely with other water management strategies that have, for example, helped reduce disease vectors in Asia and Africa (van der Hoek et al., 2001).

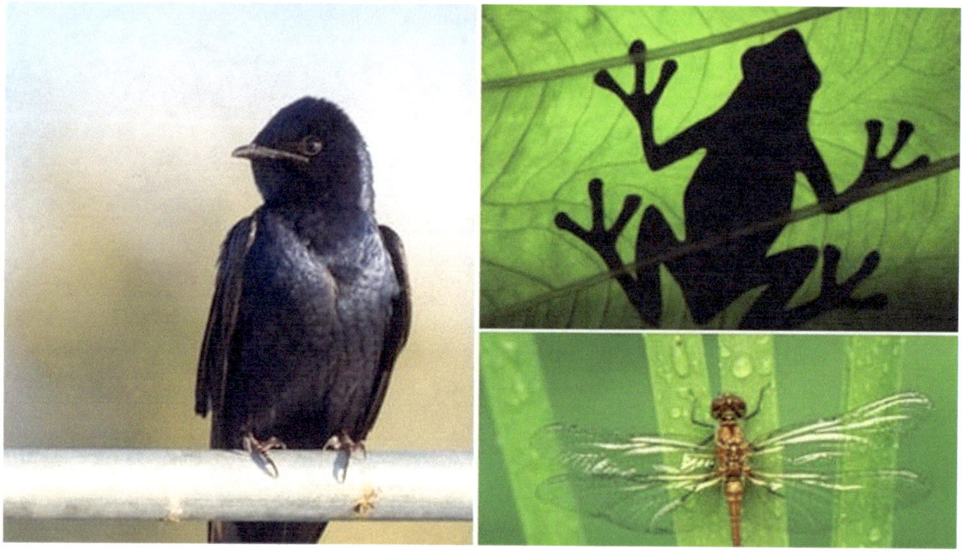

Figure 12.12. Role of natural predators in controlling mosquito populations.

Source: LinkedIn. (2024). *Natural Mosquito Control Using Predators.*

So, boosting the conservation and restoration of these natural enemies is an environmentally friendly partner to chemical or physical control methods. It isn't just about eating mosquitoes, though; natural enemies also mess with the mosquito's usual routines in mosquito habitats, which affects disease dynamics in unexpected ways. For instance, predatory arthropods like dragonflies and damselfly larvae not only decrease numbers by munching on larvae but also push survivors into choosing different egg-laying spots—an effect that shrinks accessible breeding areas. Additionally, fish introduced in select areas act as almost round-the-clock biological control agents because they consume larvae at high rates, a fact especially important in irrigated farmlands with plenty of breeding sites (van der Hoek et al., 2001). Sometimes, though, the success of these predator-based measures shifts depending on factors like environmental conditions, climate swings and human pressures; all of which mix in complex ways with malaria patterns. Generally speaking, grasping these interactions is crucial if we're to optimize natural predators in integrated vector management. Even with the obvious perks of using natural predators to cut down mosquito numbers, challenges stubbornly persist when it comes to applying these methods against malaria. Changes to habitats, pollution, or even the careless use of insecticides can harm predator communities, sometimes boosting mosquitoes and worsening disease spread. Plus, as climate change nudges temperatures and rain patterns around, predator-prey dynamics might shift, lessening the impact of these biological agents. In most cases, truly sustainable vector control has to care for the whole ecosystem so that natural predator populations stay robust. Future research should dig into the many ecological factors that shape predator success and look at how these methods might work even better when paired with habitat management and climate adaptation steps. In the end, aligning efforts to conserve natural predators with broader public health strategies can go a long way toward improving malaria control in a variety of settings (Figure 12.12).

12.4. Chemical Control Approaches

Malaria's stubborn spread pushes us to rethink how we handle mosquito control, especially by leaning on chemical options. Traditional pathogen-killers have long been the bedrock of our efforts, yet as resistance creeps in, it feels like we need a smarter, more flexible approach. Recent findings, generally speaking, hint that using agents at sub-lethal doses, such as spatial repellents that don't outright kill mosquitoes but instead alter their behavior, might lower the chance of bites while easing resistance pressures. This kind of behavior-focused alter seems to work as a good sidekick to the usual chemicals, taming mosquito activity without the heavy environmental downsides combined to intense chemical use (Achee et al., 2012). Modern computing has even nudged us past classic insecticides, opening new routes to novel compounds designed to target malaria mosquitoes more sharply. Grid computing and virtual screening let scientists sift through millions of molecules in no time at all, letting them quickly flag promising candidates. In most cases, this open-source, collaborative mix feels like the start of a fresh chapter in malaria research—pulling together global expertise to untangle some pretty complex challenges in both drug and insecticide development. By running extensive computational checks, researchers can zero in on chemical candidates that show both solid efficacy and safety before heading out into field trials (Breton et al., 2006). Even with these cool breakthroughs, relying only on chemicals won't cut it for lasting malaria control. Depending solely on chemical fixes risks upsetting local ecosystems and might even speed up resistance. That's why mixing these innovations with tried-and-true methods, like insecticide-treated nets and indoor residual spraying, and adding behavior-based adjustments is so important. Future steps should probably also give weight to tighter regulatory setups and more community input to get these tools used just right. To summarize, chemical strategies in malaria control should be seen as one piece of a bigger, layered plan—one that carefully balances effectiveness, long-term sustainability, and the need to adapt as mosquito habits evolve (Breton et al., 2006; Achee et al., 2012).

12.4.1. Types of Insecticides Used in Malaria Control

Malaria control often depends on using the right chemicals in smart, if not unpredictable, ways. People usually rely on insecticide-treated nets and indoor sprays to hit the adult Anopheline mosquitoes—the very ones that pass along the parasite. Pyrethroids, for a long time, were the go-to option; they knock down mosquitoes quickly and are relatively safe for humans. Still, because these chemicals have been overused in both farming and public health, some mosquitoes are gradually showing resistance. For instance, in Tanzania, even though pyrethroids still work well in many regions, there have been scattered signs of resistance emerging, which means individuals need to monitor the situation closely.

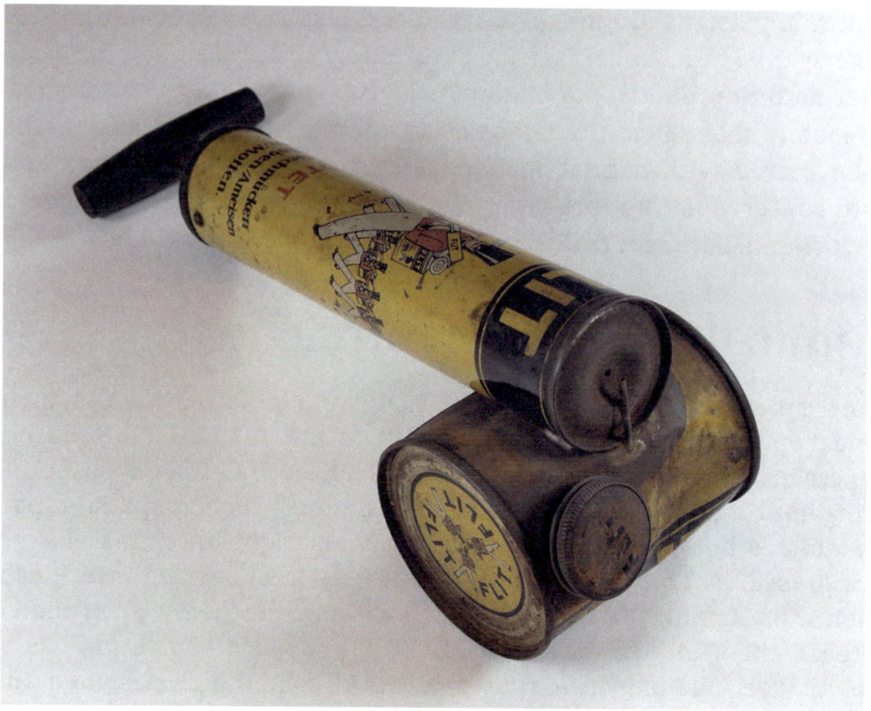

Figure 12.13. Types of insecticides used in malaria control.

Source: By Photographed by User:Bullenwächter - Museum für Hamburgische Geschichte, CC BY-SA 3.0, https://commons.wikimedia.org/w/index.php?curid=28973407

Overall, this pattern shows that mixing up insecticide choices and figuring out smart resistance management is pretty vital (Batengana et al., 2011). Even when pyrethroids have been the star of the show, other insecticide types deserve a look. Organophosphates and carbamates, for example, come into play in many indoor residual spraying programs, especially where resistance issues with pyrethroids are observed. Take pirimiphos-methyl—an organophosphate that works on mosquitoes quite differently in most cases, thereby sidestepping the usual resistance mechanisms. Some research comparing nets treated only with pyrethroids versus those used alongside other insecticides found that adding pirimiphos-methyl notably increased mosquito deaths. Generally speaking, this suggests that integrating non-pyrethroid options into control efforts could be beneficial, though the actual effectiveness can vary depending on the insecticide mix and the local mosquito species (Okumu et al., 2013). Beyond the chemical kicks, the physical barrier provided by a well-maintained LLIN remains a cornerstone of malaria prevention. Studies reveal that for vectors like *Anopheles arabiensis*, preventing bites is the primary way these nets protect people, rather than simply killing the pathogens. Pairing LLINs with indoor spraying sometimes only yields a modest bump in mosquito mortality—unless non-pyrethroid insecticides such as pirimiphos-methyl are involved. Moreover, the upkeep of these nets—ensuring they stay intact and properly fitted—plays a huge role in lowering human-mosquito contact. In the end, smart insecticide choices, good net condition, and careful resistance monitoring altogether form the backbone of effective strategies to cut down malaria transmission (Batengana et al., 2011; Okumu et al., 2013) (Figure 12.13).

12.4.2. Resistance Management Strategies

Malaria control faces a stubborn problem with mosquitoes that keep getting resistant to insecticides. LLINs and IRS have helped cut down malaria cases, yet the very same tools now struggle as more Anopheles mosquitoes learn to survive these measures. Insecticides like DDT and pyrethroids seem less reliable these days, partly because heavy pesticide use in farming adds extra pressure. West African cotton and vegetable farms, for example, show how farming practices and public health concerns end up in a complex mix. This situation suggests that tackling the problem needs both health and agricultural policies to talk with each other (Akogbeto et al., 2010). It gets even trickier when you consider the genetic tricks mosquitoes have up their sleeves. Mutations, often called kdr, which give quick resistance to pyrethroids are found in several populations, making a single insecticide fall short on multiple fronts. Molecule-based tests allow health teams to keep tabs on these markers and switch to alternatives when needed, while regular checks using WHO bioassays and residue analyses help figure out which factors are most at work. Sometimes, resistance patterns differ depending on whether they're caused by public health interventions or extra pesticide exposure from farms. The multiple resistances seen in *Anopheles arabiensis* from Ethiopia, for instance, underline the urgency for mixing various control methods (Yewhalaw et al., 2011). A smart way to fight this challenge is to mix technical know-how with practical policy steps. It's not just about rotating or mixing insecticides—methods like larval source management also deserve a spot in the plan. Bringing communities into the conversation and ensuring agricultural practices are in line with health goals are crucial moves. Strengthening pesticide regulations can help cut down those off-target exposures that push resistance, even if it means dealing with a few bumps along the way. Public health programs, by boosting their monitoring capabilities and setting up open chats with farmers, stand a better chance of keeping malaria under control. In most cases, recognizing the complex web of ecological and social factors will pave the road for strategies that work over the long run (Akogbeto et al., 2010; Yewhalaw et al., 2011).

12.4.3. Safety and Environmental Considerations of Chemical Use

Chemical methods have helped cut malaria spread, but they come with their own set of challenges. Using insecticides can crush mosquito numbers, yet if things go awry, these chemicals might harm people or other creatures nearby, even those not meant to be targeted. In many cases, inadequate training during spraying or handling means that agricultural workers and local communities face extra risks; failing to get this right can easily worsen health issues. Plus, many of these treatments persist in the environment, slowly building up in the soil and water, which can mess up the natural balance by unsettling friendly insect populations and reducing overall biodiversity. All these risks suggest that we need strict regulations and ongoing oversight to ensure that chemical use stays in line with our wider public health and environmental goals (Hawkes et al., 2025). Mixing the benefits of chemical control with caring for nature means we have to look closely at local ecosystems and adopt sustainable strategies. For instance, insecticides used in malaria fights might, in most cases, lower water quality in farmlands that communities depend upon—linking disease control with broader environmental concerns. Some individuals have even turned to GIS mapping in regions like Thailand to track where chemicals go and how they might tie in with environmental damage (Overgaard et al., 2025). There's also a move toward methods like targeted spraying paired with integrated pest management, which combine biological tools and environmental approaches to cut down on chemical use—helping to curb mosquito resistance and keep nature intact. In short, checking the environmental impact before launching these treatments is key to protecting natural resources while still fighting off malaria. Long-term progress in battling malaria relies on using chemicals carefully and responsibly. Nowadays, innovations push for insect formulations that break down quickly and reduce persisting pollution, generally aligning with sustainable development ideas. It also helps to invite local communities to monitor and share observations about chemical effects; doing so boosts transparency and lets us adjust our strategies when needed. Bringing together public health individuals, agriculturists, and environmental agencies is crucial too—they need to work side by side to ensure that chemical applications don't trigger unexpected problems beyond malaria. To summarize, better chemical safety and a mindful look at environmental issues not only bolster the ethics of our public health efforts but also protect the ecosystems that matter for everyone's well-being (Hawkes et al., 2025; Overgaard et al., 2025) (Figure 12.14).

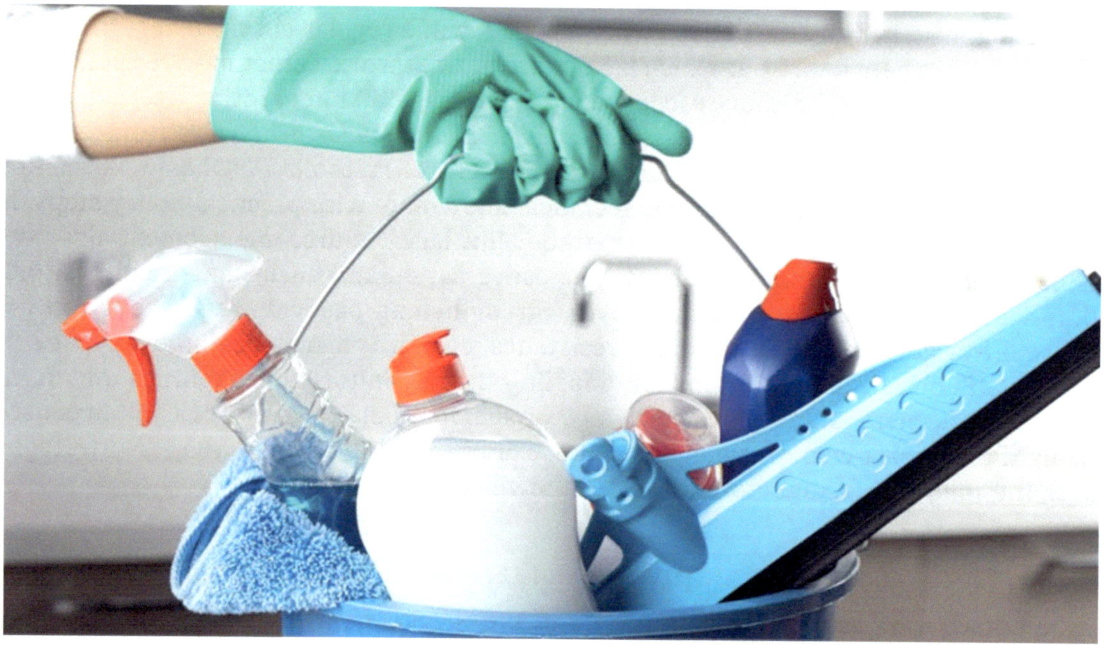

Figure 12.14. The safety and environmental considerations of chemical use.

Source: EHS. (2022). *Cleaning Products and Chemical Safety.*

12.5. Integrated Vector Management (IVM)

Malaria control isn't solved by a single trick. You've got these challenging Anopheles mosquitoes that live complex lives and keep changing their game against insecticides, so mixing up the approaches matters. IVM steps in here, it's a mash-up of chemical, biological, and environmental strategies. Instead of sticking to just one method, IVM uses what works best locally, basing decisions on how mosquitoes behave and how the disease spreads (Chanda et al., 2016). Local communities and even national groups chip in, making alters that use resources wisely while keeping nature in mind. In most cases, this evidence-led mix makes it easier to fight back against rising insecticide resistance and common operational issues, acting like a flexible toolkit to curb mosquito numbers and malaria transmission (Chanda et al., 2016).

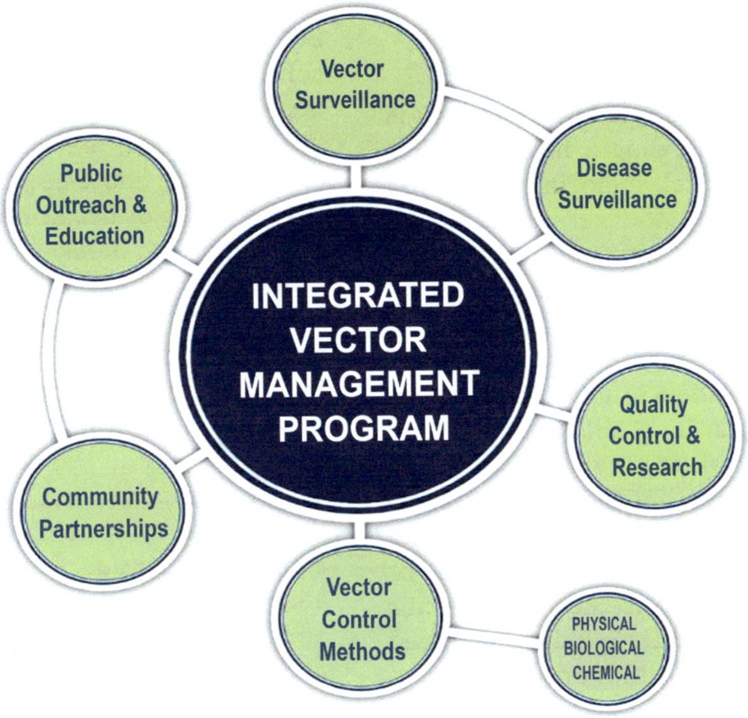

Figure 12.15. Integrated vector management (IVM).

Source: Streamline. (n.d.). *Integrated Vector Management (IVM).*

When you mix different mosquito control tools, things start falling into place on many levels. Natural methods, like using fish that munch on larvae or microbial larvicides—work hand in hand with chemical ones such as insecticide-treated nets and indoor spraying. Throw in some physical fixes like changing up breeding habitats, and you're less dependent on one single measure, which can slow down the mosquitoes' development of tolerance. New devices, such as those automated mosquito traps with infrared sensors, emerge too, hinting at fresh ideas within the IVM mix that reach right into homes and communities (Shuguang et al., 2021). This kind of mix, which loosely follows WHO hints for keeping malaria control sustainable, shows how innovation and tradition can co-mingle (Shuguang et al., 2021). Rolling out IVM isn't as simple as putting together a neat plan, it needs a real team effort. Health officials, environmental agencies, and local individuals all have to be in sync. Generally speaking, the idea works best when political commitment and proper funding set in, making regular checks on resistance and policy alters a must. Communities also need the know-how and sometimes a bit of patience to adopt these measures properly. Without that kind of grassroots and official backing, even the smartest ideas risk falling flat, which means the hard-won gains in malaria control might slip away (Chanda et al., 2016) (Figure 12.15).

12.5.1. Definition and Principles of Integrated Vector Management (IVM)

Managing vector populations isn't as straightforward as following a neat checklist. It takes many ecological, biological, and even sociopolitical thinking to get a handle on disease spread. IVM—is one way people have come up with to bring together different control methods, each altered for the local scene. , this approach is all about wisely spending resources, checking out solid evidence, and letting groups from public health, farming, and environmental fields share the load. It may seem a bit all over the place at times, but the idea is to keep interventions working well without causing extra trouble like environmental messes or speeding up insecticide resistance. Since vector behavior can change on a dime, individuals need to continually monitor situations and adjust their game plan as new challenges crop up. In most cases, IVM ends up being more than just a kit of options, it's a kind of overall strategy to steadily cut down diseases like malaria by mixing local insights on transmission and resistance (Dusfour et al., 2019). Sustainability and looking after the environment play a big role in this whole game plan. If vector control isn't handled carefully, things like chemical overuse can mess up nature or even hurt species that weren't meant to be affected, which in turn makes public health problems stick around longer. For example, when insecticides are used without thinking twice, they not only pollute but also push insects to build up resistance, cutting short the effectiveness of any intervention. So, IVM leans more on practices that are gentle on nature—using biological agents, altering habitats, and only resorting to chemicals when it seems absolutely necessary. Generally speaking, this eco-friendly mindset works hand-in-hand with broader issues like how we manage our waste, which can also feed into problems with disease vectors. By tackling these overlapping issues, the whole vector control effort becomes more sustainable and helps communities remain resilient (Ferronato et al., 2019). Nothing beats the local touch when it comes to tackling these challenges. IVM relies heavily on getting communities involved and breaking down barriers between different sectors. Local know-how, like understanding the ins and outs of urban growth, waste routines, and everyday behaviors, often turns out to be the secret ingredient for effective control. When public health officials, environmental agencies, and community groups join forces, their combined approach can cover many angles of vector proliferation. Plus, a built-in part of IVM is keeping an eye on insecticide resistance, ensuring that chemicals don't lose their bite over time. Fueled by up-to-date surveillance data and a proactive attitude, this strategy is designed to adapt quickly and prevent new problems from emerging, all in the name of keeping malaria and similar diseases in check. In essence, when diverse elements work together, even if their coordination can be a bit imperfect—the outlook for long-lasting control improves (Dusfour et al., 2019).

12.5.2. Benefits of Combining Multiple Control Strategies

Malaria transmission has dropped dramatically in some regions, which reminds us that we must keep our control measures in place, even when the risk seems low. In most cases, continuing the wide use of tools like LLINs and IRS stops the resurgence of malaria as areas near elimination. Take Zanzibar, for example; care takers of young children stuck with these interventions even when malaria didn't feel like an immediate threat. This steady use meant nearly every child under five got protection, and it shows that mixing different coverage strategies makes a difference. Overall, these observations suggest that integrating several vector control methods boosts long-term impact, largely thanks to ongoing community engagement and high intervention use (Beer et al., 2013). Combining vector control strategies also brings biological advantages that you just don't get from a single method. Experiments with replicated mesocosms generally show that while LLINs cut down adult mosquito survival significantly, they might not wipe out the entire population on their own. When LLINs are paired with treatments, like giving cattle Ivermectin—the mosquito reproduction rate drops sharply, almost eradicating the pests. This kind of synergy takes aim at different mosquito life stages and behaviors, thus improving the overall effectiveness of control. In short, using these mixed approaches multiplies the negative effects on both survival and reproduction, leading to a more effective suppression (Ng'habi et al., 2018). Mixing different tools can also help ease the issues of limitations and resistance that come along with relying on just one method. Relying solely on insecticides, for instance, might speed up resistance in mosquito populations over time, lessening long-term effectiveness. By incorporating diverse interventions with varying modes of action, the selective pressure drops and the measures tend to hold up better against adapting mosquitoes. Also, since mosquito behavior and local ecology can vary widely, mixing house-based interventions like IRS with personal protection via bed nets and treatments aimed at vectors outdoors or those that target livestock-feeding mosquitoes covers more bases. This adaptable, multi-pronged approach not only ramps up suppression but also helps sustain control gains by counteracting behavioral changes and insecticide resistance, leading to a more robust and lasting vector management (Figure 12.16).

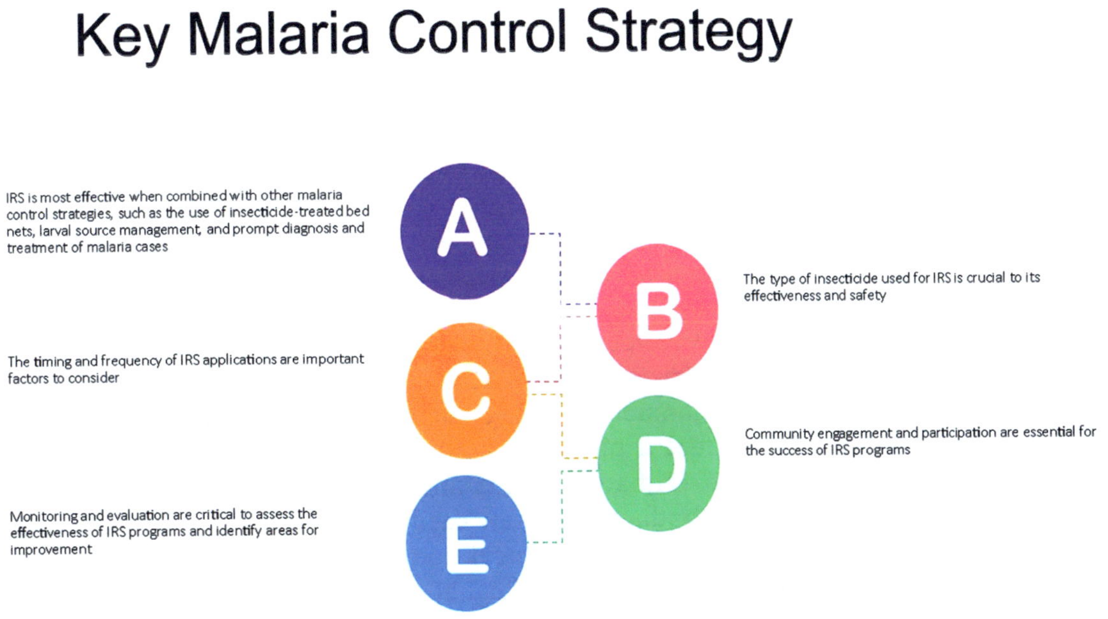

Figure 12.16. Key malaria control strategy.

Source: FasterCapital. (n.d.). *Global Health Initiatives for Malaria.*

12.5.3. Case Studies Demonstrating Successful Integrated Vector Management (IVM) Implementation

Integrated Vector Management has turned into a fundamental part of fighting malaria today, mixing natural insights with simple, tailored actions that depend on local know-how. In one case from Tanzania, for example, a program teamed up larval source management with active community engagement – a move that cut mosquito numbers and malaria cases down noticeably. The method leaned on what locals understood about their surroundings and, in most cases, built a sense of ownership that helped keep the efforts going over time. This approach sidesteps the problems of being locked into just insecticide-heavy strategies, offering instead a path for malaria control that can adjust and scale up as needed (Intergovernmental Panel on Climate Change, 2023). Over in Kenya's highlands, a somewhat different mix took hold where environmental alters and improved housing added up to lower malaria risk. Local teams worked on things like draining stagnant water and installing window screens, and meanwhile different sectors – health, housing, and environmental agencies – got involved. Such cross-sector teamwork shows that when you mix ideas from various angles, you end up with a more resilient way to keep malaria at bay. Generally speaking, syncing up these measures not only reduces contact between people and mosquitoes, but it also fits with broader plans for climate-resilient development, even if the process can sometimes feel a bit patchy (Intergovernmental Panel on Climate Change, 2023). In parts of rural Cambodia in Southeast Asia, the fight against malaria took on an especially community-driven flavor. Local people were trained to spot and clean up mosquito breeding spots, and in an unexpected twist, larvivorous fish were introduced in rice paddies to keep the larvae numbers low. At the same time, insecticide-treated nets were handed out to tackle the issue of mosquitoes that bite outdoors. This mix of education, natural controls, and practical interventions – though not always perfectly executed – shows that sustainable vector control isn't a one-size-fits-all deal. Instead, it's about mixing different tools that match the specific behavior of vectors and local conditions, ultimately paving the way for long-lasting reductions in malaria (Anne et al., 2020).

12.6. Challenges in Vector Control

Malaria vector control is a complex business. Mosquitoes keep finding ways to dodge insecticides—they simply evolve resistance against the chemicals we've long depended on. You end up with nets and indoor sprays that just don't work as well as they should, so the whole plan has to be repeatedly rethought and retooled. Environmental features, like different regional climates and habitats, mean that mosquitoes behave and breed in ways that defy a one-size-fits-all fix. And when you throw in the fact that many places battling malaria also face unpredictable healthcare systems and limited community support, things only get more complex. All these issues together point toward a need for an adaptable, all-in-one strategy—a plan that keeps up with the ever-changing habits and habitats of these pests (Christopher et al., 2022). Politics and geography add another layer of chaos. Take border zones like Yunnan Province in China—the porous boundaries and constantly moving populations there show just how easily malaria can slip through even when local control measures seem to be working. Neighboring countries, each with its own levels of malaria trouble, force us to think about joint, cross-border monitoring and quick-response systems. In many rural or lower-income pockets, fragile healthcare systems further delay reporting and intervention, which lets mosquito numbers return or simply hang around. Stronger local surveillance, a bit more political drive, and a willingness to team up across borders seem essential for truly lasting control (Li et al., 2021). Then there's the problem of missing data and scarce resources, an issue that hits low-income areas where malaria is worst. Without solid entomological checks and fresh, real-time data, making quick, targeted decisions becomes nearly impossible. Limited lab capacity and outdated data systems only add to the difficulty of tracking how well interventions are working or of catching new resistance trends in time. In most cases, these gaps call out for better investments in capacity building, tech upgrades, and creative ways to monitor mosquito activity that deliver real, actionable insights. Addressing these infrastructure faults is key if we're ever going to keep malaria transmission in check with evidence-based, flexible strategies (Li et al., 2021; Christopher et al., 2022) (Figure 12.17).

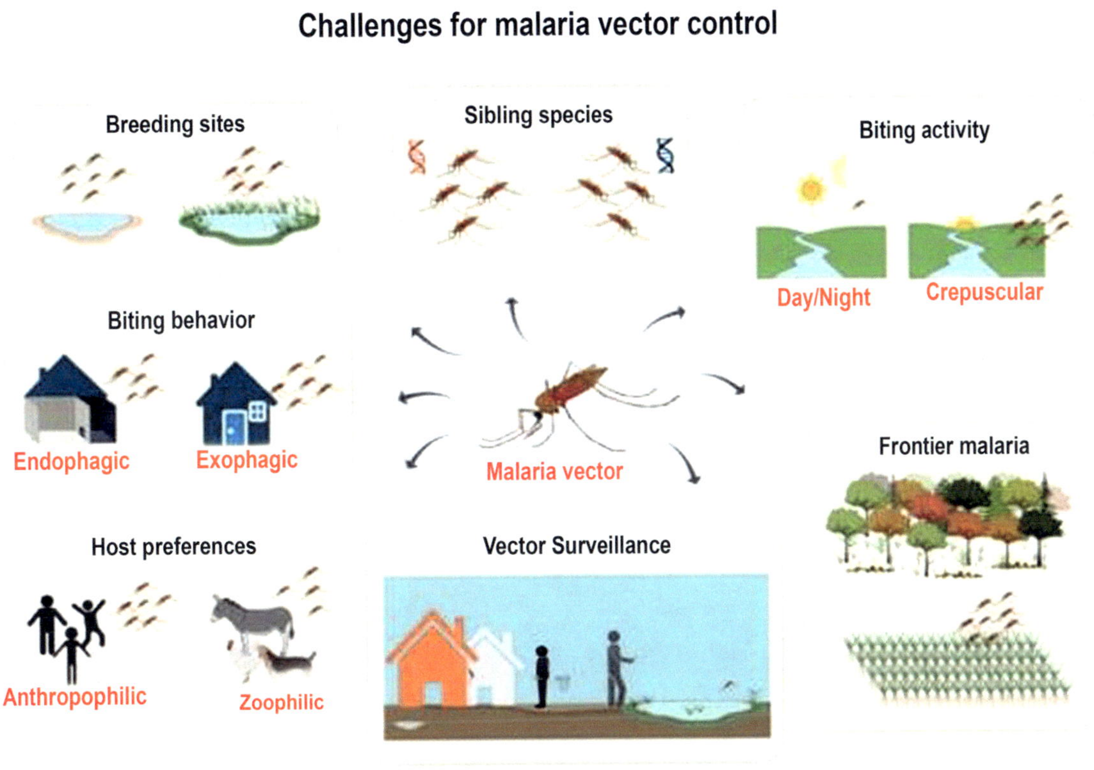

Figure 12.17. Challenges in vector control.

Source: Hadebe MT, Malgwi SA, Okpeku M. Revolutionizing Malaria Vector Control: The Importance of Accurate Species Identification through Enhanced Molecular Capacity. *Microorganisms*. 2024; 12(1):82. https://doi.org/10.3390/microorganisms12010082

12.6.1. Insecticide Resistance and Its Implications

Insecticide-treated nets and indoor residual spraying have helped bring down malaria – they're aimed right at those mosquitoes that usually bite indoors. In some parts of East Africa, even though nets aren't perfectly spread out, these methods have cut down local numbers of notorious species like *Anopheles gambiae*. Still, constant exposure to these chemicals means mosquitoes start to adapt, slowly picking up traits that make them resistant. Even with this hurdle, there's room for hope. If we switch strategies to mess with all the things mosquitoes need to survive instead of just stopping their blood meals, we might slow down resistance and keep populations low — maybe even clear them out eventually (Killeen et al., 2013). , understanding how these malaria carriers live and evolve is key if we want to beat the challenge of insecticide resistance. The standard tools, like nets and sprays, haven't managed to break the cycle of *Plasmodium falciparum* transmission in areas where the disease runs wild, which shows just how darn adaptable these pathogens can be. They alter their behavior and sometimes even change their internal chemistry so they can handle the toxins, keeping the disease moving along. In most cases, it may pay off to dive deeper into the less obvious parts of mosquito life – figuring out where they prefer to dwell, how their larvae behave, and their reproduction rhythms could open new doors to intervention. To summarize, a strategy that covers every stage of a mosquito's life seems like our best long-term hope for getting rid of malaria (Ferguson et al., 2010). When mosquitoes become resistant, it isn't just a win for them – the problem starts to spill over into bigger public health issues. Tackling these tougher populations often means cranking up the insecticide dose or switching to different chemicals, both of which can hike costs and even hurt the environment. And there's this ongoing arms race; our control efforts and the pathogens' quick adaptations keep canceling each other out unless we cover all the bases fast enough. Keeping an eye on mosquito movements, with some vigilant monitoring, is important to catch any signs of reinvasion, whether the mosquitoes are still vulnerable or have become resistant. In the end, completely eliminating the mosquitoes rather than just keeping them in check might cut down the chance for resistance to develop, underscoring why we need innovative and varied strategies to take these pests head-on (Killeen et al., 2013) (Figure 12.18).

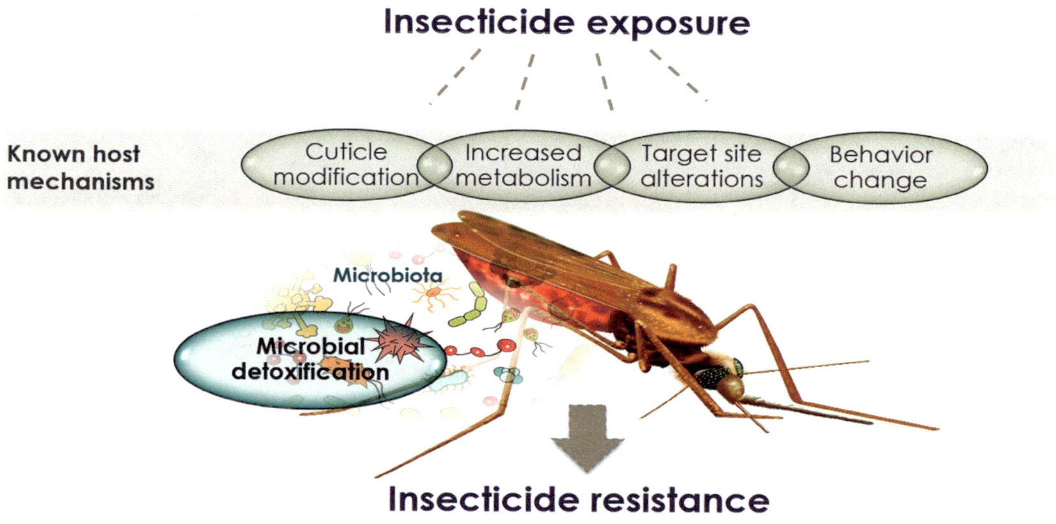

Figure 12.18. Insecticide resistance.

Source: NSADADA. (n.d.). *Microbes and Insecticide Resistance.*

12.6.2. Socioeconomic Factors Affecting Control Efforts

Malaria control isn't just a matter of spraying nets or chemicals, it's tangled up with the everyday realities of communities. Education, for one, plays a surprisingly large role. People with a bit more schooling often know why malaria crops up and how to fend it off. They're likely to stick to using ITNs or agreeing to indoor spraying because they kind of get the whole disease spread thing. Without a boost in education, control efforts can stumble under misconceptions or simple neglect. In most cases, communicating in a way that fits different reading levels makes a difference—helping everyone pitch in to cut down malaria numbers. At the same time, socioeconomic factors are hard to ignore. Households with more money can usually afford better preventive tools and keep their homes in conditions that naturally curb mosquito breeding spots. On the flip side, those with fewer dollars may have to resort to cheaper, often less effective, methods—or even informal agricultural pesticides. This sometimes ends up fueling insecticide resistance, partly because proper guidance isn't always around, and the resources just aren't. Generally speaking, this economic split means that while some individuals face a lower risk, others end up more exposed, highlighting the need for approaches that boost both local finances and a fair spread of vector control supplies (Intergovernmental Panel on Climate Change, 2023). Then there's the farming angle. In many rural spots, pyrethroid insecticides are used on crops; but these chemicals often spill over to affect mosquito populations too, sometimes in unpredictable ways that speed up resistance issues. It shows that vector control can't be pulled out of the broader mix of daily economic practices. Tackling these challenges means policies have to think about farmers' real lives, mixing in tailored education and keeping chemical use in check so that it stays sustainable. All these overlapping issues point to the need for a flexible, human-centered framework—one that juggles climate concerns and human development while keeping malaria at bay (Intergovernmental Panel on Climate Change, 2023).

12.6.3. Climate Change and Its Impact on Malaria Transmission

Environmental factors and insect-spread diseases rarely behave in a neat, predictable manner. When you look at malaria, weather shifts like rising temperatures, uneven rainfalls, and fluctuating humidity impactto the works by nudging mosquito habits in unexpected directions. A slight uptick in heat can speed up the life cycles of both the mosquitoes and the *Plasmodium* parasites they carry — in some cases, which means more transmission. On the flip side, these same changes might throw off our usual fixes like ITNs or IRS. Sometimes, mosquitoes start acting differently or even build some resistance, which kind of undercuts our standard approaches. To summarize, climate change isn't just redrawing the map of where malaria shows up; it's also putting our existing control plans to the test (Ferguson et al., 2023). People's actions and local conditions also mix things up quite a bit. Rapid urban sprawl and shifts in land use often end up creating new mosquito hangouts or twisting well-known ones into something unrecognizable. Political instability and regional migrations further muddle the picture, especially in areas that thought they had malaria under control however let their guard down. Generally speaking, climate variability can sometimes set the stage for malaria to reappear in places that were once quiet, by making the environment more inviting for both mosquitoes and parasites. And while methods like IRS or even space spraying might work well in certain settings, their success tends to vary depending on local weather features and the specific malaria strains around (Adrian et al., 2020). Figuring out, and fighting—the indirect effects of climate change on malaria control calls for some broad, flexible planning. It's not simply a matter of keeping mosquito numbers down; these weather changes can ripple through health systems, affect budgets, and even shift how people go about their daily lives. For instance, hotter days might generally lead individuals to change their outdoor routines, altering exposure risks in subtle ways. At the same time, shifts in land use and economic pressures spurred by climate changes can steer resources away from ongoing malaria efforts. Building what some call a "climate-proof" strategy means leaning on improved forecasting tools and trying out methods that can shift gears when things get unpredictable. In many cases, this proactive adaptation might be just what we need to lock in long-term malaria control while recognizing that climate change remains a dynamic, ever-present challenge for both insect behavior and public health systems (Ferguson et al., 2023) (Figure 12.19).

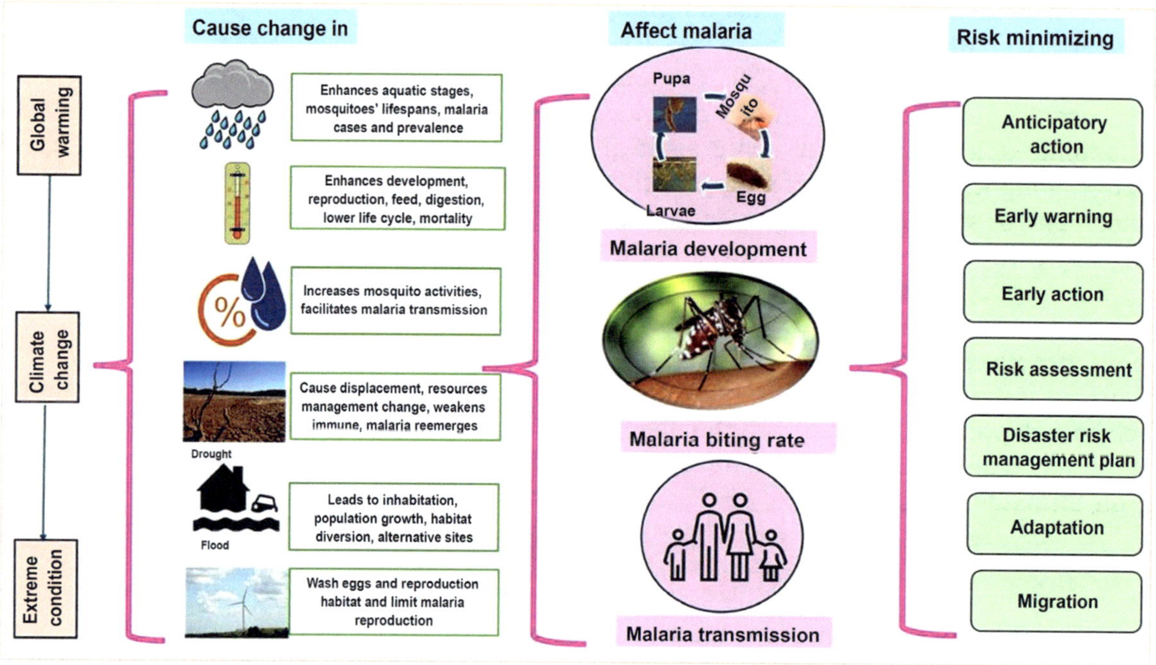

Figure 12.19. Climate change and its impact on malaria transmission.

Source: Megersa DM, Luo X-S. Effects of Climate Change on Malaria Risk to Human Health: A Review. *Atmosphere*. 2025; 16(1):71. https://doi.org/10.3390/atmos16010071

CLOSER LOOK

MEROZOITE SPILL

Merozoite spill refers to the release and spread of merozoites, which are a stage in the life cycle of the *Plasmodium* parasite responsible for malaria. This process plays a critical role in the pathogenesis of the disease and is a central component of the parasite's ability to infect red blood cells and proliferate within the host. Understanding merozoite spill is crucial for both understanding malaria's mechanism and for developing effective treatments.

Malaria is caused by several species of the *Plasmodium* genus, with *Plasmodium falciparum* being the deadliest. The parasite undergoes a complex life cycle that involves two hosts: the female *Anopheles* mosquito and the human. The cycle begins when an infected mosquito bites a human, injecting sporozoites into the bloodstream. These sporozoites travel to the liver, where they infect liver cells and mature into schizonts, a stage that produces thousands of merozoites.

Once the liver schizonts rupture, they release the merozoites into the bloodstream, marking the beginning of the merozoite spill. These merozoites are the infectious stage of the parasite and target red blood cells, where they invade, mature, and replicate.

The release of merozoites into the bloodstream is a critical event in the progression of malaria. It leads to the invasion of red blood cells, where the merozoites mature into trophozoites and eventually form new merozoites, which continue the cycle. This process is responsible for the cyclic nature of malaria symptoms.

As merozoites spill from the liver into the bloodstream, they cause an increase in the parasitemia (the number of parasites in the blood). This parasitemia correlates with the severity of the disease. The merozoites invade red blood cells by first recognizing specific receptors on the cell surface. After invading the red blood cells, they form a vacuole where they mature into trophozoites. These trophozoites then replicate, ultimately bursting the red blood cell and releasing new merozoites into circulation. This cycle repeats, causing the characteristic fever spikes and chills seen in malaria.

The release of merozoites from liver cells and their subsequent invasion of red blood cells contribute significantly to the clinical manifestation of malaria. The rupture of red blood cells releases cytokines and other immune signaling molecules, triggering inflammation and the immune response. This process is responsible for the fever, anemia, and other symptoms associated with the disease.

As the parasitic load increases, patients may experience severe malaria, characterized by organ failure, cerebral malaria, or severe anemia. This is particularly dangerous in young children, pregnant women, and immunocompromised individuals. The repeated cycles of merozoite invasion also contribute to the chronic nature of the disease in areas of endemic transmission.

SUMMARY

Managing malaria effectively means using many old reliable fixes alongside fresh, innovative ideas—each one altered to fit local environments and social norms. Even though progress has been made, areas like the Dembiya district show that our current plans sometimes don't cover all bases, particularly when dealing with cases that happen outdoors or don't fully clear up. The issue isn't just about tackling pathogens indoors; it's also about curbing risks outside where human habits and even local changes play their part. In most cases, keeping close tabs on vector numbers, their behavior, and even their changing resistance is key to adjusting our methods on the fly. Fostering genuine community awareness goes a long way in making these strategies stick over time. Recent studies, for instance, hint that there's no universal fix—what works is a mix of measures that jives with local realities (Tarekegn et al., 2021). People's attitudes and cultural habits shape how well these control measures work, especially among groups like the gold miners in the Amazon, who often deal with unique challenges. There's a lot of misunderstanding about how malaria spreads, and many still lean on traditional treatments or even off-label medications, which muddles the fight against the disease. These behaviors can slow down efforts like mass drug programs and sometimes even weaken public health messages. It seems pretty clear that talking to people in a way that fits local beliefs, while also making sure access to solid diagnosis and treatment isn't an issue, is absolutely vital. When health officials take time to understand local customs, they can develop more relatable, effective educational materials that pull a community together. In weaving these social insights into vector control strategies, health programs can better target those hard-to-reach or often-overlooked spots where the disease tends to hide (Murta et al., 2021). To wrap things up, knocking malaria out of the picture calls for flexible, evidence-driven approaches that mix science with genuine community input and a solid grasp of local culture. It's not enough to lean only on data about insects or infection numbers; we also need to factor in how people live and what parts of the environment may be inadvertently fueling the spread. More robust surveillance, interventions honed for outdoor or mobile communities, and educational efforts that respect cultural tastes are all crucial pieces of this puzzle. Stories from Ethiopia and the Brazilian Amazon remind us that fighting malaria isn't a one-and-done deal, it requires constantly updating our strategies to meet local hurdles. Moving forward, it's essential for policymakers and community leaders alike to team up using approaches tailored to each unique context, mixing sharp scientific insights with everyday realities so that control measures aren't just effective, but also welcomed at the grassroots level (Murta et al., 2021; Tarekegn et al., 2021).

Malaria transmission still stubbornly persists even though many communities now rely on insecticide-treated nets and indoor spraying. In places like parts of Africa and the Pacific, where *Plasmodium falciparum* keeps making life difficult, the old-school methods just don't cut it—so we're pushed to try something different. Generally speaking, the idea of nudging mosquito behavior with sub-lethal agents like spatial repellents, an approach known for decades yet still not woven into full-scale programs, offers an intriguing alternative (Achee et al., 2012). When we think about improving vector control, it seems clear that our research needs a broader lens—one that looks at mosquito ecology and evolutionary biology, for instance. The mosquito life cycle isn't just about blood meals; there are many stages, from breeding and resting spots to diverse feeding patterns, which often get overlooked but affect how the disease spreads. A closer look at these factors, even when repeated in discussions here and there, can help us design layered strategies that slow down transmission. In most cases, this ecological view hints at more focused interventions that add power to current methods, and sustained investment here remains absolutely critical for long-term success (Ferguson et al., 2010). Eradicating malaria worldwide won't hinge solely on new products but also on flexible, adaptive programs that absorb emerging scientific insights. The mix of spatial repellents with usual vector control measures reflects a shift toward using behavioral ecology in public health—an idea that, though not entirely new, is gaining traction. Success will likely depend on overcoming hurdles in product testing, regulatory approval, and getting these tools into endemic communities effectively. Plus, a long-term outlook that sometimes prioritizes insights from ecology and evolution could help address potential changes in mosquito populations and insecticide resistance. To summarize, a mixed approach that marries innovative behavioral alters with a robust look at mosquito life and habitat may well be the key to reducing malaria's global impact (Fergusson et al, 2010; Achee et al., 2012).

KEY TERMS FROM THIS CHAPTER

- Insecticide-Treated Nets
- Indoor Residual Spraying (IRS)
- Environmental Management
- Larvivorous Fish
- Bacillus sphaericus
- Genetically Modified Mosquitoes (GMMs)
- Personal Protective Measures
- Spatial Repellents
- Protective Housing (Screening/Netting)
- Cross-sectoral Collaboration
- Long-Lasting Insecticidal Nets (LLINs)
- Larval Source Management (LSM)
- Biological Control
- Bacillus thuringiensis israelensis (Bti)
- Sterile Insect Technique (SIT)
- Integrated Vector Management (IVM)
- Insecticide Resistance Management
- Mosquito Traps
- Community Participation
- Monitoring and Evaluation

References

1. Akilimali, A., Bisimwa, C., Aborode, A. T., Biamba, C., Sironge, L., Balume, A., Sayadi, R., Ajibade, S. B., Akintayo, A. A., Oluwadairo, T. O., & Fajemisin, E. A. (2022). Self-medication and Anti-malarial Drug Resistance in the Democratic Republic of the Congo (DRC): A silent threat. *Tropical medicine and health*, *50*(1), 73. https://doi.org/10.1186/s41182-022-00466-9
2. Achee, N. L., Bangs, M. J., Farlow, R., Killeen, G. F., Lindsay, S., Logan, J. G., Moore, S. J., Rowland, M., Sweeney, K., Torr, S. J., Zwiebel, L. J., & Grieco, J. P. (2012). Spatial repellents: from discovery and development to evidence-based validation. *Malaria journal*, *11*, 164. https://doi.org/10.1186/1475-2875-11-164(accessed on 13 May 2025).
3. Adeel, A. H., Burkot, T., Garner, P., Pyke, G., et al. (2013). Larvivorous fish for preventing malaria transmission. https://core.ac.uk/download/29016345.pdf (accessed on 13 May 2025).
4. Adeel, A., Burkot, T. R., Garner, P., Pyke, G., et al. (2017). Larvivorous fish for preventing malaria transmission. https://core.ac.uk/download/144997057.pdf (accessed on 13 May 2025).
5. Adrian, J., Beltran-Ayala, E., Carrasco-Escobar, G., Drakeley, C., et al. (2020). The relative role of climate variation and control interventions on malaria elimination efforts in El Oro, Ecuador: A modeling study. https://core.ac.uk/download/347773909.pdf (accessed on 13 May 2025).
6. Germain Gil Padonou, Judith G. Gbenoudon, Razaki Osse, Albert Salako, Casimir Kpanou, Herman Sagbohan, Virgile Gnanguenon, Frederick Oke Agbo, Olivier Oussou, Martin Codjo Akogbeto Knowledge-attitudes-practices about malaria among communities in Southern Benin. International Journal of Public Health Science (IJPHS) Vol. 7, No. 3, September 2018, pp. 186~193 ISSN: 2252-8806, DOI: 10.11591/ijphs.v7i3.14395 (accessed on 13 May 2025).
7. Ahmed, A., Cissé, G., Moirano, G., Moraga, P., et al. (2024). *Spatio-temporal dynamics of malaria in Rwanda between 2012 and 2022: A demography-specific analysis*. https://core.ac.uk/download/621202947.pdf (accessed on 13 May 2025).
8. Yewhalaw D, Wassie F, Steurbaut W, Spanoghe P, Van Bortel W, Denis L, et al. (2011) Multiple Insecticide Resistance: An Impediment to Insecticide-Based Malaria Vector Control Program. PLoS ONE 6(1): e16066. https://doi.org/10.1371/journal.pone.0016066
9. Schairer CE, Taitingfong R, Akbari OS, Bloss CS (2019) A typology of community and stakeholder engagement based on documented examples in the field of novel vector control. PLoS Negl Trop Dis 13(11): e0007863. https://doi.org/10.1371/journal.pntd.0007863
10. Akogbeto, M., Baldet, T., Chandre, F., Djogbenou, L., et al. (2010). Impact of human activities on the dynamics of insecticide resistance in Anopheles gambiae: Case of Benin (West Africa). http://agritrop.cirad.fr/558196/1/document_558196.pdf (accessed on 13 May 2025).
11. Dlamini, N., Hsiang, M. S., Ntshalintshali, N., Pindolia, D., Allen, R., Nhlabathi, N., Novotny, J., Kang Dufour, M. S., Midekisa, A., Gosling, R., LeMenach, A., Cohen, J., Dorsey, G., Greenhouse, B., & Kunene, S. (2017). Low-Quality Housing Is Associated With Increased Risk of Malaria Infection: A National Population-Based Study From the Low Transmission Setting of Swaziland. *Open forum infectious diseases*, *4*(2), ofx071. https://doi.org/10.1093/ofid/ofx071
12. Batengana, B., Chacha, M., Emidi, B., Kabula, B., et al. (2011). Detection and monitoring of insecticide resistance in malaria vectors in Tanzania Mainland. https://core.ac.uk/download/pdf/11307282.pdf.

13. Bauer, I. L. (2023). The oral repellent–Science fiction or common sense? Insects, vector-borne diseases, failing strategies, and a bold proposition. https://core.ac.uk/download/577868641.pdf (accessed on 13 May 2025).

14. Bauwens, I., Deleu, J., Franke, J., Gebreslasie, M., et al. (2015). Earth observation in support of malaria control and epidemiology: MALAREO monitoring approaches. https://core.ac.uk/download/216471605.pdf (accessed on 13 May 2025).

15. Protopopoff, N., Van Bortel, W., Speybroeck, N., Van Geertruyden, J. P., Baza, D., D'Alessandro, U., & Coosemans, M. (2009). Ranking malaria risk factors to guide malaria control efforts in African highlands. *PloS one*, *4*(11), e8022. https://doi.org/10.1371/journal.pone.0008022(accessed on 13 May 2025).

16. Beier JC, Wilke ABB, Benelli G. Newer Approaches for Malaria Vector Control and Challenges of Outdoor Transmission [Internet]. Towards Malaria Elimination - A Leap Forward. InTech; 2018. Available from: http://dx.doi.org/10.5772/intechopen.75513 (accessed on 13 May 2025).

17. Beer, N., Ali, A. S., Shakely, D., Elfving, K., Al-Mafazy, A. W., Msellem, M., Petzold, M., Björkman, A., & Källander, K. (2013). High effective coverage of vector control interventions in children after achieving low malaria transmission in Zanzibar, Tanzania. *Malaria journal*, *12*, 38. https://doi.org/10.1186/1475-2875-12-38 (accessed on 13 May 2025).

18. Okumu, F. O., Mbeyela, E., Lingamba, G., Moore, J., Ntamatungiro, A. J., Kavishe, D. R., Kenward, M. G., Turner, E., Lorenz, L. M., & Moore, S. J. (2013). Comparative field evaluation of combinations of long-lasting insecticide treated nets and indoor residual spraying, relative to either method alone, for malaria prevention in an area where the main vector is Anopheles arabiensis. *Parasites & vectors*, *6*, 46. https://doi.org/10.1186/1756-3305-6-46 (accessed on 13 May 2025).

19. OnbFerguson HM, Dornhaus A, Beeche A, Borgemeister C, Gottlieb M, Mulla MS, et al. (2010) Ecology: A Prerequisite for Malaria Elimination and Eradication. PLoS Med 7(8): e1000303. https://doi.org/10.1371/journal.pmed.1000303 (accessed on 13 May 2025).

20. van der Hoek, W.; Sakthivadivel, R.; Renshaw, M.; Silver, J. B.; Birley, M. H.; Konradsen, F. 2001. Alternate wet/dry irrigation in rice cultivation: a practical way to save water and control malaria and Japanese encephalitis? Colombo, Sri Lanka: International Water Management Institute (IWMI). v, 30p. (IWMI Research Report 047) (accessed on 13 May 2025).

21. Breton, V., Hofmann-Apitius, M., Jacq, N., Kasam, V., et al. (2006). Grid added value to address malaria. https://core.ac.uk/download/49302955.pdf (accessed on 13 May 2025).

22. Cameron, A., Reece, S. E., Drew, D. R., Haydon, D. T., & Yates, A. J. (2013). Plasticity in transmission strategies of the malaria parasite, Plasmodium chabaudi: environmental and genetic effects. *Evolutionary applications*, *6*(2), 365–376. https://doi.org/10.1111/eva.12005(accessed on 13 May 2025).

23. Maheu-Giroux M, Castro MC (2013) Impact of Community-Based Larviciding on the Prevalence of Malaria Infection in Dar es Salaam, Tanzania. PLoS ONE 8(8): e71638. https://doi.org/10.1371/journal.pone.0071638 (accessed on 13 May 2025).

24. Chanda, E. (2016). *Optimizing Strategic Insecticide Resistance Management Planning in Malaria Vectors*. https://core.ac.uk/download/322425375.pdf (accessed on 13 May 2025).

25. Chaves, L. F., & Koenraadt, C. J. M. (2010). Climate change and highland malaria: Fresh air for a hot debate. https://core.ac.uk/download/pdf/29238217.pdf (accessed on 13 May 2025).

26. Chua, T. H., Drakeley, C., Ferguson, H. M., Fornace, K., et al. (2015). Seasonal and spatial dynamics of the primary vector of *Plasmodium knowlesi* within a major transmission focus in Sabah, Malaysia. https://core.ac.uk/download/42365590.pdf (accessed on 13 May 2025).

27. Dusfour, I., Vontas, J., David, J.-P., Weetman, D., Fonseca, D. M., Corbel, V., Raghavendra, K., et al. (2019). Management of insecticide resistance in the major *Aedes* vectors of arboviruses: Advances and challenges. *PLoS Neglected Tropical Diseases, 13*(10), e0007615. https://doi.org/10.1371/journal.pntd.0007615.

28. Feachem, R.G.A., with A.A. Phillips and G.A. Targett (eds) (2009). Shrinking the Malaria Map: A Prospectus on Malaria Elimination. San Francisco: The Global Health Group, Global Health Sciences, University of California, San Francisco. (accessed on 13 May 2025).

29. Ferguson, H. M., & Govella, N. J. (2023). *Impacts of Climate Change on Malaria Vector Control in Africa*. https://core.ac.uk/download/595561131.pdf (accessed on 13 May 2025).

30. Ng'habi, K., Viana, M., Matthiopoulos, J. *et al.* Mesocosm experiments reveal the impact of mosquito control measures on malaria vector life history and population dynamics. *Sci Rep* **8**, 13949 (2018). https://doi.org/10.1038/s41598-018-31805-8 (accessed on 13 May 2025).

31. Parres-Mercader, M., Pance, A., & Gómez-Díaz, E. (2023). Novel systems to study vector-pathogen interactions in malaria. *Frontiers in cellular and infection microbiology, 13*, 1146030. https://doi.org/10.3389/fcimb.2023.1146030 (accessed on 13 May 2025).

32. Hawkes, C., & Ruel, M. T. (2025). *Understanding the Links Between Agriculture and Health*. https://core.ac.uk/download/pdf/6288827.pdf (accessed on 13 May 2025).

33. Imbahale, S. S. (2025). *Integrated Malaria Vector Control in Different Agro-Ecosystems in Western Kenya*. https://core.ac.uk/download/pdf/29251092.pdf (accessed on 13 May 2025).

34. Intergovernmental Panel on Climate Change. (2023). *Climate Change 2022–Impacts, Adaptation and Vulnerability*. https://doi.org/10.1017/9781009325844.

35. Killeen, G. F., Seyoum, A., & Knols, B. G. (2004). Rationalizing historical successes of malaria control in Africa in terms of mosquito resource availability management. *The American journal of tropical medicine and hygiene, 71*(2 Suppl), 87–93. (accessed on 13 May 2025).

36. Kouamé, R. M. A., Guglielmo, F., Abo, K., Ouattara, A., Chabi, J., Sedda, L., Donnelly, M. J., et al. (2022). Education and socio-economic status are key factors influencing use of insecticides and malaria knowledge in rural farmers in Southern Côte d'Ivoire. *BMC Public Health, 22*, Article 14446. https://doi.org/10.1186/s12889-022-14446-5.

37. Killeen, G. F., Smith, T. A., Ferguson, H. M., Mshinda, H., Abdulla, S., Lengeler, C., & Kachur, S. P. (2007). Preventing childhood malaria in Africa by protecting adults from mosquitoes with insecticide-treated nets. *PLoS medicine, 4*(7), e229. https://doi.org/10.1371/journal.pmed.0040229(accessed on 13 May 2025).

38. Li, S., & Tetteh, A. K. (2021). Automatic mosquito control device using infrared motion sensor. https://core.ac.uk/download/481607880.pdf (accessed on 13 May 2025).

39. Li, X., Zhou, H., Xu, J. W., Lin, Z., Sun, X., Li, J., Lin, X. X., et al. (2021). Seven decades towards malaria elimination in Yunnan, China. *Malaria Journal, 20*, Article 3672. https://doi.org/10.1186/s12936-021-03672-8.

40. Lutrat, C., Giesbrecht, D., Marois, E., Whyard, S., Baldet, T., & Bouyer, J. (2019). Sex sorting for

pest control: It's raining men! *Trends in Parasitology, 35*, 649–662. https://doi.org/10.1016/j.pt.2019.06.001.

41. Monroe, A. (2020). Closing the malaria prevention gap: Measuring and characterizing human behavioral drivers of persistent malaria transmission in Sub-Saharan Africa. https://core.ac.uk/download/395087942.pdf (accessed on 13 May 2025).
42. Murray, C. J. L., Ikuta, K. S., Sharara, F., Swetschinski, L. R., Robles Aguilar, G., Gray, A. P., Han, C., et al. (2022). Global burden of bacterial antimicrobial resistance in 2019: A systematic analysis. *The Lancet, 399*, 629–655. https://doi.org/10.1016/S0140-6736(21)02724-0.
43. Murta, F., Marques, L. L. G., Santos, A. C., Batista, T. S. B., Mendes, M. O., Silva, E. D., Silva Neto, A. V., et al. (2021). Perceptions about malaria among Brazilian gold miners in an Amazonian border area: Perspectives for malaria elimination strategies. *Malaria Journal, 20*. https://doi.org/10.1186/s12936-021-03820-0.
44. Nakyaze, E., Van Hulle, S., Hembling, J., Arinaitwe, E., Mbodji, M., Alwano, M. G., Lamwaka, F. C., Tukwasibwe, S., Gonahasa, S., Liu, F., Grieco, J. P., & Achee, N. L. (2024). Advancing spatial repellents for malaria control: effectiveness and cost-effectiveness of a spatial repellent under operational use in Northern Uganda-study protocol for a cluster randomized controlled trial. *Trials, 25*(1), 555. https://doi.org/10.1186/s13063-024-08378-1(accessed on 13 May 2025).
45. Navarro Ferronato, V., & Torretta, V. (2019). Waste mismanagement in developing countries: A review of global issues. *International Journal of Environmental Research and Public Health, 16*(6), 1060. https://doi.org/10.3390/ijerph16061060.
46. Overgaard, H. (2025). Malaria mosquito resistance to agricultural insecticides: Risk area mapping in Thailand. https://core.ac.uk/download/pdf/6405173.pdf (accessed on 13 May 2025).
47. Ruzzante, L., Reijnders, M., & Waterhouse, R. M. (2018). Of genes and genomes: Mosquito evolution and diversity. *Trends in Parasitology, 35*, 32–51. https://doi.org/10.1016/j.pt.2018.10.003.
48. Killeen, G.F., Seyoum, A., Sikaala, C. *et al.* Eliminating malaria vectors. *Parasites Vectors* **6**, 172 (2013). https://doi.org/10.1186/1756-3305-6-172 (accessed on 13 May 2025).
49. Tarekegn, M., Tekie, H., Dugassa, S., & Woldehawariat, Y. (2021). Malaria prevalence and associated risk factors in Dembiya district, north-western Ethiopia. *Malaria Journal, 20*. https://doi.org/10.1186/s12936-021-03906-9.
50. Whittaker, C. F. (2022). Quantifying the impacts of variation in entomological and epidemiological determinants of malaria transmission. https://core.ac.uk/download/533450122.pdf (accessed on 13 May 2025).
51. Wilson, A. L., Courtenay, O., Kelly-Hope, L. A., Scott, T. W., Takken, W., Torr, S. J., & Lindsay, S. W. (2020). The importance of vector control for the control and elimination of vector-borne diseases. *PLoS Neglected Tropical Diseases, 14*, e0007831. https://doi.org/10.1371/journal.pntd.0007831.
52. Zikayo, A. R. (2025). A review of the efficacy of insecticide-treated bed nets in reducing malaria incidence among children under five in rural Sub-Saharan Africa. International Network Organization for Scientific Research https://doi.org/10.59298/INOSRSR/2025/12.1.1500(accessed on 13 May 2025).

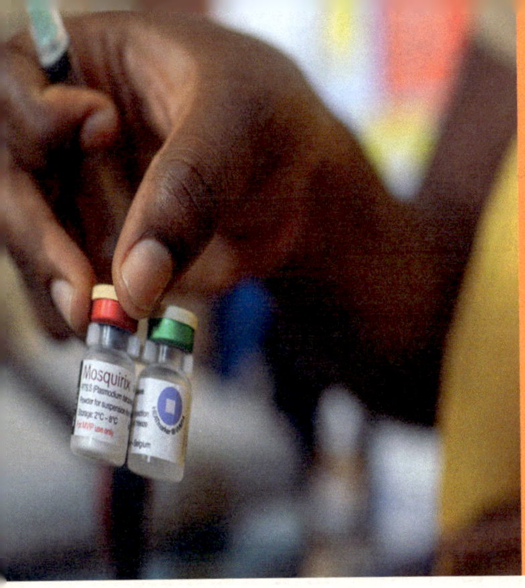

Chapter 13

CHEMOPREVENTION AND MALARIA VACCINES

Contents

Introduction

Malaria control has been a long-standing battle, trying to ease the heavy toll the disease takes, especially in regions like sub-Saharan Africa. Simple measures like insecticide-treated nets and antimalarial drugs have always been part of the mix, yet the illness still brings significant harm and loss among vulnerable groups. Lately, the introduction of malaria vaccines has kind of shifted the outlook. The RTS,S/AS01 vaccine, for instance, was the first one to win a nod from the World Health Organization (WHO)—a pretty meaningful marker. Rolling out this vaccine together with the older interventions hints at a move toward more mixed strategies against such a complex foe, particularly in areas where *Plasmodium falciparum* transmission is moderately high. Getting solid protection against malaria isn't as simple as using one tool alone. In most cases, it means pairing vaccination with other preventive measures like Seasonal Malaria Chemoprevention (SMC). This mixed approach mainly targets the riskiest times and groups, especially kids under five during peak seasons. Some clinical trials have shown that if you time the RTS,S vaccine to line up with seasonal outbreaks, its effectiveness improves noticeably, cutting down not only standard cases but also those more severe episodes. Still, putting this integrated approach into practice isn't without its challenges; many endemic areas simply don't have an established system for seasonal vaccine delivery. Pilot projects in Ghana, Kenya, and Malawi, though not flawless, offer some key insights into these logistical obstacles and point toward ways to increase both vaccination and chemoprevention efforts (Merle et al., 2023). Cost-effectiveness adds another layer of complexity when it comes to deploying malaria vaccines alongside existing interventions, especially given our limited global resources. Mathematical models generally suggest that while adding RTS,S on top of measures like treated nets and SMC can lower malaria cases and deaths, the choice of which interventions to prioritize heavily depends on local factors—transmission patterns, bed net coverage, and even insecticide resistance all play a part. The cost per dose of the vaccine is crucial, as its greatest impact seems to show in high-transmission settings where prevention tools are only moderately present. So, decision-makers must balance integrating the RTS,S vaccination with other established chemoprevention programs to get the most health benefit out of tight budgets (Hillary et al., 2023) (Figure 13.1).

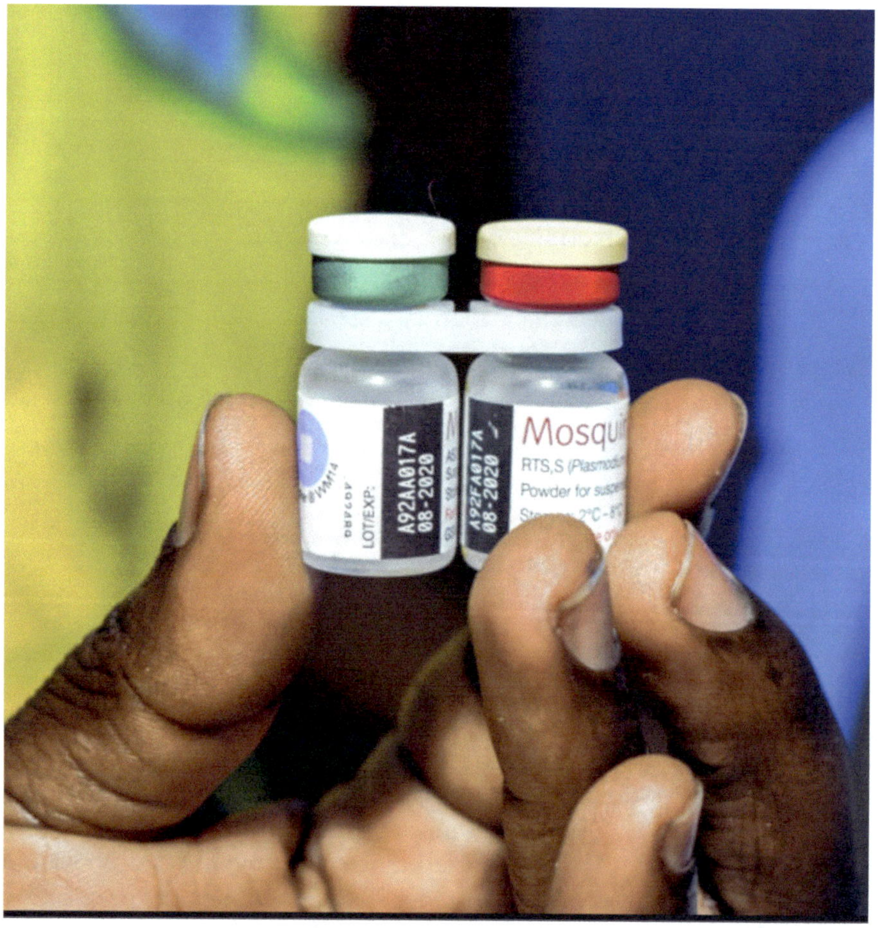

Figure 13.1. Malaria vaccines.

Source: Stat News. (2022). *Malaria Vaccines.*

Definition of Chemoprevention

When fighting malaria, people now look beyond just treating the symptoms—they try to stop the infection before it even starts. One common trick is giving antimalarial medicine to individuals who might get sick, keeping enough of the drug in the blood so that any parasite that shows up can't catch on. This method, often used for children bouncing back after a bad bout of malaria, cuts down on both deaths and repeat hospital visits. It's a shift from simply fighting an infection to breaking the cycle of disease, and in most cases, these targeted moves underline a new direction in malaria control (Kühl et al., 2025).

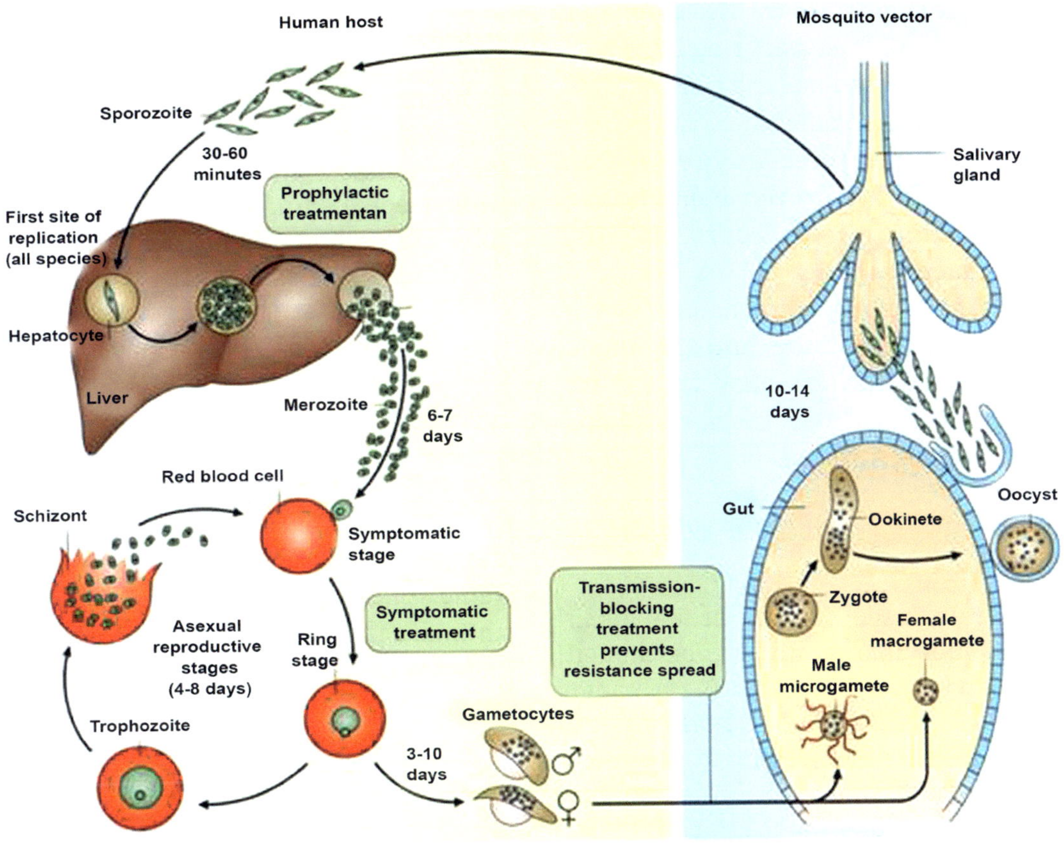

Figure 13.2. Chemoprevention.

Source: Moehrle JJ. Development of New Strategies for Malaria Chemoprophylaxis: From Monoclonal Antibodies to Long-Acting Injectable Drugs. *Tropical Medicine and Infectious Disease*. 2022; 7(4):58. https://doi.org/10.3390/tropicalmed7040058

Take, for instance, a program known as post-discharge malaria chemoprevention (PDMC). Here, preschool children, especially those knocked out by severe malaria symptoms like poor blood counts—get a monthly dose of oral antimalarials, usually over a three-month span after they leave the hospital. Drugs such as dihydroartemisinin-piperaquine, which fall under the artemisinin-based combo category, are picked not only for their power but also because they seem to sidestep the risk of resistance. Of course, none of this would matter much if the caregivers or patients didn't stick to the plan. As a result, many strategies now weigh options between community programs and hospital settings to see what best holds up under real-life challenges (Kühl et al., 2025). What makes chemoprevention stand out is how it goes hand in hand with other measures like vaccines and mosquito control. While vaccines generally gear up your immune system to fend off infections, the drugs work right away like an extra barrier that stops the parasites cold. This mix of defenses is smart, considering how drug resistance can emerge and malaria transmission can be all over the place sometimes. The WHO's support for these measures in sub-Saharan Africa reflects both the proven benefits and the workable nature of the approach. Still, keeping this success going means we need regular check-ins on drug performance, watch out for any brewing resistance, and stay tuned to whether communities are okay with these practices, especially as new vaccine options emerge (Figure 13.2).

Overview of Malaria and Its Global Impact

Malaria still remains a serious headache in many parts of sub-Saharan Africa, even though huge efforts have been made to bring it under control. Lately, instead of a one-size-fits-all approach, programs have turned to down-to-earth, data-led plans that mix local insights with hard statistics. Take Guinea, for example, their national malaria team broke the mold by splitting their strategy region by region, mixing infection numbers, details on insect resistance, and how many people are covered to decide on actions like indoor spraying, nets treated with insecticide, and seasonal drug measures. That kind of targeted plan not only lets them fine-tune prevention efforts but also managed to pull in extra funding, showing that smart data plays a critical role in fighting malaria (Diallo et al., 2024). To summarize, the ever-changing picture of malaria spread means that flexible, locally tuned strategies are needed. Looking at the big picture, malaria's toll is enormous, knocking down health and economies, especially among those already vulnerable in endemic areas. Recent models suggest that when control measures get disrupted – think of how the COVID-19 pandemic shook things up – decades of progress could unravel, leading to more cases and higher death counts. For instance, if fewer people gain access to proper antimalarial drugs or insecticide-treated nets, tens of millions more cases and hundreds of thousands additional deaths could crop up in just one year. These figures remind us that our current efforts are on a tightrope and that we must keep comprehensive control programs alive even when other public health issues call for attention (Daniel et al., 2020).

In most cases, this makes the need for prevention – whether through drugs taken in advance or the push toward vaccines – all the more urgent for long-term malaria control. When you dig into global malaria control, it becomes clear that no single solution will fix everything; mixing various approaches is the name of the game. Chemoprevention – essentially giving antimalarial drugs during peak times or to high-risk groups – has shown promise in knocking down case numbers and deaths, while recent strides in vaccine research hint at an extra layer of defense by building partial immunity to cut transmission. Mixing these modern strategies with tried-and-true vector control methods creates a more complete framework to relieve the disease burden. Local data, even when a bit uneven or complex sometimes, guide where and how these measures are rolled out to get the best bang for the buck. Ultimately, grasping the complex, complex spread and broad impact of malaria around the world is key to shaping strategies, especially in areas with unique transmission features and wildly different health system capacities (Daniel et al., 2020; Diallo et al., 2024).

Importance of Vaccines in Malaria Control

Malaria control isn't a one-track effort, it's about mixing prevention with treatment, especially where resources run thin. In many spots hit hardest by the disease, strategies like chemoprevention have cut down illness and death, even though drug resistance and rollout issues sometimes get in the way. Vaccines then emerge as a important extra measure; they increase the immune system so that infections either don't start or the parasites don't get far, helping to curb transmission and ease disease severity on a broad scale. In regions where insecticide resistance throws a wrench into traditional methods, and where prevention campaigns have taken a hit—pairing vaccines with chemoprevention seems to keep progress moving forward (Stephen et al., 2020). It's also key to note that malaria doesn't act the same everywhere. For example, in places like Cameroon, where the mix of *Plasmodium* species and a bunch of anopheline vectors complicates things, interventions need to be nimble, generally speaking. Resistance mutations in parasites and growing insecticide resistance in mosquitoes make chemoprevention alone a tougher battle, so having vaccines to target different parts of the parasite's life cycle can help lower the overall parasite load in humans. Children and pregnant women often bear the brunt, so, in many cases, added vaccination can cut down cases in these vulnerable groups. When vaccine programs run alongside chemoprevention, the whole control effort tends to be tougher and more sustainable, even in challenging settings (Antonio et al., 2019). Recent health challenges, like the COVID-19 pandemic, have shown just how fragile our malaria intervention systems can be. Interruptions in things like insecticide-treated net distributions and treatment access have left many exposed, proving that leaning on just one method isn't enough. Vaccines, offering long-lasting immunity and even some herd protection, help make up for these gaps by reducing overall transmission—plus, they ease the load on already-stretched health services by lowering clinical malaria cases. In short, rolling out effective malaria vaccines isn't just about patching up current shortcomings; it's a must for keeping control efforts steady, pushing back against disease resurgence, and, eventually, reaching elimination goals (Stephen et al., 2020).

13.1. Understanding Malaria

Environmental factors shape how malaria spreads. Temperature, humidity, and rainfall all matter — even if it's not always obvious at first glance — because they decide where and when mosquitos can thrive. When the climate warms up, for example, the parasite seems to develop faster within a mosquito, so the chance of passing it on goes up. These shifts in weather not only broaden the geographical risk but may also extend the season when transmission occurs, putting vulnerable communities at greater risk. Getting a grip on these shifting conditions is key to planning and timing treatments and vaccines, ensuring that our interventions keep up with the changing patterns of disease activity (Jan et al., 2022). Malaria's overall picture is made even more complex by the mix of parasite types and their ever-changing drug resistance. In places like Cameroon, the problem stays big despite major public health efforts, largely due to a variety of *Plasmodium* species that cause infections in ways that vary regionally. Generally speaking, artemisinin-based combination therapies — which have long been the backbone of treatment — are starting to struggle in some areas as resistance emerges. There's also the matter of gene mutations that let parasites dodge multiple drugs, highlighting the need for ongoing surveillance and regularly updated treatment plans. To summarize, successfully fighting malaria seems to rely on mixing smart chemoprevention with vaccine strategies tailored to local parasite profiles (Antonio et al., 2019). Then there's the whole issue of mosquito diversity. Different anopheline species, each with their own features and levels of resistance, complicate control measures. Some of these mosquitoes respond poorly to standard insecticidal tools like long-lasting nets, and with growing resistance to pyrethroids, DDT, and even carbamates, our current vector control programs face a real challenge. In most cases, this resistance jeopardizes the progress we've managed in reducing malaria's impact and pushes us toward a more flexible, locally responsive approach. Essentially, understanding the complex details of mosquito behavior is crucial if we're to optimize chemopreventive drug use and make vaccine-driven immunity a long-term solution for malaria control (Antonio et al., 2019) (Figure 13.3).

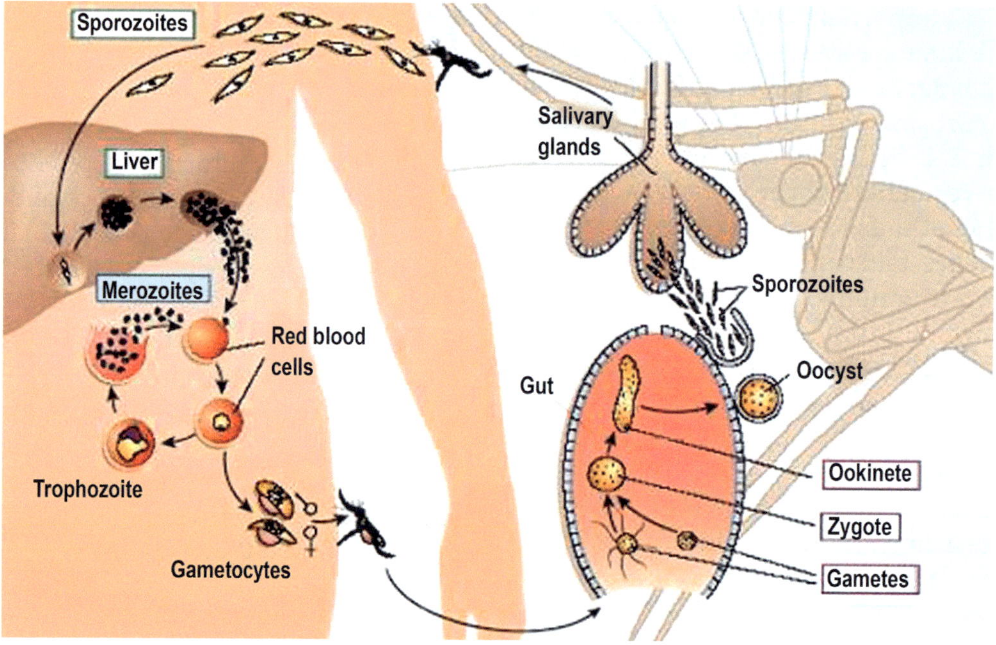

Figure 13.3. Malaria: What is it and how is it transmitted?

Source: Malwest. (n.d.). *Malaria: What is it & How is it Transmitted?* Googleusercontent.

13.1.1. Life Cycle of the Malaria Parasite

Grasping how malaria moves through its many life phases is key when fighting the disease—whether you're using vaccines or preventive drugs. The parasite doesn't follow a neat order; it bounces between mosquitoes (like those Anopheles ones) and humans in a way that often surprises you. It all starts when an infected mosquito gives a quick jab of sporozoites during a bite—these little invaders rush off to the liver, slip into liver cells without much fuss, and multiply quietly. Then, almost as if on cue, merozoites burst into the bloodstream to invade red blood cells, sparking the symptomatic blood stage. This complex journey offers plenty of opportunities for intervention, but its very complexity also muddies the waters for both vaccine creation and chemoprevention measures. Effective malaria control has to mess with these steps to cut transmission and ease the overall disease burden (Winskill et al., 2019). Much attention has settled on the liver stage—a real bottleneck in malaria's journey and a tempting target for vaccination. Whole sporozoite vaccines try to kickstart the body's defenses against the parasite both when it's floating around outside cells and when it's tucked away inside the liver. These shots, made from either weakened or natural sporozoites, stir up both antibody responses and cellular defenses, generally aiming to offer broader protection than those vaccines that focus on just one phase. Still, because the liver stage tends to hide from many treatments, it's a pretty tough nut to crack, often pushing experts to mix vaccine methods with chemoprophylaxis, especially where malaria is common (Leslie et al., 2018). Further, recent progress in lab-based cultivation of sporozoites has opened doors for mass-producing these vaccines, helping to overcome a key hurdle in current development efforts (Leslie et al., 2018). Alongside vaccine work, using preventive drugs plays a vital role in breaking the parasite's cycle, especially during the blood stage when symptoms hit hard. Anti-malaria medicines, given early on as the parasite leaves the liver, work to lower its numbers and trim its chance to spread. Often, mixing these drug strategies with mosquito control boosts the overall impact—fewer infected mosquitoes mean fewer sporozoites get into people during a bite. However, tight budgets force us to focus on the most cost-effective solutions; while vector control is still essential, adding in chemoprevention noticeably improves outcomes in high-transmission areas. Combining these drug measures with properly timed vaccine strategies offers a promising route toward cutting down malaria cases and, eventually, moving toward eradication (Winskill et al., 2019).

13.1.2. Symptoms and Health Effects of Malaria

Often, malaria kicks in with vague signs like a fever, chills, headache, and muscle aches—symptoms that can quickly turn serious if left unchecked. The culprit is a group of *Plasmodium* parasites that get transmitted by the bite of an infected Anopheles mosquito. Once inside the body, these parasites make a beeline for red blood cells, breaking them apart in a way that usually leads to anemia, one of the disease's biggest complications. This cell breakdown reduces the oxygen that organs receive, which, in turn, can result in persistent fatigue or, even more worryingly, organ failure. Kids and pregnant women, for example, are often hit much harder because their immune responses are different. And it doesn't stop there; malaria's effects run deeper, disturbing maternal and fetal health by sometimes causing stillbirths, low birth weights, and even higher maternal mortality rates (Bauserman et al., 2019). All of this underscores the complex association between parasite biology and our body's own defenses, making early diagnosis and prompt treatment absolutely vital. It's hard to overstate the toll malaria takes on children since in many areas it remains a leading cause of illness and death. Severe anemia and even cerebral malaria are among the most dangerous problems in kids—issues that often force an immediate hospital visit. In regions where the disease is common, repeated bouts of malaria can slowly pile on harmful effects like stunted growth and impaired cognitive development. Even after a child recovers from a severe episode of anemia, that post-discharge period can be a particularly risky time with a higher chance of readmission or even death. In most cases, strategies like post-discharge malaria chemoprevention (PDMC), which means giving antimalarial drugs during recovery, have shown promising results in lowering these risks (Kühl et al., 2025). These findings highlight why mixing such preventive treatments with current vaccine and medication programs may be the best way to reduce malaria's lasting impact. Beyond the immediate symptoms, malaria has a layered and multifaceted impact. The disease does not only directly damage red blood cells; it also triggers inflammatory responses that can further injure bodily tissues. In pregnant women, for instance, parasites tend to accumulate in the placenta—a process that disrupts nutrient exchange and may lead to fetal growth restrictions or even stillbirth (Bauserman et al., 2019). This type of placental malaria jeopardizes fetal health while also increasing the mother's risk of developing severe anemia, sometimes with fatal consequences.

In areas with constant exposure, repeated infections gradually wear down the immune system and make standard treatments less effective. In short, while malaria's acute effects are a major concern, its long-term, cumulative damage, especially among the most vulnerable—drives home the need for a combined prevention approach that includes both vaccines and chemopreventive measures (Figure 13.4).

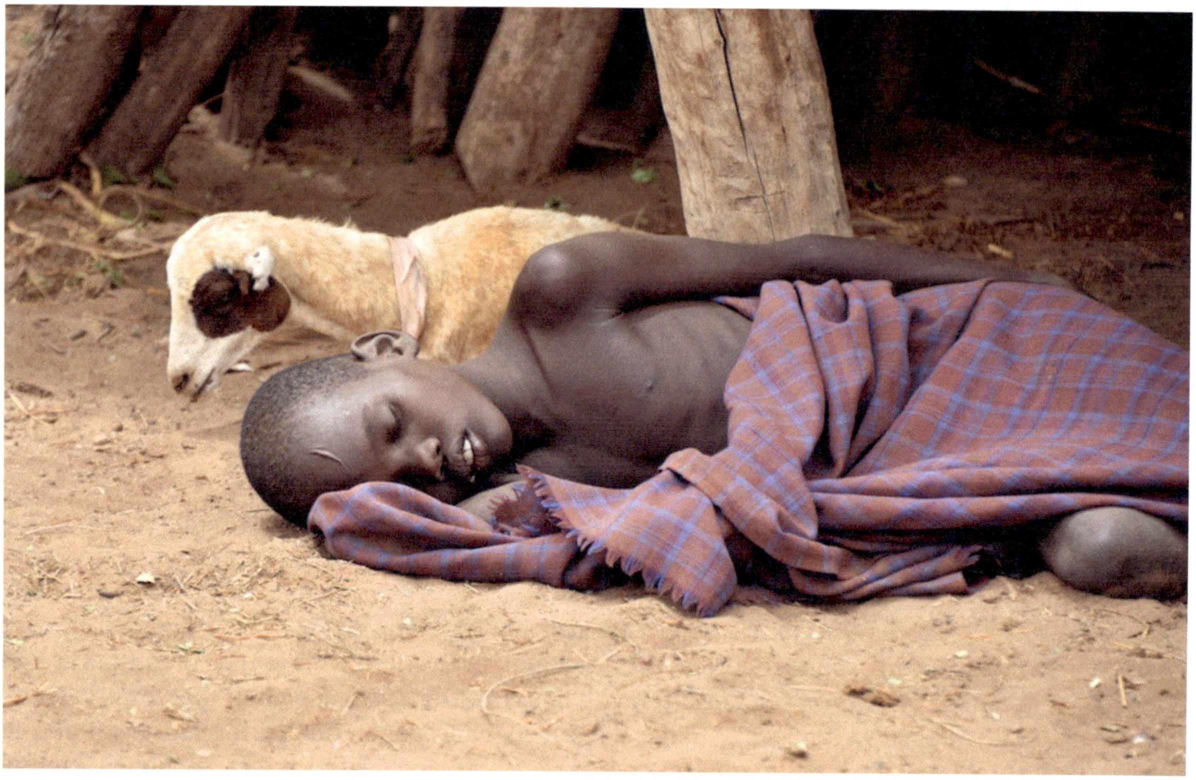

Figure 13.4. Symptoms and health effects of malaria.

Source: By Rod Waddington from Kergunyah, Australia - Malaria Patient, Nyangaton, Ethiopia, CC BY-SA 2.0, https://commons.wikimedia.org/w/index.php?curid=36667217

13.1.3. Current Statistics on Malaria Prevalence

Recent models of malaria spread have shifted our view of the disease—linking how fast it travels with what happens in patients. In tests run across different parts of Africa, simulations suggest that the rate of *Plasmodium falciparum* infection in kids between 2 and 10 can jump from around 10% to nearly 65%. That wide range shows, quite plainly, how uneven the burden can be. These numbers, which emerge repeatedly in our analyses, inform us about how much preventive work, like vaccines and drug regimens—might lower cases and save lives. One study even showed that interventions timed with seasonal patterns tend to cut down malaria cases more effectively than the usual age-based methods (Thompson et al., 2022). , having exact local transmission figures seems to be at the heart of making smarter vaccination and chemoprevention plans. Looking at the toll on young lives, illness and death statistics in sub-Saharan Africa paint a grim picture—malaria still tops the list for causing hospital stays and tragic losses among children. Post-discharge data reveals that kids coming out of a bout with severe malarial anemia often face another round of infections; these repeats also muddle efforts to stick with preventive drug schedules. Trials carried out in Kenya, Uganda, and Malawi found that using PDMC with dihydroartemisinin-piperaquine over about three months noticeably cuts both readmission and death rates among children in these regions (Kühl et al., 2025). Global health experts are now, in most cases, backing such chemoprevention steps as an essential piece of the malaria control puzzle in areas where the disease is a constant threat. In short, tracking malaria prevalence closely is directly linked to improving how we deliver these vital prevention measures. On another front, many cost-effectiveness studies and disease analyses underscores that combining different malaria-fighting strategies can yield impressive health and economic benefits. National-level models hint that teaming seasonal vaccination with chemoprevention might prevent tens of thousands of extra cases among young children over time compared to using just one method. This assessment – which factors in the ups and downs of transmission seasonality – shows that places with long, drawn-out periods of high parasite loads tend to gain the most. Moreover, economic reviews suggest that community-based delivery of chemoprevention can be more budget-friendly than hospital-based approaches, with adherence stats lending extra support to this view. These nuanced evaluations do more than just count cases; they help shape actionable policies by showing how fresh malaria stats can fine-tune tools like RTS,S vaccination and PDMC across endemic regions (Thompson et al., 2022; Kühl et al., 2025) (Figure 13.5).

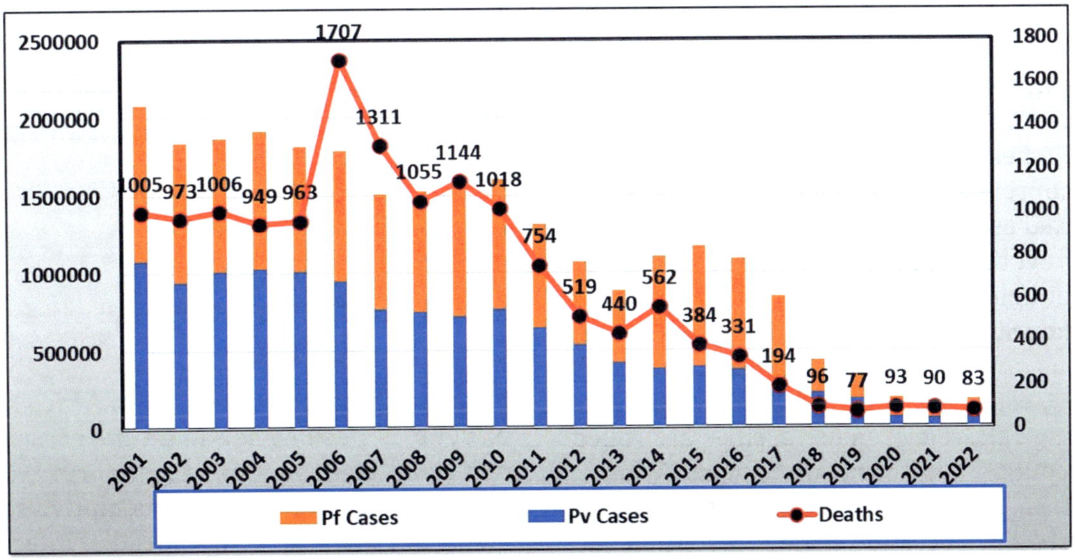

Figure 13.5. Current statistics on malaria prevalence.

Source: National Center for Vector Borne Disease Control. (n.d.). *Malaria Prevalence in India (2001–2022).*

13.2. Chemoprevention Strategies

Malaria controls these days isn't about one magic bullet, it's more of a mixed approach that combines prevention with treatment in hopes of cutting down both the number of cases and the deadly toll. Chemoprevention, for instance, has proven itself as a major player by offering antimalarial drugs beforehand, kind of like a backup to vaccination, especially for those most at risk. Take seasonal malaria chemoprevention (SMC): it primarily focuses on kids under five in areas where malaria spikes occur only during certain times of the year. During those high-risk months, children receive monthly doses that, when paired with insecticide-treated nets (ITNs), help keep the infection at bay. Mathematical models even suggest that when you mix chemoprevention with vaccines such as RTS,S, there's a notable extra boost in protection (Hillary et al., 2023). To summarize, chemoprevention has become a must-have piece in a layered strategy against malaria. Sometimes though, when the system stumbles, like when treatments and prevention efforts get interrupted—the consequences can be severe. The COVID-19 pandemic, for example, showed us that even brief disruptions in accessing these crucial interventions can quickly unravel all the hard-won progress against malaria. Models generally speak to the potential perils: if supplies of chemopreventive drugs drop or ITNs aren't distributed as needed, malaria cases and deaths can skyrocket, with some scenarios hinting at nearly doubled fatalities (Daniel et al., 2020). This underlines how fragile our gains can be, urging us to keep chemoprophylaxis running smoothly, especially for those most vulnerable like young children, even as vaccines are rolled out to counter any backward steps. When it comes to juggling limited resources, figuring out the best balance between chemoprevention and vaccination isn't exactly a walk in the park, it calls for some careful cost-effectiveness work. Generally speaking, vaccines offer that long-term protection, while chemoprevention gives an immediate, seasonal shield. Studies imply that putting more emphasis on interventions like SMC, ramping up ITN coverage, and using the RTS,S vaccine in the right areas can slash case numbers and boost overall health outcomes (Hillary et al., 2023). Still, getting the most bang for our buck depends on knowing the local ins and outs: how malaria spreads in a given spot, the patterns of insecticide resistance, and whether the health infrastructure can keep pace. In short, chemoprevention needs to be woven into broader malaria control programs in a flexible and adaptive way to ensure that every investment helps tackle this persistent public health challenge (Figure 13.6).

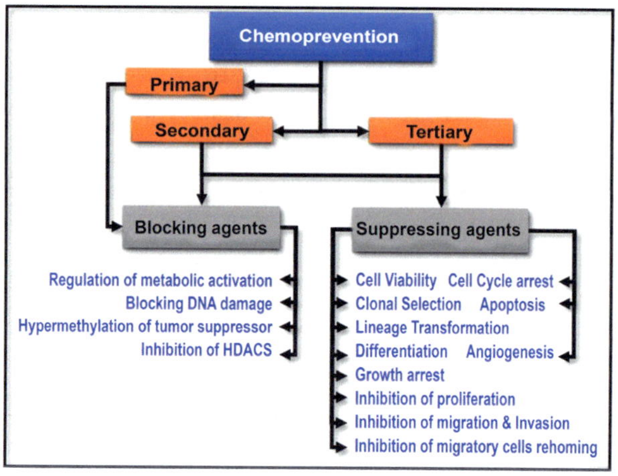

Figure 13.6. Chemoprevention strategies.

Source: ResearchGate. (n.d.). *Classification of Chemopreventive Strategies.*

13.2.1. Definition and Purpose of Chemoprevention

Malaria's impact in sub-Saharan Africa keeps us on our toes, pushing new ideas into play alongside our usual control steps. Chemoprevention, for instance, offers a kind of preemptive strike by giving antimalarial drugs ahead of infections or during sudden surges in transmission. Instead of waiting for symptoms subsequently reacting, this approach aims to stop fresh cases from emerging, which in turn helps cut down both sickness and fatal outcomes. It zeroes in on the individuals most at risk, like little kids bouncing back from a serious bout or pregnant women facing extra danger—by providing ongoing protection right when it's most needed. The World Health Organization's (WHO) support for

PDMC hints at real potential for lowering deaths and hospital readmissions among preschoolers in especially hard-hit areas (Kühl et al., 2025). Digging a bit deeper, the method works by giving antimalarial meds in a routine way to break the parasite's cycle inside humans. Generally speaking, keeping steady drug levels through repeated doses shrinks the number of parasites able to mature and spread, which helps reduce transmission at a community level. It's not just about protecting one person, it's about shifting the overall balance, with factors like timing, dosage, and how the medicine is delivered playing a big role in its success. Some recent studies point to household-based oral regimens after a hospital stay; these have proven both cost-effective and notably impactful when community delivery models are in play. In this sense, mixing chemoprevention with broader strategies, like vector control and new vaccine efforts—adds an extra layer to our fight against malaria (Kühl et al., 2025). Then there's the added benefit of chemoprevention working hand-in-hand with vaccines. While vaccines primarily aim to build a long-lasting immune response, chemoprevention jumps in immediately to tamp down the parasite, especially during high-risk periods when vaccine immunity might still be coming up to speed. In most cases, it becomes crucial to iron out key details—how effective the intervention needs to be, how long it lasts, and what coverage is required—to match health goals. Researchers, combining mathematical modeling with machine learning insights, have begun to nail down these essential properties, moving the idea from theory to a tailored intervention. This kind of fine-tuning not only boosts the overall impact but also helps guide resource choices and the coordinated roll-out alongside newer vaccine candidates, all of which adds up to a more connected strategy against malaria.

13.2.2. Types of Chemopreventive Agents Used for Malaria

Worldwide efforts to cut down on malaria have pushed researchers to come up with all kinds of chemopreventive tools, often, these tools work by targeting different parts of how the *Plasmodium* parasite develops. Drugs like chloroquine, mefloquine, doxycycline, and the atovaquone-proguanil mix are used as a kind of shield for both travelers and those living in areas where malaria is common. Often these treatments block the parasite's growth inside red blood cells so that the nasty symptoms never show up as clearly; subsequently, there are newer hybrid compounds that merge treatment benefits with improved ways of getting the medicine to the right spot. Generally speaking, this creative mixing takes advantage of conjugate chemistry, which lets scientists design molecules that end up being more stable and easier for the body to absorb. Overall, these sophisticated approaches hint that future chemopreventive agents could offer more targeted, long-lasting protection against malaria (Abdulaziz et al., 2022). Beyond the traditional antimalarials, research has also begun to mess with the parasite at earlier stages or even interfere with the pathogens that carry it; in many cases, this leads to a more rounded prevention strategy. For example, primaquine is commonly used to clear out those dormant liver forms in *Plasmodium vivax* infections—a move that helps prevent relapse and further spread. Researchers are even looking at repurposing drugs that already have a solid safety record (which might, you know, bring new options to the table faster). Of course, it's still a challenge to ensure that enough drug reaches the bloodstream and tissues to work effectively without tipping into toxicity; balancing efficacy and safety, often via detailed pharmacokinetic studies—is absolutely key, as seen in various antiviral drug evaluations that check both how active a drug is and how much of it gets to the target organs (Arshad et al., 2020). This kind of integrative research not only repeats the focus on multiple parasite forms but also helps pinpoint agents that could work alongside or boost vaccine strategies. With drug resistance on the rise and the maze-like nature of malaria transmission, combination chemoprevention regimens are catching more eyes as a way to boost effectiveness and guard against resistance.

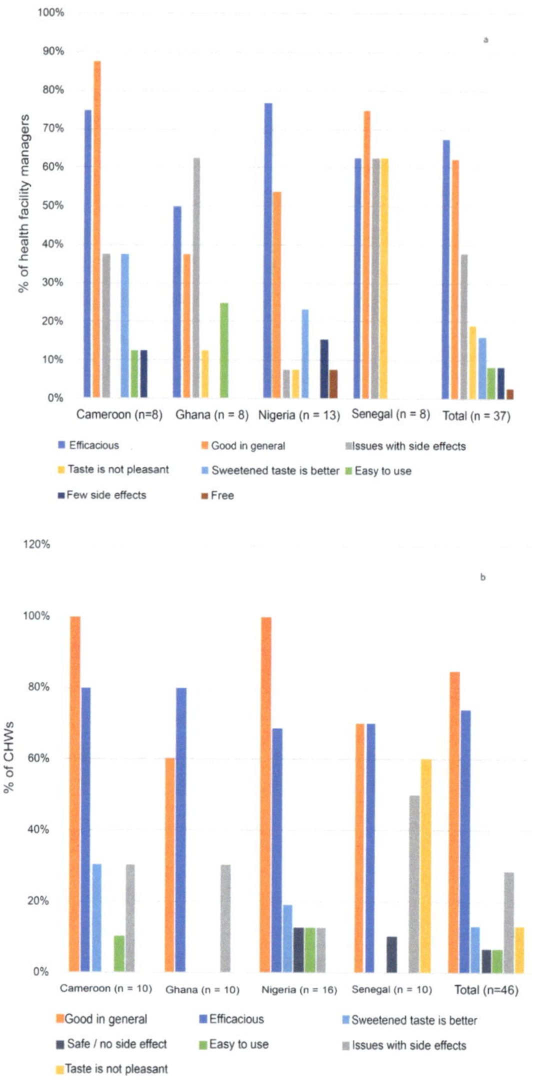

Figure 13.7. Development of new strategies for malaria chemoprophylaxis.

Source: Audibert C, Tchouatieu A-M. Perception of Malaria Chemoprevention Interventions in Infants and Children in Eight Sub-Saharan African Countries: An End User Perspective Study. *Tropical Medicine and Infectious Disease.* 2021; 6(2):75. https://doi.org/10.3390/tropicalmed6020075

These plans typically mix drugs that work in different ways, meaning the parasite is attacked on several fronts at once. Take atovaquone-proguanil, for instance, it hits the parasite by inhibiting its mitochondria and also by disrupting the folate pathway, which is a neat example of how mixing different effects can lead to better outcomes. Recent strides in medicinal chemistry have made it possible to design these multi-target solutions, often cutting down on side effects and even making it easier for patients to stick to their treatment schedules. In most cases, this strategy fits well with a broader approach where chemoprevention and vaccination go hand in hand, creating a kind of multi-layered shield against the disease. Innovations like these point toward a future where chemically optimized prophylactics mix with immunization efforts for sustained malaria control (Abdulaziz et al., 2022) (Figure 13.7).

13.2.3. Effectiveness of Chemoprevention in Malaria-Endemic Regions

Malaria tends to spike during certain seasons, and when interventions zero in on these peak moments, the overall impact can change the disease's toll. In many parts of the African Sahel, for example, young children get what's called SMC – essentially, a full treatment course given monthly when risks are highest. This method works by knocking out existing infections and keeping new ones at bay during these vulnerable periods, which generally cuts down both malaria cases and related deaths. Still, it isn't foolproof; practical issues like keeping up with drug delivery and ensuring patients stick with the regimen can weaken its impact. Plus, the use of drugs such as sulfadoxine-pyrimethamine and amodiaquine carries its own risk, as resistance might eventually develop and undermine long-term effectiveness (Greenwood et al., 2017). Recent progress in malaria vaccine research now adds some fresh hope to the mix, especially in places where transmission is seasonal. Take the RTS,S/AS01 vaccine, it went through intense trials and regulatory checks, and while it shows high efficacy at the start, that protection tends to drop off fast, which creates a little bit of a challenge for long-lasting coverage. Aligning vaccination efforts with the beginning of the malaria season can tap into the vaccine's peak performance, offering timely immunity.

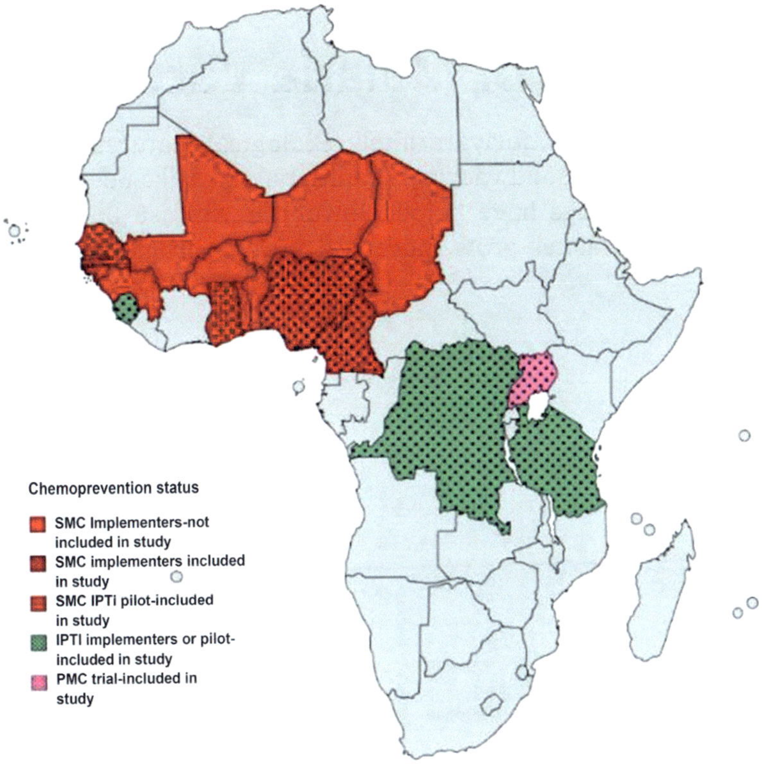

Figure 13.8. Effectiveness of chemoprevention in malaria-endemic regions.

Source: Audibert C, Tchouatieu A-M. Perception of Malaria Chemoprevention Interventions in Infants and Children in Eight Sub-Saharan African Countries: An End User Perspective Study. *Tropical Medicine and Infectious Disease*. 2021; 6(2):75. https://doi.org/10.3390/tropicalmed6020075

Mathematical models built on both epidemiological and immunological data generally indicate that matching seasonal vaccine campaigns with chemoprevention can boost overall public health benefits. In fact, this combined approach might even alter how these drugs work in the body—potentially enhancing their power and pushing back the rise of resistance (Greenwood et al., 2017). Merging chemoprevention with vaccination isn't as simple as it sounds, though. It calls for a detailed look at local malaria trends and the capacity of nearby healthcare systems. New modeling studies suggest that when RTS,S vaccination is rolled out during the season alongside regular SMC, the immediate benefits can be impressive, and there's promise for a more lasting drop in malaria cases. However, factors like local endemicity, possible coverage levels, and how perfectly the timing aligns play a critical role in whether these interventions hit the mark. There's also some real-world evidence hinting at a beneficial synergy when drug-based prevention and vaccine-induced immunity join forces, meaning that together they might do more than the sum of their parts. For these reasons, policy makers need to weigh local seasonality, current intervention reach, and the robustness of health systems when they design strategies to combat malaria (Figure 13.8).

13.3. Development of Malaria Vaccines

Fighting malaria hasn't been straightforward lately. Biological features and practical issues have muddied our attempts at crafting a solid vaccine. Traditional fixes like keeping mosquito populations in check or using preventive drugs have helped lower the disease burden, but they're running into trouble as *Plasmodium* parasites grow more resistant to drugs and mosquitoes get tougher against insecticides.

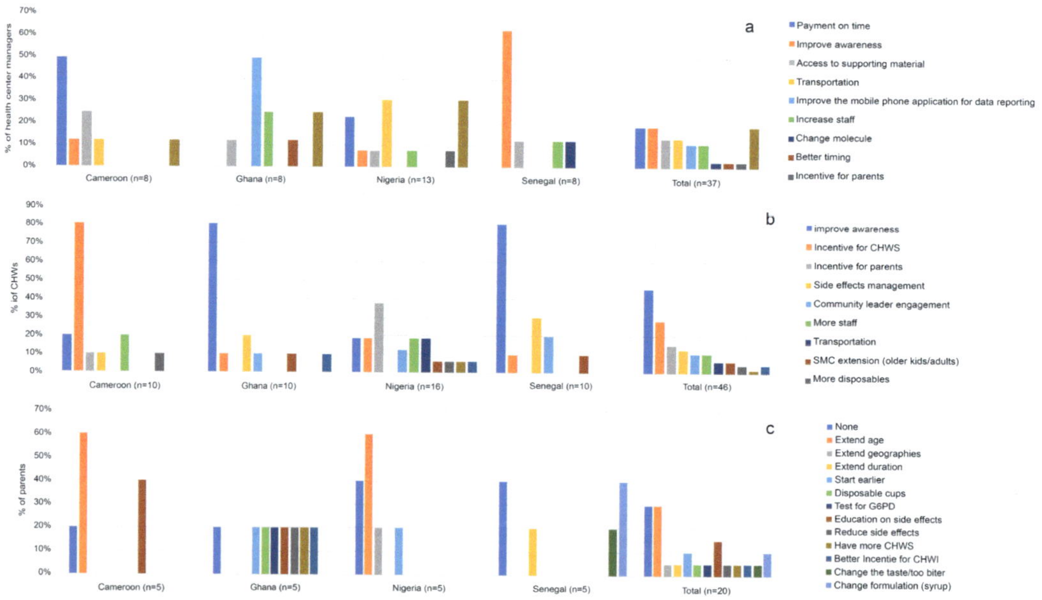

Figure 13.9. Development of malaria vaccines.

Source: Audibert C, Tchouatieu A-M. Perception of Malaria Chemoprevention Interventions in Infants and Children in Eight Sub-Saharan African Countries: An End User Perspective Study. *Tropical Medicine and Infectious Disease*. 2021; 6(2):75. https://doi.org/10.3390/tropicalmed6020075

Global events, such as the COVID-19 pandemic, only added to the mix by disrupting public health work focused on malaria. So, the idea of a long-lasting vaccine is especially appealing. Unlike regular chemoprevention that demands constant dosing, a good vaccine could give sustained immunity, cutting back on the need for repeated treatments. Of course, hurdles remain: the parasite can change its makeup, and triggering a strong, lasting immune response still proves to be a major challenge (Winter et al., 2023). Given all these twists, coming up with an effective malaria vaccine pushes researchers to think outside the box in dealing with the parasite's winding life cycle and crafty immune evasion. *Plasmodium falciparum*, the nastiest variant we face, can dodge our body's defenses thanks to its many antigenic disguises, which makes simple subunit vaccines fall short. That's why scientists are now altering with multi-stage, multi-antigen formulations, trying to get the immune system to recognize a broad slice of the parasite. These approaches show promise, but they can fade in strength over time, meaning we need better adjuvants and improved delivery methods to boost the immune kick. Interestingly, merging these vaccine efforts with existing chemopreventive strategies could offer a more robust defense, as relying on vaccines alone might not provide the quick, widespread coverage needed in high-risk areas (Winter et al., 2023).

On a somewhat different track, researchers are also digging into the idea of repurposing existing drugs for malaria prevention. This strategy comes with its own set of puzzles compared to vaccines. Investigating how these drugs behave in the body—looking at things like pharmacodynamics and pharmacokinetics—is crucial to ensure they reach key spots (like plasma or even lung tissues) at therapeutic levels. Although much of this work originally zeroed in on viral threats like SARS-CoV-2, the lessons learned are proving useful for malaria too. Understanding how well a drug becomes available in the body and how it interacts with its host is essential—whether we're dealing with tried-and-true antimalarial meds or new compounds that might one day ride along with vaccine programs.

These varied, overlapping approaches, when wedded together, seem set to shape a future where malaria prevention is smarter and more effective (Figure 13.9).

13.3.1. Historical Context of Malaria Vaccine Research

Malaria still stands as a tough public health issue that has steered vaccine research for many years. In the past, efforts mostly centered around using drugs to prevent infection and cutting down on mosquitoes, mainly because we didn't fully grasp the *Plasmodium* parasite's life cycle. Lately, breakthroughs in molecular biology and immunology have opened up fresh ways to attack the enemy, leading researchers to target the parasite at various stages. The old methods, although they did their part, ran into problems like drug resistance and shifting weather patterns that play havoc with transmission. For instance, climate changes have stretched out mosquito breeding seasons and broadened where the disease can spread, which just doesn't help (Jan et al., 2022). So, vaccines have come back into the spotlight as a promising partner for drug prevention, offering the hope of longer-lasting, more stable control against malaria's ever-changing threat. The journey of malaria vaccine research unfolds like a layered story, revealing an evolving grasp of the parasite's challenging biology and the hard work involved in building solid immunity. Early on, the focus was on stopping *Plasmodium falciparum* before it could take hold in the liver, but those first vaccine attempts didn't hold up under testing. That shortfall made it clear that the complex interplay between host and parasite calls for attacking the problem from multiple angles. Next, scientists tried to develop vaccines that work during the blood stage, aiming to lower parasite loads and ease the severity of the illness. Even with all the progress, a widely available, rock-solid vaccine has remained just out of reach, largely due to genetic differences among parasite strains and the many twists in our immune responses. At the same time, chemopreventive methods have kept moving forward. Take *Plasmodium vivax*, for example, preventing relapses here means dealing with challenging drugs like 8-aminoquinolines, which underscores the ongoing struggle to mix pharmaceutical strategies with immunological insight (Cindy et al., 2021). When you take a step back, the whole history of malaria vaccines reflects more than just scientific hurdles, it also mirrors global health priorities and funding shifts. Money and support have helped boost other tools, such as rapid tests and solid treatments, while vaccine work sometimes stumbled because of uneven funding and practical challenges. In most cases, however, the 21st century has seen real breakthroughs, like when RTS,S/AS01 (Mosquirix) earned its regulatory nod—a milestone that, generally speaking, turned decades of research into an actual intervention. Alongside these gains, there's been a growing recognition that environmental shifts and population movements are major players in how malaria spreads, making it clear that combining drug prevention and vaccines is key to the long haul (Cindy et al., 2021; Jan et al., 2022).

13.3.2. Key Milestones in Vaccine Development

Effective vaccines have been a game-changer in our battle against infectious diseases worldwide. Edward Jenner's work with smallpox back in the late 1700s showed that getting the body used to a weakened form of a virus could help it fight off the real thing without causing the full-blown illness. That early insight set off a chain reaction—vaccines for polio, measles, and so on began shaping public health. It's interesting how those breakthroughs not only slashed rates of sickness and death but also proved that creating a vaccine for every kind of microbe is no small task.

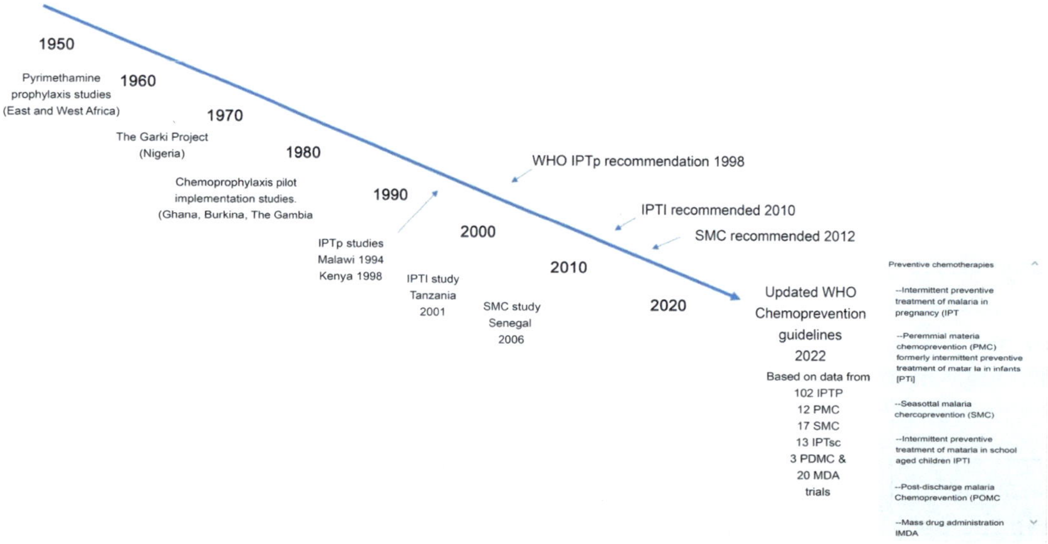

Figure 13.10. Key milestones in vaccine development.

Source: Greenwood B, Schellenberg D. Chemoprevention for the Populations of Malaria Endemic Africa. *Diseases*. 2022; 10(4):101. https://doi.org/10.3390/diseases10040101

Take malaria: the ever-shifting life cycle of *Plasmodium* parasites has made it especially challenging, so researchers had to bring in extra strategies like chemoprevention alongside vaccines (Kühl et al., 2025). Later on, in the second half of the 20th century, the whole field kind of transformed. Recombinant DNA techniques and new adjuvant formulas upped the game, letting scientists build subunit vaccines that zero in on specific antigens while cutting down on side effects. This more targeted approach was a big leap—though for malaria, the parasite's ability to dodge the immune system and its varied antigens meant an effective vaccine kept slipping away for years. Recently, however, the introduction of the RTS,S/AS01 vaccine for *Plasmodium falciparum* marked a real turning point. Sure, it only offers partial protection, yet it hints at what could happen when vaccination is paired with chemoprevention, working together to tackle transmission and disease burden (Kühl et al., 2025). Still, malaria remains an uphill struggle, with over 200 million cases each year and a heavy toll in sub-Saharan Africa. The WHO, for instance, now supports combined strategies like PDMC for those most at risk. Generally speaking, the journey of vaccine innovation—step by step—shows us that gradual, flexible gains are key. Merging PDMC with immunization efforts has even helped cut down on hospital readmissions and mortality in kids recovering from severe anemia. In short, the fight against malaria has shifted from a narrow, vaccine-only approach to a broader, more mixed strategy that combines chemoprevention, vaccination, and stronger healthcare systems, capturing the complex, ongoing progress in vaccine development (Kühl et al., 2025) (Figure 13.10).

13.3.3. Current Vaccines Available and Their Efficacy

Malaria vaccine research has come a long way—recently, the WHO even gave its nod to the RTS,S/AS01E shot for use in children. This decision, coming after roughly 30 years of heavy, ongoing study, speaks to our desperate need to tackle malaria, especially since the situation got a whole lot worse when COVID-19 shook things up. The vaccine, simply put, works by using a specific protein from *Plasmodium falciparum* (the circumsporozoite protein) to spark an immune response that steers clear of liver-stage infections. Its overall effectiveness is only moderate but has been boosted by trying new dosing strategies, like delaying or splitting doses and timing shots around the seasons. These alters seem to improve the quality of the immune reaction, such as, such as it as making antibodies stick better, without necessarily cranking up the numbers. Trials have shown that these new schedules, by increasing what scientists call antibody avidity, open up extra ways to use the vaccine effectively in malaria-prone areas (Thompson et al., 2022). Looking a bit closer, recent work hints at more public health wins when vaccination schedules are matched with local malaria seasons. Mathematical models based on phase three trial data generally suggest that vaccinating seasonally, rather than simply based on age, lowers malaria cases in kids more efficiently. Getting the vaccine in just before the worst of the transmission season tends to max out immunity right when children need it most. And there's a neat twist—pairing the seasonal RTS,S vaccination with well-known chemoprevention strategies (sulfadoxine-pyrimethamine plus amodiaquine, SP+AQ) seems to create a kind of synergy. Together, these interventions tend to beat each one on its own, cutting down on both regular and severe malaria episodes, particularly in regions where the disease tends to stick around longer (Thompson et al., 2022). It looks like mixing vaccine and drug strategies could shake up our battles with malaria. That said, the effectiveness of RTS,S isn't a one-size-fits-all story. Generally speaking, how well the vaccine does can depend on factors like local transmission rates, seasonal variations, and even how the rollout is handled locally. Models indicate that while adding RTS,S to chemoprevention plans usually brings big health gains, the actual benefits vary a lot based on the local epidemiology and the reach of existing health services. Plus, altering these vaccine efficacy models, with more immunological and field data—is key to making precise predictions and solid policies. These ongoing adjustments highlight how crucial it is to keep deployment strategies flexible so that they account for regional differences and let chemoprevention and vaccination work together in a balanced malaria control plan (Thompson et al., 2022).

13.4. Challenges in Vaccine Implementation

Even with the strides made in battling malaria, putting vaccines into play hasn't been all smooth sailing. In many areas of moderate to high malaria transmission, early breakthroughs have stalled—or even backed off—so while vaccines shine in controlled setups, they can lose steam when spread across different settings. Uptake is all over the place too; sometimes health systems aren't up to par, and cultural attitudes only add to the mix. Limited public awareness, a fair share of misinformation, and hurdles like keeping the cold chain intact only complicate things further. Plus, malaria's own challenging life cycle means vaccines must hit multiple parasite stages for broad protection. To summarize, combining vaccines with other strategies like chemoprevention and long-acting antimalarial drugs might be the only way to tackle these layered problems (Nambatya et al., 2025). Looking ahead, the success of malaria vaccine programs seems tightly complex with the strength and readiness of local health networks. Malawi's work with post-discharge malaria chemoprevention, for instance, shows that new methods need to gel with what's already in place. Generally speaking, even though many supporters are on board with adopting vaccines, they point out that solid policies, reliable supply lines, and consistent monitoring systems are crucial. Issues like lagging policy updates, clunky approval processes, and weak follow-up capacities can impact large-scale vaccine delivery. Health worker training and genuine community involvement also weigh in heavily, suggesting that scientific innovation alone won't cut it without a robust health system to back it up (Ndambo et al., 2025).

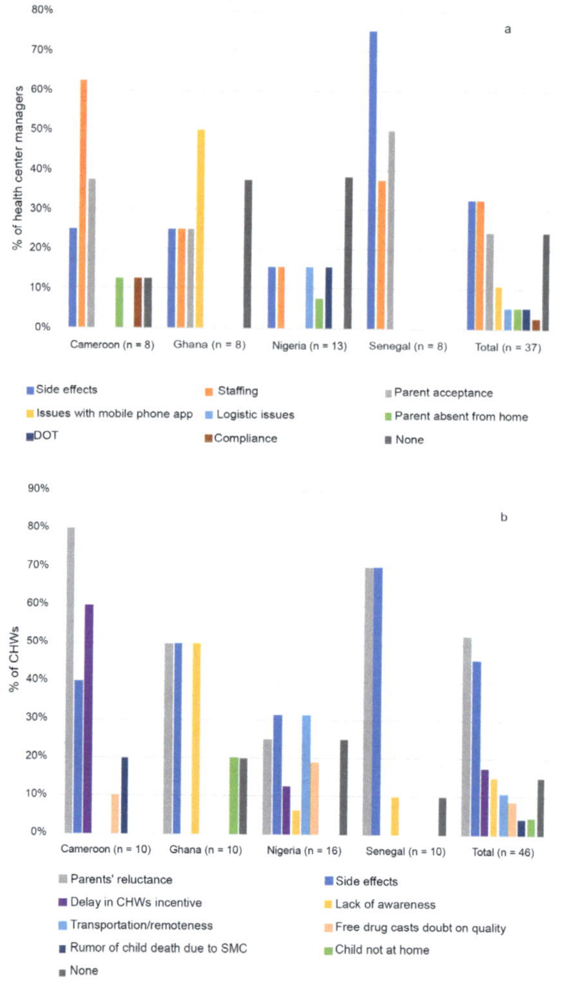

Figure 13.11. Challenges in malaria vaccine implementation.

Source: Audibert C, Tchouatieu A-M. Perception of Malaria Chemoprevention Interventions in Infants and Children in Eight Sub-Saharan African Countries: An End User Perspective Study. *Tropical Medicine and Infectious Disease.* 2021; 6(2):75. https://doi.org/10.3390/tropicalmed6020075

Then there's the challenge of fairness and funding, which keeps rearing its head when trying to scale up vaccines and chemoprevention. Regions hit hardest by malaria almost always have the poorest healthcare setups and scant resources, deepening access gaps. Factors like drug resistance and surprise stock-outs further shake community trust. Ensuring steady funding for vaccine purchases, distribution, and boosting health services is critical, even if it often has to compete with other priorities. Plus, targeting vulnerable groups, especially kids under five, calls for approaches that appreciate cultural, geographic, and economic nuances. Without tackling these issues head-on, the promise of vaccines and chemoprevention may not fully come through, and the cycle of malaria harm might continue accordingly. In most cases, future strategies will need to balance cost-effectiveness, community engagement, and fresh, innovative measures to clear these hurdles (Nambatya et al., 2025) (Figure 13.11).

13.4.1. Logistical Issues in Vaccine Distribution

Malaria control depends on getting preventative measures into people's hands, but day-to-day hurdles keep slowing down vaccine delivery. In many areas hit hard by seasonal malaria, the trick is to time the shots just before the worst part hits, this method tends to work better than simply vaccinating based on age. Getting the schedule right demands a dependable system and plenty of resources, which, let's be honest, are often scarce where they're needed most. Then there's the RTS,S vaccine that requires several doses, meaning kids under five must return to healthcare spots repeatedly—a process that only adds to the complications.

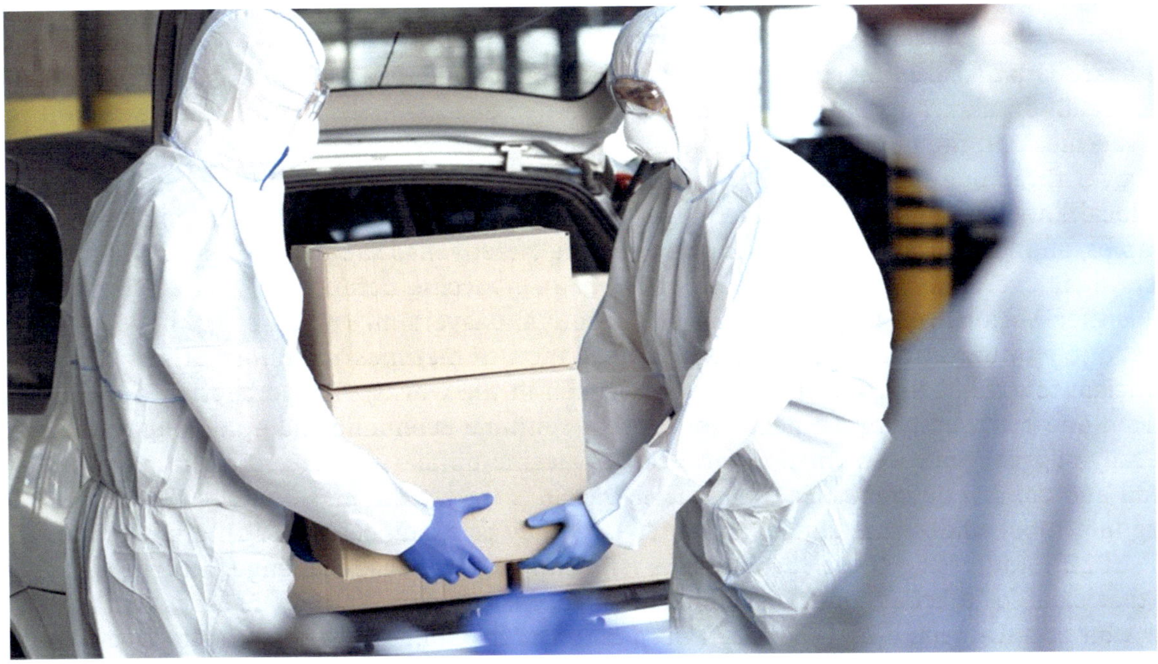

Figure 13.12. Logistical issues in vaccine distribution.

Source: Maersk. (2021). *Global Distribution of Vaccines.*

Issues like keeping the vaccines cold, moving them around safely, and not having enough trained staff all stack up, reducing both the reach and regularity of the shots. Some models even show that pairing seasonal vaccines with chemoprevention can highlight the importance of getting the logistics right (Thompson et al., 2022). When it comes to chemoprevention, the challenges are no less real. Take PDMC: kids recovering from severe anemia need to get full antimalarial treatment courses, which depends a lot on caregivers sticking with the plan and a steady stream of drugs. Many factors, like family income and past infection rates, often makes this adherence unpredictable and harder to manage. In some instances, community-based models that hand treatment directly to caregivers at discharge help cut down on travel and extra clinic visits. This not only tends to boost adherence but also lowers costs when compared to traditional facility-based methods, showing just how crucial adaptable logistics are for local needs. In most cases, PDMC can only work well if these bumps in distribution and adherence are smoothed out (Kühl et al., 2025). Cost studies also tell a similar story: the economic success of malaria prevention rides on how efficient the delivery network is. Analyses comparing community-run PDMC programs with those run-in clinics consistently show that community delivery is more cost-effective, hinting at decentralization as a smart move for regions battling malaria. That said, persisting uncertainties about adherence levels and varying impacts on mortality still complicate decisions on funding and policy. Generally speaking, while further research might help refine these estimates, it may not be worth the extra expense based on current data. Ultimately, it seems that improving existing logistics—by boosting infrastructure, better educating caregivers, and fine-tuning delivery methods—is the way to make long-lasting progress against malaria (Kühl et al., 2025) (Figure 13.12).

13.4.2. Public Perception and Acceptance of Vaccines

Healthcare trust makes or breaks efforts to curb infectious diseases. In areas where malaria is widespread, breakthroughs in the lab don't guarantee success unless communities are on board with vaccines and chemoprevention. Take Burkina Faso—people there seem to know their malaria stuff; over three out of four don't hesitate and head right to a health facility when symptoms hit. This local know-how kind of sets the stage for adopting newer strategies like multiple first-line therapies, and, frankly, the way individuals view the effectiveness and ease of getting antimalarials affects their overall acceptance (Kaboré et al., 2024). Vaccine acceptance isn't a straightforward story either. Various cultural, social, and even economic layers mix together to shape how people feel about immunization, often leading to hesitancy. Sometimes misinformation, or even just skepticism toward health officials, throws a wrench in the works; risk perception can also vary a lot from one community to the next. Models that combine economic and epidemiological insights generally suggest that even small differences in vaccine uptake can have a big impact on disease spread and control outcomes. So, for malaria vaccines to hit the mark, public health plans need to dig into those underlying doubts and alter how they communicate with different groups (Mesa et al., 2022). Addressing these vaccine fears isn't simply a medical challenge, it turns into a social one that calls for a broad, multidisciplinary approach. Looking at other diseases, we notice that even a bit of anti-vaccine sentiment can keep an outbreak simmering despite effective treatments being available. With malaria, where we're pushing forward with innovative prevention and vaccine methods, it becomes crucial to engage the public openly and clearly. Efforts to build confidence, even if it means accepting a few minor missteps in communication or punctuation here and there, are key to overcoming persisting doubts. Merging solid epidemiological data with an understanding of how people think and feel will help ensure that both chemoprevention and vaccinations lead to a real drop in malaria cases (Mesa et al., 2022) (Figure 13.13).

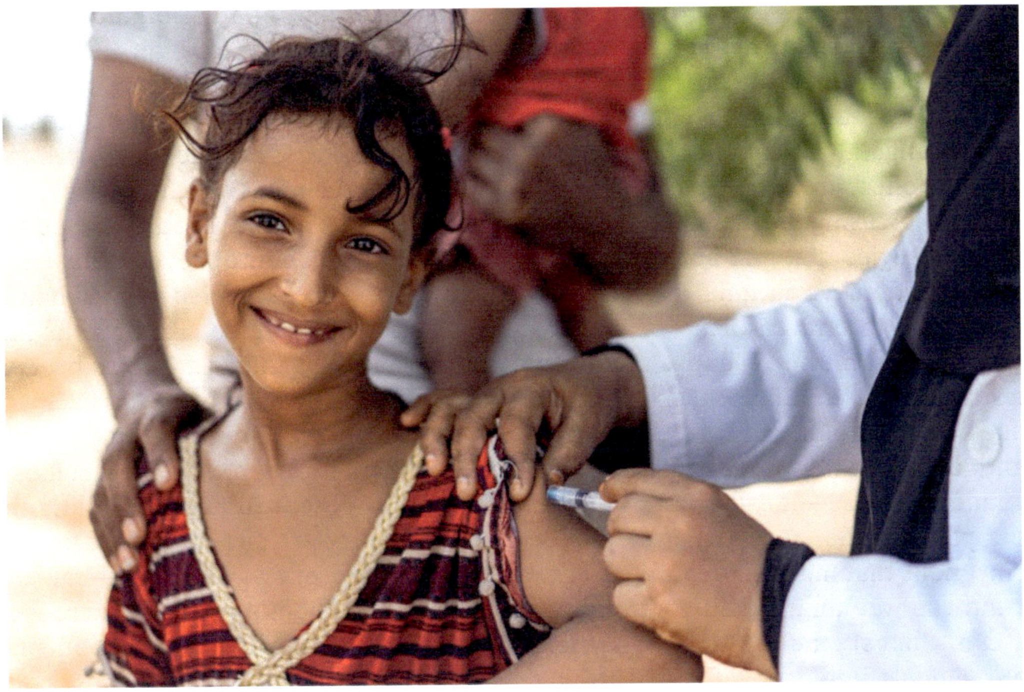

Figure 13.13. The public perception and acceptance of vaccines.

Source: UNICEF. (n.d.). *Public Acceptance of Vaccines.*

13.4.3. Variability in Malaria Strains and Vaccine Effectiveness

Malaria isn't easy to beat, it's not just that the disease simply hangs around, but the parasite itself shows off an incredible knack for changing. The *Plasmodium* species, with its diverse genetic makeup, makes it challenging to pin down a one-size-fits-all solution. Different malaria strains flaunt various antigen profiles, which messes with how our immune systems recognize them, in most cases lowering how well vaccines perform. Take RTS,S, for example; it targets one particular protein in *P. falciparum*, yet that protein can shift from one parasite population to the next, meaning that in some regions the vaccine does its job better than in others. Because the strains are always on the move, continuous molecular checking is needed to fine-tune vaccine designs and decide when and where they should be used. Plus, the way our body's defenses mix with this parasite diversity makes for a complex, if you will, picture—one that can affect both the strength and the reach of the protection vaccines are supposed to confer (Burgert et al., 2020). Lately, with the rollout of RTS,S and other advances, it's become clear that dealing with malaria means juggling strain variability along with other factors like seasonal changes and how fast the disease spreads. There's evidence suggesting that when vaccine schedules are altered to line up with seasonal transmission peaks, the immune protection syncs better with when people are most at risk. Some immunological studies even hint that fine-tuning the quality of antibodies—rather than just their number—could be the real game-changer in outsmarting the many parasite variants. And, mixing up vaccination efforts with drug-based preventive measures, like SP+AQ regimens, has shown some pretty neat, combined effects that might help counterbalance the varied ways in which different strains react. Mathematical models, which factor in all these complexities, end up painting a more realistic picture of how vaccine-driven immunity meshes with different malaria profiles; this insight then guides more tailored public health interventions in areas steeped in malaria challenges (Thompson et al., 2022). The ongoing association of strain variability and its effect on vaccine performance underscores the pressing need for adaptable public health strategies that mix both vaccines and chemoprevention. Variations in parasite genetics often lead to uneven drug resistance and unexpected immune escapes, which complicates the idea of a universal fix. In this light, vaccine designs should consider the broad range of antigens and aim to boost the quality of the immune response—ideally by targeting parts of the parasite that rarely change. Also, using vaccine plans that match the local pattern of strains and the way an affected community responds can boost the overall benefits. Keeping our models updated with this strain heterogeneity allows for more accurate forecasts on how different interventions might play out, and in turn, helps decision-makers hand out resources in the most effective way possible. At the end of the day, embracing the complex complexity of malaria's ever-changing strains is pretty much key to setting up long-term successes when combining chemoprevention with vaccination strategies (Burgert et al., 2020; Thompson et al., 2022).

13.5. Role of Chemoprevention in Vaccine Strategy

Malaria control is now at a kind of crossroads—recent progress in lessening the disease's impact has nearly stalled. Traditional methods, though they've helped a lot over the years, run into issues like insecticide and drug resistance that could undo long-earned gains. Combining drugs that prevent malaria with vaccines now seems like a promising fix. Some individuals have been using math and population models, which look at things like how long an intervention lasts, its effectiveness, and how it's rolled out—to figure out how best to mix these tools. In many cases, these models help pinpoint which features vaccines and chemopreventive drugs need to move the needle for public health. Essentially, chemoprevention isn't just a standalone fix— it also works hand in hand with vaccines to create a more lasting, robust impact against malaria (Nekkab et al., 2023). Some simulation studies even back up the idea that joining forces with chemopreventive drugs and vaccination pays off. Vaccines on their own do a decent job at controlling illness, but their ability to cut transmission, especially among different age groups—can be limited. Meanwhile, chemoprevention zeroes in directly on the parasite during its blood phase, so it helps cut down the number of infections. When these two measures are rolled out together, they often seem to do more than simply add up; they create a kind of synergy that brings about a marked drop in malaria cases. This combo not only delays the disease's rebound but also lengthens the period with low transmission after campaigns. In many cases, this means fewer mass rounds of intervention are needed, which is a clear operational win for an integrated chemoprevention-vaccine strategy (Camponovo et al., 2019). Looking ahead, the benefit of weaving chemoprevention into vaccine plans isn't limited to an immediate dip in cases. By delaying transmission's return once interventions wind down, the combined effect of chemoprevention and vaccines tends to break the malaria cycle more effectively than when either is used alone. This partnership is especially important in specific hotspots where keeping parasite levels low is crucial for long-term elimination. Moreover, mixing these approaches allows for more flexible public health responses—teams can focus on those residual pockets of transmission with both drug and vaccine measures, guided by real-world model insights. Such targeted strategies help balance resources against achieving the biggest health impact possible. Ultimately, chemoprevention boosts the vaccine effect not merely through an extra layer of protection, but also by leading to more durable, long-term drops in malaria spread, underscoring its essential role in today's malaria control paradigms (Camponovo et al., 2019; Nekkab et al., 2023) (Figure 13.14).

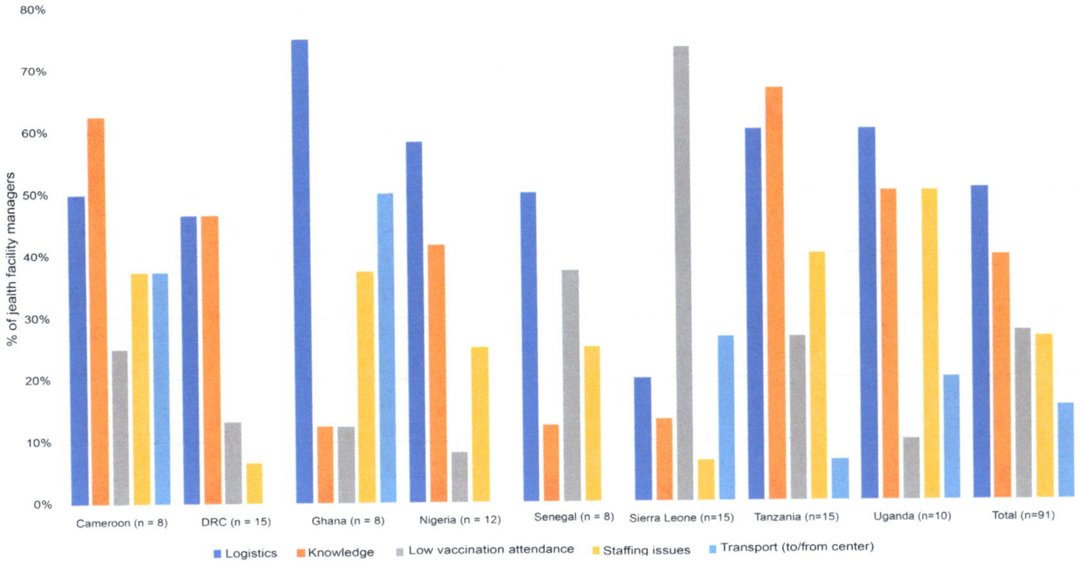

Figure 13.14. Role of chemoprevention in vaccine strategy.

Source: Audibert C, Tchouatieu A-M. Perception of Malaria Chemoprevention Interventions in Infants and Children in Eight Sub-Saharan African Countries: An End User Perspective Study. *Tropical Medicine and Infectious Disease*. 2021; 6(2):75. https://doi.org/10.3390/tropicalmed6020075

13.5.1. Complementary Use of Chemoprevention and Vaccination

Malaria control isn't solved by a single fix, it usually takes mixing several ideas together. Pregnant women, for example, often face extra danger since parasites love to gather in the placenta, which can cause anemia, low birth weight, and even higher risks for both mom and baby. Using preventative medicine, like chemoprevention, offers a quick chemical shield during those risky times. At the same time, vaccines help build longer-lasting defenses. Pairing these two approaches creates a kind of glue that covers both immediate and future threats, since neither tactic works as well on its own (Bauserman et al., 2019). Seasonal shifts in malaria transmission throw an extra wrench in efforts, making the timing of treatments a real challenge. Research generally shows that a vaccine's protection can fade, so shots often need to be given just before peak infection periods. Meanwhile, chemopreventive treatments can be timed to set in right when the risk is highest, providing prompt, direct action while the vaccine's benefits slowly build. This overlap isn't always neat, but it tends to cut down the number of clinical malarias cases and helps manage those sharp seasonal spikes (Han et al., 2017). Mixing chemoprevention with vaccination in a full-blown malaria control plan seems to offer a better path forward for public health. Vaccines get the immune system roused, while direct parasite blockers add another layer of defense, and together they build a stronger barrier than either one alone. This combined strategy can be tuned for different groups—infants, children, and others might need their own adjustments based on local climate and exposure patterns. As global health agencies look to expand vaccine programs, they're also weaving in chemopreventive strategies to shore up protection. Ongoing research remains key, helping to fine-tune these dual methods for cost, resistance, and long-term impact, all aimed at easing the brutal toll of malaria (Bauserman et al., 2019; Han et al., 2017) (Figure 13.15).

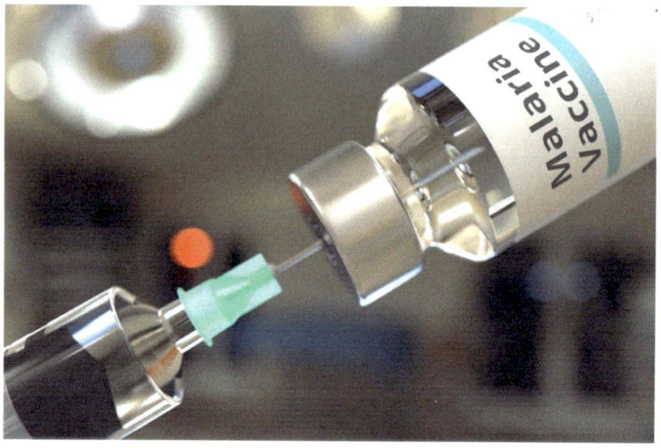

Figure 13.15. Complementary use of chemoprevention and vaccination for malaria.

Source: Gavi. (2021). *Chemoprevention and Vaccination for Malaria.*

13.5.2. Case Studies Demonstrating Combined Approaches

Recent work on malaria control now leans toward mixing vaccines with chemoprevention—a shift that's especially relevant in areas where transmission shows seasonal spikes. Take the RTS,S/AS01E vaccine, for example. It's widely seen as a breakthrough, thanks to a lot of research testing various immunization timings. One study even dug into using delayed, smaller doses paired with vaccination aimed at the season, showing that it wasn't just about more antibodies but rather the quality of those antibodies that boosted the vaccine's performance. Updated survival analysis of the drug combo sulfadoxine-pyrimethamine plus amodiaquine (SP+AQ) has also underlined its effectiveness for SMC. Researchers, by running math-based transmission models, simulated what happens when these two measures are combined, hinting at a kind of synergy that makes SP+AQ even more protective when given with RTS,S (Thompson et al., 2022). Altogether, this mix of immunological ideas and real-world data drives home how combining these strategies can fight malaria more effectively. Building on those early insights, later studies have looked at long-term, community-wide impacts of different RTS,S vaccination schedules in regions hit by seasonal malaria. Using individual-based transmission models (backed up by clinical data from Mali and Burkina Faso), researchers compared age-based vaccination plans with those timed to the season. Generally speaking, for a 15-year period, the seasonal approach produced a noticeably larger drop in clinical cases and deaths than sticking with age guidelines alone. When monthly chemoprevention through SMC with SP+AQ is added during the transmission peak, the double intervention cuts down the malaria burden in kids under five. Interestingly, the extra edge provided by RTS,S appeared to shift depending on how long the malaria season lasted and on local factors (Thompson et al., 2022); a reminder that context matters in public health decisions. This body of evidence, in most cases, supports the idea of lining up vaccine schedules and chemoprevention for the best community health outcome. These case studies drive home a clear point: malaria interventions have to fit local transmission patterns to be truly effective. In areas with long or intense malaria seasons, combining RTS,S vaccination with seasonal chemoprevention works kind of like a two-layer defense—both lowering the risk of infection and keeping immunity steady during the worst times. Models also suggest that decision-makers need to factor in regional differences, such as existing intervention coverage and realistic vaccine uptake, when planning these combined efforts. As has been shown, the teamwork between vaccination and chemoprevention not only enhances protection on an individual level, but it also shows promise as a major public health tool to cut down malaria cases and deaths considerably. Ongoing evaluations using both modeling and field trials will remain key to altering and perfecting these strategies (Thompson et al., 2022) (Figure 13.16).

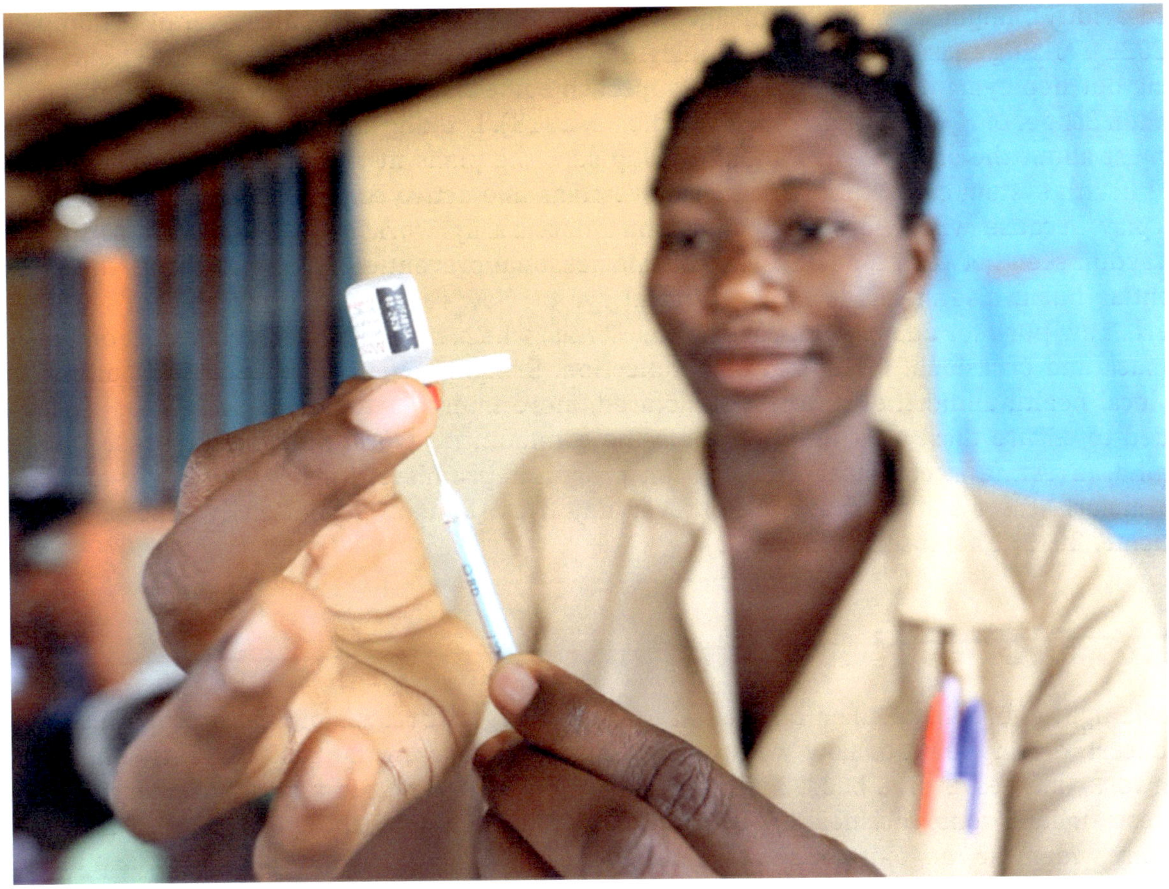

Figure 13.16. The case studies demonstrating combined approaches.

Source: WHO. (n.d.). *Case Studies on Malaria Vaccine Implementation.*

13.5.3. Future Directions for Integrated Strategies

Decades of work have pushed the fight against malaria into a new era – one where combining vaccines with regular doses of preventive drugs is starting to take center stage. Researchers have been altering with the timing and delivery of these measures, trying to match them up with the wily, seasonal peaks of malaria transmission. In many cases, tailoring vaccine schedules with rounds of chemopreventive treatments seems like a smart, if sometimes complex, way to handle the disease's ever-changing face; in other words, making sure that each region's unique malaria profile is reflected in how these tools are used. A fresh idea involving delayed-fractional vaccination paired with seasonal chemoprevention looks especially promising (Thompson et al., 2022) – it might even cut malaria cases down while stretching already thin health resources (London School of Hygiene and Tropical Medicine, 2013). Some researchers are also deep into refining the models that help map out these strategies. Mathematical and immuno-epidemiological models, for instance, aren't just abstract exercises – they let us simulate different vaccine dosing and drug schedules to see what works best for areas with unpredictable transmission patterns. In most cases, these models even give us clues about how the immune system gets a little extra kick; for example, findings suggest that antibody quality, that is, how strongly they bind (a measure sometimes called avidity), might be more important than just having more antibodies overall (Thompson et al., 2022). Mixing these immunological insights with broader epidemiological data helps in fine-tuning our deployment plans, even if the approach sometimes feels a bit rough around the edges (London School of Hygiene and Tropical Medicine, 2013). Looking ahead, defending against malaria isn't just about the science – it's about making sure the plans fit the people and places involved. Local health system capacities, realistic rollout plans and active community involvement all come into play because what works on paper won't necessarily work in resource-poor settings. The interaction seen between the RTS,S vaccine and seasonal prevention strategies points to some real potential, but it also means keeping a careful eye on how resources are used. That's why many experts now push for adaptive management systems, which can shift strategies based on real-time feedback and occasional hiccups in data collection. Bringing together researchers, policymakers, and local health authorities in a less structured, more improvisational way might be just what's needed to ensure these breakthroughs help the communities worst hit by the disease. With that in mind, investing in combined intervention programs promises a meaningful, long-term dip in both malaria cases and its heavy toll on everyday lives (London School of Hygiene and Tropical Medicine, 2013; Thompson et al., 2022).

13.6. Global Health Initiatives

Malaria fight efforts have taken off around the globe largely because of health programs working in concert, driving forward new ways to prevent the disease. In the past 10 years, international teamwork, and yes, even a boost in funding—has sparked growth in a range of malaria products like tests, medications, vaccines, and even methods to control mosquito populations. These strides not only widen the range of options for field workers, but generally speaking, they also add hope for eliminating and later eradicating malaria altogether. Quick spread of these innovations is key, making sure that breakthroughs in chemoprevention and vaccine science can reliably reach at-risk communities. Of course, if political or financial support wanes, progress might stall, which underlines the need for ongoing global cooperation (Hemingway et al., 2016). Alongside developing new products, many global health efforts are now giving extra attention to better monitoring and handling of data. With improved data collection and faster response setups, health agencies can adjust their strategies to match local disease trends and sort out resource allocation more sensibly. This mix of approaches, even pairing chemopreventive methods with vaccines—offers a more rounded and flexible shield against malaria's spread. In most cases, continual investment in research, reinforced by worldwide partnerships, keeps an environment where next-generation solutions are frequently tried out and fine-tuned. The whole balancing act of vigilant data tracking coupled with modern technology seems to mark a clear move from merely treating malaria to actively staving it off (Hemingway et al., 2016). Closer examination of annual reports from leading research institutions also reveals a broader picture of these global initiatives. They often don't just trumpet scientific breakthroughs; they also point out the administrative and financial supports that are vital for long-term success. You can see interdisciplinary achievements and cross-faculty collaborations—basics of science, clinical progress, and public policy all wedded together in these documents. Investments in both novel chemopreventive compounds and emerging vaccine candidates not only reflect a unified approach to disease management but also rely on solid institutional backing. In essence, the interplay between scientific creativity and structured support clearly sketches out the overall landscape of global initiatives aimed at controlling malaria (Figure 13.17).

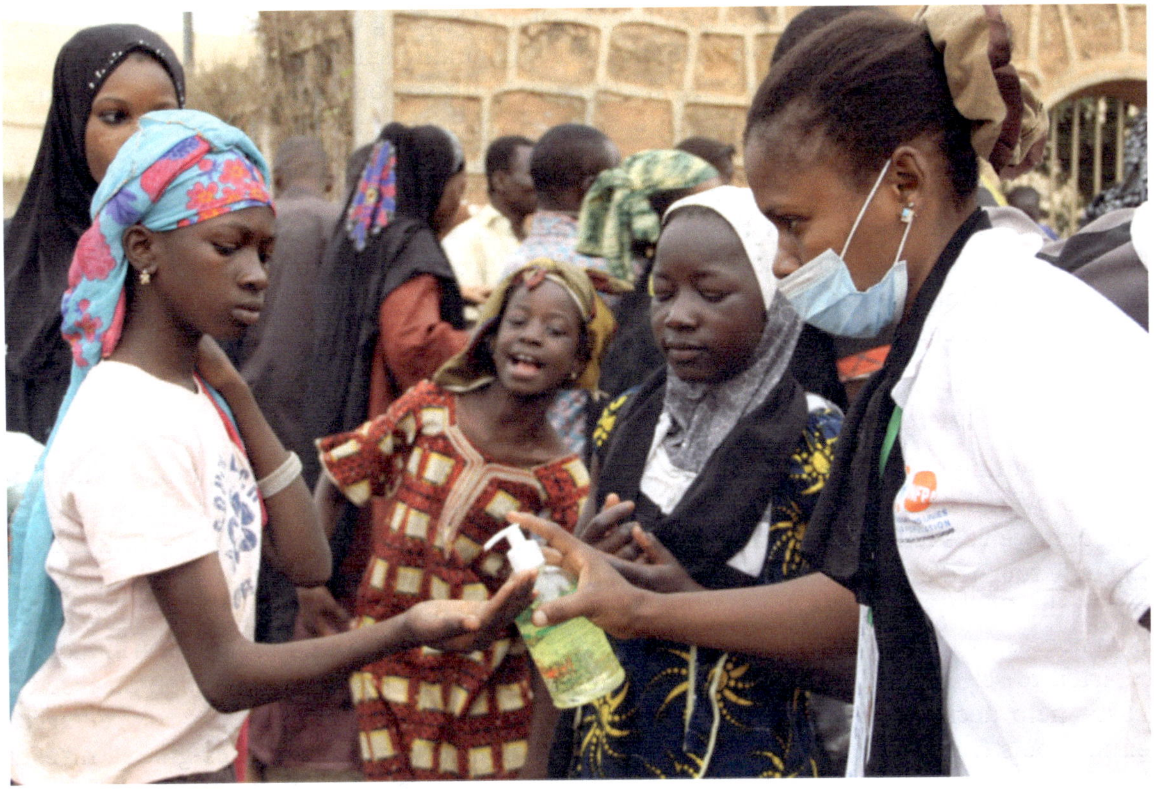

Figure 13.17. Global health initiatives.

Source: The Borgen Project. (n.d.). *Global Health Initiatives.*

13.6.1. Organizations Involved in Malaria Prevention

Malaria prevention isn't a simple challenge. A number of groups now get involved, each testing a different route, from developing vaccines to using chemoprevention. International agencies mix it up with local governments, often working in ways that fit the region's unique disease patterns rather than following a strict formula. For example, in northern Nigeria community-led seasonal malaria chemoprevention projects emerged after local research helped decide on the best delivery methods. Trusted community health workers and local leaders play a central role here by boosting drug use and keeping people on track with treatments. These efforts, in most cases, help bridge gaps in health services and nudge past cultural hurdles that might otherwise limit chemoprevention's appeal (Strachan et al., 2016). Organizations also tend to adjust their programs continuously using ongoing qualitative feedback to maximize impact. Support for malaria prevention reaches beyond just handing out treatments; it involves keeping an eye on future hurdles like drug resistance. In Burkina Faso, studies led by health ministries and their partners have looked into the feasibility of using multiple first-line therapies (MFT) to better manage uncomplicated malaria. Generally speaking, the idea is to slow the rise of artemisinin resistance by mixing up the antimalarial drugs—an approach backed by rounds of feedback from both stakeholders and patients. Those involved stress the importance of accessibility and efficient treatment management, including steady drug supplies and proper stock control, which are key to sustainable malaria control programs (Kaboré et al., 2024). This mix of careful monitoring and ready adaptation highlights a genuinely proactive stance toward keeping chemoprevention effective. Global and regional partnerships also boost the impact of malaria vaccines and preventive measures by joining scientific know-how with practical delivery methods. Major players like the WHO, along with various NGOs, team up with national health systems to shape policies and decide on resource distribution. Their role is crucial when addressing issues like how people seek care and intrinsic weaknesses in the health system. These collaborations naturally tackle challenges such as cultural acceptance and the need to explain treatment benefits, often in ways that feel grounded and relatable. By weaving together local insights with international expertise, these groups ensure that innovative methods like seasonal chemoprevention and multi-therapy approaches remain both scientifically sound and well-suited to local needs (Strachan et al., 2016; Kaboré et al., 2024).

13.6.2. Funding and Resource Allocation for Malaria Control

Progress in fighting malaria depends on having steady funding and spending money smartly, but the world's overall financial picture still leaves important gaps that could roll back recent gains. Even though we've seen malaria cases drop, the money coming in has stalled – in 2020, global funding only touched about 3.3 billion USD, which is way short of the roughly 6.8 billion USD target laid out in the Global Technical Strategy for malaria elimination. This lack of funds puts a serious strain on necessary measures like chemoprevention and vaccine rollout. Researchers, in most cases, have started to rely on optimization models that, by using locally gathered data on disease trends and costs, help decision-makers zone in on high-risk populations and work on fairer access to prevention tools (Ngwafor et al., 2024). Generally speaking, a careful, evidence-guided investment strategy is essential if we want to keep the momentum and push chemoprevention efforts further. New methods in chemoprevention also remind us that it's not just about spending money – it's about spending it in ways that count in regions where malaria is a constant worry. Take PDMC for instance. This approach gives oral antimalarial treatments to kids recovering from severe anemia, and studies have shown it can markedly cut down death rates and hospital readmissions. Some economic evaluations, comparing community-based PDMC with more institution-centered programs in sub-Saharan Africa, indicate that using local community channels is more cost-effective – offering not only better adherence but also slashing program costs. Essentially, these findings push us to invest in community-oriented interventions that boost access and ensure treatments are completed, which in turn leads to better health outcomes while making the most of limited funds. In many cases, these cost–benefit insights naturally feed into strategies that make sure chemoprevention stays in tune with the local infrastructural and social setups (Kühl et al., 2025). Still, things aren't completely cut and dried. There are persisting doubts about how reliably caregivers stick to treatment routines and exactly how much mortality falls when chemoprevention is used—a complexity that clouds funding decisions even further. Although factors influencing adherence are often complex and vary widely by context, modeling generally keeps pointing to community-based PDMC as the top cost-effective move, even if adherence takes a bit of a hit when simulated. It turns out that performing a "value of information" analysis can clarify these uncertainties—pinpointing exactly how much treatment adherence and mortality rates change, but diving deep into further research might not be the best bet given what we already know. In short, while it's important to keep backing implementation and adherence support, we must also balance that with smart research investments. Ultimately, aligning targeted funding with thorough economic and epidemiological modeling appears to be the best way forward for sustaining chemoprevention and vaccine programs, especially when budgets are tight (Ngwafor et al., 2024; Kühl et al., 2025) (Figure 13.18).

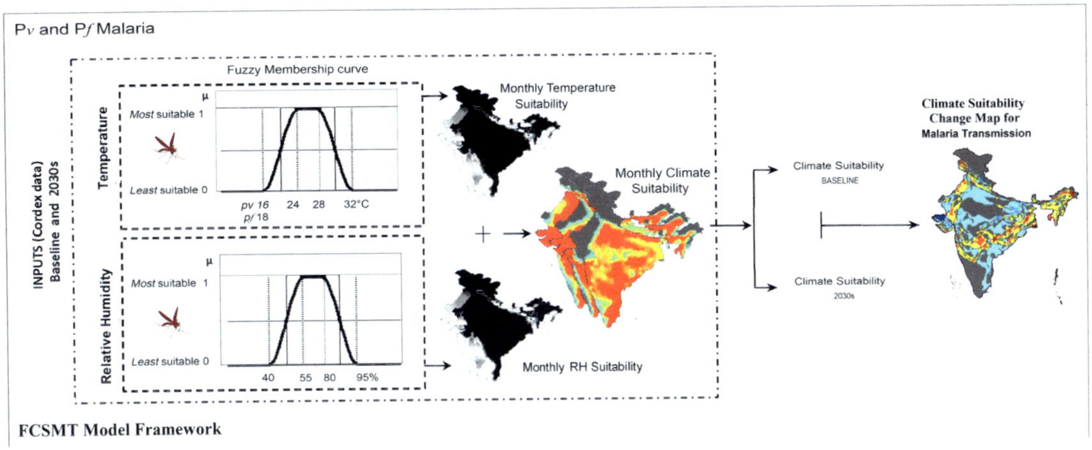

Figure 13.18. Funding and resource allocation for malaria control.

Source: Sarkar S, Gangare V, Singh P, Dhiman RC. Shift in Potential Malaria Transmission Areas in India, Using the Fuzzy-Based Climate Suitability Malaria Transmission (FCSMT) Model under Changing Climatic Conditions. *International Journal of Environmental Research and Public Health.* 2019; 16(18):3474. https://doi.org/10.3390/ijerph16183474

13.6.3. Collaborative Efforts Between Countries and Institutions

Malaria controls these days depends on many efforts that link countries and institutions in ways that aren't always straightforward. The virus's complex nature means that no single group can handle it alone, so experts often mix chemoprevention with vaccine trials—an approach that, generally speaking, speeds up progress towards cutting down cases. International bodies, research centers, and governments sometimes casually overlap their efforts by designing, testing, and eventually rolling out vaccines, all while dealing with both lab puzzles and day-to-day obstacles. Different strengths from various regions get thrown together in unexpected ways, with vaccine studies happening in areas where the disease is rampant and preventive treatments getting out at the same time. This kind of combined approach, which looks at both immune responses and well-tested drug plans, is seen as key, especially in places like sub-Saharan Africa where malaria still looms large (David et al., 2024). Community involvement plays a big role too, it's the bridge between high-level science and everyday action. It isn't only about picking the right vaccine or the perfect drug regimen; local leaders, healthcare workers, and community groups are repeatedly recognized for making a difference. In most cases, chemoprevention and vaccine programs thrive when locals take part, lending their trust and hands-on knowledge to the project. Research repeatedly reminds us that when local voices are heard, vaccination efforts and the uptake of preventive medicine become more effective. These joint initiatives not only alter health services to better suit local needs, but they also help manage the environment in smart, community-friendly ways (Awasthi et al., 2024).

Sustained partnerships among countries and institutions add another layer to this collaborative mix by pooling the funds and know-how needed for broader vaccine and drug distribution. Coordinated funding, often, admittedly, a bit complex at times—avoids too much duplication and helps ensure that resources are shared fairly with underserved populations. In many cases, working together across sectors even sparks innovations in supply chain strategies, data sharing, and monitoring systems that guide policy shifts along the way. Efforts that cross national borders bolster surveillance, especially where malaria doesn't respect boundaries and drug resistance starts showing up. To summarize, this broad cooperation doesn't just boost scientific progress; it builds a tougher, more resilient health system that can keep malaria in check for the long haul (Awasthi et al., 2024; David et al., 2024).

CLOSER LOOK

SEASONAL MALARIA CHEMOPREVENTION (SMC)

SMC is a public health strategy designed to prevent malaria in children living in regions where malaria transmission is highly seasonal, typically in the Sahel region of sub-Saharan Africa. This preventive approach involves administering full treatment courses of antimalarial drugs at regular intervals during the peak malaria transmission season, regardless of whether the child is infected at the time. SMC is endorsed by the WHO as an effective and cost-efficient method of reducing malaria-related illness and death among young children.

SMC is particularly effective in areas where malaria transmission is concentrated within a few months of the year, usually during or just after the rainy season when mosquito populations surge. In such settings, the disease burden among children under five years of age is especially high. Since these children have not yet developed sufficient immunity to malaria, they are most vulnerable to severe illness and death.

The primary goal of SMC is to maintain therapeutic concentrations of antimalarial drugs in the blood during the period of greatest risk, thereby preventing infection or halting the progression of disease in its early stages. The strategy has been shown to significantly reduce both clinical episodes of malaria and severe outcomes, including hospital admissions and mortality.

The standard drug regimen for SMC consists of sulfadoxine-pyrimethamine (SP) and amodiaquine (AQ). This combination is administered once a month for up to four months, depending on the length of the transmission season. The treatment is usually given over three consecutive days: one dose of SP on the first day, and a dose of AQ on each of the three days.

These drugs are chosen for their safety profile, long half-lives, and effectiveness in preventing malaria infection. However, the development of drug resistance is a concern, which is why SMC is typically limited to regions where SP and AQ remain effective.

SMC is usually delivered through community-based programs, often led by community health workers who go door-to-door administering the drugs. This approach ensures high coverage and adherence, particularly in rural and hard-to-reach areas. Parental involvement and community engagement are also critical components of successful implementation.

Since its introduction, SMC has been widely scaled up in West and Central Africa, protecting millions of children each year. It is estimated that SMC can reduce malaria cases in children by about 75% during the transmission season.

Despite its success, SMC faces several challenges. These include logistical difficulties in reaching remote areas, ensuring adherence to the multi-day regimen, and managing the risk of increasing drug resistance. Moreover, SMC does not replace other malaria control measures such as ITNs or indoor residual spraying (IRS); rather, it complements them.

Future strategies may involve expanding SMC to older children or integrating it with other health services such as nutrition or vaccination programs. Research is also ongoing to explore alternative drugs for use in areas with resistance to SP or AQ.

SUMMARY

Malaria control keeps changing, and it shows that tackling the disease means mixing strategies without sticking to a single playbook. The RTS,S/AS01E vaccine, for example, marks a real turning point after years of work mixing what we know about the immune system with how the disease spreads. With this new tool in hand, experts are trying out different immunization plans – sometimes delaying smaller doses or timing shots by season – which, rather unexpectedly, seem to boost protection beyond our first guesses. Mixing preventive medicines with the vaccine brings a kind of synergy that hints at more enduring, overall control. It turns out the focus isn't solely on having more antibodies, but on improving their quality while matching treatment timing with local spread patterns. In most cases, fine-tuning both vaccine methods and drug prevention strategies will be key to staying ahead of malaria, especially with global challenges shaking things up (Thompson et al., 2022). Even with these clear advances, malaria stubbornly stays on the list of tough public health problems, particularly for kids bouncing back from severe anemia. PDMC – where treatment is given during a critical recovery window , has slashed death rates and readmissions, yet rolling this out isn't without hurdles. Issues like whether caregivers consistently follow the guidelines and how best to deliver the treatment make things messier than they first appear. Some studies suggest that community-based PDMC not only keeps costs low but also helps with sticking to the treatment, unlike when it's managed solely in a hospital. Interestingly, economic and social factors sometimes mix in unpredictable ways, affecting how well people adhere to the regimen. All this points to the importance of mixing social insights with clinical strategies when refining these prevention programs. Practically speaking, especially in sub-Saharan Africa, such approaches could prove instrumental in tackling both the immediate and lasting impacts of malaria (Kühl et al., 2025). Bringing together vaccine breakthroughs with drug-based prevention creates a broad strategy against malaria, even though a few uncertainties still need clear answers through more studies and policy modifications. Vaccines like RTS,S lay the groundwork for reducing infections, but getting the best results means understanding just how effective they are in different settings and how they work hand-in-hand with other preventive measures. At the same time, data-driven economic evaluations remind us that smart choices about delivery and boosting adherence are crucial – costs have to be balanced with improving health outcomes. The modest yet important gains seen in lowering death rates and raising adherence make it clear that targeted studies, which also consider economic realities, are needed to fully iron out these issues. Ultimately, integrating vaccine use with well-thought-out chemoprevention strategies – informed by both cost-effectiveness and human behavior – offers a hopeful route to reducing malaria cases and fatalities. Policymakers, therefore, must lean on adaptable, evidence-based plans that mirror local transmission patterns and available resources if we're to keep up these hard-won benefits (Thompson et al., 2022; Kühl et al., 2025).

New strides in fighting malaria have put the spotlight on chemoprevention as a handy mid-term tactic to ease the burden on those most at risk – especially little kids in areas where the disease runs high. Even though the WHO has recommended various chemoprevention methods for years, they haven't taken off. Recent work generally shows that stepping up chemoprevention not only saves costs but also cuts down severe malaria cases and deaths; this kind of evidence nudges us toward making these measures a default in protecting vulnerable kids. The shift to include chemoprevention in overall malaria policy marks a turning point—one that aims to tackle stalled progress by using proven, preventative moves to blunt seasonal spikes and boost health in endemic regions

(Littmann et al., 2024). Vaccines, meanwhile, are playing a vital role alongside chemoprevention. The RTS,S/AS01 vaccine, for example, won strong support from the WHO after impressive pilot program results. Data from Ghana, Kenya, and Malawi tell us that hospital admissions for severe malaria dropped by about 30% in vaccinated children, and those earlier safety concerns seem to have faded away. When the RTS,S vaccine joins forces with Seasonal Malaria Chemoprevention in areas with clear seasonal peaks, the combined effect noticeably slashes clinical malaria cases. Still, making the vaccine available everywhere isn't so simple challenges like missing seasonal delivery systems and uneven immunization coverage beyond infancy mean that strategies need to be fine-tuned for different local realities (Merle et al., 2023). All these insights together show that chemoprevention and vaccination work hand in hand in the fight against malaria. Mixing these approaches—tailored to local transmission patterns and the strengths of existing health systems—holds real promise for a more effective and lasting control strategy. Boosting program delivery will involve working through practical hurdles like developing better vaccine distribution models and building community trust, while also sharpening surveillance so interventions can adapt as needed. In short, chemoprevention offers quick, immediate protection and vaccines bring a longer-term immunological boost; pairing them up is key to comprehensively lowering malaria morbidity and mortality in affected regions (Merle et al., 2023; Littmann et al., 2024).

KEY TERMS FROM THIS CHAPTER

- Mass Drug Administration (MDA)
- Primaquine
- Atovaquone-Proguanil Prophylaxis
- Chemoprophylaxis Adherence
- Blood-Stage Vaccines
- Vaccine Efficacy
- Cold Chain Management
- Global Vaccine Implementation
- Prophylaxis
- Mefloquine Prophylaxis
- Doxycycline Prophylaxis
- Pre-Erythrocytic Vaccines
- Transmission-Blocking Vaccines (TBVs)
- Herd Immunity
- Booster Doses

References

1. Hemingway, J., Shretta, R., Wells, T. N., Bell, D., Djimdé, A. A., Achee, N., & Qi, G. (2016). Tools and Strategies for Malaria Control and Elimination: What Do We Need to Achieve a Grand Convergence in Malaria?. *PLoS biology*, *14*(3), e1002380. https://doi.org/10.1371/journal.pbio.1002380 (accessed on 13 May 2025).
2. Ngwafor, R., Pokharel, S., Aguas, R. *et al.* Models for malaria control optimization—a systematic review. *Malar J* **23**, 295 (2024). https://doi.org/10.1186/s12936-024-05118-3(accessed on 13 May 2025).
3. Alkhzem, A. H., Woodman, T. J., & Blagbrough, I. S. (2022). Design and synthesis of hybrid compounds as novel drugs and medicines. *RSC Advances, 12*, 19470–19484. https://doi.org/10.1039/d2ra03281c.
4. Antonio-Nkondjio, C., Ndo, C., Njiokou, F., Bigoga, J. D., Awono-Ambene, P., Etang, J., Same Ekobo, A., et al. (2019). Review of malaria situation in Cameroon: Technical viewpoint on challenges and prospects for disease elimination. *Parasites & Vectors, 12*. https://doi.org/10.1186/s13071-019-3753-8.
5. Arshad, U., Pertinez, H., Box, H., Tatham, L., Rajoli, R. K. R., Curley, P., Neary, M., et al. (2020). Prioritization of anti-SARS-CoV-2 drug repurposing opportunities based on plasma and target site concentrations derived from their established human pharmacokinetics. *Clinical Pharmacology & Therapeutics, 108*, 775–790. https://doi.org/10.1002/cpt.1909.
6. Awasthi, K. R., Jancey, J., Clements, A. C. A., Rai, R., & Leavy, J. E. (2024). Community engagement approaches for malaria prevention, control and elimination: A scoping review. *BMJ Open, 14*, Article e081982. https://doi.org/10.1136/bmjopen-2023-081982.
7. Strachan, C. E., Kana, M., Martin, S., Dada, J., Wandera, N., Marasciulo, M., Counihan, H., Kolawole, M., Babale, T., Hamade, P., Meek, S. R., & Baba, E. (2016). The use of formative research to inform the design of a seasonal malaria chemoprevention intervention in northern Nigeria. *Malaria journal*, *15*, 474. https://doi.org/10.1186/s12936-016-1526-9 (accessed on 13 May 2025).
8. Bauserman, M., Conroy, A. L., North, K., Patterson, J., Bose, C., & Meshnick, S. (2019). An overview of malaria in pregnancy. *Seminars in perinatology*, *43*(5), 282–290. https://doi.org/10.1053/j.semperi.2019.03.018(accessed on 13 May 2025).
9. Burgert, L. (2020). Modelling to guide the development of pharmaceutical interventions against malaria. https://core.ac.uk/download/552405732.pdf (accessed on 13 May 2025).
10. Greenwood, B., Dicko, A., Sagara, I., Zongo, I., Tinto, H., Cairns, M., Kuepfer, I., Milligan, P., Ouedraogo, J. B., Doumbo, O., & Chandramohan, D. (2017). Seasonal vaccination against malaria: a potential use for an imperfect malaria vaccine. *Malaria journal*, *16*(1), 182. https://doi.org/10.1186/s12936-017-1841-9 (accessed on 13 May 2025).
11. Thompson, H. A., Hogan, A. B., Walker, P. G. T., Winskill, P., Zongo, I., Sagara, I., Tinto, H., Ouedraogo, J. B., Dicko, A., Chandramohan, D., Greenwood, B., Cairns, M., & Ghani, A. C. (2022). Seasonal use case for the RTS,S/AS01 malaria vaccine: a mathematical modelling study. *The Lancet. Global health*, *10*(12), e1782–e1792. https://doi.org/10.1016/S2214-109X(22)00416-8(accessed on 13 May 2025).

12. Cameron, E., Camponovo, F., Chitnis, N., Golumbeanu, et al. (2022). Leveraging mathematical models of disease dynamics and machine learning to improve development of novel malaria interventions. https://core.ac.uk/download/552124235.pdf (accessed on 13 May 2025).

13. Camponovo, F., Ockenhouse, C., Lee, C., & Penny, M. A. (2019). Mass campaigns combining antimalarial drugs and anti-infective vaccines as seasonal interventions for malaria control, elimination and prevention of resurgence: A modelling study. *BMC Infectious Diseases, 19*, Article 4467. https://doi.org/10.1186/s12879-019-4467-4.

14. Chu, C. S., & White, N. J. (2021). The prevention and treatment of *Plasmodium vivax* malaria. *PLOS Medicine, 18*, e1003561. https://doi.org/10.1371/journal.pmed.1003561.

15. Diallo, O., Diallo, A., Toh, K. B., Diakité, N., Dioubaté, M., Runge, M., Symons, T. L., et al. (2024). Subnational tailoring of malaria interventions to prioritize the malaria response in Guinea. *medRxiv*. https://doi.org/10.1101/2024.06.26.24309532.

16. Han, L., Hudgens, M. G., Emch, M. E., Juliano, J. J., Keeler, C., Martinson, F., Kamthunzi, P., Tegha, G., Lievens, M., & Hoffman, I. F. (2017). RTS,S/AS01 Malaria Vaccine Efficacy is Not Modified by Seasonal Precipitation: Results from a Phase 3 Randomized Controlled Trial in Malawi. *Scientific reports, 7*(1), 7200. https://doi.org/10.1038/s41598-017-07533-w

17. (accessed on 13 May 2025).

18. Itsara, L. S., Zhou, Y., Do, J., Grieser, A. M., Vaughan, A. M., & Ghosh, A. K. (2018). The development of whole sporozoite vaccines for *Plasmodium falciparum* malaria. *Frontiers in Immunology, 9*. https://doi.org/10.3389/fimmu.2018.02748.

19. Kaboré, J. M. T. (2024). Piloting multiple first-line artemisinin-based combination therapies as an innovative approach for managing uncomplicated malaria in the health district of Kaya, Burkina Faso. https://core.ac.uk/download/636766039.pdf (accessed on 13 May 2025).

20. Kühl, M. J. (2025). Addressing implementation uncertainty in post discharge malaria chemoprevention: Determinants of adherence, cost-effectiveness, and the value of further research in Malawi and other malaria-endemic African countries. https://core.ac.uk/download/596353573.pdf (accessed on 13 May 2025).

21. Littmann, J., Achu, D., Laufer, M. K., Karema, C., & Schellenberg, D. (2024). Making the most of malaria chemoprevention. *Malaria Journal, 23*. https://doi.org/10.1186/s12936-024-04867-5.

22. London School of Hygiene & Tropical Medicine. (2013). *Annual Report 2013*. https://core.ac.uk/download/19452766.pdf (accessed on 13 May 2025).

23. Merle, C., Badiane, N. A., Affoukou, C., Affo, S. Y., Djogbénou, L., Ogouyemi Hounto, A., Kompaoré, S., et al. (2023). Implementation strategies for the introduction of the RTS,S/AS01 (RTS,S) malaria vaccine in countries with areas of highly seasonal transmission: Workshop meeting report. *Malaria Journal, 22*. https://doi.org/10.1186/s12936-023-04657-5.

24. Mesa, O. D. (2022). Estimating the impact and economic trade-offs of infectious disease control strategies using metapopulation models. https://core.ac.uk/download/533450132.pdf (accessed on 13 May 2025).

25. Nambatya, W., Ocan, M., Robberstad, B., Achan, J., & Idro, R. (2025). Malaria chemoprevention and vaccination strategies for children living in endemic areas of Africa: A review. *Frontiers in Malaria*. https://www.semanticscholar.org/paper/b65968aa90f3ea2e1fbdd33b6a1540e055e6d862 (accessed on 16 May 2025).

26. Ndambo, M. K., Bærøe, K., Phiri, K. S., Chiumia, I. K., Teig, I. L., Robberstad, B., Kaarbøe, O. M., Kühl, M. J., Chinkhumba, J., Nkosi-Gondwe, T., Tizifa, T. A., Mamani-Mategula, E., Munthali, L., & Manda-Taylor, L. (2025). Conceptualizing the implementation of post-discharge malaria chemoprevention in Malawi using a co-design approach. *Malaria journal, 24*(1), 51. https://doi.org/10.1186/s12936-025-05265-1(accessed on 13 May 2025).

27. Nekkab, N., Malinga, J., Braunack-Mayer, L., Kelly, S. L., Miller, R. S., & Penny, M. A. (2023). Modelling to inform next-generation medical interventions for malaria prevention and treatment. *Communications Medicine, 3*. https://doi.org/10.1038/s43856-023-00274-0.

28. Okoth, W. A., Ho, M. F., Zaman, M., Cooper, E., Som, P., Burgess, M., Walton, M., et al. (2023). A CAF01-adjuvanted whole asexual blood-stage liposomal malaria vaccine induces a $CD4^+$ T-cell-dependent strain-transcending protective immunity in rodent models. *mBio, 14*. https://doi.org/10.1128/mbio.02547-23.

29. Olawade, D. B., Wada, O. Z., Ezeagu, C. N., Aderinto, N., Balogun, M. A., Asaolu, F. T., & David-Olawade, A. C. (2024). Malaria vaccination in Africa: A mini-review of challenges and opportunities. *Medicine, 103*, e38565. https://doi.org/10.1097/md.0000000000038565.

30. Rogerson, S. J., Beeson, J. G., Laman, M., Poespoprodjo, J. R., William, T. W., Simpson, J. A., Price, R. N., et al. (2020). Identifying and combating the impacts of COVID-19 on malaria. *BMC Medicine, 18*. https://doi.org/10.1186/s12916-020-01710-x.

31. Semenza, J. C., Rocklöv, J., & Ebi, K. L. (2022). Climate change and cascading risks from infectious disease. *Infectious Diseases and Therapy, 11*, 1371–1390. https://doi.org/10.1007/s40121-022-00647-3.

32. Thompson, H. A. (2022). Modelling the public health impact of second-generation malaria vaccines. https://core.ac.uk/download/541722294.pdf (accessed on 16 May 2025).

33. Topazian, H. M., Schmit, N., Gerard-Ursin, I. C. G., Charles, G., Thompson, H., Ghani, A. C., & Winskill, P. (2023). Modelling the relative cost-effectiveness of the RTS,S/AS01 malaria vaccine compared to investment in vector control or chemoprophylaxis. *Vaccine, 41*, 3215–3223. https://doi.org/10.1016/j.vaccine.2023.04.011.

34. Weiss, D. J., Bertozzi-Villa, A., Rumisha, S. F., Amratia, P., Arambepola, R., Battle, K. E., Cameron, E., et al. (2020). Indirect effects of the COVID-19 pandemic on malaria intervention coverage, morbidity, and mortality in Africa: A geospatial modelling analysis. *The Lancet Infectious Diseases, 21*, 59–69. https://doi.org/10.1016/s1473-3099(20)30700-3.

35. Williams, S. (2018). Evaluating effective altruism and its implications on the fight against malaria. TC 660H Plan II Honors Program The University of Texas at Austin May 10, 2018 (accessed on 16 May 2025).

36. Winskill, P., Walker, P., Cibulskis, R., & Ghani, A. C. (2019). Prioritizing the scale-up of interventions for malaria control and elimination. *Malaria Journal, 18*. https://doi.org/10.1186/s12936-019-2755-5.

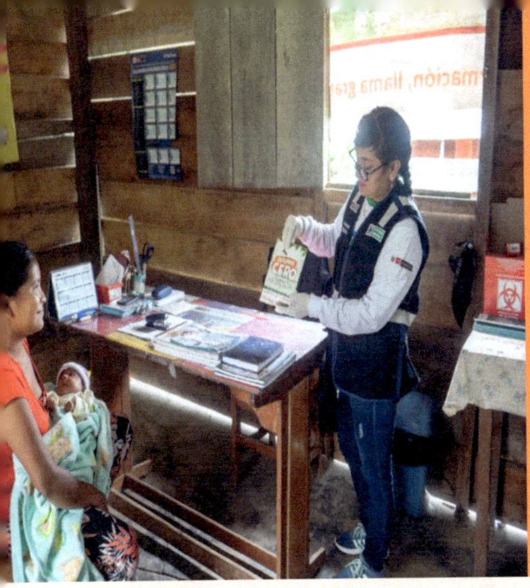

Chapter 14

MALARIA IN SPECIAL POPULATIONS

Contents

Introduction

Malaria is still a huge global problem, often hitting hardest where hospitals and clinics are few and far between. In many cases, even with prevention and treatment efforts rolling on, the toll remains high in terms of illness and death, especially among those already at risk. The parasite spreads in ways that are not straightforward, and its knack for dodging drugs only adds to the mess. That makes it clear, generally speaking, that we need to focus more on groups facing unique challenges. , getting a grip on these communities, with all their biological, social, and environmental features—is key to crafting interventions that work (Christopher et al., 2022). Some groups, like expectant mothers, kids under five, and individuals with weakened immunity, tend to bear malaria's fiercest impact. Pregnant women, for example, face extra hazards because the parasite can mess with the placenta, sometimes leading to low birth weights or even infant loss. Little children, whose immune systems are still getting up to speed, often end up fighting off much more severe illnesses. And if someone is already dealing with conditions such as HIV/AIDS, managing malaria gets even trickier, making the overall picture far grimmer. These overlapping risks mean that integrating healthcare and boosting surveillance efforts becomes pretty much indispensable (Christopher et al., 2022). Further, malaria control is up against the parasite's growing resistance to antimalarial drugs and even the insecticides used against its carriers, not to mention the uneven distribution of healthcare resources in many affected areas. This drug resistance forces us to keep altering treatment plans and preventive strategies, often in response to new challenges. Then there's the added strain from other diseases, like COVID-19, which can overwhelm systems and pull resources away at critical times. All of these factors point to an urgent need for flexible, locally tuned control programs that make sure vulnerable groups have fair shot at prevention, diagnosis, and treatment (Figure 14.1).

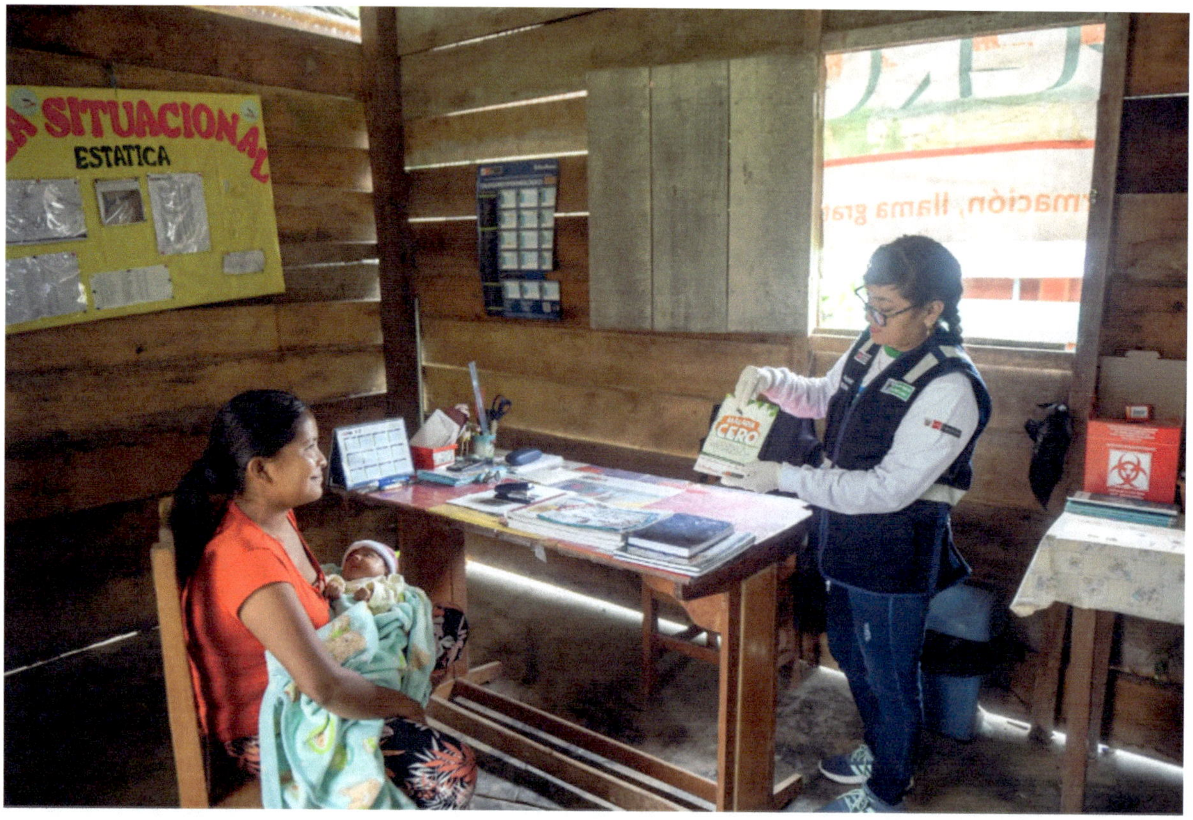

Figure 14.1. Malaria in special populations.

Source: Vivax Malaria. (2024). *Population at Risk of Malaria.*

Plasmodium parasites cause malaria when an infected female Anopheles mosquito bites someone. In most cases, as soon as these tiny invaders enter the bloodstream they head off to the liver, multiply, and eventually return to the blood to attack red blood cells, often sparking fevers, chills, and even anemia. The illness isn't cut-and-dried; sometimes it's just a fleeting fever, yet other times it can spiral into severe complications or even death. Local conditions, genetic differences, and the state of one's immune system all play roles, especially for groups like pregnant women, infants, or those with weaker defenses. In essence, grasping how these biological steps play out is key for managing malaria's heavy toll. The local environment and socio-economic conditions also mix into how malaria spreads. Climate features and weather changes can alter mosquito breeding patterns and speed up the parasite's development, which reshuffles where and how intensely the disease appears. At the same time, communities with fewer health resources often face delays in diagnosis and treatment, nudging the disease into more severe forms.

This mix of natural drivers and social challenges makes it clear that understanding malaria involves more than just tracking a parasite, it demands looking at how environmental, economic, and healthcare factors collide, as noted in several global health assessments (Intergovernmental Panel on Climate Change, 2023). Adding to the challenge, drug resistance has thrown an extra wrench in the works, particularly for already at-risk groups. As malaria parasites grow resistant to antimalarial drugs, medicines that once worked start to lose their effectiveness, leaving resource-strapped areas and vulnerable populations like children and expectant mothers in an even tougher spot. This resistance not only escalates rates of illness and death but also complicates treatment efforts overall. Keeping a close eye on these evolving patterns and tailoring treatments accordingly is crucial, since fighting malaria now means battling a cascade of interconnected issues (Christopher et al., 2022).

Importance of Studying Malaria in Special Populations

Pinning down how diseases move around in our ever-changing environment matters for public health. Take malaria, for example, it's now showing up in highland areas that never used to see it, a sign that shifts in climate and local ecology can mix things up in unexpected ways. Often, the individuals living in these outlying zones, with fewer hospitals and poorer infrastructure—end up at greater risk. Generally speaking, it isn't just the weather at play; economic woes and biological factors come into the picture, jointly influencing both how likely someone is to get infected and how severe the infection might turn out. Recognizing this mixed bag of factors paves the way for more specialized measures and helps prepare us for the chance that climate change will push malaria into new areas (Chaves & & Koenraadt, 2010). Looking at the economic and developmental side of things, the relationship between disease and poverty can't be ignored. In regions like Sub-Saharan Africa, where natural resources may be plentiful but persistent poverty still sticks around—malaria plays a big part in hampering education, labor output, and even the strength of local institutions. Essentially, the constant presence of the disease seems to sap human capital and slow down regional progress.

In most cases, studying malaria in these communities uncovers how closely intertwined health struggles are with broader socioeconomic challenges, which in turn shapes policies that tie health interventions to economic development strategies (Carmignani et al., 2011). In short, linking malaria control with social and economic factors gives us a more complete picture for planning effective public health responses. It's also important to look at malaria's toll on particular groups, such as pregnant women, young kids, and those with weakened immune systems. These groups have their own unique ways of dealing with the disease, often in ways that a standard, one-size-fits-all approach might not catch. For instance, the changes in a woman's immune system during pregnancy can boost her chances of facing severe malaria, calling for care that's specifically designed for that situation. Similarly, observing how malaria unfolds among children plays a key role in shaping vaccine strategies and deciding where to channel resources. By zeroing in on these special populations, our research not only works toward more fairness in healthcare but also sharpens overall malaria control efforts—ensuring that each group gets the tailored attention it needs for better outcomes (Figure 14.2).

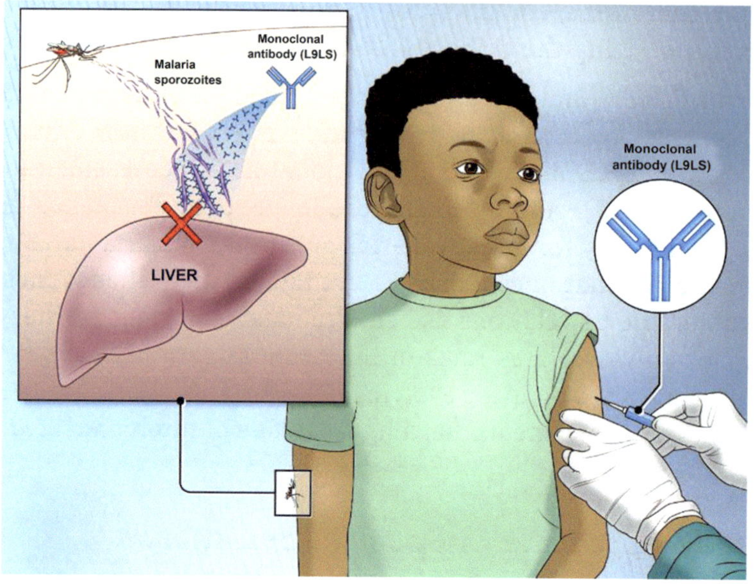

Figure 14.2. Importance of studying malaria in special populations.

Source: NIAID. (2024). *Malaria Research in Special Populations*.

14.1. Epidemiology of Malaria

Malaria spreads in ways that are shaped by the land, the weather, and how communities' live day to day. In many parts of sub-Saharan Africa—places where healthcare often falls short—the disease still hits hard, made worse by issues like growing drug resistance and weak diagnostic setups (Christopher et al., 2022). Drug-resistant strains of *Plasmodium falciparum* tend to push up death rates and muddle treatment plans, especially for groups such as pregnant women and little kids. Sometimes malaria even shows up alongside other infections that wear down the immune system, making people even more vulnerable. Generally speaking, knowing how the numbers change from one region to the next and among different groups is key to crafting the right kind of help. This kind of epidemiological insight calls for stronger health systems, better surveillance, and treatment plans that fit the local needs. When it comes to people at higher risk, malaria is a whole different ball game. Kids under five, for example, mostly because their immune defenses are still getting ready, end up facing serious health issues and higher chances of death. Pregnant women are in a similar tough spot; catching malaria can lead to problems like low birth weight, maternal anemia, and increased infant mortality. The risks aren't the same everywhere either—the mix of urban sprawl, shifting populations, and local mosquito habits means that even in areas known for malaria, its impact can vary a lot (John et al., 2020). To summarize, a one-size-fits-all strategy just won't work. Instead, health programs need to pin down who's most at risk so that they can direct resources, distribute tools like insecticide-treated nets, and put in place effective preventive drug measures where they're needed most. Mixing malaria with other global health challenges makes controlling the disease even trickier. For instance, the steady rise of antimicrobial resistance tends to undermine standard treatments, which forces constant reassessment of which drugs are still effective (Christopher et al., 2022). In some cases, when healthcare systems are overly burdened by crises such as COVID-19, routine monitoring of malaria gets pushed apart—further increasing risks for vulnerable groups (John et al., 2020). This complex mix of issues calls for strategies that are robust yet flexible, mixing malaria control efforts with broader plans to handle infectious diseases. The ever-changing patterns in how malaria spreads, evolves resistance, and meets gaps in healthcare access clearly show why a resilient, adaptable approach is needed to protect those who are most at risk from a disease that, despite its ancient roots, keeps reinventing itself (Figure 14.3).

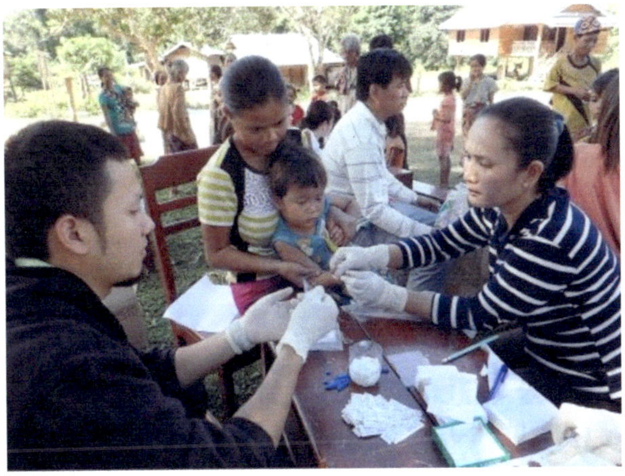

Figure 14.3. Epidemiology of malaria.

Source: Institut Pasteur du Laos. (2017). *Malaria Epidemiology Research.*

14.1.1. Global Prevalence and Incidence Rates

Infectious diseases around the globe hit hard for many reasons; environment, social setup, and cash problems all play a part. Malaria, for instance, isn't just about a pesky mosquito bite; it flips its behavior depending on shifts in weather, bustling city life, or even how people move about. Kids and pregnant women tend to get hit harder, partly because of the way their bodies handle these infections. Urban sprawl and a warming climate reshape where mosquitoes dwell, which in turn bumps up risk in communities that are already struggling. When you mix in our increasingly connected world, malaria proves to be complex with broader social and environmental issues. In most cases, if we don't dig into these underlying factors, our current fixes might not make a lasting dent in reducing malaria cases worldwide (Bradley et al., 2001). Different parts of the world show malaria in very different lights, especially in regions also wrestling with other tropical diseases. In sub-Saharan Africa, for example, the burden is even heavier thanks to many neglected tropical diseases that make communities extra vulnerable. Ethiopia serves as a clear example—here, the overlapping presence of malaria with illnesses like hookworm, lymphatic filariasis, and leishmaniasis makes public health problems even more complex. This kind of overlap tends to increase the risks for those already facing poverty, and even ongoing control efforts can feel a bit overwhelmed by so many layers of disease. Generally speaking, it's clear that a one-dimensional approach won't be enough; what's needed is a more integrated strategy aimed at both malaria and the other parasitic infections hitting special populations (Deribe et al., 2012). When checking out global malaria trends, it turns out that economic and geographic factors have a lot to do with who gets exposed and who can access healthcare. Refugees, displaced individuals, and people stranded in remote areas often deal with extra risks—not only do they often lack proper shelter and preventative tools, but weak health systems don't help either. Noticeably, the groups most affected, small children, pregnant women, and those with weakened immunity, usually end up in these vulnerable spots, which pushes up the incidence even further. In most cases, effective strategies need to account for both the biological side of things and the broader socioeconomic conditions driving malaria's reach among these at-risk groups (Bradley et al., 2001; Deribe et al., 2012).

14.1.2. High-Risk Regions and Demographics

Many regions get hit harder by infections, and many local ecology, financial challenges, and limited healthcare often sets the stage. For example, malaria still wreaks havoc in parts of western sub-Saharan Africa—places already short on resources for basic disease surveillance and treatment. In these spots, rising drug resistance messes up our usual fixes, pushing death rates even higher. A global look even points to western sub-Saharan Africa as having the highest fatality rates related to bacterial resistance (Christopher et al., 2022).

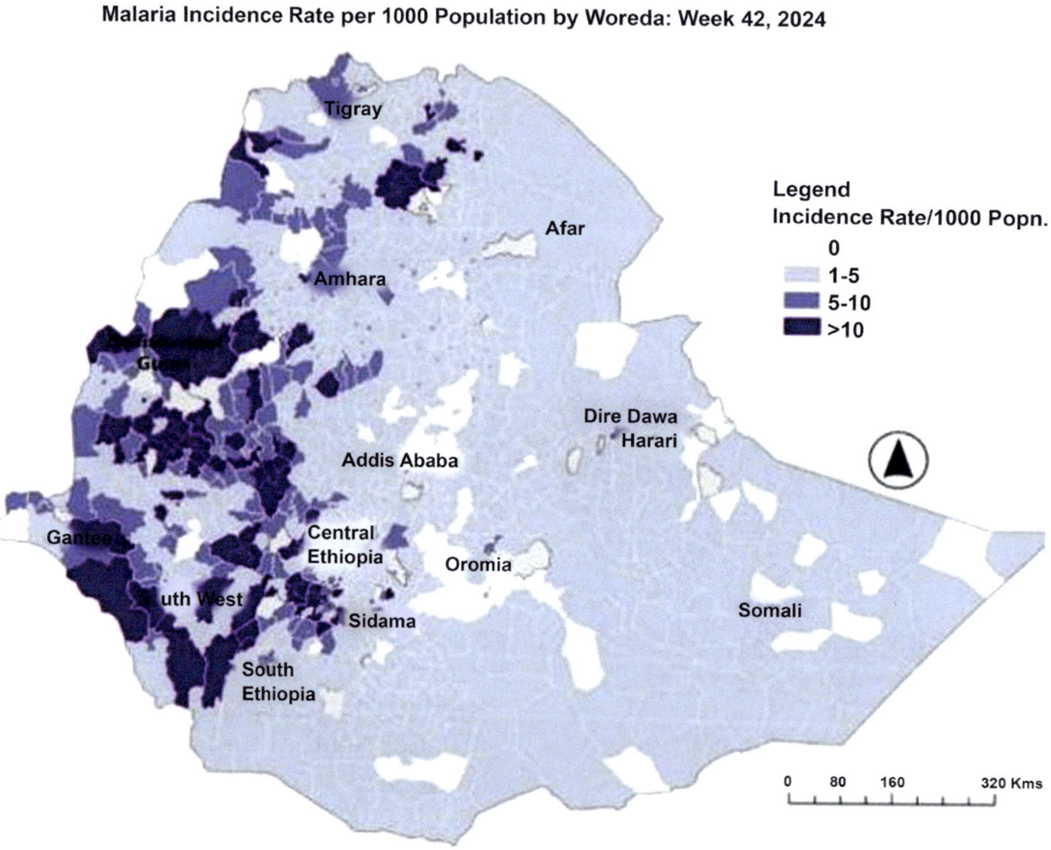

Figure 14.4. High-risk regions and demographics of malaria.

Source: World Health Organization. (n.d.). *Geographical Distribution of Malaria Cases.*

It's a stark reminder that when microbial resistance and endemic diseases tag-team together, the effects are both direct and indirect. Essentially, digging into these local health conditions is crucial if we're to shape interventions aimed at easing malaria's harsh impact on the most vulnerable. Different groups within malaria zones don't face the same level of risk either. Take forest workers in Southeast Asia, say, those in Cambodia, who spend so much time in mosquito-infested wild areas because they rely on the forest for a living. Research in Cambodia's forests shows that a large percentage of these individuals end up with infections from *Plasmodium falciparum* and *Plasmodium vivax* (Kunkel et al., 2021). There isn't a single, clear risk marker based on age or gender here; rather, the risk seems to sprinkle itself around unpredictably across the group. Generally speaking, this makes carving out targeted prevention plans all the trickier, highlighting how fresh, adapted strategies become essential for people who live in persistent transmission zones. Even the standard diagnostic and control approaches often stumble with these high-risk individuals. Look at the forest-goers again: rapid diagnostic tests (RDTs) don't always catch low-density or asymptomatic malaria infections, and underestimation can delay proper treatment. In most cases, mass screening and treatment programs run into trouble because the tests just aren't sensitive enough for the subtle signs these populations show (Kunkel et al., 2021). This pushes us to rethink our strategies, may be trying intermittent preventive measures specifically tuned to high-risk groups, so that, when merged with regional and demographic insights, our efforts hit closer to home (Figure 14.4).

14.1.3. Impact of Climate Change on Malaria Distribution

Vector-borne diseases are shifting in ways that show how mixed-up our environment and public health can be, especially for individuals like pregnant women and little kids. Climate change, by altering temperature and rainfall, ends up giving Anopheles mosquitoes (the malaria carriers) a leg up in areas that used to be off-limits for the disease. Suddenly, borders we used to rely on blur, and communities in highlands or temperate spots—once thought to be safe—might now see outbreaks that strain already stretched health services. In most cases, figuring out exactly how weather and mosquito behavior mix is a must for creating interventions that truly protect these at-risk groups (Intergovernmental Panel on Climate Change, 2023). At the same time, changes in mosquito breeding grounds brought on by climate shifts can increase both the intensity and timing of malaria outbreaks. When rain falls heavier and temperatures rise, mosquitoes develop faster and the parasites inside them seem to speed through their life cycle.

This quicker turnaround ups the chance of infection, putting children under five and those with weakened immune defenses at greater peril. Unpredictable weather swings can also throw off established control plans, forcing local officials to experiment with more flexible, adaptive strategies. And when factors like pesticide use get thrown into the mix—since climate-driven pest changes may mean more frequent applications—the ecological balance can be upset, sometimes even leading to resistance issues (Tudi et al., 2021). Social factors also get combined with climate's impact on malaria, hitting marginalized or resource-poor communities especially hard. When climate changes mess with food security and everyday livelihoods, it not only weakens immune responses but also limits access to essential tools like insecticide-treated nets and antimalarial drugs. This uneven burden on vulnerable populations reminds us that ethical, fair public health policies are crucial. It helps when experts from climate science, epidemiology, and social policy work together to tackle the spread of malaria amid these shifts. Ultimately, mixing climate adaptation into malaria control plans seems like one solid path toward long-lasting health improvements (Intergovernmental Panel on Climate Change, 2023) (Figure 14.5).

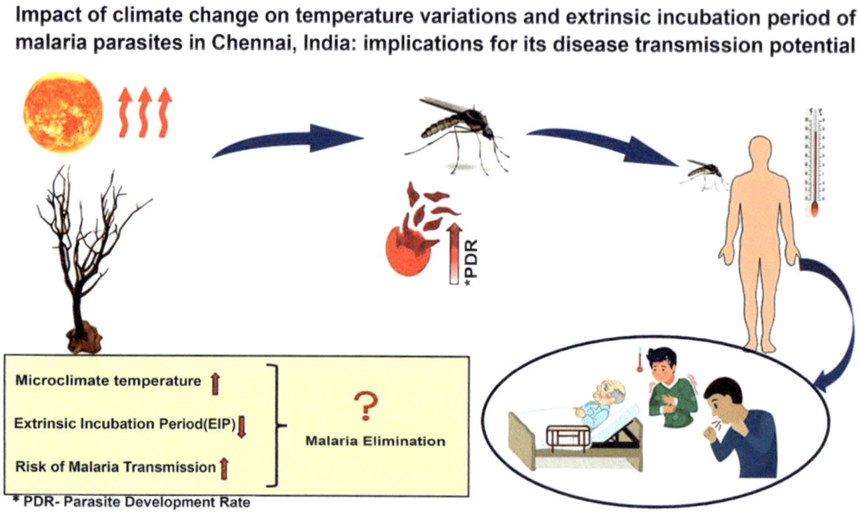

Figure 14.5. Impact of climate change on malaria distribution.

Source: Springer Nature. (2024). *Climate Change Impact on Malaria.*

14.2. Vulnerable Populations

Environmental factors and individual vulnerability mix in ways that aren't always predictable. Shifts in weather, sudden changes in rainfall or odd temperature swings, can stir up mosquito populations and hit some people harder than others. Pregnant women, young kids, and those with weakened immune systems often live in areas where health services are pretty sparse, which only adds to their risk. When the climate warms or rain patterns shift, fresh hideouts for malaria-carrying pathogens appear, letting the disease creep into new regions. Poverty, malnutrition, and limited access to basic care further complicate matters, and in most cases, recognizing these complex issues is crucial for designing interventions that tackle both the disease itself and the social backdrop (Intergovernmental Panel on Climate Change, 2023). Malaria's impact on at-risk groups gets even trickier with the rise of antimicrobial resistance (AMR)—a genuine headache for treatment efforts. In many high-infection areas, it's not just the malaria parasite causing trouble; resistant strains make standard medicines less effective, leading to longer illnesses and more spread. Fewer treatment options and an uneven distribution of healthcare mean that proper diagnosis and care are hard to come by, especially in low-income settings. On top of this, malaria sometimes shows up alongside other infections, so the burden of AMR further undermines treatment success. Generally speaking, battling AMR calls for integrated strategies; robust surveillance, upgraded lab setups, and new therapies aimed squarely at those who are most vulnerable (Christopher et al., 2022). Social and economic struggles also lower at defenses, making malaria's toll even more uneven. Children under five, pregnant women, and individuals with compromised immune systems tend to face more severe bouts of the disease. Limited education, crumbling housing, and a lack of things like insecticide-treated bed nets only add fuel to the fire. Often, these marginalized communities run into hurdles like geographic isolation and tight budgets, which delay both diagnosis and treatment. Plus, malnutrition, a common issue in poor regions, weakens natural defenses even more, paving the way for worse outcomes. All these overlapping challenges point to a clear need for public health strategies that mix community support with fair healthcare access and locally driven interventions, offering a real chance to ease malaria's impact and move toward better health equity.

14.2.1. Pregnant Women and Maternal Health

Malaria and pregnancy mix in a worrisome way, especially in regions where infectious diseases hit hard. Pregnant women seem to be extra susceptible to *Plasmodium falciparum*, likely because their bodies change and parasites tend to settle in the placenta. This often leads to problems like maternal anemia and babies coming into the world too small, issues that ripple out into long-term challenges for child development. In many parts of sub-Saharan Africa, where malaria transmission is intense, these risks multiply. Targeted efforts to prevent and manage malaria in expectant moms have become a top priority, given how much the disease contributes to newborn deaths PATH, 2014). When you step back and look at the situation, it's clear that tackling malaria in pregnant women isn't just about treating one disease on its own. Generally speaking, mixing maternal health programs with wider infectious disease strategies, like linking reproductive health services with HIV/AIDS care—has proven valuable.

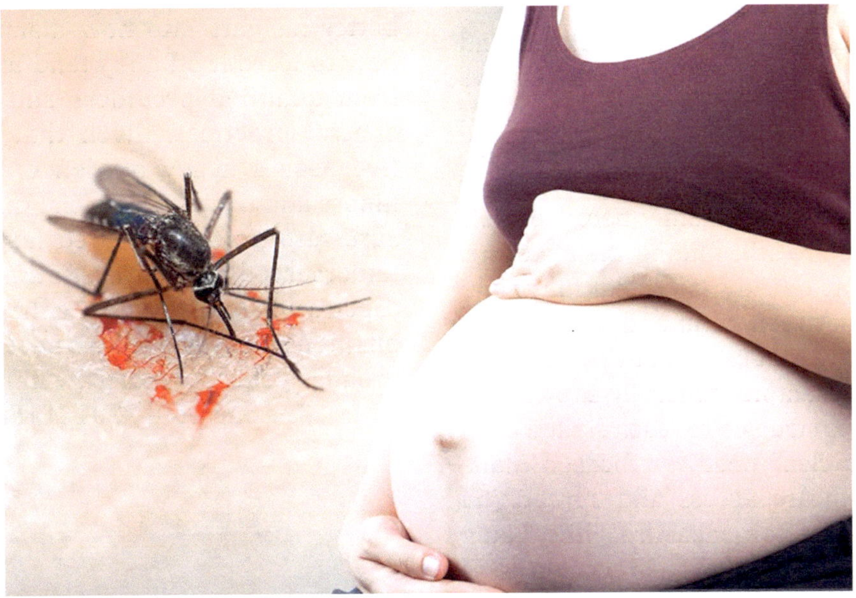

Figure 14.6. Pregnant women and maternal health.

Source: Parenting FirstCry. (2017). *Pregnancy and Malaria.*

Co-infections have a way of making things worse, so integrating care helps catch missed opportunities for diagnosis and treatment. This approach also touches on overlapping social issues, such as healthcare access and even gender-based violence, issues that sometimes get sidelined. In most cases, country-specific data and tailored policy adjustments are key for making these broad strategies stick (Dunn-Georgiou et al., 2009). But taking care of pregnant women facing malaria goes beyond just clinical treatment. It also means giving them the tools and knowledge they need through health education and community engagement. Empowering women with simple insights about malaria prevention, recognizing infection signs, and sticking with antenatal care can make a big difference in reducing risks. Preventive methods like intermittent preventive treatment in pregnancy (IPTp) and the use of insecticide-treated nets (ITNs) are core parts of these programs, though they call for steady resources and ongoing political backing. At the same time, improving the local healthcare setup so that testing and treatment happen on time is crucial. All these aspects, clinical care, education, and infrastructure, come together to form an overall plan aimed at protecting maternal health from malaria's ongoing threat (PATH, 2014) (Figure 14.6).

14.2.2. Children Under Five Years Old

Young kids face a heavy risk from malaria, and this challenge strains public health efforts – especially in places where healthcare isn't always consistent. Even with all the work done to control the disease, children under five still come out worst, mainly because their immune systems are still finding their footing. Getting treatment quickly is crucial for them; yet differences between rural and urban areas often lead to delays that can cost lives. Research in Myanmar, for example, generally shows that rural communities struggle to reach skilled care. This points to a clear need for focused plans that boost healthcare access and spread the word about prevention measures like using insecticide-treated bed nets, which seem to sway treatment-seeking habits in a positive way (Aung et al., 2016). In many regions where malaria rates have plunged, keeping up prevention among caretakers of little ones still matters a lot to block any comeback. Studies in Zanzibar reveal that, although many caretakers no longer see malaria as an immediate threat, tools like long-lasting insecticidal nets (LLINs) and indoor residual spraying (IRS) continue to be widely used. Generally speaking, this ongoing care is due to caretakers recognizing the value of these methods and planning to stick with them even as the disease appears less frequent. It seems that success in malaria programs depends not only on having the right tools available but also on keeping that community commitment alive and a shared understanding of the risks (Beer et al., 2013). Maintaining high usage of these measures, even when the immediate threat feels lower—is vital for preventing outbreaks among vulnerable kids. How caretakers manage malaria risk in young children comes down to what they know, how easily they can get help, and how they view the danger. In many malaria-endemic regions, families with little ones can benefit from many health strategies that mix prevention education, better healthcare delivery, and community involvement. Evidence generally indicates that when caretakers gain better insights into how malaria spreads and how to ward it off, they tend to seek treatment from qualified providers and stick to vector control practices. Given that children under five bear a heavy burden of malaria-related illness and death, it's crucial that policies make sure resources are shared fairly, especially in underserved rural areas. Strengthening these aspects will not only reduce the disease's impact on these vulnerable groups but also help advance broader goals for malaria elimination (Beer et al, 2013; Aung et al., 2016) (Figure 14.7).

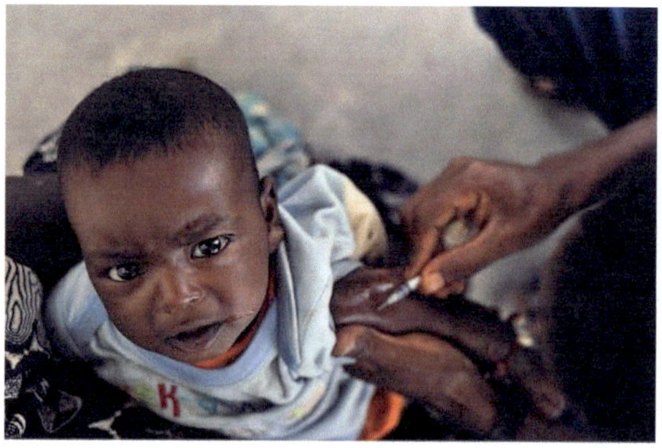

Figure 14.7. Children under five years.

Source: The Borgen Project. (n.d.). *Malaria and Child Mortality.*

14.2.3. Immunocompromised Individuals

People with weak immune systems face tough challenges when malaria strikes. Conditions like HIV/AIDS, cancer treatments, or organ transplants can drag down natural defenses so much that fighting malaria almost becomes a battle uphill. In regions where malaria is common, these individuals often see higher parasite levels and sometimes have trouble clearing the infection altogether, which can drag out the illness and open the door to extra complications. Even typical treatments sometimes need to be altered—almost like a delicate balancing act—to make sure medications don't interact in ways that worsen their weakened state. When you look at how a fragile immune system jives with infectious diseases, it highlights some key issues for both preventing and treating malaria in these populations. Take vaccines, for instance; generally speaking, the usual live-attenuated types might be too risky because they can set off problems in those with diminished defenses. Although malaria vaccines are still in development, the basic ideas on how vaccines signal the immune system remain pretty important. Figuring out how different vaccines work with the body can help design safer ways to build immunity in these individuals (Vetter et al., 2017). This perspective even points to the potential need for extra therapies alongside regular treatments, with a close watch on results. Managing malaria in someone with a compromised immune system isn't a one-person job, it demands extra vigilance and a real team effort across different medical fields. Other health issues, like diabetes, can further muddy the waters. For example, diabetic patients, whose blood sugar levels need careful control, face even more risk when their immune systems are already struggling, since metabolic swings affect both immunity and drug performance (Hussain et al., 2020). In a nutshell, several overlapping conditions can increase the danger, making it crucial to integrate care plans that address all aspects of health. Ongoing research remains vital, as it gradually reveals how exactly immunosuppression and malaria connect, ultimately helping tailor targeted therapies and management strategies for these vulnerable groups (Figure 14.8).

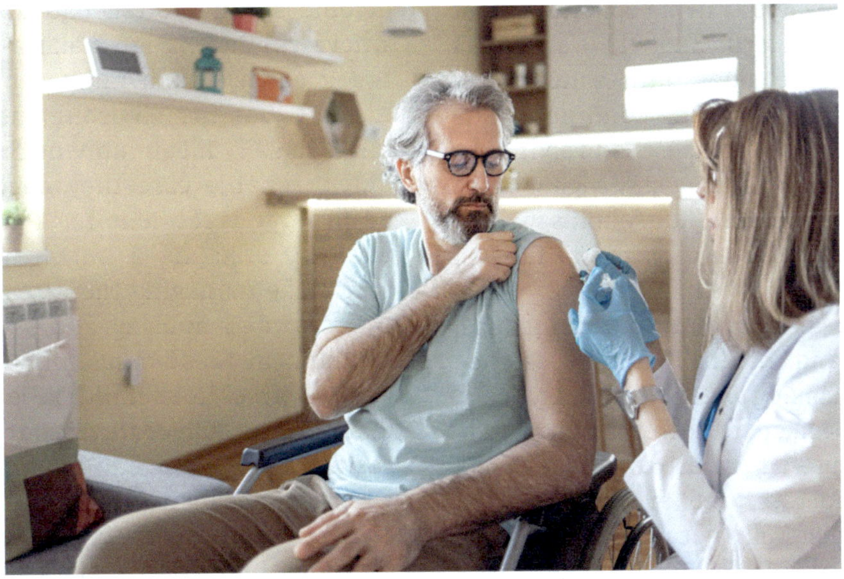

Figure 14.8. Immunocompromised individuals.

Source: Maxim Healthcare. (2023). *Malaria Risk in Immunocompromised People.*

14.3. Socioeconomic Factors

Different groups often deal with malaria prevention in ways that trace back to deeper social and economic conditions. A study in Ghana, for example, found that people living in the countryside tended to use ITNs more than their urban counterparts. It turns out that factors like how educated the family leader is and their overall financial situation play a big part in whether households can and do use these nets. Generally speaking, families with more money are more likely to invest in ITNs, while those struggling financially end up missing out on this critical protection. The research also makes it clear that public health efforts need to look at these social and economic layers since urban and rural areas each face their own set of challenges in regions where malaria is common (Yeboah et al., 2023). In a sense, the gaps in income and education end up making certain populations more vulnerable to the disease. Economic status doesn't just shape the kind of tools people use; it also sticks into everyday living conditions that can raise malaria risk. In Zimbabwe's Mutasa District, for instance, one study noticed that households with poorer living conditions, like having livestock kept too close or relying on old animal-drawn carts, often saw higher rates of malaria. Lower-income households, which usually have fewer resources, seem to face an extra burden, inadvertently increasing their exposure to the insects that spread malaria. On the other hand, having basic necessities nearby, such as drinking water within easy reach of the home, is linked to lower malaria risk. It's a mixed picture where economic hardship, environmental factors, and everyday life all come together; generally speaking, it suggests that fixing infrastructure is just as important as improving economic conditions to curb malaria spread (Zinyengere et al., 2018). It isn't just about having nets or better homes—wider issues like education and community involvement also weigh in heavily. Households led by someone with a stronger education tend to be better at picking up prevention habits, grasping health messages, and getting treatment when needed. Economic strength, too, gives families the means to buy ITNs or access health services when necessary. In most cases, these social factors highlight that any malaria-control plan has to bring together things like better schooling, more jobs, and improved living standards along with medical efforts. Policymakers need to see that cutting down on malaria means dealing with poverty, boosting education, and making homes safer. Skip out on these broader social improvements, and you risk leaving vulnerable groups behind, which might just stall malaria elimination attempts in the long run (Zinyengere et al., 2018; Yeboah et al., 2023).

14.3.1. Poverty and Access to Healthcare

Poverty and healthcare access end up shaping the health outcomes for those most at risk of malaria in a pretty tangible way. People in low-income settings often end up living in spots where conditions let malaria-carrying insects breed easily, which ramps up their exposure. It's not just the environment either; limited funds usually mean individuals can't afford the quick, reliable care they need, like bed nets or prompt treatment for infections. Poverty ends up stacking a bunch of little barriers that make managing the disease even tougher. Overcrowded housing and sketchy sanitation, common in these areas, only fuel the spread. With scarce household resources and long distances or high costs discouraging them from seeking care, many end up delaying treatment, which can lead to much more severe illness or even death. In short, poverty not only ups the odds of getting malaria but also cuts off access to the critical care needed, especially for children and pregnant women (Shadmi et al., 2020). Truth be told, weak health systems in low-income regions only add to the mess, particularly when dealing with malaria. Clinics in these struggling areas often lack even the basic quality required for solid diagnosis, treatment, and follow-up care; studies in low- and middle-income countries generally show that issues like low clinical expertise, meager resources, and a poor patient experience hit marginalized groups the hardest (Margaret et al., 2018). This poor quality can lead to misdiagnoses, wrong treatments, and missed chances to stop the disease from taking hold. So, the people most at risk face a double whammy—few facilities exist, and even when they do, the care often falls short. These system-wide weaknesses seriously undercut efforts to lower both sickness and death from malaria, highlighting a pressing need for strategies that tackle economic hurdles and boost health system quality alike (Margaret et al., 2018). Handling the complex mix of poverty and limited healthcare access calls for multifaceted solutions that speak to malaria-prone communities' everyday struggles. Policymakers must, in most cases, work to spread resources more fairly, this means things like subsidies for prevention and investing in sturdier healthcare infrastructure in impoverished areas. Care providers must offer not just technically sound treatment but also respectful and timely service; such efforts help build trust and get people to seek out help (Margaret et al., 2018). At the same time, community-run initiatives, even with their occasional imperfections, can empower individuals with the knowledge and tools to fend off malaria, softening some aspects of entrenched poverty. Broader socioeconomic crises also tend to throw more challenges into the mix, stressing the need for flexible, resilient health systems ready to adapt as conditions change (Shadmi et al., 2020). By centering fairness and gradually improving overall system quality, malaria control programs can better ease the burden on those hit hardest by poverty and limited healthcare access (Figure 14.9).

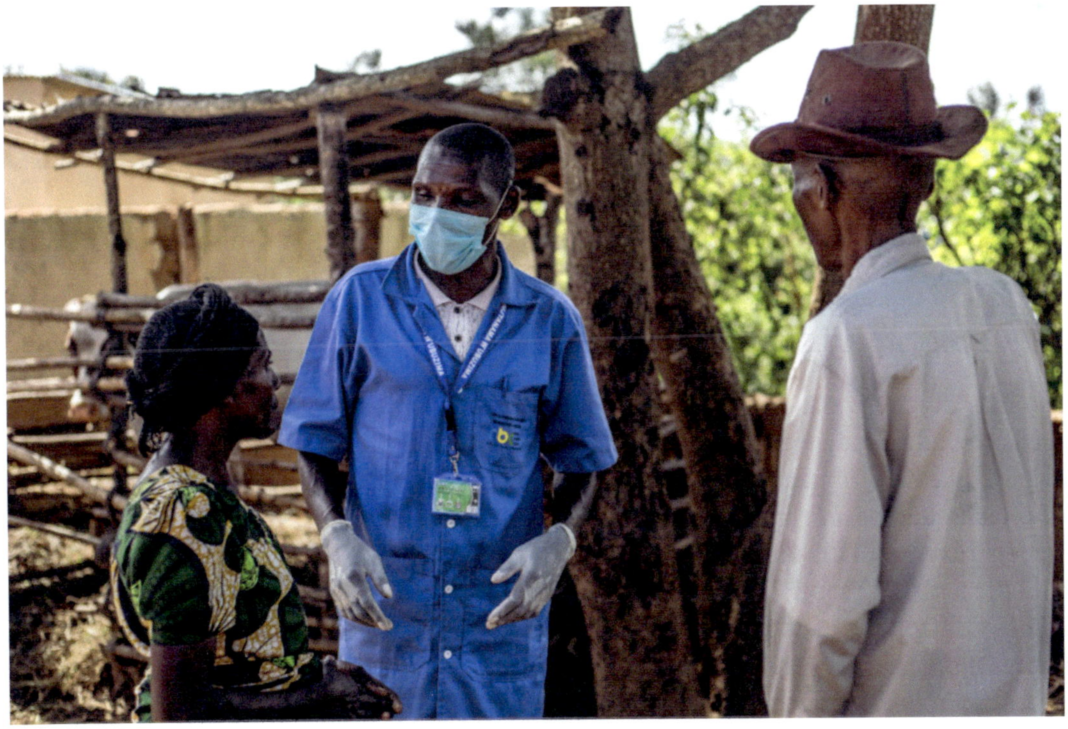

Figure 14.9. Community health workers lead the fight against malaria.

Source: WHO Africa. (2023). *Community Health Workers and Malaria Control.*

14.3.2. Education and Awareness of Malaria Prevention

Accurate, culturally tuned health details stand at the heart of our fight against malaria, especially for groups like pregnant women, kids, and individuals with weakened immunity. It isn't enough to simply dish out generic health tips; messages need to be shaped for real-life situations and address the specific vulnerabilities each community faces. Solid education bumps up knowledge and nudges attitudes, whether that's through encouraging the regular use of insecticide-treated bed nets or prompting timely visits to health services. When communities are given the right kind of local insight, they naturally take charge, which helps break down barriers from stigma, misinformation, and delays in seeking care. In most cases, combining these education drives to wider health system improvements makes care more accessible and sustainable a must for populations frequently left on the sidelines (Margaret et al., 2018).

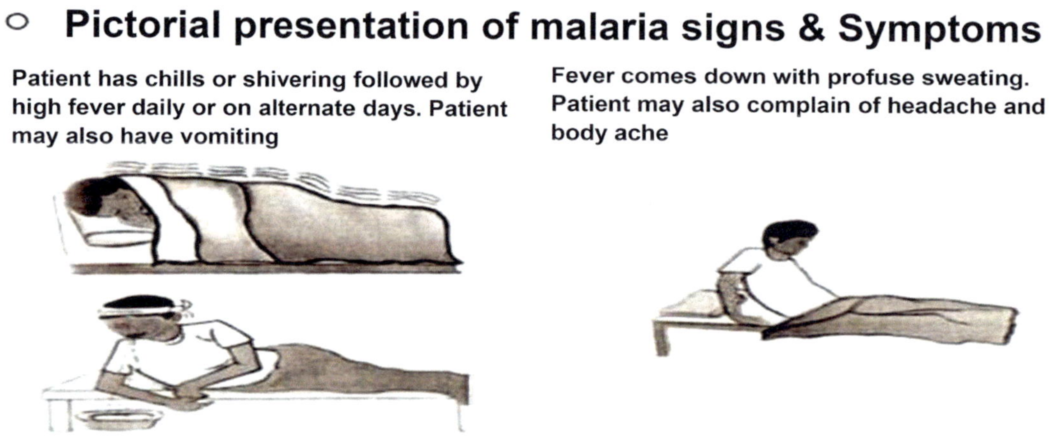

Figure 14.10. The education and awareness of malaria prevention.

Source: Mohammed Katagum Y, Binti Kadir Shahar H, Bin Ibrahim F, Baharom A, Baharudin R. Using an Educational Training Module to Increase Knowledge, Attitudes and Practices of Malaria among Medicine Vendors in Yobe, Nigeria [Internet]. Infectious Diseases. IntechOpen; 2021. Available from: http://dx.doi.org/10.5772/intechopen.98512

To summarize, these mixed strategies play a key role in reducing malaria's heavy toll on those most at risk. Tackling malaria prevention means raising awareness on both a personal level and within larger systems. For example, pregnant women benefit from focused interventions that clearly explain the risks during pregnancy and emphasize intermittent preventive treatment, which can lead to fewer adverse birth outcomes (KFF Policy Brief, 2016). Local community health workers, trusted in their own neighborhoods, help bridge the gap between official health providers and at-risk populations by sharing consistent, evidence-based info in everyday language. It also helps to weave malaria education into school lessons and community meetups, so that knowledge gets passed down naturally and keeps everyone in the loop. These layered efforts should work hand in hand with responsive health systems that treat these groups with care – since, quite frankly, poor-quality care tends to hit those already struggling even harder (Margaret et al., 2018). Sustained, clear awareness not only aids prevention but also encourages faster diagnoses and better treatment adherence, all of which can make a big difference in survival. Beyond teaching individuals or small groups, building an environment where health smarts mix with strong, transparent governance boosts malaria prevention among special populations. Getting policymakers to back investments in health education, and to keep a close eye on quality—ensures that prevention messages are supported by a dependable health infrastructure. Equitable and responsive health systems build trust with the public, encouraging those who've often felt sidelined to take advantage of available preventive services (Margaret et al., 2018). Plus, continually revieing and adjusting education efforts goes a long way toward tackling new challenges and specific local roadblocks. Training health workers to communicate in respectful and culturally sensitive ways can enhance the overall experience, making people more likely to adopt preventive measures. In the end, mixing education with strong health systems and an understanding of social dynamics creates a fuller picture for cutting malaria's impact on vulnerable groups (Figure 14.10).

14.3.3. Impact of Migration and Displacement

People moving around changes how diseases like malaria stick around, especially for those forced to leave home. Conflict or economic hardship drives many to new areas with different malaria risks, and these vulnerable individuals often end up in places where conditions shift unexpectedly. Border regions, for example, turn into hotspots as transient groups mix with locals, keeping the disease's cycle alive. Recent studies generally point out that setting up test-and-treat hubs at international borders might catch infections among migrants and help curb cross-border cases, but such steps alone just aren't enough for total elimination. Instead, we need integrated, adaptive strategies that consider how mobile and hard-to-reach communities live (Topazian et al., 2024). In many cases, understanding the ebb and flow of people is key to breaking the chains of transmission. Building new settlements through ecological migration programs is another twist in the tale of malaria risk. In southern Yunnan Province, one study compared a native village with a freshly established migration settlement and found noticeable changes. The new village had a spike in *Anopheles minimus* mosquitoes—the main culprits for malaria, and recorded cases that the old village never saw. This clear contrast shows that shifting human habitats and altering the environment can create just the right conditions for malaria to spread. The findings imply that public health planning for displaced groups needs to keep vector monitoring and control in mind, especially where environmental changes tip the scales in favor of these mosquitoes (Liu et al., 2024). In most cases, such insights push us to adopt context-sensitive interventions that work with the local vector ecology. Besides natural factors, displacement messes with access to malaria prevention and treatment services. People on the move often hit barriers like weak healthcare infrastructure, language gaps, and social exclusion, which can delay proper diagnosis and care. Add in migratory flows across high-transmission border areas, and the exposure risks just keep mounting—making it hard for public health teams to stick to consistent surveillance and intervention routines. These layered challenges stress the need to mix malaria control within broader humanitarian responses designed for displaced populations. Bringing together different sectors is crucial if we want to deliver culturally tuned health education, ensure insecticide-treated nets are on hand, and boost cross-border health efforts to reduce malaria's toll on mobile groups (Topazian et al., 2024). In most cases, truly addressing the link between migration, displacement, and malaria proves vital for fair and effective disease control outcomes (Figure 14.11).

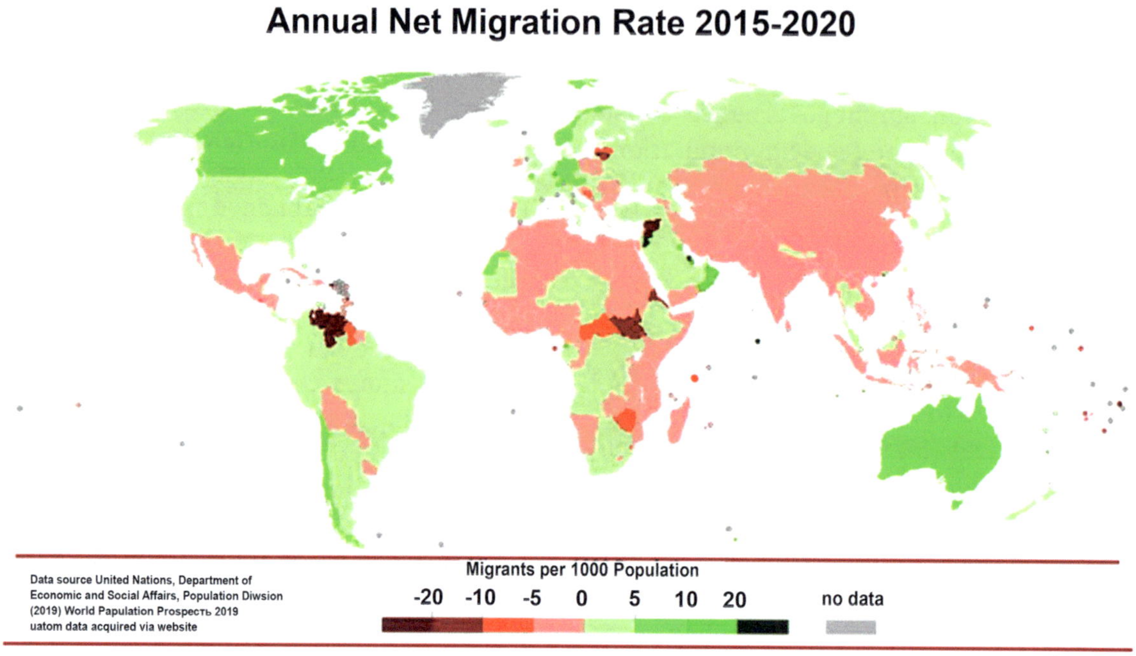

Figure 14.11. Migration and displacement.

Source: By A11w1ss3nd - Own work, CC BY-SA 4.0, https://commons.wikimedia.org/w/index.php?curid=82819695

14.4. Cultural Beliefs and Practices

Culture and health mix in ways that shape disease outcomes, especially for people facing malaria. In many tribal areas, age-old customs and rituals play a huge role; folk beliefs and the trust in traditional healers using magic-like rites and local herbal remedies can both help and sometimes hold back proper treatment. Different tribes hold their own ways of seeing things, and these ideas determine whether individuals are willing to try modern medicine at all. , fighting malaria isn't just about the drugs or vaccines on offer; it's also about understanding and working with familiar traditions. Without tuning health strategies to these unique cultural settings, reducing illness might miss the mark (Balgir et al., 2011). Local environments and social habits also throw another wrench into managing diseases like malaria, particularly where everyday living, work, and ancient customs intersect with shifting ecologies. Take Indonesia, for example; here, local groups and international organizations often join forces to tackle diseases that jump from animals to people, generally speaking. When local communities share their own insights on animal-human encounters, and their unique attitudes to disease—the effect on malaria prevention can be huge. Training sessions and community-led efforts, sometimes labeled as participatory epidemiology, weave indigenous knowledge into broader health surveillance in a way that builds trust and makes campaigns feel more relevant (Bourhy et al., 2012). Getting healthcare to fit cultural needs means looking at both the gifts and the hurdles found in traditional practices. Sure, a heavy trust in folk medicine might slow down formal treatment schedules, but these practices also pack valuable wisdom, like herbal cures that can sometimes work well with standard therapy. In many cases, health experts and community healers need to chat and work side by side, united by the shared goal of knocking out malaria. Local health plans must also stay flexible, because even within one community, beliefs can vary a lot. Clear, tailored communication can help sort out misunderstandings about how malaria spreads and is treated, leading to better results. In short, bridging the gap between local views and modern medicine stands out as a key strategy if we're serious about beating malaria in vulnerable groups (Balgir et al., 2011) (Figure 14.12).

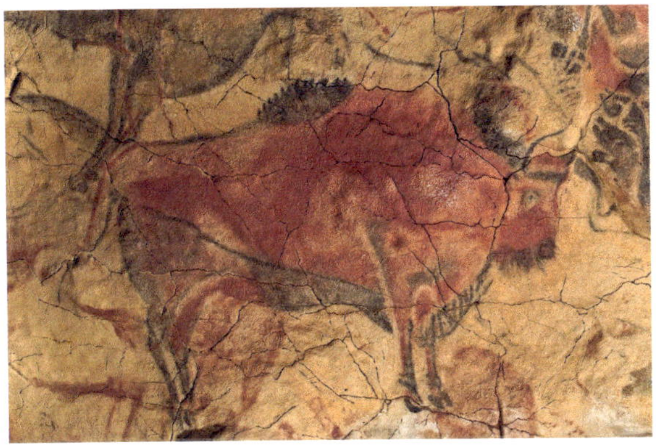

Figure 14.12. Cultural beliefs and practices.

Source: By Museo de Altamira y D. Rodríguez, CC BY-SA 3.0, https://commons.wikimedia.org/w/index.php?curid=24512679

14.4.1. Traditional Medicine and Malaria Treatment

In many parts of the world where formal healthcare is hard to reach, traditional medicine has been grabbing more attention for treating malaria. There's a long-standing habit of turning to plant-based remedies—remedies deeply woven into local culture and often practically effective for dealing with fever and similar ailments. Often, particularly in low-income areas, people rely on these age-old treatments either on their own or alongside modern medicine. This trend comes partly from the difficulties of accessing structured healthcare, and partly from a genuine, inherited trust in traditional wisdom. Still, it's important to note that the safety and effectiveness of these remedies can vary a lot, with many lacking the rigorous tests you'd expect in modern clinical settings. Generally speaking, fitting traditional treatments into malaria care calls for thoughtful attention to evidence-based methods and a close link-up with established health systems; a move that might help mend gaps in care quality and access seen in resource-poor settings (Margaret et al., 2018; World Health Organization, 2020). In essence, while these practices hold promise, there remains a clear need for care that is both safe and reliably effective. Many local remedies hinge on botanicals like Artemisia annua, the plant behind artemisinin—a compound that has played a pivotal role in modern antimalarial drugs. Even though pharmaceutical drugs have nowadays set a high bar for malaria treatment, numerous communities persist in using raw extracts or simple mixtures brewed from nearby plants. This ongoing reliance not only underscores a lasting cultural preference but also points to cracks in the healthcare system that prevent widespread access to the best therapies. Unregulated use of these traditional methods sometimes raises real concerns about inconsistent dosing, potential toxicity, and unwanted interactions with conventional antimalarials. In most cases, rolling out traditional treatments safely demands strong quality control, clear and standardized protocols, and better education for both local healers and patients. Addressing these issues tends to align closely with broader health goals aimed at delivering fair and high-quality care that respects local beliefs while keeping risks in check (Margaret et al., 2018; WHO, 2020). When we look at strategies to better combat malaria in vulnerable groups, the mix between traditional methods and contemporary treatment plans becomes especially complex. Groups like pregnant women, young children, and other at-risk individuals face added dangers—not only from the disease itself but also from treatment approaches that may not be properly managed. Recognizing this, many experts suggest a more collaborative approach, where traditional healers join forces with modern medical professionals, sharing insights and building trust along the way. It also seems key to beef up surveillance and data collection on how these traditional treatments perform over time. As health systems gradually shift toward a model that emphasizes both quality and fairness, weaving traditional medicine into malaria treatment protocols might boost acceptance and adherence, as long as safety and effectiveness stay front and center. Altogether, such an inclusive framework could help reshape healthcare delivery in malaria-endemic regions, ensuring that even the most vulnerable get care that's both competent and thoughtful (Margaret et al., 2018; WHO, 2020) (Figure 14.13).

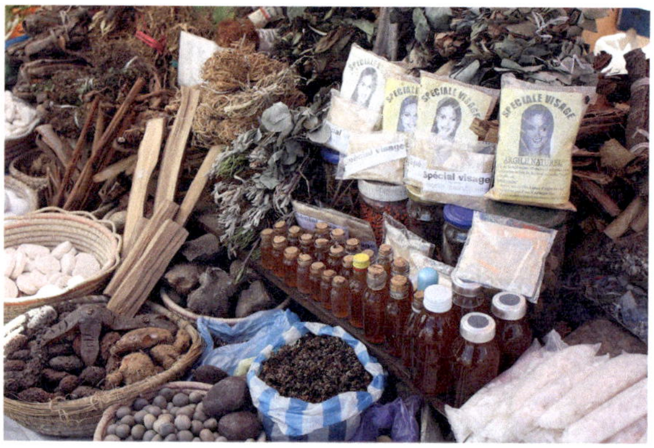

Figure 14.13. Traditional medicine and malaria treatment.

Source: By Marco Schmidt [1] - Own work, CC BY-SA 3.0, https://commons.wikimedia.org/w/index.php?curid=10554987

14.4.2. Community Attitudes Towards Malaria Prevention

Community feelings about fighting malaria aren't shaped by just one thing—they're swept along by bigger social and economic currents as well as by how local health services work. In many cases, people with fewer resources and those pushed to the margins end up facing higher malaria risks because they don't get the same easy access to prevention tools or healthcare. Often, this imbalance gets worse when basic health education is missing and when a cultural take on the disease steers individuals away from modern prevention. Even simple measures like using treated nets or inviting indoor spraying might meet with doubt, mixed-up information, or even simply be pushed apart by day-to-day survival challenges. To get what's behind these attitudes, you need to look at the social backdrop and the way public health messages are shared in places with scarce resources (Shadmi et al., 2020). This mix of challenges calls for interventions that tune in to local values and respect structural limits if malaria is ever to be controlled long-term. How communities deal with malaria also rests a lot on their trust in the local health services. In low- and middle-income settings, for instance, bad experiences, whether it's unskilled staff or disrespectful care, tend to erode confidence and make people less willing to adopt prevention practices. When the health system can't deliver reliable, courteous, or timely help, community engagement takes a hit, and widespread adoption of malaria control methods becomes a struggle. In most cases, improving the quality of care through smarter governance, better training of health workers, and more effective delivery systems goes a long way toward rebuilding that trust. If individuals see that their system is keeping up with expectations and providing fair access to prevention tools, they're more likely to join in the effort (Margaret et al., 2018). Further, broader social and political factors also play a big role in shaping local attitudes toward preventing malaria. Issues like social isolation, economic instability, and obstacles combined to gender or education can all keep certain groups from fully participating in malaria programs. Trying to get communities involved means grappling with these realities and working shoulder-to-shoulder with local leaders to create strategies that feel both culturally relevant and accessible. When communities are given clear, practical info about malaria risks and prevention, it sparks a sense of ownership that's crucial for lasting behavior change. Strengthening inclusive, high-quality care isn't just about meeting today's health demands, it also builds the kind of resilience needed to face future challenges in malaria control among those most at risk (Margaret et al., 2018; Shadmi et al., 2020).

14.4.3. Role of Cultural Practices in Disease Transmission

Malaria risk in special populations isn't only a matter of nature, it's also very much about long-held cultural habits. In many communities, how a household is set up and the way people choose to sleep are closely combined to traditions, and these choices can either heighten or lower the chance of getting bitten by mosquitoes. Poverty often makes matters worse by limiting access to effective prevention, meaning that everyday customs—whether it's shared bedrooms or particular house designs—play a bigger role than we might expect.

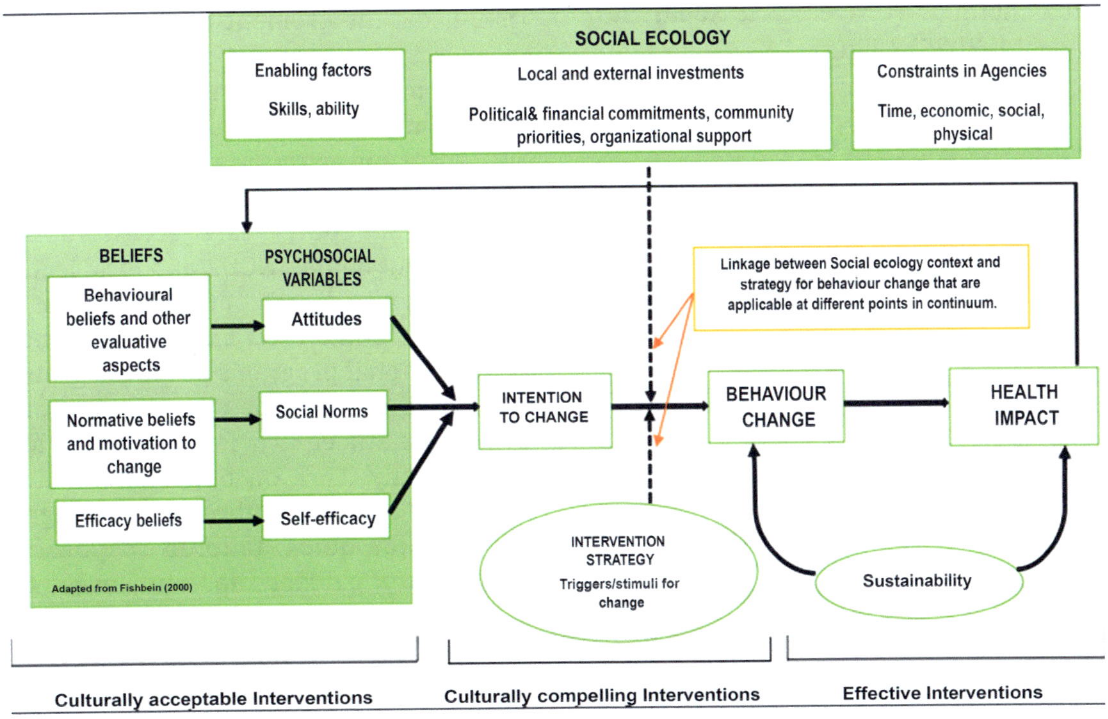

Figure 14.14. Role of cultural practices in disease transmission.

Source: Springer Nature. (2018). *Cultural Practices and Malaria Transmission.*

Generally speaking, these intertwined factors pose a real challenge for keeping the disease at bay (Nwaobi, 2025). Cultural practices go beyond just the layout of a home. Often, nighttime collections or community ceremonies take place outdoors, right when mosquitoes are most active, thereby upping the infection risk. At the same time, some individuals lean on traditional healers instead of formal medical services, which can delay proper care, especially impacting groups like pregnant women and children. In most cases, one finds that the mix of social rituals and environmental influences creates a layered problem, nudging experts to consider several angles in understanding how the disease spreads (Chaves & & Koenraadt, 2010). Trying to cut down on malaria means that public health strategies need to work hand-in-hand with cultural norms. With the risk landscape constantly shifting due to factors like climate variability and changes in land use, health programs must appreciate how local customs shape exposure and treatment habits. In short, mixing modern biomedical advances with a sensitive understanding of traditional ways not only makes sense but can also lead to more sustainable, community-approved prevention methods (Chaves & & Koenraadt, 2010; Nwaobi, 2025) (Figure 14.14).

14.5. Prevention Strategies

Special populations facing malaria prevention need extra care. Pregnant women, infants, and individuals with weakened defenses have their own hurdles because of immune changes or bodily shifts that make them prone to harsh disease. Sometimes the answer lies in mixing specific measures like IPTp with ITNs designed for these particular groups , and that combo can cut down both illness and death. A solid public health setup and community outreach that respects local ways are key to making these plans stick. Teaching people to use ITNs reliably and get quick access to tests can help spot issues early on. In most cases, these strategies must flex to local realities, since global differences – much like what we see with other infections – call for protocols that are tuned to individual communities (Christopher et al., 2022). Beyond just controlling mosquito vectors and using drugs as prevention, bolstering health systems is crucial for protecting these groups. Improving surveillance, refining diagnostic checks, and offering the right treatments seem essential when facing challenges like drug resistance and concurrent infections. Recent public health events generally remind us of the benefits of coordinated, continent-wide readiness and resource planning that speak directly to high-risk people (John et al., 2020). Strengthening lab work and making sure antimalarials are on hand can lower the chance of serious complications. Plus, merging malaria prevention into maternal and child health programs gives a more rounded care approach which, in many cases, also addresses socioeconomic issues that worsen vulnerability. In short, balancing fast-acting control with long-term reduction can build a resilient health system for those at risk. Local involvement and supportive policy measures also turn out to be major players in keeping malaria down among vulnerable groups. Health initiatives often focus on raising general awareness and getting the community to embrace prevention, despite hurdles like misinformation, stigma, and spotty care access. Sometimes government bodies, NGOs, and local leaders join forces in a way that smooths out the distribution of resources like ITNs and prophylactic drugs. When national programs put these groups first, it tends to boost fairness and even strengthens overall health equity. Policymakers, for their part, usually work on better surveillance and reporting tools so outbreaks get caught early, allowing for quick, tailored responses. With cross-sector partnerships and investments in education and infrastructure – not always a neat process – lasting progress can be made to ease malaria's toll and meet broader public health ambitions John et al., 2020; Christopher et al., 2022).

14.5.1. Use of Insecticide-Treated Bed Nets

Keeping malaria progress going isn't an easy feat, especially in areas that shift from high to low transmission. As cases drop, many people start feeling like the threat's mostly gone, and that can lead to skimping on prevention.

Zanzibar, for instance, shows a surprising twist: even when caretakers seem less alarmed, over 70% of kids under five still sleep under those long-lasting treated nets. Add a dose of indoor spraying and almost every child finds some protection. This steady commitment to prevention, even when fear is downplayed— speaks to the nets' importance in guarding our most vulnerable, like little ones who remain at risk (Beer et al., 2013). Bed nets protect best when they're not just available but also used properly, day in and day out. Seasonal changes, which affect how malaria spreads, sometimes nudge caretakers into using nets only during so-called high-risk periods. In Zanzibar, around 25% of caretakers admit they switch nets on seasonally. This mix of shifting weather and everyday habits underlines a core point: people still generally plan to stick with net use, which is a hopeful sign for ongoing efforts. It also means there's a solid need for regular community chats and education to keep the habit alive, especially among those who face bigger risks if malaria comes knocking again (Beer et al., 2013). Bed nets have long been the backbone of the fight against malaria, but new moves are on the horizon too. Researchers are testing ideas like genetically altered parasite vaccines which, in early studies, have shown promising signals for future malaria control. Until these vaccines become a regular option, though, keeping ITNs in use remains absolutely essential, especially for young kids and others with weakened immunity who bear a heavier share of the disease's toll. Maintaining high net coverage, paired with vigilant monitoring and flexible policies, is our best bet to sustain progress and, in most cases, finally push toward eliminating malaria.

14.5.2. Indoor Residual Spraying and Environmental Management

In areas where malaria is on the decline but still a worry, keeping up the protections is a must to prevent a comeback. Take Zanzibar for instance, caretakers there stick with measures like IRS and long-lasting insecticidal nets for kids under five, even if many see the disease as a distant problem. IRS means simply spraying insecticides on walls inside homes, which cuts down the mosquito count; mixed in with basic environmental clean-ups to remove mosquito breeding spots, it builds a solid defense. Communities seem to understand—repeating these steps over time shows just how much they value avoiding a malaria comeback (Beer et al., 2013). Switching gears, eliminating malaria calls for rethinking old control programs. Generally speaking, it's not enough just to keep using familiar methods—in most cases, improved surveillance and altering spray schedules to better match local needs are now in play. Instead of a one-size-fits-all plan, spraying frequency and coverage are adjusted based on specific local factors, like various mosquito types and their breeding grounds. Environmental management, which could involve draining stagnant water or clearing areas where mosquitoes hide, works hand in hand with IRS. This whole approach, integrated into a broader health system that can adapt to issues like insecticide resistance, relies on steady investments and cooperation between sectors, sometimes even across borders (Feachem et al., 2009). For special groups such as young children and those with weaker immunity, mixing indoor spraying with environmental clean-ups brings extra benefits. Simply, IRS reduces the number of mosquitoes inside the house during peak times, lowering the chance of a bite from an infected insect. At the same time, cleaning up around homes cuts back on the overall mosquito population. These combined actions—working both directly and indirectly—are crucial in settings where people have not built up full protection, and, honestly, where complacency might be creeping in as malaria cases fall. Continuous community education, along with slightly inconsistent but persistent use of both measures, helps keep everyone vigilant. All of this means that local ecological and cultural nuances are factored in, ensuring that the fight against malaria stays on track, even when it seems less urgent (Feachem et al., 2009; Beer et al., 2013) (Figure 14.15).

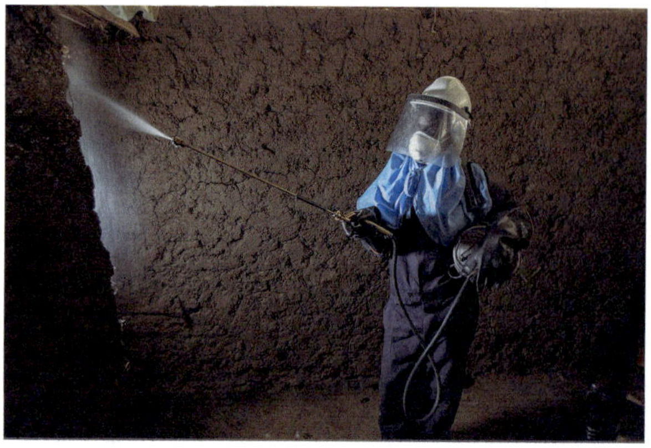

Figure 14.15. Indoor residual spraying.

Source: By President's Malaria Initiative - House IRS Kenya 7, Public Domain, https://commons.wikimedia.org/w/index.php?curid=72083473

14.5.3. Vaccination Efforts and Research

Eradicating malaria isn't a straight shot, it's been a winding road, one that's taken plenty of cues from past battles against diseases like smallpox, polio, and measles. Vaccines have stood at the heart of these struggles, generally speaking, and they've been central to turning the tide on infections. Research isn't confined to pristine lab settings; actually, it spills over into real-world fieldwork too, helping alter vaccine formulas, delivery styles, and even the timing of doses for different communities. Ongoing study not only sharpens vaccine performance but also sorts out issues unique to each epidemiological setting. With malaria's convoluted life cycle and the way, it shows up differently from one region to the next, flexible, adaptable research plans become absolutely necessary. Robust surveillance—mixed with modern molecular tools that track how the parasite evolves—is key to keeping vaccination efforts on target, especially for groups like pregnant women and immunocompromised individuals (Breman et al., 2011). When you dig into how malaria affects special populations, things get even more varied; immune responses can shift noticeably in people such as pregnant women or those with other health conditions. They need vaccines that are safe and strong enough to provide real protection. It's not only about measuring vaccine efficacy in sterile tests—human factors matter too. Cultural beliefs, local health practices, and even the everyday way people think about and access vaccines play a heavy role in designing immunization programs that can reach a broad audience and keep up the fight against malaria. In most cases, as the final stages of eradication come into view, persisting spots of transmission will force us to innovate in vaccine delivery and keep rechecking our strategies to match changing realities (Breman et al., 2011).

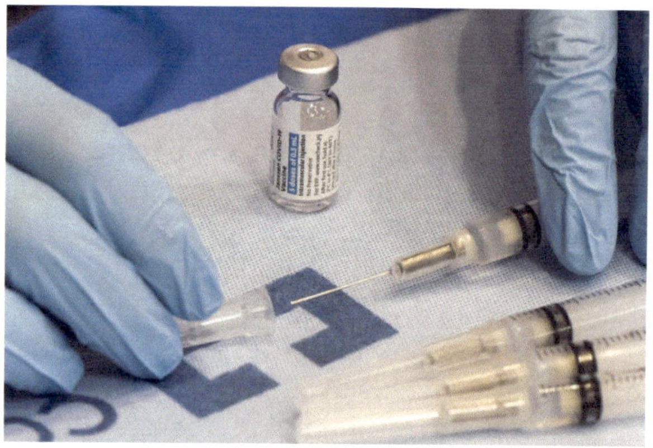

Figure 14.16. Vaccination efforts and research.

Source: The Washington Post. (n.d.). *505TSXVBZUI6XMYUF2MTXWB6GE. https://external-content.duckduckgo.com/iu/?u=https%3A%2F%2Fwww.washingtonpost.com%2Fwp-apps%2Fimrs.php%3Fsrc%3Dhttps%3A%2F%2Farc-anglerfish-washpost-prod-washpost.s3.amazonaws.com%2Fpublic%2F505TSXVBZUI6XMYUF2MTXWB6GE.jpg%26w%3D1440&f=1&nofb=1&ipt=a1c0103d7a1441cb8df054b8cbfa44880f169197c755d7a4e5efc597d8796303.*

Even if malaria shares some traits with other zoonotic diseases like rabies, rolling out vaccines in resource-thin settings is still a huge challenge. Look at African canine rabies campaigns—these efforts show that huge vaccination drives can work when detailed data and sharp operational insights come into play, like nailing down target group estimates and fine-tuning logistics to reach everyone. Translating those lessons into malaria vaccination means beefing up surveillance systems and directing resources toward high-risk areas. Economic assessments, too, hint that getting ahead with vaccination is cost-effective, underscoring the importance of rolling out comprehensive immunization programs to protect those most hit by malaria's heavy burden (Figure 14.16).

14.6. Treatment Challenges

Treating malaria in certain groups isn't as simple as following a set protocol. When you work with populations like pregnant women, infants, or people juggling other health issues, the body's own features tend to throw off how drugs are absorbed and used. This means that setting up just the right dose, and checking in on patients regularly—is a must. Rising antimicrobial resistance further messes with the usual treatments, often causing therapies to fall short and illnesses to worsen. Further, limited access to proper diagnostics and treatment centers in many low-resource areas only deepens the trouble (Christopher et al., 2022). To summarize, you need a strategy that mixes clinical know-how, local disease trends, and practical logistics. Another tough nut to crack is how fast drug-resistant malaria strains are spreading. It's frustrating because these altered *Plasmodium* strains not only weaken the primary drugs but also tend to prolong sickness and boost the risk of severe outcomes. Kids and immunocompromised individuals, in particular, struggle more since their bodies just can't handle extra side effects or clear infections as efficiently. Just like what we've seen with bacteria, this kind of resistance in malarial parasites calls for serious investment in new medications and better monitoring practices (Christopher et al., 2022). Plus, when issues like HIV or tuberculosis are already on the table, careful juggling of medications becomes even more critical, piling on to an already complex treatment landscape. In many malaria-prone regions, scarce resources and uneven health services add another layer of difficulty. Often there aren't enough well-equipped labs or seasoned practitioners, meaning that catching and managing the disease quickly turns into a guessing game. This gap sometimes forces a reliance on presumptive treatments, which can backfire by promoting improper drug use and further fueling resistance. Moreover, problems with procuring and distributing medicines can make it tough to keep treatments consistent. Experiences from other infectious diseases in resource-strapped settings show that ramping up surveillance, training staff, and getting ready for emergencies are crucial steps. Strengthening these areas in malaria-endemic places is vital if we're going to overcome these challenges and truly help those hit hardest.

14.6.1. Drug Resistance and Its Implications

Drug resistance has become a challenging problem for global health, especially when it comes to handling malaria in those most at risk. Not too long ago, breakthroughs in biomedical science had many of us believing that we could finally nip infectious diseases in the bud with new drugs, however those pesky malaria strains evolved in ways that defied our hopes. In many cases, the heavy use of antimalarial treatments puts enough pressure on parasites that some manage to slip past therapy. This twist in evolution not only threatens decades of progress but also forces us to rethink our treatment methods. The mix of uneven drug exposure and the parasite's own clever biological maneuvers (think both molecular and metabolic alters) makes it hard to figure out lasting fixes. So, generally speaking, understanding the trade-offs and costs in this evolutionary race is key for keeping treatments effective, especially for those like pregnant women and immunocompromised individuals who are hit the hardest (Findlater et al., 2018). When you look beyond just the individual patient, drug resistance in malaria ripples out to affect whole communities. Partially treated or untreated infections can become hidden reservoirs that help spread the disease even further. And mind you, the way people move around internationally only speeds things up, as resistant parasites hitch a ride into areas that were once under control (Findlater et al., 2018). For special groups—children or individuals with other health issues—the problem often leads to higher sickness and even greater risk of fatality, complicating how clinicians try to manage the cases. Moreover, our heavy reliance on a very limited set of antimalarial drugs ups the stakes, making it almost inevitable that resistance becomes widespread unless we mix in both new drug ideas and prevention steps like enhancing vector control. To summarize, the complex interplay between drug resistance and the environment demands cooperative monitoring and cross-border teamwork to tackle these emerging threats effectively (Echaubard et al., 2018; Findlater et al., 2018). Keeping malaria in check among vulnerable populations calls for strategies that take the parasite's evolving nature into account. Some research suggests that alternating drug regimens, using combination therapies, or even varying how and when treatments are given—be it across different places or times—can help slow down resistance. Studies on parasite life-history trade-offs have even hinted that the selection pressures from our drugs might be nudging these organisms to change their transmission traits, which then affects disease patterns across whole populations. Mixing these insights might just pave the way for new treatment protocols that are fine-tuned to the special needs of high-risk groups, balancing short-term wins with long-term durability (Echaubard et al., 2018). Ultimately, dealing with drug resistance calls for an adaptive, flexible management plan that considers the complex association between host, parasite, and environment; thus building a bit of extra resilience into our malaria control programs in these ever-changing epidemiological landscapes (Figure 14.17).

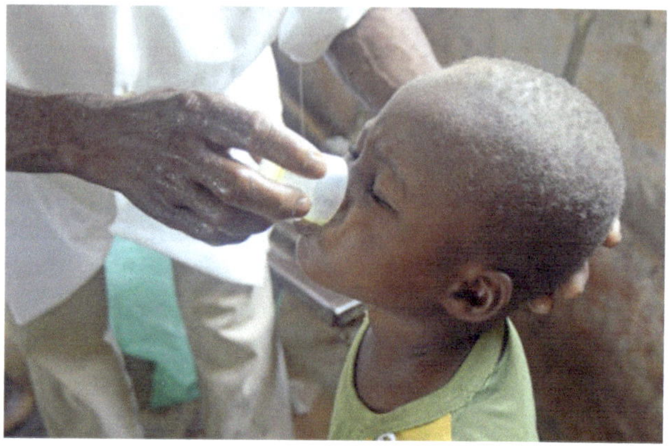

Figure 14.17. Drug resistance and its implications in malaria.

Source: The New York Times. (2014). *Drug Resistance in Malaria.*

14.6.2. Access to Effective Treatment in Special Populations

Access to proper malaria treatment in certain groups isn't as straightforward as it seems. Social, cultural, and even environmental issues mix together and make getting a quick diagnosis and care challenging. Take gold miners in the Amazon, for example, they often live in rough conditions with almost no nearby medical help. Their mobile way of life and a deep-seated wariness of formal clinics push many to depend on old-fashioned remedies or unchecked medications, which in most cases ends up with poor treatment and extended periods of being contagious. Further, these miners often hold on to outdated ideas about how malaria spreads, a view that frequently stops them from using prevention measures or following treatment plans consistently. To get things right, interventions need to appreciate these unique lifestyles and dig into how these miners think and act, so that outreach can be both culturally respectful and effective (Murta et al., 2021). Older adults face a whole different set of hurdles when it comes to treating malaria. For many seniors, other health issues can mask or even worsen malaria symptoms. Cognitive issues, like dementia, or at times even a bout of delirium—can make it hard for them to quickly spot the signs of illness or stick to treatment instructions. In hospitals, where older patients are especially at risk, delirium may worsen cognitive decline and cloud the diagnostic picture further. It becomes essential, then, to ensure proper sensory stimulation, hydration, and strict infection control in these settings. Generally speaking, melding malaria care with broader geriatric treatment isn't a luxury, it's a necessity to help these vulnerable individuals recover properly (Livingston et al., 2020). This multifaceted challenge calls for a team effort that targets both the infection and the complications arising from aging. Making sure that everyone gets fair access to malaria treatments, especially in remote or marginalized communities, means facing many logistical and systemic challenges. Health systems have to adjust on the fly, whether that means sending out mobile clinics or setting up community-based check-ups to catch and treat malaria earlier. Although programs that distribute drugs widely hold promise for lowering malaria rates, these efforts sometimes hit a wall because of local fears and cultural beliefs surrounding medication safety. By involving local stakeholders and acknowledging indigenous practices while still backing evidence-based solutions, a better balance can be struck that promotes trust and cooperation. In most cases, this integrative approach, drawing on both social insights and rigorous medical efforts, helps bridge the gap between official healthcare services and the community's lived realities (Murta et al., 2021) (Figure 14.18).

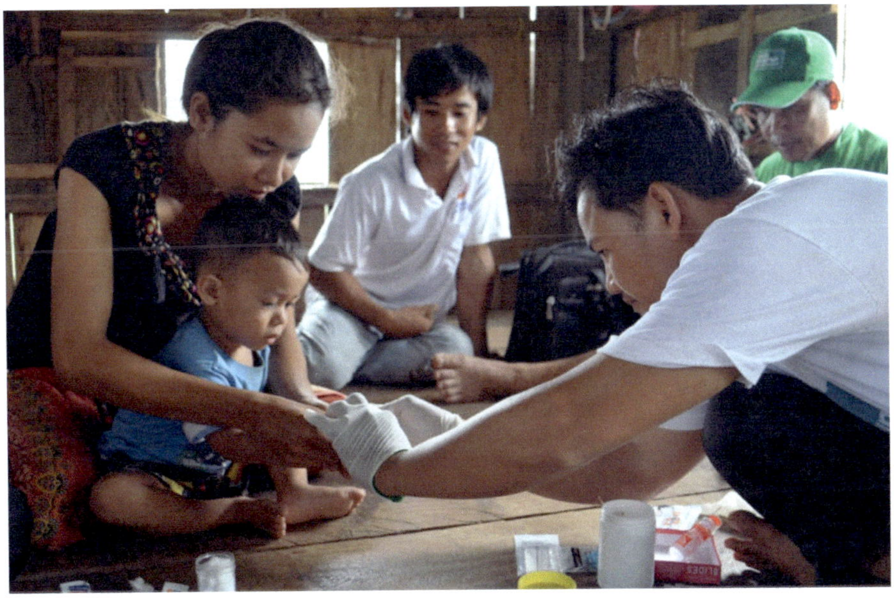

Figure 14.18. Access to effective treatment in special populations.

Source: University of Melbourne. (n.d.). *Access to Malaria Treatment.*

14.6.3. Barriers to Healthcare Services

In many parts of the world where malaria is common, getting proper healthcare is a real struggle. Teens and young adults, for example, often find themselves stuck in school settings where the available health services just don't cut it for what they need. Sure, there might be basic clinics offering malaria tests and treatments, but most young people aren't aware of more specialized care. Limited supplies, not enough trained staff, and a lack of privacy all add up to create big obstacles to effective treatment. Social stigma, mixed with a general misunderstanding of what patients need, only worsens the situation. And when key services don't reach those who are already marginalized, efforts to fight malaria take an even bigger hit. In most cases, boosting funding and improving training can help break down these barriers and make care fairer for everyone (Jacobs et al., 2023). Inequalities in healthcare for communities dealing with malaria go well beyond just the limits of a single institution; they mirror deeper economic and societal divides. Low-income and minority groups, squeezed into crowded living conditions with few quality healthcare resources, find themselves at greater risk and receive slower diagnoses and treatments as a result. Then you have global crises like the COVID-19 pandemic throwing extra wrenches into the works—resources get pulled away and travel becomes a problem, so routine services take a back seat. The economy takes a hit too, which makes it even tougher for those already struggling to pay for healthcare. All these structural roadblocks mean that targeted policies and community-based programs are needed to lessen malaria's impact on these special populations (Shadmi et al., 2020). It isn't just money or logistics at play either—cultural or communication barriers also make it tough for many to access malaria care. In lots of regions, local health systems don't adapt to the diverse needs of their communities, partly because there isn't enough emphasis on cultural understanding. Young people, for instance, might hold back from seeking help over worries about privacy or judgment. Similarly, individuals with disabilities or from marginalized backgrounds often face discrimination that discourages them from even trying to get care. In most cases, making services not only available but also friendly and adapted to different cultural contexts is key. Mixing in peer education and approaches that respect cultural nuances could build trust and boost the use of malaria prevention and treatment options among these vulnerable groups (Jacobs et al., 2023).

CLOSER LOOK

PLASMODIUM VIVAX

Plasmodium vivax is one of the five species of malaria-causing parasites known to infect humans, alongside *P. falciparum, P. malariae, P. ovale*, and *P. knowlesi*. While it is generally less deadly than *P. falciparum, P. vivax* is the most geographically widespread species and presents unique challenges to malaria control and elimination efforts due to its ability to cause recurrent infections.

P. vivax is predominantly found in Asia, Latin America, and parts of the Middle East and Oceania. Unlike *P. falciparum*, which thrives mostly in sub-Saharan Africa, *P. vivax* can develop in cooler climates and higher altitudes, allowing it to exist in a broader range of ecological zones. It accounts for a significant proportion of malaria cases outside Africa, particularly in South and Southeast Asia.

Like all *Plasmodium* species, *P. vivax* is transmitted through the bite of an infected female Anopheles mosquito. Once in the human host, sporozoites travel to the liver, where they develop into liver-stage parasites called schizonts. A unique and important feature of *P. vivax* is its ability to form dormant liver-stage parasites known as hypnozoites. These hypnozoites can reactivate weeks, months, or even years after the initial infection, causing relapses without a new mosquito bite. This ability makes *P. vivax* particularly difficult to eliminate.

After the liver stage, parasites enter the bloodstream and infect red blood cells. Infected individuals may experience fever, chills, headache, vomiting, and fatigue—classic symptoms of malaria. Though *P. vivax* typically causes milder illness than *P. falciparum*, it can still lead to severe disease, especially in children and pregnant women, and contributes to significant morbidity.

The relapsing nature of *P. vivax* makes it harder to control than *P. falciparum*. Many national malaria programs focus more heavily on *P. falciparum*, and diagnostic and treatment tools are less tailored to *P. vivax* infections. The need for G6PD testing before administering primaquine or tafenoquine further complicates treatment delivery in resource-limited settings.

Additionally, *P. vivax* often causes low-density infections that are harder to detect, contributing to ongoing transmission by asymptomatic carriers. These factors make surveillance, treatment, and elimination efforts more complex.

SUMMARY

Malaria control for certain communities isn't a simple medical challenge, it's wrapped up in our environment and social fabric. Climate change, for instance, keeps shifting where and when malaria pops up, affecting not only local ecosystems but everyday lives too. Experts now have to mix insights from natural and social sciences to help vulnerable areas build some resilience. In most cases, the idea of climate-resilient development gives us some clues; it pushes for sustainable changes that look after nature and our own health. You can't separate the fight against malaria from global efforts to tackle climate change and its domino effects on disease patterns (Intergovernmental Panel on Climate Change, 2023). To summarize, this broad and, at times, complex approach matters if we're going to spot and ease new risks for those hit hardest by the disease. It's not just the environment that plays a role—how accessible and solid our health systems are equally key. Sure, some regions are making headway, but many still see pregnant women, kids, and immunocompromised individuals getting shortchanged by inconsistent care. When quality drops, inequalities increase and trust takes a hit, especially among those already up against a lot of systemic barriers. Pushing for universal health coverage that focuses on improving quality is pretty much a must if we want to cut down on malaria's toll. Some existing frameworks, often born out of resource-strained settings—offer a kind of rough guide on boosting services for at-risk communities (Margaret et al., 2018). , putting these vulnerable groups first remains essential to turning progress in treating malaria into real, tangible health benefits. If you take a step back, the bottom line is clear: fighting malaria in special populations means tackling issues from all angles, mixing environmental strategies with a strong healthcare push. Climate shifts and social inequities are so intertwined nowadays that old, one-dimensional strategies just won't cut it. Future gains depend a lot on political commitment to build high-quality health infrastructure, fair policies, and community-driven initiatives that match the unique needs of each group. This kind of all-around strategy not only promises to ease the malaria burden but also nudges us closer to broader health fairness and sustainable progress. In the end, sticking with a unified, flexible plan is crucial to making sure our malaria control efforts stay effective and responsive in an ever-changing global scene (Margaret et al., 2018; Intergovernmental Panel on Climate Change, 2023).

Malaria's toll on at-risk groups isn't just about the parasite itself; it comes from many factors that collide in unpredictable ways. Pregnant women, children, people with weakened immune systems, and travelers all face their own ups and downs because their bodies can react differently, sometimes their natural defenses aren't up to par and exposure risks vary widely. These individuals usually bear a heavier burden of illness and death, which shows we need special ways to test for, treat, and prevent malaria. Social and economic challenges paired with inconsistent healthcare only make things tougher in areas where the disease is common. In most cases, when you throw in elements like shifting climate patterns and the ever-changing face of infection outbreaks, the need for strategies that flexibly address both biological and environmental issues becomes clear (Intergovernmental Panel on Climate Change, 2023). The growing problem of drug resistance is another twist in the malaria story, especially for these vulnerable groups. We're now seeing resistant strains of the *Plasmodium* parasite, which generally hit populations that already struggle with limited access to care even harder. As these resistant strains cause infections to persist longer, they end up fueling the spread of malaria, leading to worse outcomes overall. It's a bit of a double-edged sword: as treatments lose their punch, infections take longer to clear, complicating recovery and driving up transmission rates. Understanding this resistance is pretty crucial if we're to make smart policy moves about drug distribution and come up with better treatment plans. Strengthening ways to watch for these trends, like boosting lab facilities and surveillance—is key, especially in resource-challenged settings where these at-risk groups live (Christopher et al., 2022). Putting it all together, it seems tackling malaria in these special segments means mixing clinical care, outbreak tracking, and social-environmental insights into one mixed approach. Preventive steps such as using insecticide-treated nets, giving pregnant women intermittent preventive treatments, and even rolling out vaccines can cut down infection rates and bad outcomes. Better diagnostic tools and treatments that fit individual needs would boost care for the most vulnerable. It also takes working together across different fields, such as climate resilience efforts and careful management of antimalarial drugs—to adapt to the challenges coming from both environmental shifts and growing drug resistance. In most cases, a broad, continuous push focusing on these at-risk communities is essential if we want to control malaria worldwide, which means we have to keep investing in research, better healthcare systems, and stronger community ties (Christopher et al., 2022; Intergovernmental Panel on Climate Change, 2023).

KEY TERMS FROM THIS CHAPTER

- Pregnant Women
- Low Birth Weight
- Children Under Fi ve
- Seasonal Malaria Chemoprevention (SMC)
- HIV Co-infection
- Imported Malaria
- Refugees and Displaced Persons
- Elderly Populations
- Co-morbid Conditions
- Placental Malaria
- Infants
- Severe Malaria in Children
- Immunocompromised Individuals
- Non-immune Travelers
- Migrant Populations
- Occupational Risk Groups
- Asymptomatic Carriers
- High-Risk Populations

References

1. Deribe, K., Meribo, K., Gebre, T., Hailu, A., Ali, A., Aseffa, A., & Davey, G. (2012). The burden of neglected tropical diseases in Ethiopia, and opportunities for integrated control and elimination. *Parasites & vectors*, *5*, 240. https://doi.org/10.1186/1756-3305-5-240
2. Aung, T., Lwin, M. M., Sudhinaraset, M., & Wei, C. (2016). Rural and urban disparities in health-seeking for fever in Myanmar: findings from a probability-based household survey. *Malaria journal*, *15*(1), 386. https://doi.org/10.1186/s12936-016-1442-zBalgir, R. S. (2011). Genetic disease burden, nutrition and determinants of tribal healthcare in Chhattisgarh State of Central-East India: A status paper. https://core.ac.uk/download/pdf/332892.pdf.
3. Lembo, T., Hampson, K., Kaare, M. T., Ernest, E., Knobel, D., Kazwala, R. R., Haydon, D. T., & Cleaveland, S. (2010). The feasibility of canine rabies elimination in Africa: dispelling doubts with data. *PLoS neglected tropical diseases*, *4*(2), e626. https://doi.org/10.1371/journal.pntd.0000626
4. Beer, N., Ali, A. S., Shakely, D., Elfving, K., Al-Mafazy, A. W., Msellem, M., Petzold, M., Björkman, A., & Källander, K. (2013). High effective coverage of vector control interventions in children after achieving low malaria transmission in Zanzibar, Tanzania. *Malaria journal*, *12*, 38. https://doi.org/10.1186/1475-2875-12-38 (accessed on 13 May 2025).
5. Bourhy, H., Gaidet, N., & Molia, S. (2012). Mission to Indonesia to participate in the 1st Indonesia-France Seminar in Medicine & Public Health and investigate potential collaborations on animal health: 2nd–9th of November 2012. http://agritrop.cirad.fr/567354/1/document_567354.pdf (accessed on 13 May 2025).
6. Bradley, D., Cairncross, S., Haines, A., & Stephens, et al. (2001). Health and sustainable development. https://core.ac.uk/download/13110836.pdf (accessed on 13 May 2025).
7. Breman, J. G., de Quadros, C. A., Dowdle, W. R., Foege, W. H., Henderson, D. A., John, T. J., & Levine, M. M. (2011). The role of research in viral disease eradication and elimination programs: lessons for malaria eradication. *PLoS medicine*, *8*(1), e1000405. https://doi.org/10.1371/journal.pmed.1000405 (accessed on 13 May 2025).
8. Carmignani, F., & Chowdhury, A. (2011). The development effects of natural resources: A geographical dimension (WP 2011-09). https://core.ac.uk/download/67751462.pdf (accessed on 16 May 2025).
9. Chaves, L. F., & Koenraadt, C. J. M. (2010). Climate change and highland malaria: Fresh air for a hot debate. https://core.ac.uk/download/pdf/29238217.pdf (accessed on 16 May 2025).
10. Dunn-Georgiou, E., Gay, J., & Hardee, K. (2009). *A Practical Guide to Integrating Reproductive Health and HIV/Aids into Grant Proposals to the Global Fund.* A Practical Guide to Integrating Reproductive Health and HIV/AIDS into Grant Proposals to the Global Fund. https://core.ac.uk/download/71342654.pdf (accessed on 13 May 2025).
11. Echaubard, P., Rudge, J. W., & Léfèvre, T. (2018). Evolutionary perspectives on human infectious diseases: Challenges, advances, and promises. *Evolutionary Applications, 11*, 383–393. https://doi.org/10.1111/eva.12586.
12. Feachem, R.G.A., with A.A. Phillips and G.A. Targett (eds) (2009). Shrinking the Malaria Map: A Prospectus on Malaria Elimination. San Francisco: The Global Health Group, Global Health Sciences, University of California, San Francisco. (accessed on 13 May 2025).

13. Findlater, A., & Bogoch, I. I. (2018). Human mobility and the global spread of infectious diseases: A focus on air travel. *Trends in Parasitology, 34*, 772–783. https://doi.org/10.1016/j.pt.2018.07.004.

14. Hussain, A., Bhowmik, B., & do Vale Moreira, N. C. (2020). COVID-19 and diabetes: Knowledge in progress. *Diabetes Research and Clinical Practice, 162*, 108142. https://doi.org/10.1016/j.diabres.2020.108142.

15. Intergovernmental Panel on Climate Change. (2023). *Climate Change 2022–Impacts, Adaptation and Vulnerability*. https://doi.org/10.1017/9781009325844.

16. Jacobs, C., Mwale, F., Mubanga, M., Kasonde, M., Saili, A., Mukonka, R., Mwilu, L. M., et al. (2023). Perceptions of youth-friendly sexual and reproductive health services in selected higher and tertiary education institutions of Zambia: A qualitative study on the perspectives of young people and healthcare providers. *PLOS Global Public Health, 3*, e0002650. https://doi.org/10.1371/journal.pgph.0002650.

17. Okumu, F. O., Sumaye, R. D., Matowo, N. S., Mwangungulu, S. P., Kaindoa, E. W., Moshi, I. R., Madumla, E. P., & Lwetoijera, D. W. (2013). Outdoor mosquito control using odour-baited devices: development and evaluation of a potential new strategy to complement indoor malaria prevention methods. *MalariaWorld journal*, *4*, 8. https://doi.org/10.5281/zenodo.10894810 (accessed on 13 May 2025).

18. Kruk, M. E., Gage, A. D., Arsenault, C., Jordan, K., Leslie, H. H., Roder-DeWan, S., Adeyi, O., et al. (2018). High-quality health systems in the Sustainable Development Goals era: Time for a revolution. *The Lancet Global Health, 6*, e1196–e1252. https://doi.org/10.1016/S2214-109X(18)30386-3.

19. Kunkel, A., Nguon, C., Iv, S., Chhim, S., Peov, D., Kong, P., Kim, S., et al. (2021). Choosing interventions to eliminate forest malaria: Preliminary results of two operational research studies inside Cambodian forests. *Malaria Journal, 20*. https://doi.org/10.1186/s12936-020-03572-3.

20. Liu, MD., Li, CX., Wang, XZ. *et al.* Impact of ecological migration village construction on vector mosquito and mosquito-borne disease in the southern Yunnan Province, China. *Int J Trop Insect Sci* **44**, 1117–1123 (2024). https://doi.org/10.1007/s42690-024-01226-4(accessed on 16 May 2025).

21. Livingston, G., Huntley, J., Sommerlad, A., Ames, D., Ballard, C., Banerjee, S., Brayne, C., et al. (2020). Dementia prevention, intervention, and care: 2020 report of the Lancet Commission. *The Lancet, 396*, 413–446. https://doi.org/10.1016/S0140-6736(20)30367-6.

22. Murray, C. J. L., Ikuta, K. S., Sharara, F., Swetschinski, L. R., Robles Aguilar, G., Gray, A. P., Han, C., et al. (2022). Global burden of bacterial antimicrobial resistance in 2019: A systematic analysis. *The Lancet, 399*, 629–655. https://doi.org/10.1016/S0140-6736(21)02724-0.

23. Murta, F., Marques, L. L. G., Santos, A. C., Batista, T. S. B., Mendes, M. O., Silva, E. D., Silva Neto, A. V., et al. (2021). Perceptions about malaria among Brazilian gold miners in an Amazonian border area: Perspectives for malaria elimination strategies. *Malaria Journal, 20*. https://doi.org/10.1186/s12936-021-03820-0.

24. PATH (2014). *Community-Based Approach to Intermittent Preventive Treatment for Malaria in Pregnancy in Kisumu, Kenya*. https://core.ac.uk/download/75781810.pdf (accessed on 16 May 2025).

25. Nkengasong, J. N., & Mankoula, W. (2020). Looming threat of COVID-19 infection in Africa: Act collectively, and fast. *The Lancet, 395*, 841–842. https://doi.org/10.1016/S0140-6736(20)30464-5.

26. Nwaobi, G. C. (2025). *Modelling the Health Sector Policy Reforms for Nigeria: A Phased Project Study*. https://core.ac.uk/download/pdf/9312772.pdf (accessed on 13 May 2025).

27. Shadmi, E., Chen, Y., Dourado, I., Faran-Perach, I., Furler, J., Hangoma, P., Hanvoravongchai, P., et al. (2020). Health equity and COVID-19: Global perspectives. *International Journal for Equity in Health, 19*. https://doi.org/10.1186/s12939-020-01218-z.

28. Topazian, H., Charles, G. D., Schmit, N., Pianella, M., Marshall, J. M., Kleinschmidt, I., Hauck, K., et al. (2024). Estimating the potential impact of surveillance test-and-treat posts to reduce malaria in border regions in sub-Saharan Africa: A modelling study. *Malaria Journal, 24*. https://www.semanticscholar.org/paper/931dc278d46fc72018b0fca8940026086a535684 (accessed on 13 May 2025).

29. Tudi, M., Ruan, H. D., Wang, L., Lyu, J., Sadler, R., Connell, D., Chu, C., et al. (2021). Agriculture development, pesticide application and its impact on the environment. *International Journal of Environmental Research and Public Health, 18*, 1112. https://doi.org/10.3390/ijerph18031112.

30. United Nations. (2016). *The Millennium Development Goals Report*. https://doi.org/10.18356/98544aa9-en.

31. Vetter, V., Denizer, G., Friedland, L. R., Krishnan, J., & Shapiro, M. (2017). Understanding modern-day vaccines: What you need to know. *Annals of Medicine, 50*, 110–120. https://doi.org/10.1080/07853890.2017.1407035.

32. World Health Organization. (2020). Clinical management of severe acute respiratory infection (SARI) when COVID-19 disease is suspected: Interim guidance. *Pediatria i Medycyna Rodzinna, 16*, 9–26. https://doi.org/10.15557/pimr.2020.0003.

33. Yeboah, A. (2023). Comparative analysis of factors associated with insecticide-treated net utilization between rural and urban areas in Ghana: Implication for malaria control and prevention. https://core.ac.uk/download/580972573.pdf (accessed on 13 May 2025).

34. Zinyengere, D. T. (2018). Household determinants of malaria in Mutasa District of Zimbabwe. https://core.ac.uk/download/217230200.pdf (accessed on 13 May 2025).

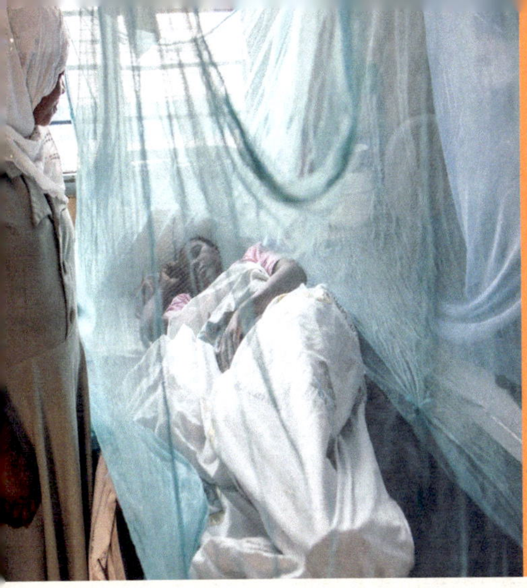

Chapter 15

HEALTH SYSTEMS AND MALARIA CONTROL

Contents

Introduction

Malaria still holds its ground as a nagging problem across many parts of the world, and global health hurdles only add to the mix. In many areas, improvements in technology and treatments haven't completely overpowered the fact that health services aren't always up to par – clinics, hospitals, and local outreach programs all play a role, and sometimes, these links falter unexpectedly. It isn't only about tackling the parasite; it's also about looking closely at the whole network that brings diagnosis, prevention, and treatment to people. This overlap between effective health service delivery and controlling malaria gives us clues about where things might be slipping, and in many cases, it sparks ideas for better, more resilient strategies to lower both the number of cases and the fatalities. New treatments have opened up fresh possibilities for managing malaria. Take tafenoquine, for instance – a single-dose drug that works to clear those hard-to-reach parasites hidden in the liver (specifically *Plasmodium vivax* hypnozoites), which are often responsible for relapses that hurt treatment success.

Of course, no breakthrough drug can work in a vacuum; its effectiveness hinges on the health system's capacity, which has to include proper diagnostics, like testing for glucose-6-phosphate dehydrogenase deficiency before tafenoquine is given. Modeling studies generally show that when patients stick to their treatment plans and when these new drugs are woven into existing strategies, transmission rates can be reduced significantly (Nekkab et al., 2021). But it all comes down to whether local health setups can keep up with these innovations. In places on the brink of wiping out malaria, staying alert and ready to respond is even more critical. Fewer cases can sometimes lull both communities and health workers into a false sense of ease, which risks undoing years of hard work. Research in low-transmission settings tells us that keeping a sharp eye on every potential case – even when they seem rare – is essential to prevent any resurgence (Azizi et al., 2020). Ensuring that case management routines remain sharp and that the healthcare workers are actively engaged can make all the difference. In the long run, fusing gradual health system strengthening with malaria-specific efforts is seen as the backbone of any sustainable push toward total disease elimination (Figure 15.1).

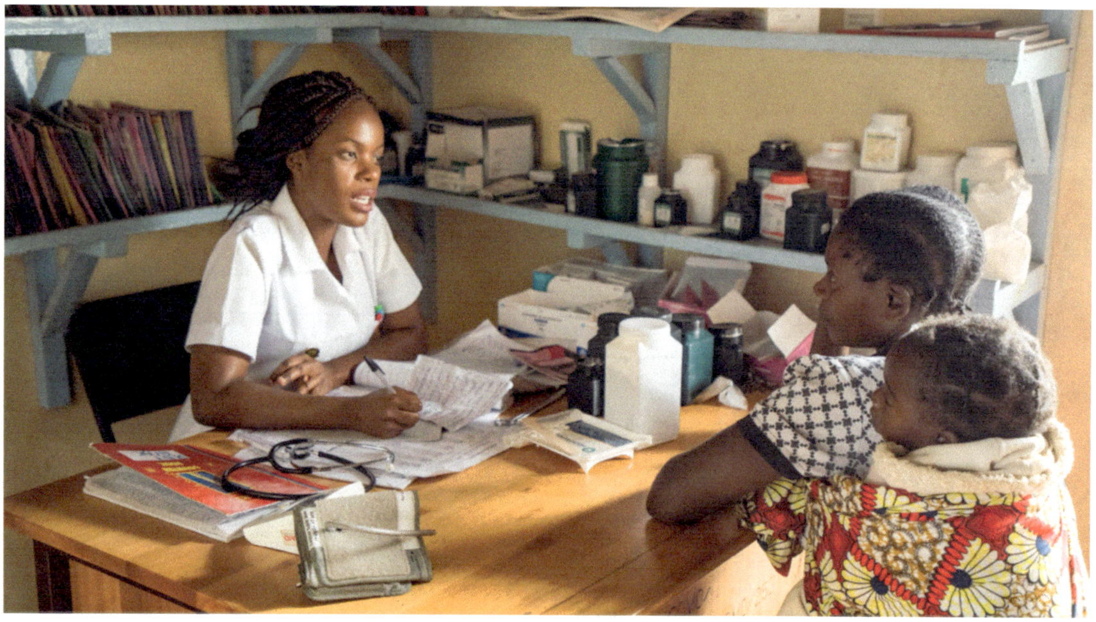

Figure 15.1. Health systems and malaria control.

Source: Bill & Melinda Gates Foundation. (n.d.). *GH malaria GA1780641 JH539869. https://external-content.duckduckgo.com/iu/?u=https%3A%2F%2Fwww.gatesfoundation.org%2F-%2Fmedia%2Fgfo%2F4our-work%2Fprograms%2Fglobal-health%2Fgh_malaria_ga1780641_jh539869new3200x1800.jpg%3Fh%3D726%26iar%3D0%26mw%3D1290%26w%3D1290%26hash%3D810230DFE97E97B58429C10FEA9DEFD2&f=1&nofb=1&ipt=d36c6f0fdd1e9a2807859159d636ba57189d8021366a71cf6632e94d683eaa12.*

Definition of Health Systems

Health systems are a bit like the many layers of a pie, it's not just hospitals or clinics, but groups, individuals, and all sorts of actions aimed at keeping us healthy, restoring health when needed, and generally keeping things in balance. Instead of being solely about treating patients, there's also the money side, the rules, and even information sharing that keep the whole thing ticking. They sort of exist in a wild mix of social and economic settings where each part bumps against another. You might say their success shows up in fewer illnesses or a longer life for people, thanks to everything from keeping problems at bay to patching things up. Look at global disease trends, and you notice that these systems are always having to shift gears to handle challenges like malaria, where success hinges as much on organized care as on community involvement (Spencer et al., 2018). The strength of a health system matters, especially where malaria is still a big worry. It's not enough to have flashy buildings or heaps of cash; the care given needs to be spot-on, prompt, and delivered with a respectful tone—qualities that build trust and encourage people to seek help. In practical terms, good care means keeping patients safe, nailing down correct diagnoses, offering treatments that work, and sticking with patients over time. When any of these bits drop the ball, malaria tends to stick around and cause even more trouble. Plus, these systems must also juggle good management, a skilled team, and clever data use that can pivot as malaria's spread shifts over time. If a health system can weave malaria control into its overall work, it shows its central role in the fight against the disease (Margaret et al., 2018). Digging even deeper, one has to look at fairness and how easy it is for everyone to use these health services—two things that are especially key for beating malaria. Health coverage should have no gaps, making sure that even the people on the edge get the prevention and treatment they need. Economic inequalities, remote locales, and even cultural features can shape who gets help, which is why solutions must be wide-ranging and involve local voices. Plus, there's a need for solid ways to measure how well services are doing, from tracking quality and spending to seeing improvements in health related to malaria. Good systems keep an eye on the numbers to learn and adapt, ensuring that efforts fit local realities. In short, when you think about health systems with malaria in mind, you see they're not just the loose parts that hold everything together—they're the driving force behind fair, quality care for everyone (Margaret et al., 2018; Spencer et al., 2018).

Overview of Malaria as a Global Health Issue

The global health community has pushed hard against infectious diseases, yet malaria still proves stubborn in many resource-poor areas. In sub-Saharan Africa, for instance, the mix of local weather, economics, and weak infrastructure spurs its spread. It's not just about illness—malaria digs into economies and stretches out fragile health systems juggling other diseases. And with COVID-19 in the picture, things get even messier; the overlapping signs like fever, fatigue, or breathing issues make it hard to tell one from the other, especially when labs aren't fully equipped. This overlap calls for screening methods that mix well into existing routines so that misclassifications are kept to a minimum, ensuring care that's both prompt and fitting (Chanda et al., 2020). Systemic holes in the health setups of many low- and middle-income countries only add to the malaria burden. Often, these areas lack enough funding, skilled staff, and essential supplies, which means efforts like regular surveillance, quick diagnostic tests, vector control, and solid patient management can fall short. In most cases, when emergencies like pandemics hit, they pull away precious resources, sometimes undoing all the progress made against malaria. The international community is increasingly aware that our health systems need to be more resilient and flexible. Even with broader access to rapid tests and treatments, the unpredictable nature of outbreaks means that ongoing investments in readiness (and addressing root social issues like poverty and rapid urban growth) are absolutely critical (Madhav et al., 2017). Then again, the fact that malaria often shows up alongside new infectious threats weaves a complex picture of environmental, epidemiological, and system challenges. People on the move, whether due to travel or migration, can unintentionally spread malaria and other pathogens, further complicating control efforts. Strengthening our health systems becomes key here, it's about preventing illness, catching it early, and managing not only malaria but its co-infections, too. Coordinating community efforts with facility-level services may sound simple, but it can help stretch limited resources while improving outcomes. Integrated health approaches should push for easily available testing and treatment to lower both transmission and severe cases. In a broader sense, dealing with malaria through the lens of pandemic readiness boosts overall health security and renews our collective drive toward universal health coverage and sustainable disease control (Madhav et al., 2017; Chanda et al., 2020) (Figure 15.2).

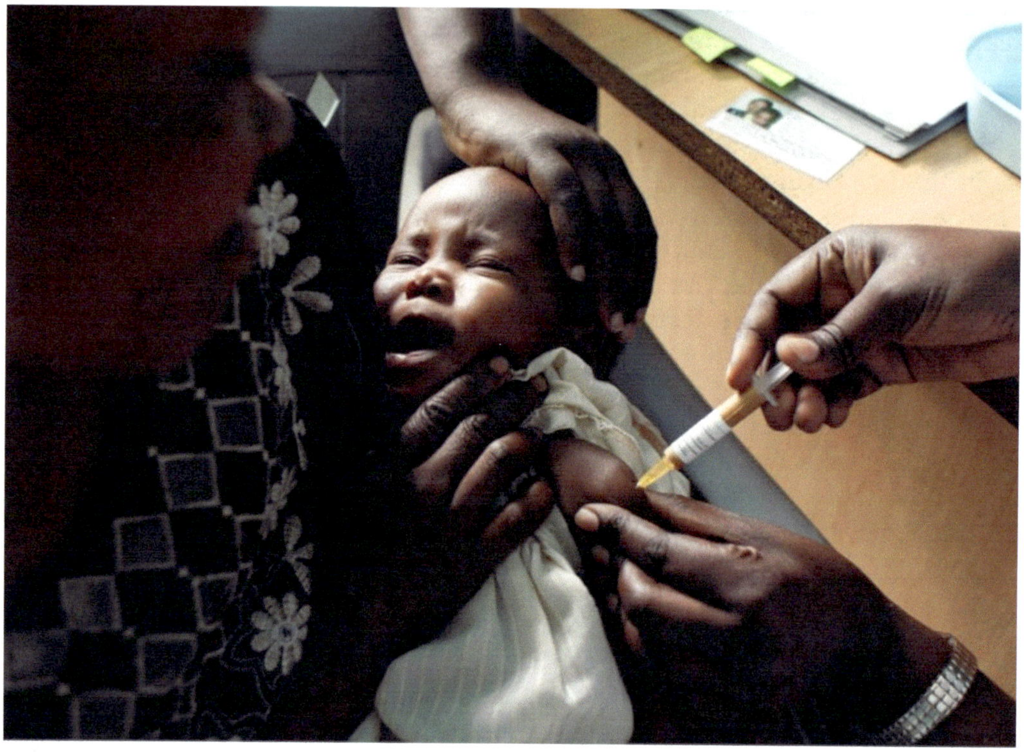

Figure 15.2. Malaria deaths still at "unacceptably high levels" worldwide.

Source: Global News. (2019). *Malaria Deaths Remain High Globally.*

Importance of Effective Malaria Control Strategies

Malaria control is a must, especially in places where stretched health systems can barely keep up. The spread of the disease isn't fixed, it twists and turns with local environments, social habits, and money issues. Old evaluation methods, in most cases, miss the long-term ripple effects of interventions, so resources sometimes end up used in less helpful ways. Sometimes mixing math-based simulations with everyday health setups brings out insights that wouldn't otherwise appear. For example, modeling how a new malaria vaccine might roll out alongside regular immunization programs can reveal both its effectiveness and cost issues across different settings. This kind of approach tends to mirror real-life complexities, nudging interventions toward more fitting and sustainable action in affected areas (Tediosi et al., 2010). Using modern data-driven tools lets policymakers handle the unpredictability of malaria more nimbly. Techniques like stochastic multi-armed bandit models and Gaussian Process regression open up new ways to test various policy options, yielding strategies that respond to simulated outcomes. Unlike traditional expert judgment, these computer-driven methods keep refining recs continuously as new data, and the disease's unpredictable twists—come in. This flexible approach means that health systems can better adapt their control strategies to distinct local situations, ultimately improving coverage, boosting adherence, and driving down the risks and fatalities linked with malaria (Bent et al., 2017). Beyond immediate health outcomes, well-coordinated and context-aware malaria strategies have a wider impact on social and economic fronts. Effective measures can ease the heavy financial strain malaria places on low-income countries, where budgets are tight and competing health needs run high. Combining efforts, like vaccines, solid case management, and vector control—help stretch benefits across both health and financial sectors. Taking a long, hard look at the cost-effectiveness of different delivery methods further reveals which strategies sustainably cut transmission while best using available resources. This comprehensive, albeit sometimes complex, planning is key to moving from basic control toward eventual elimination in the right areas. Overall, these dynamic, evidence-informed approaches show real promise for lasting health improvements and building stronger, more resilient systems (Tediosi et al., 2010).

15.1. Historical Context of Malaria

Malaria has troubled humanity for centuries, its history woven into early records that capture our clumsy attempts to fight a little-understood foe. In those days, treatments often missed the mark, and children, among others, suffered tremendous losses. Even regions like Italy—once thought clear of the disease—have started seeing local cases emerge, a sign that our health systems can sometimes be caught off guard. This stubborn persistence is partly because the parasite develops resistance to our treatments and mosquitoes even shrug off insecticides. Generally speaking, such challenges call for better surveillance and more resilient health services in low-resource settings, and a real mix of social, political, and cultural insights must complement our scientific efforts to address malaria's deep and ongoing public health impact (Buonsenso & Cataldi, 2010). It isn't all about money, either; political will or strong institutions have had their say over the years. Comparisons from sub-Saharan Africa, say between Tanzania and Uganda, reveal a striking contrast. While both countries faced similar economic pressures, Tanzania invested thoughtfully in health infrastructure and malaria policy—efforts that noticeably reduced child mortality. Uganda, on the other hand, often stumbled over political instability and weakened health governance, which in turn undermined its control programs. In most cases, this tells us that sturdy governance and protected, merit-based health institutions are as crucial as any fiscal resource. Even if the details differ, one thing remains clear: history shows us that political and institutional strength must join economic considerations to fight malaria effectively (Croke et al., 2011). Looking back, the forces shaping malaria's spread have always been more than just scientific challenges. Social factors—how communities live, how power is shared, even the scars left by wars—can tip the scales in unexpected ways. Past eradication efforts often fell short because they ignored the complex mix of cultural, political, and economic influences on local populations. Resource imbalances and power struggles, for instance, consistently frustrated even our brightest scientific advances. Nowadays, building health systems with an eye on history means tailoring malaria strategies to local realities, ensuring that technical fixes are paired with policies aimed at reducing social inequities. In the end, this long view of malaria pushes us toward a comprehensive, multidisciplinary approach that pairs medical science with real-world socio-political complexities in order to protect those most at risk (Buonsenso & Cataldi, 2010) (Figure 15.3).

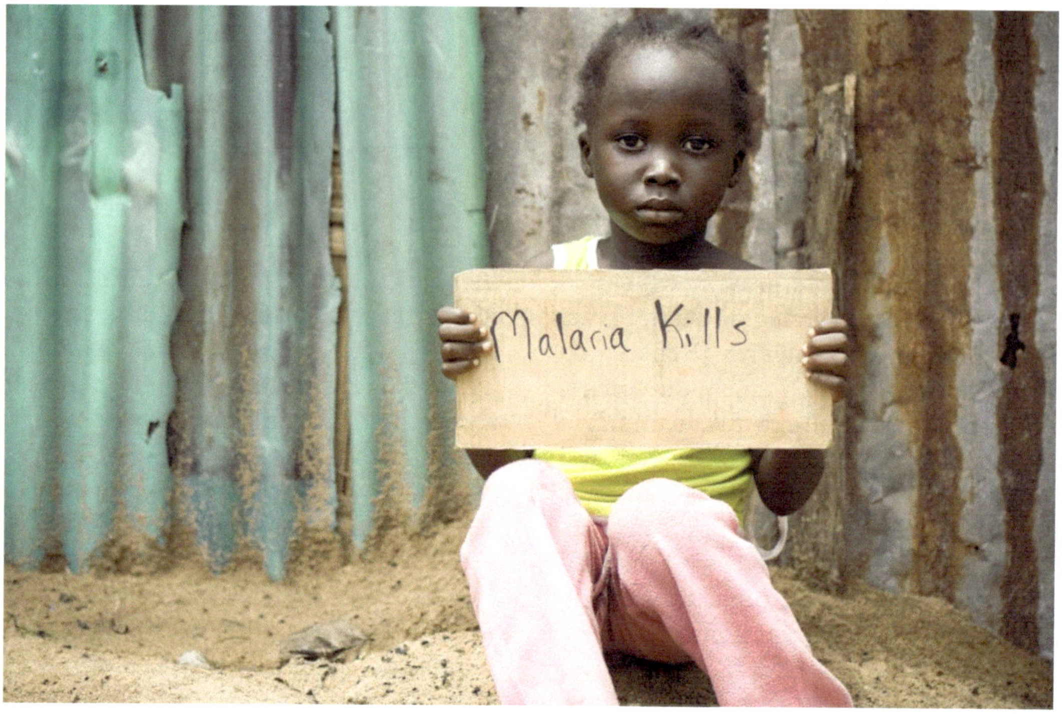

Figure 15.3. The historical context of malaria.

Source: Cambridge Independent. (n.d.). *Historical Perspective on Malaria.*

15.1.1. Historical Prevalence of Malaria Worldwide

Malaria's struggle has spanned centuries—evidence shows it was widespread long before our modern treatments even existed. Vast stretches of Africa, Asia, Europe, and the Americas hosted this relentless disease, not simply because it was an inevitable visitor but largely due to climates that made life easy for Anopheles mosquitoes, those prime carriers. People moving from place to place, shifts in the environment, and harsh socio-economic setbacks all helped keep malaria around, even when early control efforts stumbled. Its effects weren't only on health; the disease also reshaped economies and social habits, influencing where individuals settled and how work was organized. To summarize, the continuing fight against malaria reminds us why strong, adaptable health systems—ones that both prevent and treat such infections—are so critical to global public health priorities (Bever et al., 2016). Understanding how malaria ebbs and flows over time and across different places is key to crafting effective control methods. Historical records tell us that transmission rates could swing wildly between neighboring areas, shaped by natural settings and the everyday movements of people. Sometimes, small, but stubborn—pockets kept the disease alive even when nearby regions saw drops in cases, making a complete wipeout a real headache.

In most cases, recent insights from regions like Lake Kariba in Zambia have shown that pairing mass drug administration with extra measures, such as insecticide-treated nets, can seriously alter these patterns. Generally speaking, malaria's historical footprint isn't fixed; it flexes in response to our interventions and daily behaviors, reminding us to mix scientific know-how with practical health strategies to lessen the disease burden regionally and globally (Bever et al., 2016). Looking back at malaria control, our health systems have gradually grown more flexible in facing this ongoing challenge. Advances from research, policymaking, and community outreach have wedded together in ways that often reveal just how complex malaria transmission can be. Annual reports and institutional reviews, while sometimes a bit repetitive, consistently show that both academic circles and health organizations have dug deep into these trends—helping mold strategies on local and international levels. The mix of data-rich modeling with on-the-ground field work reflects today's modern approach to understanding and curbing malaria's spread. Clearly, progress depends on steady investments in health infrastructure and fresh ideas, as past control efforts have shown both memorable wins and stubborn obstacles when it comes to finally breaking malaria's cycle worldwide (Figure 15.4).

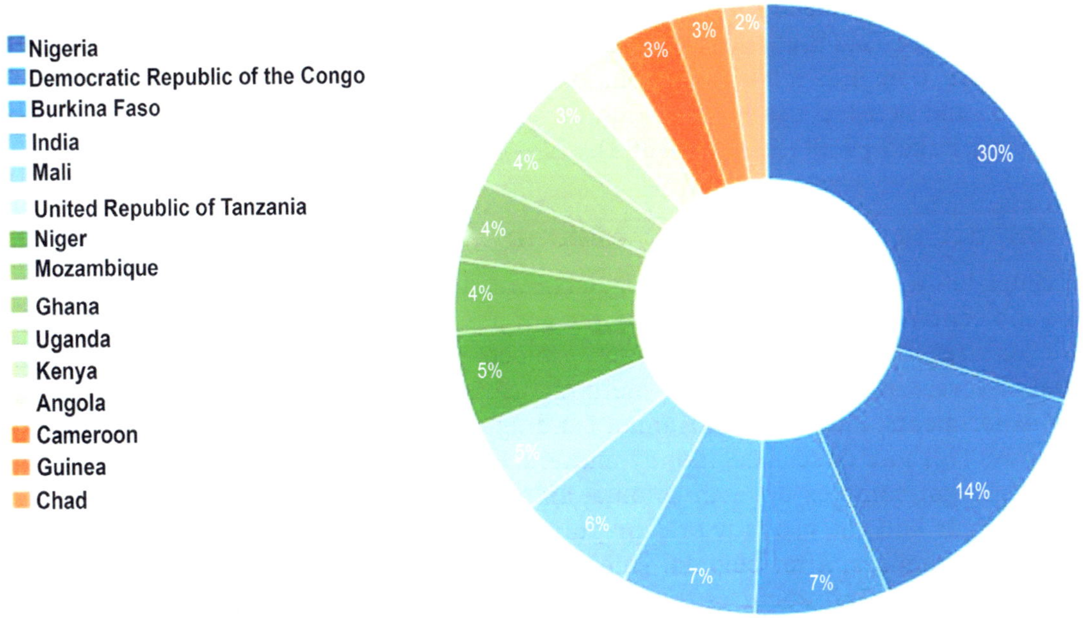

Figure 15.4. Historical prevalence of malaria worldwide.

Source: Down To Earth. (2017). *Global Malaria Prevalence Map.*

15.1.2. Evolution of Malaria Control Measures

Malaria control has been on quite the rollercoaster ride for nearly a century. Early on, people mainly tackled the problem by messing with the environment—draining swamps and clearing mosquito hangouts, even though they only had a basic idea of how the parasite, mosquito, and people all fit together. Then, around the mid-1900s, chemical tools like DDT came along and suddenly indoor spraying was the big thing, cutting down transmission in many parts of the world. Still, putting too much trust in chemicals soon showed mosquitoes aren't so easily tricked; they began to adapt in unexpected ways. All of this history, in most cases, highlights that fighting malaria isn't just a chemical or biological challenge, it's many understanding local social conditions, environmental shifts, and the ever-changing tricks of the pathogens (Wallace et al., 2003). Nowadays, the emphasis has shifted to methods like insecticide-treated nets and indoor spraying because, generally speaking, they work well against mosquitoes that tend to stick indoors. But as these tools got rolled out on a larger scale, it also became clear that not all mosquitoes play by the same rules. Some types have learned to bite outdoors or even switch to non-human creatures, which means the transmission isn't halted entirely despite our best efforts. This isn't to say that outright resistance has taken over; rather, it's more like an ecological reshuffling where the smarter, adaptable mosquitoes end up surviving. Keeping a close, if somewhat casual, eye on these behavioral twists is pretty key for health teams trying to stay ahead of the game (Govella et al., 2013). At the same time, the way we treat malaria has morphed along with our growing grasp of how medicine mixes with everyday life. It turns out that how well a treatment works isn't just about genetics or drugs, it also reflects social stresses and deeper inequalities that affect patients. Instead of pigeonholing the issue as merely a genetic fate, newer views (and, yes, even Lewontin's so-called "triple helix" idea) nudge us toward thinking in broader, messier terms. Factors like early development, environmental features, and even daily social pressures get complex up in treatment outcomes. In most cases, this broader look suggests that a one-dimensional approach simply won't cut it. Successful malaria control, therefore, demands a health system overhaul that meshes together biomedical fixes with socioeconomic and political changes—a kind of real-world mix where medicine and social justice are inseparably linked (Wallace et al., 2003).

15.1.3. Impact of Colonialism on Malaria Management

Colonial times left a deep stamp on how malaria was handled from the very start. Settler health was front and center while indigenous concerns got pushed apart, all in the name of protecting big economic ventures like massive infrastructure projects and plantation setups that needed a steady, healthy labor force. In many cases, the methods used were heavy-handed, such as forced labor and risky experiments, like that odd Human Landing Catch technique where individuals were put in harm's way. This mix of science, money matters, and power plays shows a complex mix where fighting disease got complex up with colonial ambitions (Chakraborty et al., 2013). Even though these early efforts laid the groundwork for public health, they were also steeped in exploitation and ethical compromises. After colonial rule, newly independent nations found themselves stuck with old systems and infrastructures that didn't quite match their diverse needs. Health programs built under colonial rules typically zoomed in on one disease at a time, leaving broader public health issues by the wayside. Generally speaking, this narrow focus made it tough to achieve lasting improvements, because it barely scratched the surface of social and economic factors that let malaria stick around. Studies remind us of that poverty and disease often feed off each other, suggesting that without a boost in living conditions, the push for better preventive practices stays weak. In most cases, the shadow of colonial legacies continues to warp health priorities and overall malaria control strategies (Chakraborty et al., 2013). Today, teams fighting malaria still wrestle with hangovers from those old colonial systems that keep shaping policy decisions. Outside funding agencies often steer research and interventions in ways that echo past dominance, and it's not unusual to see a reliance on outdated methods such as labor-intensive mosquito checks using human volunteers—strategies that feel all too familiar. While these approaches do yield useful entomological data, they also spark uneasy questions about labor ethics and whether human life is properly valued in research settings. Generally speaking, acknowledging these historical threads is key to crafting malaria control strategies that lean more on local know-how rather than external dictates. A closer look at this legacy may help build approaches that are fairer and more in tune with the real needs of communities (Ann et al., 2011) (Figure 15.5).

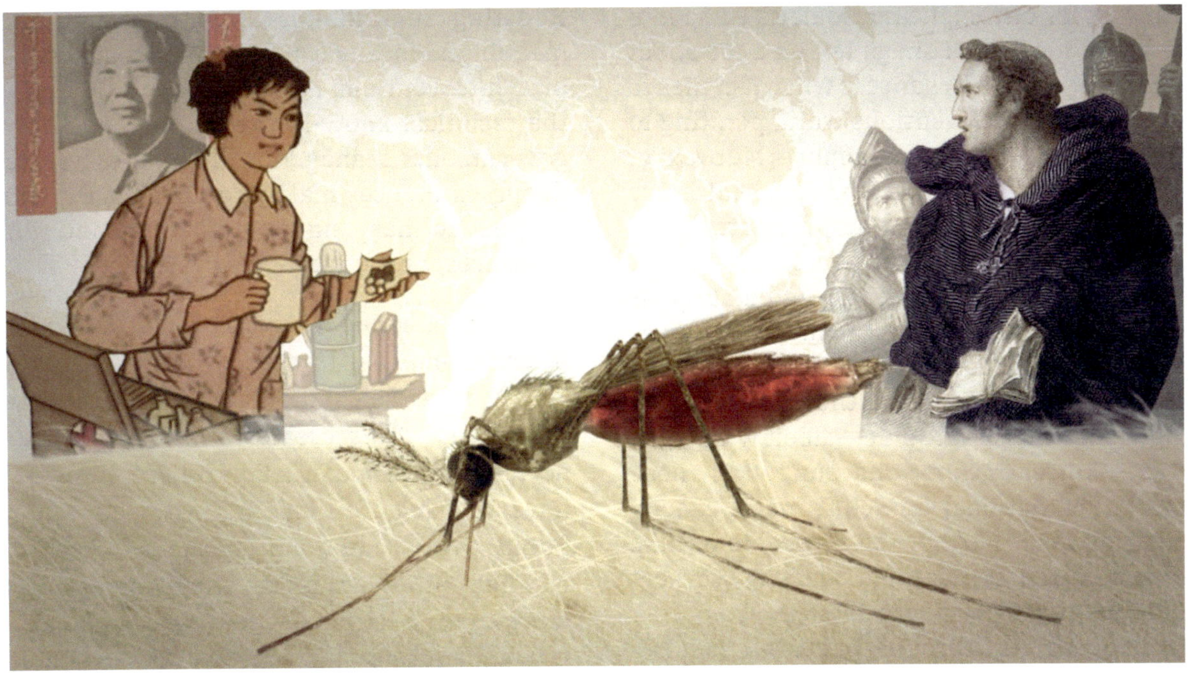

Figure 15.5. Colonialism on malaria management.

Source: NPR. (2012). *Colonial History and Malaria.*

15.2. Current Global Health Systems

Malaria control isn't simple at all. Global health systems are tangled up in challenges that emerge all over the place—in some cases, not just medicine but many sturdy infrastructure, steady governance, and people who know their stuff makes the difference. In many parts of the world, getting quality healthcare remains an uneven game. When resources run dry, broken systems can't keep supplies steady or hold on to trained staff, so treatments and tests often don't arrive on time. You see these links everywhere, since moving drugs around and putting policies into practice lean heavily on efficient government and proper money management, even though these factors shift from one country to the next. Generally speaking, knowing these behind-the-scenes parts helps us figure out why malaria control makes progress sometimes and stumbles at other moments (London School of Hygiene and Tropical Medicine, 2013). At the local level, district health management teams turn out to be a big deal, bridging the gap between national plans and the details on the ground. The story of District Council Health Management Teams (CHMTs) in parts of Africa shows both some wins and plenty of bumps along the way, especially when it comes to giving pregnant women malaria prevention treatments. Even with some financial backing and training aimed at better antenatal care, things like funding delays, too-few people working, and supply hiccups keep holding them back.

Subsequently, there's intermittent preventive treatment with sulfadoxine-pyrimethamine (SP) – its popularity keeps shifting because drug policies change and the public isn't always on board, particularly after new first-line treatments for uncomplicated malaria came into play. These local-level snags tell us a lot about how crucial good governance is when it comes to making malaria interventions work, pointing to the need for more tailored support (Mubyazi et al., 2013). Mixing public and private healthcare even further muddies the waters. Private clinics often run almost on their own, rarely syncing up well with government programs, and that opens up gaps in coverage which can mean fewer opportunities for people to get free or subsidized malaria meds. District authorities usually acknowledge the private side—albeit with some caution—since tracking and supplying these drugs under national guidelines isn't exactly straightforward. Further, basic problems like unreliable water sources and a lack of workers sometimes force providers to stray from best practices, such as directly observed malaria therapy. Local political will, shown when extra resources are thrown into the mix, proves pretty important for easing these issues. To summarize, boosting health systems means juggling better governance, smarter resource distribution, and working together across every corner of healthcare delivery (Mubyazi et al., 2013).

15.2.1. Structure of Health Systems in Malaria-Endemic Regions

Robust malaria control in areas where it's common depends a lot on health systems that can deliver prevention, diagnosis, and treatment. National programs often sketch out the big plan while local clinics and regional centers bring the ideas to life, sometimes in surprising ways. Community health workers, for example, play a huge role, reaching out into far-flung areas to spot malaria signs early and jump on treatment without delay. Of course, things aren't always smooth: unpredictable infrastructure, too few staff, and unpredictable supply chains tend to get in the way. All these issues, mixed with shifting political will and funding, generally point to the need for flexible health frameworks that can keep up with malaria's ever-changing patterns. Boosting surveillance and using data that's meaningful locally can help steer resources and plan interventions more effectively. It isn't just the technical know-how that matters; the way governments manage and fund these systems deeply influences malaria outcomes. Decisions, shaped by many national agendas and global pressures, aren't made in a vacuum.

For countries with tight budgets, incoming international aid is crucial, but it sometimes comes with rules that don't quite jibe with local needs. This creates a bit of a balancing act for National Malaria Control Programs—they have to navigate demands from government bodies, NGOs, and donor agencies, occasionally running into overlapping efforts or duplicated work. When choices are made only at the top, subnational differences in malaria spread can get lost, showing that more collaborative, context-sensitive approaches are needed to turn global ambitions into real, sustainable change (Intergovernmental Panel on Climate Change, 2023). Climate changes and environmental factors throw yet another wrench into how health systems work in malaria-endemic regions. With weather patterns shifting and mosquito behaviors evolving, systems need to be nimble—able to adjust when malaria risk rises unexpectedly. Global studies tell us that planning for climate resilience is key if malaria interventions are to stay effective over time. This kind of planning calls for team efforts across health, environmental monitoring, and community outreach (sometimes things get a little complex in practice). When health planners put climate info to work, they can target efforts like indoor spraying and insecticide-treated net distribution much more precisely. In the end, mixing ecological insights with societal needs creates a tougher system that can hold its own, even when the environment throws some unpredictable challenges our way (Intergovernmental Panel on Climate Change, 2023) (Figure 15.6).

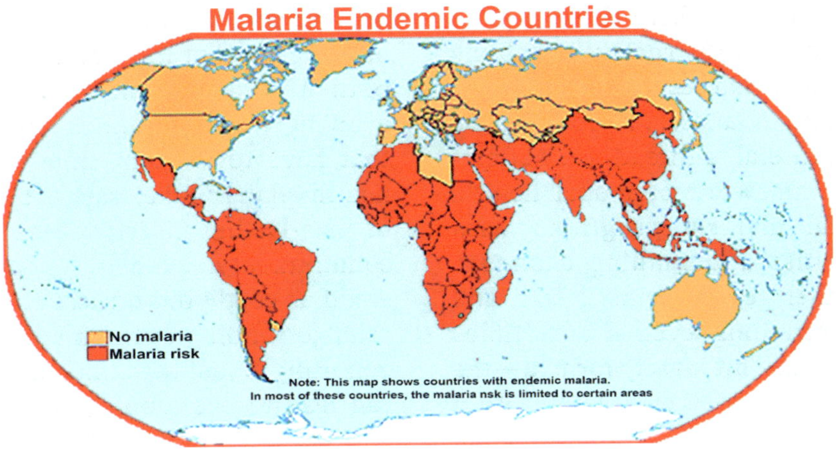

Figure 15.6. Structure of health systems in malaria-endemic regions.

Source: Penn State University. (n.d.). *Malaria Distribution and Health Systems.*

15.2.2. Role of International Organizations in Malaria Control

Managing infectious diseases in areas with struggling healthcare systems isn't as simple as it might seem, it takes many coordinated plans and multiple strategies. International players jump in here, boosting local health efforts against malaria by creating partnerships that cross borders and traditional limits. They bring together funds, skills, and technology so that countries facing malaria head-on can roll out better ways to prevent, diagnose, and treat the disease. Take the WHO, for instance; it often steps up as a central hub setting global standards and rallying efforts to improve surveillance and response strategies. In most cases, their leadership helps ensure that the measures are rooted in evidence yet tailored to fit various local conditions. Plus, many of these global agencies remind us issues like poverty and limited education, which can heavily impact health that need to be addressed too (Juvekar & Hegde, 2024). In short, their influence isn't just technical; it also shapes smart policies to push for fairer health access around the globe. Beyond just juggling policies, international organizations also roll out innovative capacity-building projects that empower local health systems to manage malaria better. They often set up collaborative programs that focus on transferring knowledge and honing skills for both seasoned healthcare providers and community workers alike. You can see this in partnerships where Chinese public health experts work directly with African teams, an example often dubbed "Paired Learning by Doing." This kind of hands-on collaboration, where experts from different backgrounds learn and implement solutions together—sparks the adoption of methods like the "1,7-malaria Reactive Community-based Testing and Response" model. Such efforts not only lead to noticeable drops in malaria rates but also boost the long-term resilience of local institutions when facing public health challenges (Lu et al., 2023). Generally speaking, these international endeavors act as a driving force behind sustainable progress through shared expertise and creative learning approaches. At the same time, international groups also fuel South-South and triangular cooperation, letting developing countries swap know-how and resources more fluidly. This trend has become especially important as emerging economies like China get more involved in global health, particularly in regions where malaria is a major hurdle. These partnerships help fill in gaps in both experience and infrastructure, enabling targeted interventions that respect local disease patterns and cultural nuances. Moreover, these organizations are careful to thread these efforts into the larger framework of global health, aligning national malaria programs with worldwide priorities and funding channels. By knitting together governments, NGOs, and community organizations, even if sometimes the connections seem a bit loosely formed—the result is a more cohesive healthcare system. With a push toward shared responsibility and global health fairness, international organizations are proving essential in widening the reach of malaria control measures, thereby lowering the illness and death rates linked to the disease (Lu et al., 2023; Juvekar & Hegde, 2024).

15.2.3. Funding and Resource Allocation for Malaria Initiatives

Malaria control kicks off with the need for strategic cash that fits both local health goals and global funding norms. It isn't as straightforward as just spending money; different players like international donors, governments, and local implementing groups must work together in unpredictable ways so that efforts don't overlap but rather boost one another. Global Health Initiatives (GHIs) play a big role here—their way of running things tends to shape exactly where the funds end up, ensuring that key interventions such as insecticide-treated nets, indoor spraying, and antimalarial treatments get the boost they need. When a country takes charge, it not only taps into sustainability but also weaves malaria control into the bigger picture of health system improvements. International partnerships, especially those aimed at uplifting marginalized communities (women and girls, for instance), are another piece of the puzzle (KFF Policy Brief, 2010). To summarize, pairing up proper funding with smart governance and these kinds of teamwork moves turns out to be essential for enduring malaria control. Money matters in malaria control are all about looking closely at how every dollar flows and counting up impacts, both now and later. New technologies and evolving WHO guidelines stir up budget needs that have to slide in smoothly with national health plans. Take, say, the constant supply of long-lasting insecticide-treated nets or the commitment needed for indoor spraying—both stand as costly but critical strategies that need reliable funding over time. Studies show that, generally speaking, uncoordinated spending can lead to overlapping costs and fragmented efforts, which in turn trim down efficiency and cost-effectiveness. In most cases, developing a cost model that covers both direct spending and extra expenses, like staffing and infrastructure—helps health planners anticipate financial needs better, making a case for more sensible funding. Subsequently there's the potential entrance of new tools like malaria vaccines (Mtui & Osoro, 2011), which will shake up how resources have to be distributed. In short, a robust approach to fiscal planning is crucial if malaria control is to stick around even when budgets are tight. Getting the resources for malaria programs isn't a walk in the park. There's a heavy reliance on outside aid and the noisy unpredictability of donor money, and that can mess with steady program rollouts. Even though international development partners do chip in significantly, leaning too hard on them can sap a nation's ability to set its own priorities, making the whole approach a bit patchy. Several long-range strategy documents show just how fragmented funds can get, often, the available cash is only a small slice compared to what's needed. This mismatch forces countries into thinking outside the box, sometimes ramping up domestic financing strategies, like sticking to the Abuja Declaration's call for a 15% health budget in African nations. Strengthening costing skills, regularly checking what's driving expenses, and mixing financial planning across various programs all help streamline the process. Ultimately, sustainable malaria control isn't just about amassing enough funds; it's about deploying them through a coherent, interconnected framework that boosts the overall health system (KFF Policy Brief, 2010; Mtui & Osoro, 2011) (Figure 15.7).

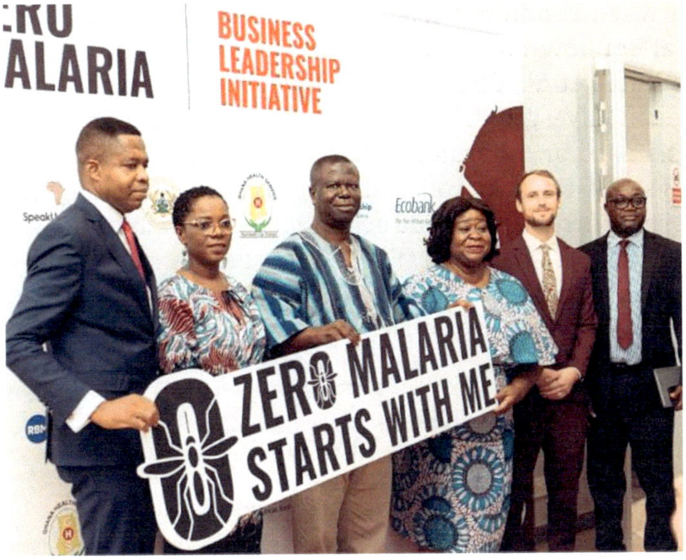

Figure 15.7. Funding and resource allocation for malaria initiatives.

Source: Zero Malaria. (2023). *Funding Malaria Elimination Programs.*

15.3. Malaria Transmission and Epidemiology

Grasping how malaria moves around is key if we're to come up with real health responses. Usually, it all starts when an infected Anopheles mosquito bites a person and transfers those *Plasmodium* parasites—yes, the very ones that set the stage for infection. It's not just one single factor; mosquito numbers, how our bodies naturally fight off sickness, weather features, and even economic and social conditions all mix together, creating a patchwork of disease patterns that differ from place to place. This jumble makes control efforts a real challenge. Health systems need to adjust to these local vibes because one solution rarely fits all. Dynamic math models have popped up as handy tools—they take in all these measures so policymakers can sort out what might happen when they try different interventions (Tediosi et al., 2010). In general, mixing how the disease spreads with how health systems work gives us a more textured picture of wisely using our resources and aims to go beyond those quick, short-term fixes toward something lasting. Looking closer, it isn't only about the parasite itself but also about how both the parasites and their mosquito carriers mix with communities. Transmission intensity can swing from very low to high, and these swings not only affect how many people fall ill and how badly but also how well interventions perform. For example, while pre-erythrocytic vaccines tend to do better when malaria levels are low, blood-stage vaccines might pack a stronger punch in areas where the disease runs rampant (Tediosi et al., 2010). These subtle differences matter a lot for health systems trying to fine-tune where every buck goes. Plus, seeing how malaria spreads and how well a local health setup can manage cases helps shape strategies to cut down on both sickness and death. Mixing real-world epidemiological data with health infrastructure details lets programs even predict bumps in healthcare demand as transmission patterns evolve. To summarize, this kind of integrated view underlines how control measures need to be shaped to fit local realities. Health systems aren't just about one-off fixes; they're expected to keep an eye on disease hotspots, treat cases as they emerge, and rally communities even when conditions keep changing. Some studies even suggest that shifts in malaria levels directly affect how much service demand there is and how cost-effective different interventions can be (Tediosi et al., 2010). Generally speaking, holding onto the gains in malaria control means continuously investing in health facilities and training, especially when faced with challenges like drug resistance or mosquitoes that seem to adapt on the fly. When countries build flexible, robust health systems that can roll with the punches of shifting malaria trends, they're in a better spot for long-term control and maybe even eventual elimination. In essence, understanding the ever-changing association of malaria transmission goes hand in hand with strengthening our health systems for sustainable control (Figure 15.8).

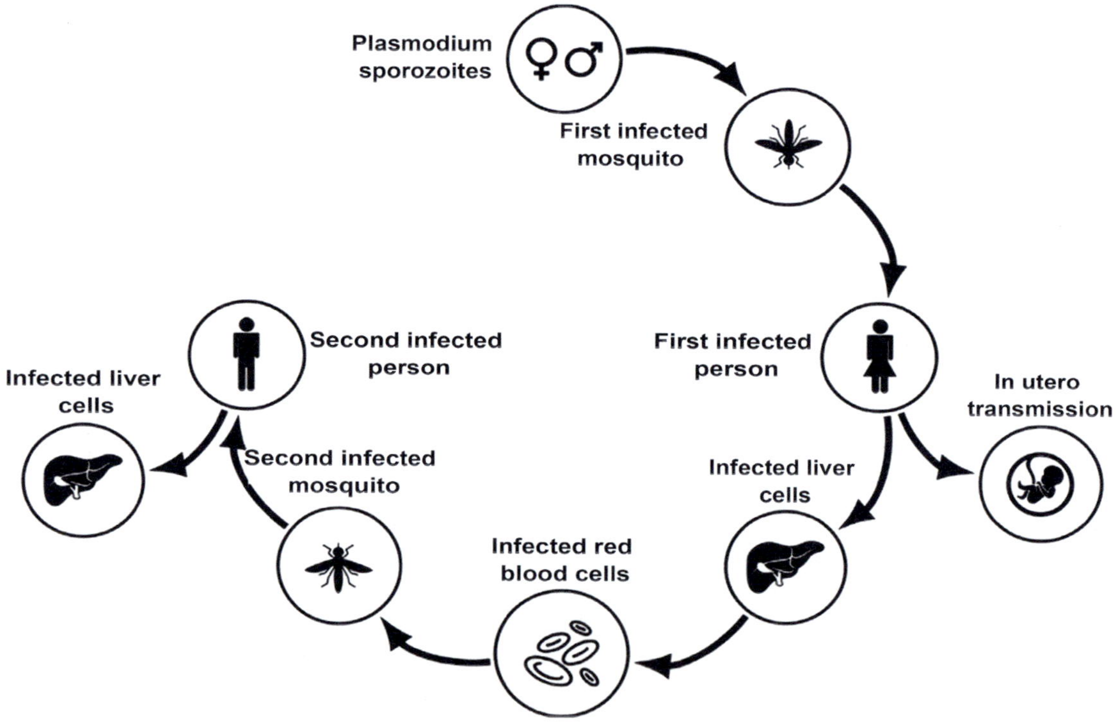

Figure 15.8. Malaria transmission and epidemiology.

Source: Ibrahim, M. (2020). *Malaria Transmission Cycle*. ResearchGate.

15.3.1. Life Cycle of the Malaria Parasite

The malaria parasite's journey is a complex one that significantly shifts how health systems tackle the disease. It starts when an infected female Anopheles mosquito bites a person, releasing sporozoites that quickly rush to the liver. There, these little invaders slip into liver cells and reproduce asexually, eventually forming merozoites. Once they burst out into the blood, these merozoites invade red blood cells, starting repetitive cycles that bring on symptoms like fever and anemia. This part of the cycle, in most cases, is pretty challenging since treatments have to hit more than one stage of the parasite's development. Knowing all these steps helps explain why tools like insecticide-treated nets—designed to disrupt mosquito bites—are so important in keeping transmission low. Expanding such measures among vulnerable groups remains a top priority for many health systems (Killeen et al., 2007). On another note, progress in malaria control also depends a lot on understanding the parasite's sexual reproduction, which takes place inside the mosquito. Some of the merozoites eventually transform into male and female gametocytes that float around in the human bloodstream until a mosquito happens to feed. Once inside the mosquito's gut, these gametocytes come together to form zygotes that then turn into ookinetes and later oocysts, and by the end, new sporozoites are produced. This mosquito stage is a key player in keeping the transmission going, highlighting why vector control measures are needed alongside clinical treatments. Health systems generally must support combined actions that include managing mosquito populations, spotting infections early, and getting treatment to people promptly, even if it sounds like assembling a complex puzzle (Tonna, 2006). Facing malaria means health systems need to cover all angles, from preventing infections to treating illness once it starts. Every phase in the parasite's cycle opens up a different chance to intervene, whether it's by reducing mosquito bites or by using antimalarial drugs that target the parasite in the bloodstream. Of course, pulling off these efforts depends on having strong, flexible health services that can reach those in need, day in and day out. Meanwhile, developing vaccines and other innovative strategies is super important, though the parasite's convoluted cycle makes the whole task extra challenging. In most cases, a solid malaria control plan ends up requiring a mix of approaches that digs deep into the parasite's biology while also handling broader issues like access and sustained coverage (Killeen et al., 2007; Tonna, 2006).

15.3.2. Factors Influencing Malaria Transmission

Malaria's spread ties closely with many environmental features and biology that drives the life cycles of both the Anopheles mosquito and the *Plasmodium* parasite. Weather factors like temperature, humidity, and even unpredictable rainfall influence where mosquitoes breed and how many there are. Sometimes a spike in heat speeds up the parasite's growth in the mosquito, which can boost the chance of infections getting passed on. Poor housing and not having enough preventive measures only add to the risk. Health systems try to cut down on mosquito bites with methods such as insecticide-treated nets and indoor spraying, but rising insecticide resistance in key mosquito groups has become a challenging problem, pushing us to develop new approaches and tighten up surveillance (Gansan et al., 2022). There's also the ever-changing nature of the mosquitoes and parasites themselves, which further jumbles the picture. For example, when pyrethroids—the main insecticides used in bed nets—start losing their punch in high-burden areas, it undermines the nets' protective role. This issue is made even more complicated by the slow rollout of alternative control tools in many places hit hardest by malaria. Newer innovations like dual active ingredient nets show promise against those resistant pathogens, yet high costs and uneven evidence about their added benefits keep them from being widely adopted. Health infrastructures, often in tandem with gradually evolving surveillance systems, work to keep an eye on these resistance trends and assess whether new tech makes economic sense (Gansan et al., 2022). Besides these entomological and environmental puzzles, social and economic factors also play a big role in steering malaria's course. Take, for instance, how crises like COVID-19 disrupted malaria services—shifting focus, stressing healthcare resources, and putting a damper on everyday control activities. Interruptions in supply chains and reduced community outreach sometimes mean that nets aren't distributed on time or diagnoses aren't made quickly, which in turn can raise the risk of transmission. Moreover, issues such as poverty, education gaps, and lack of access to healthcare add layers of vulnerability. All this means that health systems not only have to tackle the biological side of malaria but also beef up their response to wider public health challenges and social inequities to keep the disease in check (Gansan et al., 2022) (Figure 15.9).

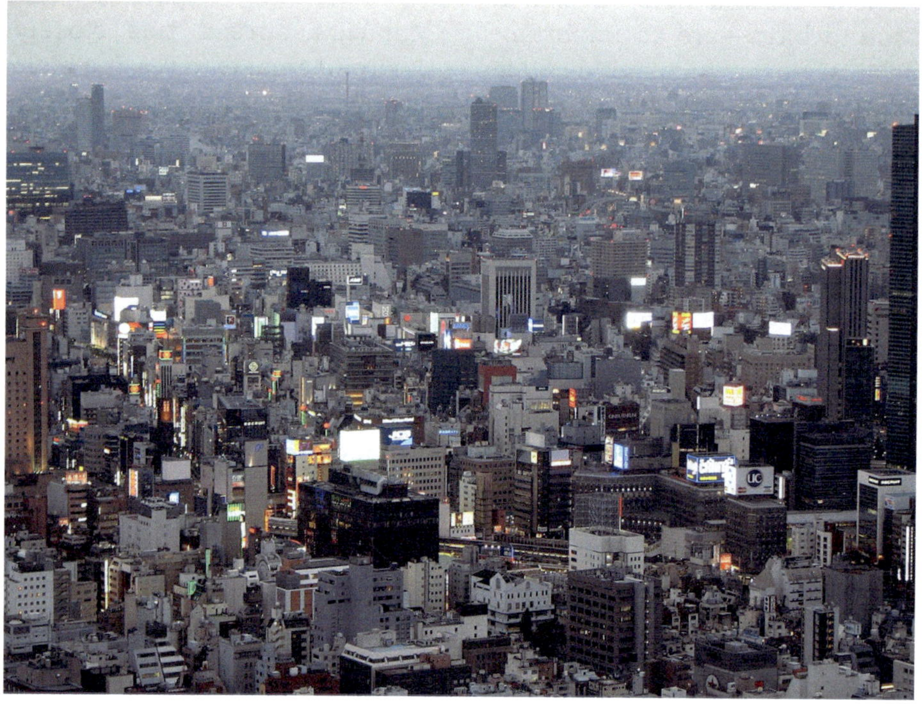

Figure 15.9. Influence of urbanization on the prevalence of malaria.

Source: By Chris 73 / Wikimedia Commons, CC BY-SA 3.0, https://commons.wikimedia.org/w/index.php?curid=1004215

15.3.3. Demographic and Geographic Distribution of Malaria Cases

Understanding malaria isn't as simple as checking a few numbers, it's about digging into who's affected and where they live. In many parts of sub-Saharan Africa, where the disease hits hard, local access to health services and the everyday conditions people face end up making a big difference. Rural areas, for instance, often have weak health systems, meaning individuals wait too long for treatment and don't get the right medicines, which ramps up the risk. Age and economic status, too, play a role—little kids and soon-to-be moms show up as especially vulnerable. When the health system stumbles, cases go untreated or aren't managed right, causing the disease to spread even more (Galactionova et al., 2015). All these human details have to be part of any malaria-fighting strategy so that the help given is both fair and on target. Where you live matters almost as much as who you are. Regions that get heavy rains, have plenty of water, and boast thick patches of greenery tend to be natural hubs for Anopheles mosquitoes. Think about spots along Kenya's coast or near Lake Victoria—these areas keep showing stubbornly high rates of malaria, while places like Nairobi, with more modern infrastructure, generally see much lower numbers (Gopal et al., 2019). This kind of patchwork spread tells us that a one-size-fits-all approach just won't work. Using local maps and geospatial details, health systems can spot the trouble areas, work out how best to distribute resources, and even plan for changes linked to events like El Niño (Gopal et al., 2019). Mixing demographic features with geographic factors makes malaria control a pretty complex problem. Different crowd densities, common behaviors, and the local environment all mix together to influence who falls ill and how well treatments work. When certain groups or areas don't get enough coverage, they become pockets where malaria just keeps surviving, undercutting wider prevention efforts (Galactionova et al., 2015). In most cases, health systems need to combine local community insights with spatial data to stay ahead of the disease. Recognizing and working with these mixed patterns can boost the ability to craft flexible, responsive policies—a key move in the long journey toward wiping out malaria by 2030 (Gopal et al., 2019).

15.4. Prevention Strategies

Malaria control hinges on mixing prevention strategies with the workings of our health systems. Often, check-ups during pregnancy become key moments for providing things like intermittent preventive treatment (IPTp) and insecticide-treated nets (LLINs) to those who need them most—pregnant women, for instance. There's no doubt these interventions help, yet practical hurdles emerge along the way. People might steer clear because of doubts about the quality of providers, scant drug supplies, or even the high cost of care. Plus, when patients aren't given enough clear info on how safe and effective antimalarial treatments are, they sometimes lean on herbal remedies or unregulated drugs. In most cases, health systems need to put patient-focused care first—care that's affordable, reachable, and mindful of cultural differences so that women and other high-risk groups keep getting steady, effective protection (Hill et al., 2015). Besides the usual protective measures, fresh biomedical ideas are showing promise as added support to traditional malaria control tools. Researchers are working on live attenuated malaria vaccines—using genetically engineered *Plasmodium falciparum* sporozoites that stall the parasite's growth in the liver, and this development is seen as a breakthrough. Early tests with genetically attenuated parasites (GAP) have even shown what some might call full protection in animal studies, hinting at a bright future for human vaccines. The idea is to kickstart immunity before the blood-stage parasites, which cause the worst symptoms, even appear—a pretty crucial step in cutting down both spread and severity. In most cases, weaving vaccination into everyday malaria prevention, especially when backed by solid clinical trials and a strong health infrastructure, could lower the number of cases (Okumu et al., 2013). What's needed overall is a prevention strategy that juggles community involvement, innovative biotech, and sturdier health services, all working together for long-term malaria control. Ensuring everyone has fair access to prevention tools means making big, sometimes complex, changes that consider socio-economic and cultural factors influencing how people seek care. For instance, building trust between healthcare providers and local communities, tightening up supply chains for antimalarial drugs and tests, and rolling out targeted education can all help individuals use these interventions better. It also makes sense to bring in new vaccines gradually keeping a close eye on their impact and altering how they're delivered within our existing health systems. To summarize, mixing time-tested methods with emerging technology, and sometimes even repeating key ideas, can ease the burden of malaria and help keep outbreaks at bay (Okumu et al., 2013; Hill et al., 2015) (Figure 15.10).

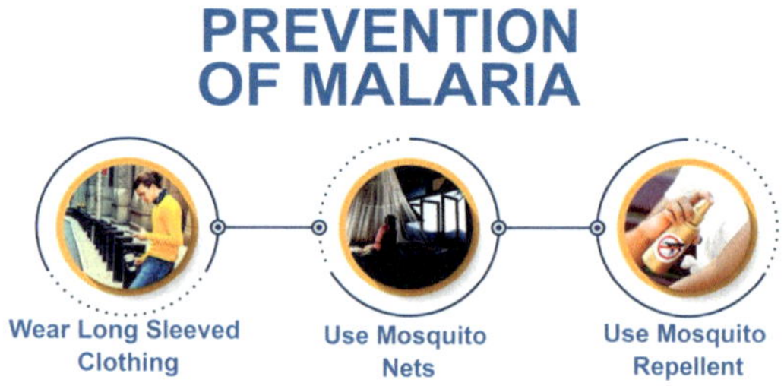

Figure 15.10. Prevention strategies of malaria.

Source: Dr. Lal PathLabs. (2023). *Malaria Prevention Tips.*

15.4.1. Use of Insecticide-Treated Bed Nets (ITNs)

Efforts to cut down malaria have lately leaned into preventive moves that help individuals and entire communities simultaneously. Insecticide-treated bed nets have become a favorite tool in the fight; these nets shield not just the most vulnerable, like little kids and expecting mothers, but also curb mosquito numbers and disturb malaria's spread. Getting a broad share of the population covered is pretty key. A number of studies generally say that if you manage to hit about 80% coverage among high-risk individuals, you can lower the overall malaria load (Killeen et al., 2007). How mosquitoes behave matters a lot for this approach. Most of the pathogens that carry malaria tend to bite humans and dwell indoors, so they're more likely to come in contact with the chemicals on these nets. That said, mosquitoes can be clever sometimes, switching up their feeding hours or even where they settle down, which makes indoor methods less effective at times. , it's less about a total failure of the nets and more about the pathogens showing a kind of behavioral resilience—, the less adaptable species get wiped out while the ones that can adjust keep on going (Govella et al., 2013). It's a shifting battle, meaning regular checks and flexible strategies are needed. Mixing bed nets into wider malaria control plans calls for a health system that can handle not just distribution, but also clear education and dealing with everyday obstacles. Maintaining community interest and overcoming social and economic hurdles is pretty much essential if you want frequent, proper use. Plus, ongoing insect monitoring should naturally inform changes in control strategies as mosquito behaviors vary. This sort of all-in-one, evidence-driven approach doesn't just keep the nets working, it also boosts the system's ability to roam, adapt, and challenge malaria's changing game (Killeen et al., 2007; Govella et al., 2013) (Figure 15.11).

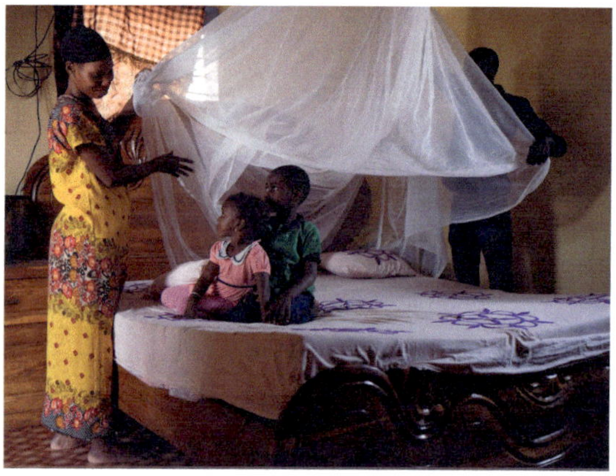

Figure 15.11. Use of insecticide-treated bed nets (ITNs).

Source: Medium. (n.d.). *Bed Nets for Malaria Prevention.*

15.4.2. Indoor Residual Spraying (IRS)

Malaria control often kicks off with a focus on the very insects that spread it. Many programs target adult mosquitoes indoors by spraying chemicals on walls and surfaces, this is the crux of IRS. Rather than relying on overly complex ideas, the method simply depends on getting rid of mosquitoes that brush past these treated spots. IRS works best when mosquitoes are still easily affected by the insecticides; if they start resisting, things can quickly go off course. In most cases, ongoing checks become necessary, especially in areas where many mosquito species and varied chemical exposures exist (Okumu et al., 2013). This kind of steady look-over helps keep IRS a key part of stopping malaria both right away and in the long run. Some programs have even mixed IRS with other tools, like LLINs—to boost protection. Research combining hut trials with computer models has shown that pairing IRS with certain chemicals (organophosphates such as pirimiphos methyl, for instance) can, generally speaking, give communities a bit of an edge. On the flip side, using pyrethroid-based IRS along with nets might sometimes end up being overkill, and, oddly enough, even using DDT for IRS in tandem with nets can reduce the overall benefit in some cases. Local mosquito behavior, differences in chemical properties, and pre-existing insecticide coverage all play into these mixed results (Okumu et al., 2013). In practical terms, it means that IRS is best not seen as a lone hero, but rather as one element in a broader, carefully considered strategy. Keeping IRS effective for the long haul means taking insecticide resistance head-on. The more we use pyrethroids in IRS, especially when similar chemicals are used in agriculture—the more mosquitoes (like *Anopheles gambiae*) can develop resistance. Field observations at several national sites have noted that these vectors no longer respond as readily as before, which calls for constant and careful monitoring. In many cases, switching to other chemicals or even rotating different options might help to keep the spray potent a bit longer. Such forward-looking moves, built into solid health policies (and sometimes, admittedly, a bit complex in their execution), are essential for ensuring that IRS continues to play its part in reducing malaria transmission in regions hit hardest by the disease (Batengana et al., 2011).

15.4.3. Vaccination Efforts and Research

Generally speaking, vaccines play a crucial role in fighting infections around the world. We might be all caught up on the latest viruses like SARS-CoV-2, yet the fight against old enemies like malaria still boils down to developing and using effective shots. Science has lately peeled back layers of malaria's winding life cycle, which let researchers craft vaccines aimed at specific parasite stages. Still, challenges, like making these vaccines reliably effective, ensuring smooth delivery setups, and winning over community trust—hang around, thanks in part to broader health system limits. The rapid vaccine rollouts during emergent outbreaks remind us of that sturdy health systems and cross-border teamwork matter, especially in poorer regions where malaria sticks around (Hu et al., 2020). Boosting these systems could not only widen malaria vaccine reach but also kick overall disease control into a higher gear, combining together research, policy, and care delivery. New research tricks have been shaking up the whole vaccine development scene with the promise to transform how we tackle malaria. Tools such as genomic sequencing and bioinformatics are revealing fresh antigen targets that help create vaccines with longer-lasting, more vigorous immunity. At the same time, field trials in malaria-hit areas stress the need to mix these vaccines into local healthcare setups so that coverage and practical impact are maximized. Since pathogens seem to keep changing their playbook, vaccines—along with better diagnostic and treatment methods—must evolve too. Recent global health hiccups have shown, in most cases, which aligning resource allocation and evidence-based policymaking is key to keeping vaccination drives on track without sidelining other vital services for the most vulnerable (Yoshikawa et al., 2020). All things considered, with sustained investment in research and system capacity, vaccine innovations can turn into real, tangible wins in the battle against malaria. Rolling out vaccination programs means tackling not just scientific hurdles but also economic, cultural, and logistical messes within our health systems. Chatting with community leaders and using communication that genuinely respects local customs can help lower at vaccine hesitancy and the swirl of misinformation. At the same time, ensuring fair access demands stronger cold chain systems and tailored training for health workers working in the challenging environments typical of malaria-endemic areas. If we look back at responses during recent pandemics, it's clear that multisectoral teamwork, from governments to NGOs and international groups—can seriously boost immunization efforts. Building these kinds of partnerships into malaria control plans may well add the resilience and flexibility needed when other health challenges and tight resources come into play. Encouragingly, evidence-based frameworks that naturally integrate service delivery will fortify health systems' abilities to keep vaccination programs running over time, thereby playing a key role in cutting down malaria cases (Hu et al., 2020; Yoshikawa et al., 2020) (Figure 15.12).

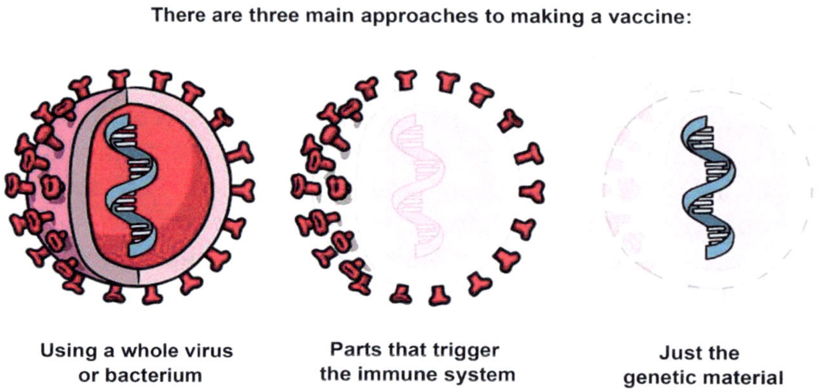

Figure 15.12. The vaccination efforts and research.

Source: By World Health Organization, CC BY-SA 3.0 IGO, CC BY-SA 3.0 igo, https://commons.wikimedia.org/w/index.php?curid=98863612

15.5. Treatment Approaches

Timely treatment plays a huge role in beating malaria and depends a lot on how strong health systems are. Rwanda, for example, has long wedded antimalarial drugs to its fight against the disease—a move that in the early 2000s helped bring down numbers. Yet, malaria isn't a static enemy; its shifting transmission and resistance patterns call for treatment plans that can change on the fly. Rwanda overhauled its health services so that quick diagnosis and care happen at many levels, including right in the community, which cuts wait times and improves patient outcomes. This spread-out care serves to lower the overall infectious pool, although, generally speaking, ongoing investments in surveillance, supply chains, and skilled healthcare workers remain crucial (Karema et al., 2020). Health crises today often overlap in unexpected ways. The recent COVID-19 outbreak, for instance, has thrown new challenges into malaria treatment, especially in sub-Saharan regions. Both diseases share symptoms like fever, fatigue, and breathing problems, which muddles the diagnosis process and sometimes skews treatment decisions. Health systems now have the dual job of using lab tests to confidently tell them apart, while also facing supply hiccups and resource shortages driven by pandemic pressures. Running tests that spot both infections at once can help make the most of limited resources, cutting down on misdiagnosis that might leave malaria untreated or push back COVID-19 care. In most cases this shows that systems need to be flexible and coordinated during public health emergencies (Chanda et al., 2020). Besides muddled diagnoses, sticking to treatment and having drugs available are key to keeping malaria in check. Supply interruptions, especially during lockdowns and travel restrictions—can quickly undo progress. Asymptomatic or low-level infections further complicate things, letting undetected cases keep the disease going. Health systems must not only ensure that effective antimalarial therapies reach those who need them but also increase community engagement and education to boost timely care-seeking and adherence to doses. Even with COVID-19 hogging the global spotlight, malaria care shouldn't be pushed apart; mixing services to cover both diseases can widen treatment reach and cut down on sickness and death. Strategic shifts like pooling resources and co-locating diagnostic services for both conditions are essential for keeping the malaria fight on track (Chanda et al., 2020; Karema et al., 2020).

15.5.1. Antimalarial Medications and Their Effectiveness

Malaria control heavily depends on how our health systems perform and how well people can get effective treatments. Getting treated isn't just about curing an infection or stopping it from getting worse; it also cuts down on the chance that stubborn, drug-resistant parasites will spread. Still, the journey from spotting the disease to finishing treatment is often bumpier than it should be. Many individuals struggle to even get into care, and sometimes health providers don't strictly follow the guidelines. Further, the quality of the medication might not be great and patients might miss doses, chipping away at the overall benefits. All these scattered system hiccups tend to lead to treatment failures and end up putting sustainable malaria control in jeopardy, which clearly calls for targeted fixes in our health systems (Galactionova et al., 2015). Getting access to antimalarial medicines is only half the battle—sticking to the prescribed treatment regimen makes the difference. Studies looking at how well patients follow these regimens often show a split when comparing widely used Artemisinin-based combinations like artemether-lumefantrine (AL) and amodiaquine-artesunate (AQAS). Generally speaking, caregivers tend to stick more reliably with AL, and many clinical sites report that AL is easier on patients. Still, it isn't an all-or-nothing picture; in some settings, there's evidence that people manage to dose AQAS correctly more often. This inconsistency in both sticking to schedules and following dosage instructions highlights the complex reality: it isn't enough for health systems to simply supply the drugs, they also need to make sure that patients use them properly to get the best outcomes and stave off resistance (Banek et al., 2018). You can't judge the power of antimalarial drugs apart from the bigger picture of our health systems. In sub-Saharan Africa, effective case management rates swing wildly, from as low as 8% to as high as 72%, and that gap comes from several sources. Often, people delay seeking treatment, providers don't always toe the line with established protocols, patients might not stick to the treatment plan, and even counterfeit drugs sneak into the mix. Tackling these issues calls for many strategies. In most cases, making sure that supply chains deliver quality drugs, boosting the training and oversight of healthcare providers, and getting communities more involved in their own care are all vital moves. At the end of the day, turning the proven promise of these medicines into real-world success hinges on solid, practical health system improvements (Galactionova et al., 2015) (Figure 15.13).

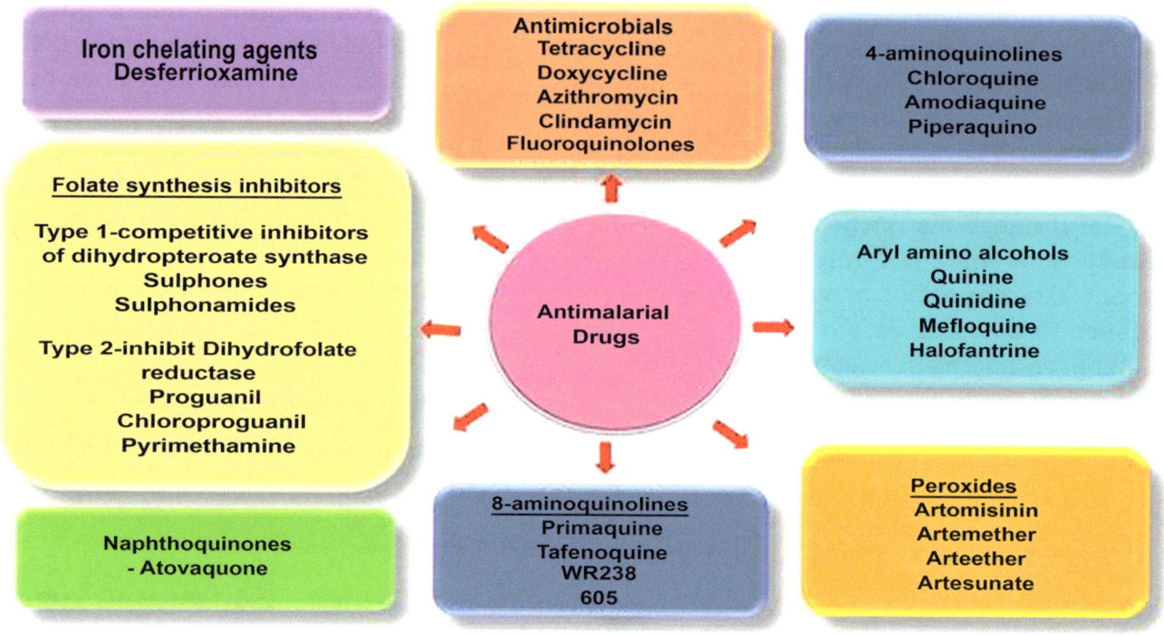

Figure 15.13. Antimalarial medications and their effectiveness.

Source: ResearchGate. (2022). *Classes of Antimalarial Drugs.*

15.5.2. Challenges in Treatment Adherence and Access

Malaria remains a heavy weight in many regions, not only because of the disease itself but due to a jumble of issues that keep treatment on unpredictable ground. Even when we have powerful drugs available, the overall impact suffers from weak health systems that just can't keep up. In central Africa and parts of Southeast Asia, the mix of poor drug quality, rising resistance, and uneven patient follow-through muddies the waters. The crux is that quality care isn't only about having medicine on hand; it's also about having providers who can guide patients and communities that understand what finishing a treatment means. Without those basics, ensuring that patients stick with their prescribed drugs remains a tough nut to crack (Rathmes et al., 2020). Getting diagnostic and treatment services out to those affected is another complex story. Even with the promise of quick, point-of-care tests that should lead to faster decisions, many facilities find themselves battling staff shortages, overwhelming patient loads, and frequent runouts of essential supplies. These challenges, in most cases, leave health workers scrambling to give proper counseling and follow-up, which are vital for keeping patients on track with their antimalarial therapies. Add to that sometimes-awkward provider-patient exchanges and worries about confidentiality and stigma, and you have a situation where reaching quality care feels almost out of reach. To summarize, effective malaria control has to fix these complex problems so that both tests and treatments become truly accessible and sustainable (Young et al., 2019). There's also a social and cultural side to the problem that overlaps with these systemic issues. How patients see their illness, how much they trust the health system, and the norms around medication all end up influencing whether they complete their treatment. Often, insufficient training and supervision of healthcare workers end up diluting what should be straightforward patient education and treatment monitoring. Meanwhile, economic pressures mean that immediate needs can sometimes override the importance of sticking with a full course of medicine. Tackling these barriers usually calls for a mix of better supply chains, improved worker competence, and engaging local communities to build real trust in the process. Without these changes, the continuous spread of drug resistance and ongoing transmission pretty much seem inevitable—a major concern for global health efforts (Young et al., 2019; Rathmes et al., 2020) (Figure 15.14).

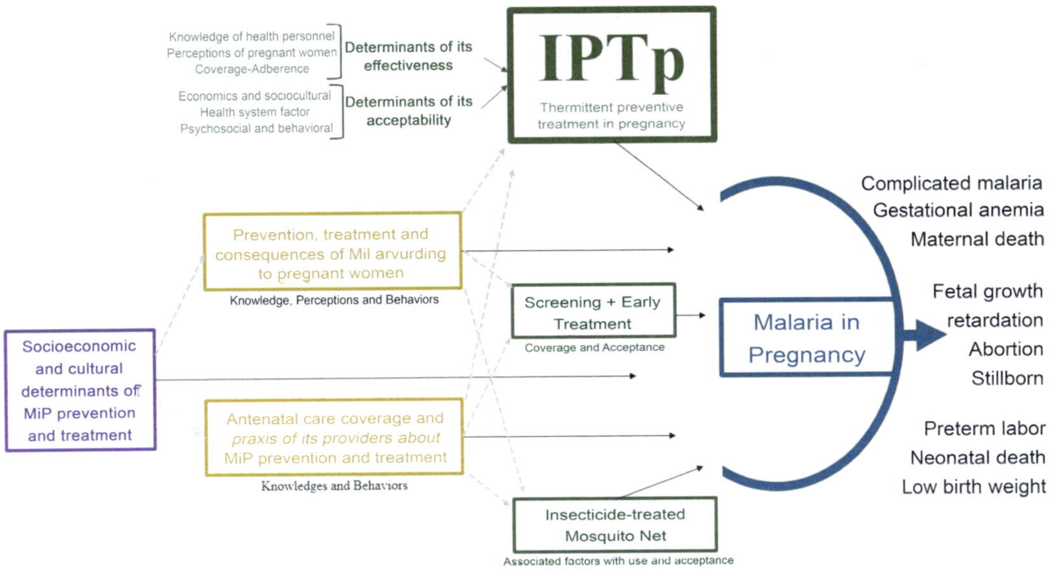

Figure 15.14. Challenges in treatment adherence and access for malaria.

Source: Cardona-Arias JA. Systematic Review of Mixed Studies on Malaria in Pregnancy: Individual, Cultural and Socioeconomic Determinants of Its Treatment and Prevention. *Tropical Medicine and Infectious Disease*. 2022; 7(12):423. https://doi.org/10.3390/tropicalmed7120423

15.5.3. Role of Healthcare Providers in Managing Malaria Cases

Malaria control depends on health workers being able to diagnose and treat patients quickly, even though uneven resources often impact that plan. In some remote spots like rural Cambodia, past turmoil and long-lasting under-investment have left clinics with barely enough tools or staff, so getting proper care becomes a real challenge. Providers here aren't just busy with treatments; they're also out there teaching individuals how to avoid the disease, keeping track of whether patients stick with their medications, and even watching for hints of drug resistance. In most cases, these overlapping duties point to how essential it is to invest in better training and resources so that health workers can manage both individual care and the broader public health issues combined to malaria control (DeHart et al., 2020). Sometimes, health workers step far outside the typical patient-care box by building partnerships that help fight malaria. For example, in Papua New Guinea, mixing public and private efforts, even teaming up, say, with mining companies—has opened up new ways to improve access to care and extra resources. Often, these professionals act like intermediaries who translate community needs into concrete health actions, all while coordinating with a jumble of other groups to boost local facilities. This kind of collaborative approach usually makes malaria control more sustainable since private know-how and funding effectively back up government projects. In many cases, when providers come on board in these partnerships, fighting malaria moves past only treating patients, morphing into a mixed strategy of prevention, education, and overall health system improvement (Thomason, 2011). As conditions around malaria continue to change, health professionals must keep up with new trends in transmission affected by everything from climate shifts to increased human movement. Generally speaking, this means updating their diagnostic and treatment methods on the fly—staying on guard for any resistant strains and reporting them right away so that national systems can react in time. Providers often lead community programs that train local frontline workers to spot symptoms, deliver antimalarial medicines safely, and send severe cases for immediate care. Their ability to mix solid, evidence-based practices with fresh, adaptive strategies influences the success of wider malaria control programs and reinforces their crucial role in efforts to strengthen the overall health system (Thomason, 2011; DeHart et al., 2020).

15.6. Challenges in Malaria Control

Malaria control depends a lot on how strong our health systems are, but they often hit serious snags. In places like Tanzania, even if case numbers have dropped, mosquitoes are getting tougher against the pyrethroids used in bed nets and indoor sprays. Mosquitoes changing what they do—switching up feeding times or picking new spots to breed—adds yet another twist. The picture isn't any simpler when you consider that many health centers are outdated, diagnosis and treatment can be slow, and funding for malaria programs comes and goes. All these bits and pieces can quickly undo progress, so in most cases, we need fresh strategies that boost our healthcare while dealing with both the pathogens' resistance and their shifting behavior (Mboera et al., 2013). Around the same time, rough environmental and climate changes muddy the water further. Global warming and unusual rainfall patterns now stretch the seasons and territories where malaria mosquitoes thrive, which might even roll back earlier gains. These weather shifts set up perfect conditions for mosquito breeding, making outbreaks even more unpredictable. Health systems are now pressured to bring in new tools like mapping tech and remote sensing to spot trouble early—yet many high-burden countries just don't have the resources for these innovations.

It seems clear that better care delivery has to go hand-in-hand with a kind of cross-sector teamwork that mixes climate adjustment plans with vector control measures, something recent reviews on the climate's impact have hinted at (Zhang et al., 2024). Meanwhile, keeping malaria at bay over the long haul also means tackling the social and community challenges head-on. People's beliefs and willingness to get involved play a huge role in how well measures like treated nets or indoor sprays work on the ground. Still, common misconceptions, limited education, and local traditions often slow down the proper use of these tools. Even everyday jobs like farming, water projects, or construction sometimes accidentally create perfect mosquito hangouts, meaning we need approaches that take local life and nature into account. Then there's money—irregular funding often stops programs in their tracks or stifles new ideas. Generally speaking, any real fight against malaria has to be woven into broader efforts that boost health systems, spark community action, link different sectors, and secure steady financing to meet the ever-changing challenges of malaria elimination (Mborera et al., 2013) (Figure 15.15).

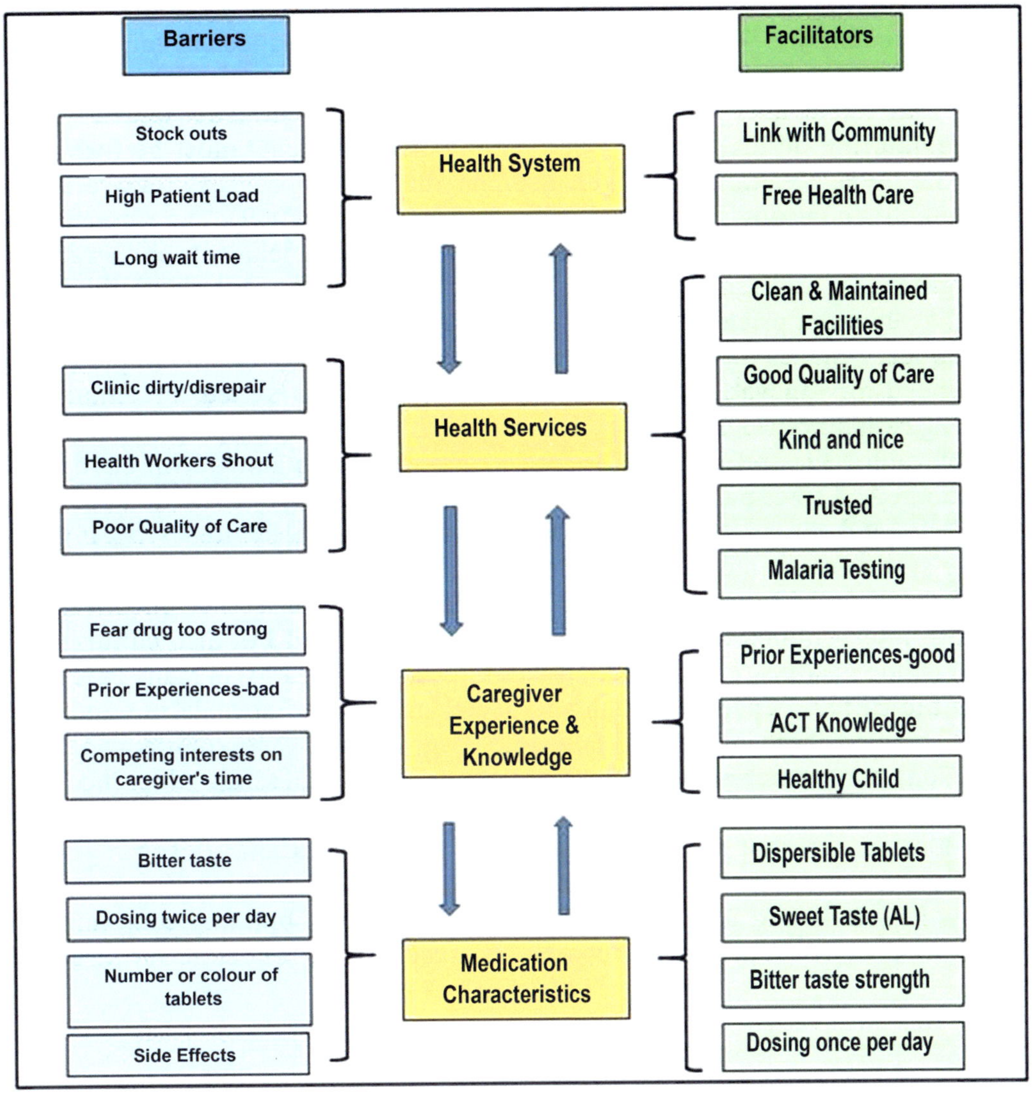

Figure 15.15. Challenges in intersectoral approaches in malaria control.

Source: Banek K, DiLiberto DD, Webb EL, Smith SJ, Chandramohan D, Staedke SG. Exploring Barriers and Facilitators of Adherence to Artemisinin-Based Combination Therapies for the Treatment of Uncomplicated Malaria in Children in Freetown, Sierra Leone. *Healthcare*. 2021; 9(9):1233. https://doi.org/10.3390/healthcare9091233

15.6.1. Drug Resistance and Its Implications

Malaria control can get challenging when drug-resistant strains of the *Plasmodium* parasite start to show up and spread. Countries on the brink of eliminating malaria now face a day-to-day reality where effective antimalarial drugs are absolutely critical – a situation that, in most cases, forces a sudden shift in strategies and surveillance systems. Drug resistance not only knocks down treatment success, but it also drags out how long someone stays sick and boosts the chances of disease spreading. Shifting focus from control to complete elimination calls for a close, all-around look at how ready a country is—both operationally and technically, especially for dealing with these pesky resistance patterns. This whole mix of challenges clearly points to the need for stronger health systems that can handle rigorous case detection, keep treatment routines on track, and conduct solid monitoring on drug safety. Quite simply, these systems must be flexible enough to alter them on the fly as resistance emerges, keeping the steady progress toward a malaria-free future and helping to dodge any sudden setbacks (Feachem et al., 2009). The ripple effects of drug resistance go far beyond clinical outcomes; they mess with the financial side and strategic planning of malaria programs. As resistance creeps in, countries suddenly find themselves facing steep costs – buying newer, often pricier drugs and setting up more robust surveillance infrastructures. This financial squeeze makes an already tough funding scene even more complex, which pretty much forces a need for innovative and stable financing methods suited for elimination efforts. Moreover, as drug resistance clogs up the works, the usually predictable patterns of malaria spread can turn erratic, calling for an integrated mix of biomedical tools along with environmental and social interventions. And since parasites and the mosquitoes that carry them don't respect borders, cooperative policies and shared resources across regions become absolutely vital. If we don't get a handle on these systemic and monetary hurdles, the hard-won gains in eliminating malaria could be at risk of slipping back (Feachem et al., 2009). Tackling drug resistance effectively also means leaning on health interventions that are not just technically sound but also culturally aware and ethically solid. Visiting healthcare professionals and international teams, in many cases, need to give real thought to the cultural, environmental, and social backdrop that malaria elimination efforts depend on. Overlooking local insights or failing to forge lasting partnerships can easily lead to miscommunications and unmet expectations, which might even mess up adherence to treatment protocols crucial for staving off resistance. Building genuine, respectful relationships—ones that are tailored to local needs—not only smooths out the implementation of drug regimens but also bolsters crucial surveillance and prevention efforts. In the end, combining international expertise with local know-how is key to optimizing antimalarial drug use, building community trust, and ultimately keeping drug resistance under control in these diverse, endemic settings.

15.6.2. Socioeconomic Factors Affecting Health Systems

Health systems' knack for fighting malaria depends on economic and social realities – they shape everything from getting a checkup to receiving the right kind of care. In many areas where malaria is prevalent, you see shortages in hospitals, a lack of trained staff, and not nearly enough insect-treated nets to go around; these issues slow down diagnosis and treatment and tend to trap communities in cycles of poverty and illness. Research out of Kenya, for example, generally shows that individuals with lower incomes experience higher rates of malaria and more severe outcomes (Nyawanda et al., 2025). It seems pretty clear that helping these communities by targeting resources directly is a major step toward building stronger, fairer health systems. Farming choices, schooling, and income gaps all mix together to influence not just how diseases like malaria spread, but also how well a community can return when outbreaks occur. Often, the way people engage with local health programs is complex up with their financial and social challenges. In places like the East African highlands – where malaria sometimes seems to reappear – everyday stresses and erratic weather join forces, making control efforts a real headache (Chaves & & Koenraadt, 2010). Even though a lot of discussion focuses on climate factors, it's important not to overlook how economic struggles strain health facilities and sap community resilience. Generally speaking, looking at both social and environmental factors together is key to understanding why malaria sticks around and how we can craft better responses. People's decisions to seek treatment are also steeped in their economic circumstances. Many in poorer communities may delay or skip getting help because the costs – from transportation fees to lost work hours – just add up. This, in turn, weakens the overall fight against malaria. These hurdles point to why social safety nets and local health initiatives that lighten the financial load matter. It isn't just about beefing up clinical services; tackling deeper issues like poverty, education gaps, and overall social fairness is just as important. In most cases, this broad, complex approach seems to be the most promising way to finally break the cycle of malaria transmission, a fact that recent public health reviews and studies have underlined (Chaves & & Koenraadt, 2010; Nyawanda et al., 2025) (Figure 15.16).

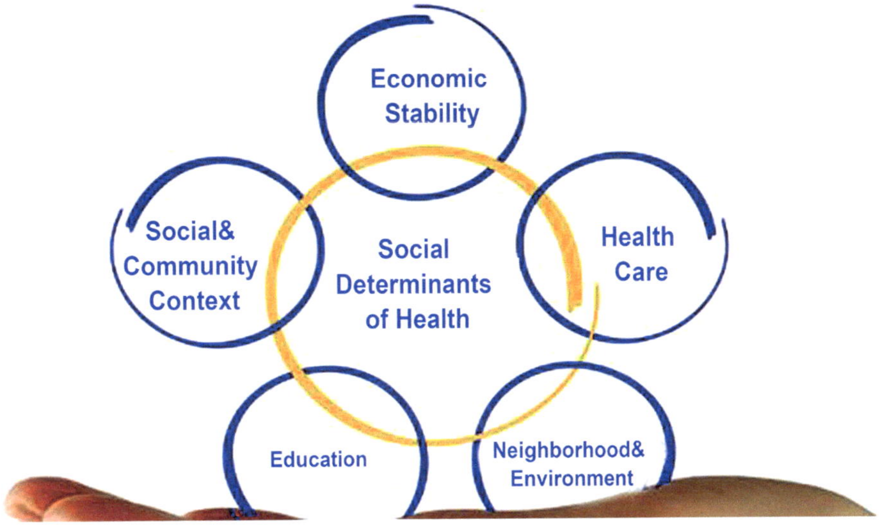

Figure 15.16. Socioeconomic factors affecting health systems.

Source: Duke Health. (n.d.). *Socioeconomic Impact on Healthcare.*

15.6.3. Political and Logistical Barriers to Effective Implementation

Health projects depend a lot on strong leadership and clear pathways. In malaria control, unpredictable politics and leaders who keep on changing their minds turn steady efforts into a bit of a mess. Without a leader that genuinely steers things in one direction, malaria programs can end up lost or off course—leaving policies scattered and funds coming in unpredictably. You often see that genuine political backing is what makes it possible to pull together different sectors like education, infrastructure, or even local efforts, all of which help tackle health issues in a rounded way (Margaret et al., 2018). In most cases, health systems are not just about clinical fixes; they also have to deal with a political scene that can either increase or choke off the flow of needed innovations and money, making this political side a tough nut to crack. Logistical hurdles add another layer to the chaos. Many malaria-prone areas are tucked away in remote spots, where delivering basics like insecticide-treated nets, rapid tests, and proper medicine feels almost like an uphill climb. Problems such as supply chain disruptions, poor transportation networks, and too few people on the ground all combine to delay or even block the timely care that communities need. Weak health data systems further complicate matters by not capturing real-time changes—so when cases spike, the response might already be late (Margaret et al., 2018). All of these missteps in the system hint at deeper, foundational issues that must be mended if policies are to translate into real improvements on the ground. Then there's the social side, which makes things even trickier. Often, individuals living in poverty or with less schooling find themselves caught in a loop of lower-quality care and little engagement from the health services designed for them. This gap not only saps trust but also means community members might skip out on prevention programs. Trying to mix malaria control with broader health services—say, mental health or maternal care—gets complex too, as the old ways of doing things don't always mesh well with new demands. Fixing these barriers means rethinking how services are delivered and ensuring governance is up for the challenge of inclusivity, so that both technical and social issues are addressed head-on (Margaret et al., 2018). To summarize, when political commitment meets a drive for fairer health services, there's a better shot at coping with the multifaceted challenges of malaria control.

CLOSER LOOK

RTS,S/AS01 MALARIA VACCINE

The RTS,S/AS01 malaria vaccine, also known by its trade name Mosquirix, is the world's first malaria vaccine to reach large-scale implementation. Developed over several decades through a partnership led by GlaxoSmithKline (GSK), in collaboration with the PATH Malaria Vaccine Initiative and funded by organizations such as the Bill & Melinda Gates Foundation, RTS,S represents a landmark advancement in malaria prevention, particularly for children in sub-Saharan Africa.

RTS,S is designed specifically to protect against *Plasmodium falciparum*, the most deadly and prevalent malaria parasite in Africa. *P. falciparum* is responsible for the majority of malaria-related deaths, particularly among children under the age of five. The vaccine targets the pre-erythrocytic stage of the parasite's life cycle, aiming to prevent the parasite from infecting liver cells after transmission through a mosquito bite.

RTS,S is a recombinant protein-based vaccine that contains a part of the *P. falciparum* circumsporozoite protein (CSP)—a protein found on the surface of sporozoites (the form of the parasite transmitted by mosquitoes). This protein is fused with a portion of the hepatitis B surface antigen (HBsAg), which helps boost the immune response. The vaccine is formulated with a proprietary adjuvant called AS01, which enhances the body's immune reaction to the vaccine.

The goal of the RTS,S/AS01 vaccine is to induce an immune response that neutralizes the parasite before it can infect liver cells and multiply, thus preventing the development of symptomatic malaria.

Clinical trials and pilot programs have shown that RTS,S provides moderate protection against malaria in young children. A large Phase III trial conducted in seven African countries found that the vaccine reduced malaria cases by around 40% and severe malaria by about 30% in children who received the full four-dose regimen.

While the efficacy is lower compared to vaccines for many other diseases, the public health impact is significant in high-transmission settings. When used in combination with other preventive tools, such as ITNs and seasonal malaria chemoprevention (SMC)—RTS,S can substantially reduce the malaria burden.

In October 2021, the World Health Organization (WHO) recommended the broad use of the RTS,S/AS01 vaccine for children in areas with moderate to high transmission of *P. falciparum* malaria. The recommendation followed successful pilot programs in Ghana, Kenya, and Malawi, where the vaccine was shown to be safe, effective, and deliverable through routine immunization systems.

The vaccine is administered in four doses: three doses given at monthly intervals starting at around five months of age, followed by a fourth booster dose approximately 18 months later.

RTS,S is not a standalone solution. Its moderate efficacy and the need for a four-dose schedule present logistical challenges, particularly in resource-limited settings. There are also concerns about the durability of protection over time. However, research is ongoing into next-generation vaccines, such as R21/Matrix-M, which may offer higher efficacy.

SUMMARY

Effective malaria control depends on health systems that can quickly take on new treatments and testing methods. Take tafenoquine, for example, paired with tests for glucose-6-phosphate dehydrogenase deficiency (G6PDd), this pairing has stirred up a fresh way to tackle *Plasmodium vivax* malaria. This new therapy not only makes it easier for patients to stick with their doses but also deals with those pesky relapsing infections that have long frustrated elimination efforts. A study based on Brazilian settings predicted that using tafenoquine could greatly cut down on transmission and drop case numbers (Nekkab et al., 2021). In many cases, mixing new drugs with older, trusted infrastructures shows how clinical breakthroughs and system improvements go hand in hand, helping to optimize resources and treatment outcomes while moving closer to wiping malaria out. Health systems, however, need to be flexible enough to face malaria's uneven challenges across different areas. The effectiveness of responses can vary a lot, which means there's no one-size-fits-all recipe for malaria control. In low-transmission areas where patients often don't finish a primaquine regimen, tafenoquine brings marked improvements in cure rates, even if it isn't a magic bullet. On the flip side, places with high transmission and lots of kids needing care signal that more well-tailored dosing might be required. Generally speaking, this situation underscores how local disease behavior and unique demographics demand adaptive approaches from health systems (Nekkab et al., 2021). Strengthening surveillance and making sure everyone can access diagnostics and treatments can let these systems handle shifting conditions, keeping malaria control efforts sustainable over time. At the end of the day, progress toward malaria elimination is tightly linked to how resilient and responsive our health systems turn out to be, especially in areas also battling other infections. While tafenoquine's rollout marks an exciting step forward, it should be seen as just one piece of a broader malaria control mix that includes prevention, diagnosis, treatment, and even logistic coordination. The COVID-19 pandemic, for example, laid bare both vulnerabilities and strengths in our health setups, reminding us that effective systems must be ready to manage multiple threats simultaneously. By learning from such global challenges, malaria programs can boost rapid response, foster community involvement, and ensure care keeps coming without a hitch. Ultimately, building stronger health systems remains the key to lasting drops in malaria transmission and better public health overall.

Malaria control is taking on a new twist as fresh ideas mix with long-established methods. New approaches often use agents that don't outright kill—devices like spatial repellents gently deter vectors by shifting their behavior, lowering contact between humans and mosquitoes without relying on heavy insecticides. This method isn't exactly a magic bullet, but it does mark a shift from traditional, kill-focused strategies to ones that modify behavior—a change that might help ease problems like insecticide resistance and environmental worries. In most cases, mixing these innovations with existing public health plans means giving them a solid place alongside tried-and-true interventions, though doing so demands careful scientific checks and thoughtful policy alters (Achee et al., 2012). Malaria vaccines continue to stand out as a pressing challenge. Even after decades of intense research, no licensed vaccine has yet emerged—a clear sign of how challenging malaria biology can be. That said, clinical trials in sub-Saharan Africa have shown promising progress, generally indicating that the region is building its research strength. High-standard trials adhering to international practices are slowly reshaping the landscape. It's interesting to note that these improved research facilities not only help test new malaria vaccines but also support the evaluation of other infectious and chronic disease interventions. Building and maintaining strong clinical trial networks, even with a few hiccups here and there, is key for long-term health improvements and bolstering global malaria elimination efforts (Nyika et al., 2013). Taking everything together, successful malaria control today calls for a mixed strategy. On one hand, newer vector management ideas, like spatial repellents—need to be woven into public health systems, while on the other, the boost in clinical research capabilities remains crucial. Local networks, especially in areas such as sub-Saharan Africa, serve as great examples of how focused capacity building can drive broader progress. In most cases, merging innovative vector strategies with robust research practices and adaptable policies pinpoints the way forward; such a combined effort is essential if we're to reduce malaria's impact and ultimately wipe it out.

KEY TERMS FROM THIS CHAPTER

- Primary Health Care
- Malaria Control Programs
- Integrated Disease Management
- Case Management
- Health Workforce
- Health Education
- Monitoring and Evaluation
- Public-Private Partnerships
- Universal Health Coverage (UHC)
- Health Infrastructure
- National Malaria Control Program (NMCP)
- Surveillance Systems
- Drug Supply Chain
- Community Health Workers
- Behavior Change Communication (BCC)
- Health Financing
- International Collaboration
- Sustainability of Malaria Control

References

1. Achee, N. L., Bangs, M. J., Farlow, R., Killeen, G. F., Lindsay, S., Logan, J. G., Moore, S. J., Rowland, M., Sweeney, K., Torr, S. J., Zwiebel, L. J., & Grieco, J. P. (2012). Spatial repellents: from discovery and development to evidence-based validation. *Malaria journal, 11*, 164. https://doi.org/10.1186/1475-2875-11-164(accessed on 13 May 2025).
2. Hill, J., Kayentao, K., Achieng, F., Diarra, S., Dellicour, S., Diawara, S. I., Hamel, M. J., Ouma, P., Desai, M., Doumbo, O. K., ter Kuile, F. O., & Webster, J. (2015). Access and use of interventions to prevent and treat malaria among pregnant women in Kenya and Mali: a qualitative study. *PloS one, 10*(3), e0119848. https://doi.org/10.1371/journal.pone.0119848 (accessed on 13 May 2025).
3. Azizi, H., Esmaeili, E. D., Farahbakhsh, M., Zeinolabedini, M., Mirzaei, Y., & Mirzapour, M. (2020). Malaria situation in a clear area of Iran: An approach for the better understanding of the health service providers' readiness and challenges for malaria elimination in clear areas. *Malaria Journal, 19*, Article 106. https://doi.org/10.1186/s12936-020-03188-7.
4. Banek, K., Webb, E. L., Smith, S. J., Chandramohan, D., & Staedke, S. G. (2018). Adherence to treatment with artemether-lumefantrine or amodiaquine-artesunate for uncomplicated malaria in children in Sierra Leone: a randomized trial. *Malaria journal, 17*(1), 222. https://doi.org/10.1186/s12936-018-2370-x(accessed on 16 May 2025).
5. Batengana, B., Chacha, M., Emidi, B., Kabula, B., et al. (2011). Detection and monitoring of insecticide resistance in malaria vectors in Tanzania Mainland. https://core.ac.uk/download/pdf/11307282.pdf (accessed on 13 May 2025).
6. Bent, O., Remy, S. L., Roberts, S., Walcott-Bryant, C., et al. (2017). *Novel Exploration Techniques (NETs) for Malaria Policy Interventions*. http://arxiv.org/abs/1712.00428 (accessed on 13 May 2025).
7. Bever, C. A., Eckhoff, P. A., Gerardin, J., Hamainza, B., et al. (2016). *Malaria Elimination Campaigns in The Lake Kariba Region of Zambia: A Spatial Dynamical Model*. http://arxiv.org/abs/1603.04773 (accessed on 13 May 2025).
8. Buonsenso, D., & Cataldi, L. (2010). Watch out for malaria: still a leading cause of child death worldwide. *Italian journal of pediatrics, 36*, 58. https://doi.org/10.1186/1824-7288-36-58Chakraborty, S., Papageorgiou, C., & Perez Sebastian, F. (2013). *Health Cycles and Health Transitions*. https://core.ac.uk/download/151157346.pdf (accessed on 13 May 2025).
9. Chanda-Kapata, P., Kapata, N., & Zumla, A. (2020). COVID-19 and malaria: A symptom screening challenge for malaria-endemic countries. *International Journal of Infectious Diseases, 94*, 151–153. https://doi.org/10.1016/j.ijid.2020.04.007.
10. Chaves, L. F., & Koenraadt, C. J. M. (2010). Climate change and highland malaria: Fresh air for a hot debate. https://core.ac.uk/download/pdf/29238217.pdf (accessed on 13 May 2025).
11. Chisholm, D., Sweeny, K., Sheehan, P., Rasmussen, B., Smit, F., Cuijpers, P., & Saxena, S. (2016). Scaling-up treatment of depression and anxiety: A global return on investment analysis. *The Lancet Psychiatry, 3*(5), 415–424. https://doi.org/10.1016/s2215-0366(16)30024-4.
12. Croke, K. (2011). *Politics, Child Mortality, And Health System Development in Tanzania and Uganda, 1995–2009*. https://core.ac.uk/download/pdf/11307595.pdf (accessed on 13 May 2025).

13. Galactionova, K., Tediosi, F., de Savigny, D., Smith, T., & Tanner, M. (2015). Effective coverage and systems effectiveness for malaria case management in sub-Saharan African countries. *PloS one, 10*(5), e0127818. https://doi.org/10.1371/journal.pone.0127818 (accessed on 13 May 2025).

14. DeHart, Ciera, "Health Concerns in Cambodia Compounded by Historical and Rural Setbacks" (2020). *Senior Honors Theses*. 967. https://digitalcommons.liberty.edu/honors/967 (accessed on 13 May 2025).

15. Drain, P. K., Drain, D., Izadnegahdar, R., Kolars, J. C., Miller, W. C., Pinto, A. D., & Suchdev, P. (2013). "We learn from them; they learn from us": Global health experiences and host perceptions of visiting healthcare professionals. *Academic Medicine, 88*(4), 483–487.

16. Feachem, R.G.A., with A.A. Phillips and G.A. Targett (eds) (2009). Shrinking the Malaria Map: A Prospectus on Malaria Elimination. San Francisco: The Global Health Group, Global Health Sciences, University of California, San Francisco.(accessed on 13 May 2025).

17. Gansané, A., Candrinho, B., Mbituyumuremyi, A., Uhomoibhi, P., N'Falé, S., Mohammed, A. B., Guelbéogo, W. M., et al. (2022). Design and methods for a quasi-experimental pilot study to evaluate the impact of dual active ingredient insecticide-treated nets on malaria burden in five regions in sub-Saharan Africa. *Malaria Journal, 21*. https://doi.org/10.1186/s12936-021-04026-0.

18. Okumu, F.O., Kiware, S.S., Moore, S.J. *et al.* Mathematical evaluation of community level impact of combining bed nets and indoor residual spraying upon malaria transmission in areas where the main vectors are *Anopheles arabiensis* mosquitoes. *Parasites Vectors* **6**, 17 (2013). https://doi.org/10.1186/1756-3305-6-17 (accessed on 13 May 2025).

19. Gopal, S., Ma, Y., Xin, C., Pitts, J., & Were, L. (2019). Characterizing the Spatial Determinants and Prevention of Malaria in Kenya. *International journal of environmental research and public health, 16*(24), 5078. https://doi.org/10.3390/ijerph16245078(accessed on 13 May 2025).

20. Govella, N.J., Chaki, P.P. & Killeen, G.F. Entomological surveillance of behavioural resilience and resistance in residual malaria vector populations. *Malar J* **12**, 124 (2013). https://doi.org/10.1186/1475-2875-12-124(accessed on 13 May 2025).

21. Hu, B., Guo, H., Zhou, P., & Shi, Z. L. (2020). Characteristics of SARS-CoV-2 and COVID-19. *Nature Reviews Microbiology, 19*, 141–154. https://doi.org/10.1038/s41579-020-00459-7.

22. Zhang, Y., Wang, M., Huang, M., & Zhao, J. (2024). Innovative strategies and challenges mosquito-borne disease control amidst climate change. *Frontiers in microbiology, 15*, 1488106. https://doi.org/10.3389/fmicb.2024.1488106 (accessed on 13 May 2025).

23. Mubyazi, G. M., Magnussen, P., Byskov, J., & Bloch, P. (2013). Feasibility and coverage of implementing intermittent preventive treatment of malaria in pregnant women contacting private or public clinics in Tanzania: experience-based viewpoints of health managers in Mkuranga and Mufindi districts. *BMC health services research, 13*, 372. https://doi.org/10.1186/1472-6963-13-372 (accessed on 13 May 2025).

24. Intergovernmental Panel on Climate Change. (2023). *Climate Change 2022–Impacts, Adaptation and Vulnerability*. https://doi.org/10.1017/9781009325844.

25. James, S. L., Abate, D., Abate, K. H., Abay, S. M., Abbafati, C., Abbasi, N., Abbastabar, H., et al. (2018). Global, regional, and national incidence, prevalence, and years lived with disability

for 354 diseases and injuries for 195 countries and territories, 1990–2017: A systematic analysis for the Global Burden of Disease Study 2017. *The Lancet, 392*(10159), 1789–1858. https://doi.org/10.1016/s0140-6736(18)32279-7.

26. Juvekar, A., & Hegde, A. (2024). *Persistent Global Health Threats: The Impact of Infectious Diseases in Resource-Limited Regions.* Conduct Science Proceedings. https://doi.org/10.55157/conductscience-proceedings.2024.1.52(accessed on 13 May 2025).

27. Okumu, F. O., Sumaye, R. D., Matowo, N. S., Mwangungulu, S. P., Kaindoa, E. W., Moshi, I. R., Madumla, E. P., & Lwetoijera, D. W. (2013). Outdoor mosquito control using odour-baited devices: development and evaluation of a potential new strategy to complement indoor malaria prevention methods. *MalariaWorld journal, 4,* 8. https://doi.org/10.5281/zenodo.10894810(accessed on 13 May 2025).

28. Karema, C., Wen, S., Sidibe, A., Smith, J. L., Gosling, R., Hakizimana, E., Tanner, M., et al. (2020). History of malaria control in Rwanda: Implications for future elimination in Rwanda and other malaria-endemic countries. *Malaria Journal, 19.* https://doi.org/10.1186/s12936-020-03407-1.

29. Kelly A. H. (2011). Will He Be There?: Mediating malaria, immobilizing science. *Journal of cultural economy, 4*(1), 65–79. https://doi.org/10.1080/17530350.2011.535336Mboera, L. E. G., Mazigo, H. D., Rumisha, S. F., & Kramer, R. A. (2013). Towards malaria elimination and its implication for vector control, disease management and livelihoods in Tanzania. *MalariaWorld journal, 4,* 19. https://doi.org/10.5281/zenodo.10928325(accessed on 13 May 2025).

30. Kruk, M. E., Gage, A., Arsenault, C., Jordan, K., Leslie, H. H., Roder-DeWan, S., Adeyi, O., et al. (2018). High-quality health systems in the Sustainable Development Goals era: Time for a revolution. *The Lancet Global Health, 6*(11), e1196–e1252. https://doi.org/10.1016/s2214-109x(18)30386-3.

31. Killeen, G. F., Smith, T. A., Ferguson, H. M., Mshinda, H., Abdulla, S., Lengeler, C., & Kachur, S. P. (2007). Preventing childhood malaria in Africa by protecting adults from mosquitoes with insecticide-treated nets. *PLoS medicine, 4*(7), e229. https://doi.org/10.1371/journal.pmed.0040229 (accessed on 13 May 2025).

32. London School of Hygiene & Tropical Medicine. (2013). *Annual Report 2013.* https://core.ac.uk/download/19452766.pdf (accessed on 13 May 2025).

33. Lu, S., Ma, X., Ding, W., Wang, D., Zhou, Z., Lin, K., Luo, F., et al. (2023). The "Paired Learning by Doing" approach for capacity building derived from the China–UK–Tanzania pilot project on malaria control during 2015–2018. *China CDC Weekly, 5,* 694–697. https://www.semanticscholar.org/paper/a3aab506a5d44673ecfeb9419e995768222b5b3f (accessed on 13 May 2025).

34. Madhav, N., Oppenheim, B., Gallivan, M., Mulembakani, P., Rubin, E. M., & Wolfe, N. (2017). Pandemics: Risks, impacts, and mitigation. In *Disease Control Priorities: Improving Health and Reducing Poverty* (3rd ed.). The World Bank. https://doi.org/10.1596/978-1-4648-0527-1_ch17.

35. Mtui, J., & Osoro, O. (2011). Aggregate cost implications of selected cost-drivers in the Tanzanian health sector. Final Report 12/1/2011. Commissioned by: Ministry of Health and Social Welfare. https://core.ac.uk/download/pdf/11307328.pdf (accessed on 13 May 2025).

36. KFF Policy Brief. (2010). *The U.S. Global Health Initiative: Key Issues.* https://core.ac.uk/download/71348666.pdf (accessed on 13 May 2025).

37. Nekkab, N., Lana, R. M., Lacerda, M., Obadia, T., Siqueira, A. M., Monteiro, W. M., Villela, D. A. M., et al. (2021). Estimated impact of tafenoquine for *Plasmodium vivax* control and elimination in Brazil: A modelling study. *PLoS Medicine, 18*(5), e1003535. https://doi.org/10.1371/journal.pmed.1003535.

38. Nyawanda, B. O. (2025). *Bayesian Spatial-Temporal Modelling to Assess the Impact of Climate Variability and Control Interventions on The Burden of Malaria in Kenya.* https://core.ac.uk/download/646239520.pdf (accessed on 13 May 2025).

39. Nyika, A., Olotu, A., Roca-Feltrer, A., Holder, A. A., Luty, A. J., Hill, A. V. S., Moonen, B., et al. (2013). Experience and challenges from clinical trials with malaria vaccines in Africa. https://core.ac.uk/download/pdf/11307788.pdf (accessed on 13 May 2025).

40. Parkhurst, J., Ghilardi, L., Webster, J., Snow, R. W., & Lynch, C. A. (2020). Competing interests, clashing ideas and institutionalizing influence: Insights into the political economy of malaria control from seven African countries. *Health Policy and Planning, 36*(1), 35–44. https://doi.org/10.1093/heapol/czaa166.

41. Rathmes, G., Rumisha, S. F., Lucas, T., Twohig, K. A., Python, A., Nguyen, H. L. T., Nandi, A., et al. (2020). Global estimation of anti-malarial drug effectiveness for the treatment of uncomplicated *Plasmodium falciparum* malaria 1991–2019. *Malaria Journal, 19*, Article 339. https://doi.org/10.1186/s12936-020-03446-8.

42. Tediosi, F. (2010). *Simulation of the Costs and Consequences of Potential Vaccines for Plasmodium Falciparum Malaria.* https://core.ac.uk/download/18234515.pdf (accessed on 13 May 2025).

43. Thomason, Jane, PNG Mineral Boom: Harnessing the Extractive Sector to Deliver Better Health Outcomes (January 1, 2011). Development Policy Centre Discussion Paper No. 2 , Available at SSRN: https://ssrn.com/abstract=1919304 or http://dx.doi.org/10.2139/ssrn.1919304(accessed on 13 May 2025).

44. Tonna, I. (2006). *Is Vaccination the Only Option for Possible Global Malaria Eradication?* Malta Medical Journal Volume 18 Issue 02 July 2006. https://core.ac.uk/download/46602052.pdf (accessed on 13 May 2025).

45. Wallace, R. (2003). *Structured Psychosocial Stress and Therapeutic Intervention: Toward A Realistic Biological Medicine.* https://web-archive.southampton.ac.uk/cogprints.org/3002/index.htmlYoshikawa, H., Wuermli, A. J., Rebello Britto, P., Dreyer, B. P., Leckman, J. F., Lye, S. J., Ponguta, L. A., et al. (2020). Effects of the global coronavirus disease-2019 pandemic on early childhood development: Short- and long-term risks and mitigating program and policy actions. *The Journal of Pediatrics, 223*, 188–193. https://doi.org/10.1016/j.jpeds.2020.05.020.

46. Young, N., Achieng, F., Desai, M., Phillips–Howard, P. A., Massougbodji, A., Aol, G., Bigogo, G., et al. (2019). Integrated point-of-care testing (POCT) for HIV, syphilis, malaria and anaemia at antenatal facilities in western Kenya: A qualitative study exploring end-users' perspectives. *BMC Health Services Research, 19*, Article 74. https://doi.org/10.1186/s12913-018-3844-9.

INDEX

L

M

N

O

P

R

S

T

V

W

Z